Organizational Behavior

STEPHEN P. ROBBINS

San Diego State University

Organizational
Concepts, Controversies,

Behavior

and Applications SECOND EDITION

Prentice-Hall, Inc., Englewood Cliffs, New Jersey   07632

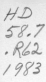

Library of Congress Cataloging in Publication Data
ROBBINS, STEPHEN P. (date)
    Organizational behavior.

    Includes indexes.
    1. Organizational behavior.   I. Title.
HD58.7.R62   1983   158.7   82-13171
ISBN 0-13-641480-X

Editorial/production supervision by Kim Gueterman
Interior design by Mark Binn
Cover design by Debra Lynne Watson
Cover art by Ruth A. Marsilio
Manufacturing buyer: Ed O'Dougherty

Organizational Behavior: Concepts, Controversies, and Applications, Second Edition
by Stephen P. Robbins

Printed in the United States of America
10 9 8 7 6 5 4 3 2 1

ISBN 0-13-641480-X

Prentice-Hall International, Inc., *London*
Prentice-Hall of Australia Pty. Limited, *Sydney*
Editora Prentice-Hall do Brazil, Ltda., *Rio de Janeiro*
Prentice-Hall Canada Inc., *Toronto*
Prentice-Hall of India Private Limited, *New Delhi*
Prentice-Hall of Japan, Inc., *Tokyo*
Prentice-Hall of Southeast Asia Pte. Ltd., *Singapore*
Whitehall Books Limited, *Wellington, New Zealand*

*To Nancy Virginia Hibert, Without
Whom This Book Would Have Been Finished
A Whole Lot Earlier*

Overview

I Introduction
  1 What Is Organizational Behavior?   3
  2 Models: Toward Explaining and Predicting Behavior   19

II The Individual
  3 Values and Attitudes   49
  4 Personality   71
  5 Perception   107
  6 Motivation   131
  7 Learning   165

III The Group
  8 Foundations of Group Behavior   199
  9 Group Dynamics   231
  10 Communication   261
  11 Leadership   285
  12 Power   313
  13 Conflict   337

IV The Organization System
  14 Organization Structure   369
  15 Job Design   401
  16 Performance Evaluation and Rewards   427
  17 Organizational Culture   453
  18 Organizational Development   475

V Organizational Dynamics
  19 Organizational Politics: An Integrating Concept

Contents

Preface   xxiii

PART I

Introduction

1   What Is Organizational Behavior?   3

Replacing Intuition with Systematic Study   5
Putting the "Organization" into Organizational Behavior   6
Is OB Worth Studying?   7
Contributing Disciplines to the OB Field   8

Psychology   8
Sociology   8
Social Psychology   10
Anthropology   10
Political Science   10

Are "OB" and "Management" Synonymous Terms?   11
There Are Few Absolutes in OB   11
The Value of Dialogue on OB Issues   12
For Discussion   13
For Further Reading   14
POINT: Strauss et al., Organizational Behavior Is
    a Social Science   15
COUNTERPOINT: Wilson, Sociobiology: Studying Behavior
    From a Biological Basis   17

2 Models: Toward Explaining and Predicting Behavior 19

Classification of Models 21

Subjective versus Objective Models 21
Static versus Dynamic Models 21
Physical versus Abstract Models 22
Normative versus Descriptive Models 22

Components of a Model 22

Objective 23
Variables 23
Relationships 24
Summary 25

Variables in Our OB Model 25

The Dependent Variables 26
The Independent Variables 28

Toward a Contingency OB Model 33
For Discussion 33
For Further Reading 34
POINT: Skinner, Control of Human Behavior 36
COUNTERPOINT: Rogers, Controlling Behavior: Proceed with Caution 38

Case IA Arnie Bentley—Househusband 40
Case IB "I Love My Work" 41
Case IC Brave New World Revisited 43
Case ID "I'm Not Always Right, But I'm Right Most of the Time" 44

PART II
The Individual

3 Values and Attitudes 49

Values 50

Importance of Values 51
Sources of Our Value Systems 51

Types of Values   52
Recent Changes in Employee Values   54

Attitudes   55

Sources of Attitudes   56
Types of Attitudes   56
Attitudes and Consistency   57
Cognitive Dissonance Theory   58
Measuring the A—B Relationship   60
An Example: Predicting Union Activity   61

Implications for Performance and Satisfaction   62

Attitudes and Productivity   62
Attitudes and Withdrawal Behaviors   63
Attitudes and Satisfaction   64

For Discussion   64
For Further Reading   65
POINT: Likert and Katz, Toward Achieving a High Level of
Job Satisfaction   66
COUNTERPOINT: Lawler and Porter, The Effect of
Performance on Job Satisfaction   68

4 Personality   71

What Is Personality?   72
Personality Determinants   73

Heredity   73
Environment   74
Situation   75

Personality Characteristics   75

Trait Approach   76
Type Approach   76
Summary   79

Two Popular Personality Development Theories   80

Maturation Theory   80
Passages Theory   80

Major Personality Attributes Influencing OB   82

Locus of Control   82
Achievement Orientation   83
Authoritarianism   84
Machiavellianism   84
Risk Taking   85

Personality—Job Fit Theories   85

Instrumental versus Expressive Orientation   85
The Six Personality Types Model   86

The Self-Concept and Defensive Behaviors   87
Personality and Stress   90

What Is Stress?   90
Facts about Stress and Work   91
Symptoms of Stress   92
Stress and Performance   93

Implications for Performance and Satisfaction   97
For Discussion   99
For Further Reading   100
POINT: Holden, Twins Raised Apart: Some Case
    Studies   102
COUNTERPOINT: Farber, Twins Raised Apart: A Review of
    the Evidence   104

5 Perception   107

What Is Perception?   109
Factors Influencing Perception   109

The Perceiver   109
The Target   112
The Situation   113

Person Perception: Making Judgments about Others   113

Attribution Theory   113
Specific Applications in Organizations   115
Frequently Used Shortcuts in Judging Others   117

Implications for Performance and Satisfaction   120

Productivity   121
Absenteeism and Turnover   122
Job Satisfaction   123
Summary   123

For Discussion   124
For Further Reading   124
POINT: Bass et al., Training Can Improve Perceptual
    Accuracy   126
COUNTERPOINT: Crow, Training May Reduce Perceptual
    Accuracy   128

6 Motivation 131

What Is Motivation? 132
Individual Needs: The Foundation of Motivation 133

Self-Interest: The Ultimate Motivating Force 133
How Many Needs Are There? 134
Maslow's Hierarchy of Needs 134
ERG Theory 136
Achievement, Power, and Affiliation Motives 137
Needs: A Summary 139
Reading an Individual's Needs 140

Extrinsic versus Intrinsic Motivators 141

Motivation-Hygiene Theory 141
Cognitive Evaluation Theory 144

Popular Process Theories of Motivation 146

Equity Theory 147
Goal-Setting Theory 150
Reinforcement Theory 151
Expectancy Theory: An Integrative Model 152

Implications for Performance and Satisfaction 156
For Discussion 158
For Further Reading 158
POINT: Strauss, Statement of the Personality-versus-
Organization Hypothesis 160
COUNTERPOINT: Strauss, Criticism of the Personality-
versus-Organization Hypothesis 162

7 Learning 165

Learning and Motivation 166
A Definition of Learning 167
Relevance of Learning to OB 168
Conditioning 169

Classical Conditioning 169
Operant Conditioning 170

Shaping: A Managerial Tool 171

Primary and Secondary Reinforcers 171
Methods of Shaping Behavior 172
Schedules of Reinforcement 173
Reinforcement Schedules and Behavior 174

Implications for Performance and Satisfaction 176
For Discussion 179
For Further Reading 180
POINT: Locke, The Myths of Behavior Mod in
Organizations 181
COUNTERPOINT: Gray, The Myths of the Myths about
Behavior Mod in Organizations 183

Case IIA Business Is Good at Consolidated—Check It
Out! 186
Case IIB Money Isn't Everything, I Guess! 187
Case IIC The Green Bay Legend 189
Case IID The Right Woman in the Wrong Job 190
Exercise IIA Value Assessment 192
Exercise IIB Attitude Measure of Women as
Managers 194
Exercise IIC Needs Test 196

PART III
The Group

8 Foundations of Group Behavior 199

Defining and Classifying Groups 200
Why Do People Join Groups? 201

Security 201
Identity, Self-Esteem, and Status 202
Affiliation 202
Power 202
Group Goals 203

Key Group Concepts 203

Roles 203
Norms 211
Status 215

Clothing and the Key Group Concepts 221
Implications for Performance and Satisfaction 222

Roles 222
Norms 222
Status 223

For Discussion   224
For Further Reading   224
POINT: Leavitt, Suppose We Took Groups Seriously   226
COUNTERPOINT: Walton, Where Groups *Were* Taken
   Seriously   228

9 Group Dynamics   231

Methods of Group Analysis   232

   Sociometry   232
   Interaction Analysis   234

Group-Behavior Model   235

   Defining the Key Components   235
   Background Factors   236
   Personal System   237
   Required and Emergent Behavior   238
   Summary   239

Contingency Variables That Affect Group Behavior   239

   Sex of Members   239
   Personality Characteristics of Members   240
   Number of Members   240
   Heterogeneity of Members   241

Characteristics of Group Decision Making   242

   Groupthink   243
   The Risky-Shift Phenomenon   245

Toward Improved Group Decision Making   247

   Nominal Group Technique   247
   Delphi Technique   247

Group Cohesiveness   248

   Determinants of Cohesiveness   248
   Cohesiveness and Group Productivity   251

Implications for Performance and Satisfaction   252
For Discussion   253
For Further Reading   253
POINT: Holder, Decision Making by Consensus   255
COUNTERPOINT: Hampton, Summer, and Webber, Group
   Decision Making Is Not Always Better   258

10 Communication 261

Communication-Process Model   262
Barriers to Effective Communication   264
Nonverbal Communication   266
Perception and the Creation of Meaning   267

Applying Equity Theory to Communication   268
Looking for Informational Cues   269

Special Group Languages   270
Communication Networks   272

The Five Common Networks   273
The Five Networks and Group Effectiveness   274
The Informal Group Communication Network   274

Implications for Performance and Satisfaction   276
For Discussion   277
For Further Reading   278
POINT: Rogers, Barriers and Gateways to
    Communication   280
COUNTERPOINT: Kursh, The Benefits of Poor
    Communication   282

11 Leadership 285

What Is Leadership?   286
Transition in Leadership Theories   286
Trait Theories   287
Behavioral Theories   288

Ohio State Studies   289
University of Michigan Studies   289
The Managerial Grid   290
Summary of Behavioral Theories   290

Contingency Theories   292

Autocratic-Democratic Continuum Model   292
Fiedler Model   294
Path-Goal Model   297
Leader-Participation Model   299
Sometimes Leadership Is Irrelevant!   302

Looking for Common Ground: What Does It All Mean?   303
Implications for Performance and Satisfaction   304
For Discussion   306
For Further Reading   306

POINT: Fiedler and Chemers, Leaders Make a
    Difference   308
COUNTERPOINT: Pfeffer, Do Leaders Really
    Matter?   310

12 Power 313

A Definition of Power   314
Contrasting Leadership and Power   315
Bases and Sources of Power   316

Bases of Power   317
Sources of Power   318
Summary   319

Dependency and Uncertainty   320
Power Tactics   324
Power in Groups: Coalitions   325
Implications for Performance and Satisfaction   326

Performance   327
Satisfaction   327

For Discussion   328
For Further Reading   328
POINT: McClelland and Burnham, A Case for the Power-
    Oriented Manager   330
COUNTERPOINT: Leavitt and Lipman-Blumen, A Case for
    the Relational Manager   332

13 Conflict 335

A Definition of Conflict   336
Transitions in Conflict Thought   337

The Traditional View   337
The Behavioral View   338
The Interactionist View   338

Differentiating Functional from Dysfunctional
    Conflicts   338
The Conflict Paradox   339
Conflict Process   340

Stage I: Potential Opposition   340
Stage II: Cognition and Personalization   342
Stage III: Behavior   342
Stage IV: Outcomes   344

Implications for Performance and Satisfaction   346
For Discussion   348
For Further Reading   348
POINT: Filley, The Case for Problem Solving   350
COUNTERPOINT: Robbins, Problem Solving: A Special
    Case   352

Case IIIA   Welcome to the School Board   355
Case IIIB   A Man Has Got to Know His Place   357
Case IIIC   Tip Says No Way   358
Case IIID   Getting Off to a Good Start   359
Exercise IIIA   Status Ranking Task   361
Exercise IIIB   Leadership Questionnaire   362
Exercise IIIC   Power-Orientation Test   363

PART **IV**
The Organization System

14 Organization Structure   367

What Is Structure?   368

Complexity   368
Formalization   370
Centralization   371

Why Do Structures Differ?   372

Size   372
Technology   373
Environment   376
Power-Control   377

How Structures Differ: A Classification Scheme   378

The Simple Structure   379
The Bureaucratic Structure   380
The Functional Structure   381
The Product Structure   382
The Adhocratic Structure   383

Key Structural Variables and Their Relevance to OB   386

Size   387
Organizational Level   387

Line versus Staff   387
Span of Control   388
Horizontal Differentiation   388
Vertical Differentiation   389
Centralization   389

Implications for Performance and Satisfaction   389
For Discussion   392
For Further Reading   392
POINT: Bennis, The Coming Death of Bureaucracy   394
COUNTERPOINT: Miewald, The Greatly Exaggerated Death
    of Bureaucracy   396

15 Job Design 399

What Is Job Design?   401
Historical Development of Job Design   401

Scientific Management   402
Job Enlargement   403
Job Enrichment   403
Sociotechnical Systems   403
Summary   404

The Job Characteristics Model   404

Core Dimensions   404
Interrelationships   405
Predictions from the Model   406
Summary   407

Current Redesign Options   408

Job Rotation   408
Work Modules   408
Job Enrichment   409
Integrated Work Teams   412
Autonomous Work Teams   412
Quality Circles   413
Shorter Workweek   414
Flex-time   416

Job Redesign Options and Job Characteristics   417
Implications for Performance and Satisfaction   418
For Discussion   418
For Further Reading   419
POINT: Hackman, A Job Design Scenario: Route One   420
COUNTERPOINT: Hackman, A Job Design Scenario: Route
    Two   422

16 Performance Evaluation and Rewards   425

Performance Evaluation   427

Purposes of Performance Evaluation   427
Performance Evaluation and Motivation   427
Performance Standards   428
Methods of Performance Evaluation   428
Problems in the Search for Objectivity   429
Sharing Performance Evaluation Results   432

Rewards   433

Effect of Rewards on Behavior   434
Perceptions of Rewards   434
Determinants of Rewards   435
Reward Determinants in Practice   438
Types of Rewards   439

Implications for Performance and Satisfaction   442
For Discussion   442
For Further Reading   443
POINT: Olsen and Bennett, Performance Appraisal as a
    Management Technique   444
COUNTERPOINT: Olsen and Bennett, Performance
    Appraisal as a Social Process   446

17 Organizational Culture   449

What Is Culture?   450

A Definition   450
Two Examples   452

Socialization: How Organizations Create Their
Cultures   454

What Is Socialization?   455
The Socialization Process   456
Socialization Methods   457
Conclusions   462

Implications for Performance and Satisfaction   462
For Discussion   463
For Further Reading   464
POINT: Powell and Butterfield, The Case for the Subsystem
    Climates in Organizations   465
COUNTERPOINT: Drexler, Climate Is Organization-
    Specific   468

18 Organizational Development 471

Change and OD 472
OD Objectives 474
Basic Approaches to OD 476

  Structural Techniques 476
  Human Process Techniques 477

Implications for Performance and Satisfaction 485
For Discussion 486
For Further Reading 486
POINT: Levinson, An Assessment of OD Practice 488
COUNTERPOINT: Sashkin, In Defense of OD
  Practice 491

Case IVA   Who's in Charge Here? 493
Case IVB   Easy Come, Easy Go! 494
Case IVC   In Search of a 50 Percent Increase in
  Efficiency 495
Case IVD   What Happened to Team Effort? 497
Exercise IVA   Bureaucratic Orientation Test 498
Exercise IVB   Rate Your Job's Motivating Potential 499
Exercise IVC   Rate Your Classroom Culture 500

PART V
Organizational Dynamics

19 Organizational Politics: An Integrating Concept 503

What Is Organizational Politics? 505
Why Use Organizational Politics as an Integrating
  Concept? 507

  The Individual 507
  The Group 507
  The Organization System 508
  Summary 508

Factors Contributing to Dysfunctional Politicking 509

Individual Factors   509
Cultural Factors   510

Predicting Dysfunctional Politicking   512
Some Concluding Thoughts   514
For Discussion   515
For Further Reading   515
POINT: Mayes and Allen, Organizational Politics Goes
Beyond the Simple Performance of Job Tasks   517
COUNTERPOINT: Robbins, All Job Behaviors Are
Political   520

Case VA   I Don't Make Decisions!   522
Case VB   It's Performance Appraisal Time   524
Case VC   Games People Play in the Shipping
Department   525
Case VD   United Manufacturing Company   527

Appendix: Scoring Keys for Activity
Exercises   531

Glossary   537

Name Index   547

Subject Index   557

Preface

The objectives of this second edition of *Organizational Behavior* are unchanged from the previous edition. I have continued to work toward creating a book that is highly readable, interesting, thought-provoking, current, goal-oriented, and integrative.

Readable. Readers should find the writing style to be clear, logical, and conversational. As in the first edition, I continue to rely on an extensive use of examples as a way to clarify and illustrate concepts.

Interesting. The chapters have been purposely designed to be moderate in length. Long discourses on topics of marginal relevance have been avoided. The result, I believe, is a book that comprehensively "covers the distance" in organizational behavior, but in a way that makes the journey enjoyable.

Thought-provoking. The education process is composed of more than merely knowing a lot of facts. It is of equal or greater importance to *understand* that which we *know*. Toward this end, each chapter closes with a "Point-Counterpoint" dialogue which debates two sides of an issue relevant to that chapter's content. To reflect the more recent controversies in the field and to better relate debate topics to chapter content, one-third of these dialogues have been changed from the first edition.

Current. In addition to updating the research base of this book, a number of topics have been expanded to reflect recent contributions. These include, but are certainly not limited to values; the attitude-behavior controversy; personality attributes influencing organizational behavior; stress; person perception and its application to organizations; goal-setting theory; why people join groups; perception, communication, and the creation of meaning; power bases, sources, and tactics; job design; socialization; organizational culture; and organizational politics.

Goal-oriented. This book is intended to aid the reader in explaining and predicting behavior in organizations. More specifically, it is concerned with those factors that influence performance (productivity, absence, and turnover) and satisfaction. To emphasize these objectives, there is a section entitled "Implications for Performance and Satisfaction" at the end of Chapters 3 through 18. This section brings together the material in each of these 16 chapters for the specific purpose of ascertaining its relevance to organizational performance and satisfaction. To further facilitate the transference from theory to practice, I've included in this edition case exercises at the end of each major part and added student application exercises at the conclusion of the Individual, Group, and Organization Systems parts.

Integrative. The last objective has been operationalized by the development of a building-block model in Chapter 2. This model, which was introduced in the first edition, has been slightly modified to more accurately reflect the key variables that affect performance and satisfaction.

In summary, I believe you'll find this book both provocative and informative. But, of course, any book can be improved upon. Your feedback can help me make the next edition better. After you've completed reading the book, please feel free to write me and let me know what you liked and didn't like about it. You can address your correspondence to: Professor Stephen P. Robbins, c/o Editor—College Division, Management and Industrial Relations, Prentice-Hall, Inc., Englewood Cliffs, New Jersey 07632.

Acknowledgments

Every author has a long list of individuals to whom he is indebted. I appreciate the comments and suggestions made by Professors Ramon J. Aldag (University of Wisconsin, Madison), Richard Blackburn (University of North Carolina), and Mark A. Mallinger (Pepperdine University).

I have learned and grown from the interactions with my departmental colleagues at San Diego State, particularly Tom Atchison, Jim Belasco, Dave Belcher, Herman Gadon, Jai Ghorpade, Dave Hampton, Natasha Josefowitz, Daryl Mitton, Del Nebeker, Alan Omens, and Penny Wright. And comments from my friends Johanna Hunsaker, Phil Hunsaker, and Cindy Pavett at the University of San Diego have improved the final product.

There are dozens of people at Prentice-Hall who contributed to this book. To acknowledge all of them is impossible. I am particularly indebted to Jayne Maerker; Jayne's assistant, Linda Albelli; my production editor, Kim Gueterman, and designer Mark Binn.

Last, but far from least, I am indebted to the support provided by my daughters, Dana and Jennifer. They understand their weird father, his bizarre priorities and preoccupation with meeting publication deadlines. They are caring, thoughtful, and responsible. They also make raising teenagers look easy.

Stephen P. Robbins

Organizational Behavior

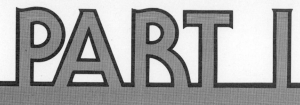

Introduction

CHAPTER 1

What Is Organizational Behavior?

AFTER STUDYING THIS CHAPTER, YOU SHOULD BE ABLE TO—

Define and explain the following key terms and concepts:

Caused behavior
Contingency variables
Intuition
Management

Organization
Organizational behavior
Systematic study

Understand:

The value of the systematic study of OB
The contributions made by major behavioral science disciplines
   to OB
The difference between OB and management
The objectives of OB education
Why managers require a knowledge of OB
The need for a contingency approach for studying OB
The value of dialogue on OB issues

> I'm not smart. I try to observe. Millions saw the apple fall but Newton was the one who asked why.
>
> —BERNARD BARUCH

Each of us is a student of behavior. Beginning seconds after our birth we become aware that certain types of behavior are linked to certain types of responses. For example, it did not take most of us long to figure out that crying usually elicited increased attention. As we matured, we expanded our observations to include the behavior of others. While much of our observing, recording, classifying, and interpreting of how certain events are related and why individuals do certain things may have been unconscious, the fact remains that we have been "reading" others for many years.

You have already developed some generalizations that you find helpful in explaining and predicting what people do and will do. But how did you arrive at these generalizations? By observing, sensing, asking, listening, and reading. That is, your understanding comes either directly, from your own experience with things in the environment, or secondhand, through the experience of others.

How accurate are the generalizations that you hold? Some may represent extremely sophisticated appraisals of behavior and prove highly effective in explaining and predicting the behavior of others. However, most of us also carry about with us a number of beliefs that frequently fail to explain why people do what they do. To illustrate, consider the following half-dozen statements:

1. People are basically lazy.
2. Everyone is motivated by money.
3. You can't teach an old dog new tricks.
4. A job is just a means of survival.
5. Everyone wants a challenging job.
6. Happy workers are productive workers.

How many of these statements are true? For the most part, they are all false, and we shall touch on each at points later in this book. But whether these statements are true or false is not really important at this time. What is important is to make you aware that many of the views you hold concerning human behavior are based on intuition rather than fact. As a result, a systematic approach to the study of behavior can improve your explanatory and predictive abilities.

REPLACING INTUITION
WITH SYSTEMATIC STUDY

The use of casual or common sense approaches for obtaining knowledge about human behavior is inadequate. In this book it will be argued that a systematic approach will uncover important facts and relationships, and provide a base from which more accurate predictions of behavior can be made.

Underlying our systematic approach is the belief that behavior is not random. It is caused, and directed toward some end which the individual believes, rightly or wrongly, is in his or her best interest.

> Behavior generally is predictable if we know how the person perceives the situation and what is important to him or her. While people's behavior may not appear to be rational to an outsider, there is reason to believe it usually is *intended* to be rational and it is seen as rational by them. An observer often sees behavior as nonrational because the observer does not have access to the same information or does not perceive the environment in the same way.[1]

Certainly there are differences between individuals. Placed in similar situations, all people do not act alike. However, there are certain fundamental consistencies underlying the behavior of all individuals that can be identified and used to alter conclusions based on individual differences.

The fact that there are these fundamental consistencies is very important. Why? Because it allows predictability. When you get into your car, you make some definite and usually highly accurate predictions about how other people will behave. You predict that other drivers will stop at stop signs and red lights, drive on the right side of the street, pass on your left, and not cross the solid double line on mountain roads. Notice that your predictions about the behavior of people behind the wheel of their cars is almost always correct. Obviously, the rules of driving make predictions about driving behavior fairly easy. What may be less obvious is that there are rules (written and unwritten) in every setting. Therefore, it can be argued that it is possible to predict behavior (obviously, not always with 100 percent accuracy) in supermarkets, classrooms, doctors' offices, elevators, and in most structured situations. To illustrate further, do you turn around and face the doors when you get into an elevator? Almost everyone does, yet did you ever read that you're supposed to do this? Probably not! Just as I make predictions about automobile drivers (where there are definite rules of the road), I can make predictions about the behavior of people in elevators (where there are few written rules). In a class of sixty students, if you wanted to ask a question of the instructor, I would predict that you would raise your hand. Why don't you clap, stand up, raise your leg, cough, or yell "Hey, teach, over here!" The reason is that you have learned that raising your hand is appropriate behavior in school. These examples support a major contention in this book: Behavior is generally predictable and the systematic study of behavior is a means to making reasonably accurate predictions.

1. Edward E. Lawler III and John G. Rhode, *Information and Control in Organizations* (Pacific Palisades, Calif.: Goodyear, 1976), p. 22.

When we use the phrase "systematic study," we mean looking at relationships, attempting to attribute causes and effects, and basing our conclusions on scientific evidence, that is, on data gathered under controlled conditions and measured and interpreted in a reasonably rigorous manner.

Systematic study replaces intuition or those "gut feelings" about "why I do what I do" and "what makes others tick." Of course, a systematic approach does not mean that those things you have come to believe in an unsystematic way are necessarily incorrect. Many of the conclusions we shall make in this book, based on reasonably substantive research findings, will only support what you always knew was true. Some of your opinions, however, will be disproved, while still others will prove to be surrounded by so much contradictory evidence as to make the drawing of conclusions highly tentative. In summary, one of the objectives of this book is to encourage you to move away from your intuitive views of behavior toward a systematic analysis, in the belief that the latter will enhance your effectiveness in accurately explaining and predicting behavior.

PUTTING THE "ORGANIZATION" INTO ORGANIZATIONAL BEHAVIOR

This chapter's title asks, "What is organizational behavior?" To this point, we have addressed only the general subject of behavior, which concerns itself with the actions people do that can be observed or measured. Now, let us turn our attention to the "organizational" context.

First, what is an *organization?* An organization is *the planned coordination of the activities of two or more people in order to achieve some common and explicit goal through division of labor and a hierarchy of authority.* Manufacturing and service firms clearly meet this definition, as do schools, hospitals, churches, military units, retail stores, police departments, and local, state, and federal government agencies.

What, then, is *organizational behavior?* Organizational Behavior (frequently abbreviated as OB) is *a field of study that investigates the impact that individuals, groups, and structure have on behavior within organizations for the purpose of applying such knowledge toward improving an organization's effectiveness.* That's a mouthful of words, so let's break it down.

Organizational behavior is a field of study. This means that it is a distinct area of expertise with a common body of knowledge. What does it study? It studies three determinants of behavior in organizations: individuals, groups, and structure. Additionally, OB is an applied field. It applies the knowledge gained about individuals, groups, and the effect of structure on behavior toward the end of making organizations work more effectively.

To sum up our definition, OB is concerned with the study of what people do in an organization and how that behavior effects the performance of the organization. And because OB is specifically concerned with employment-related environments, you should not be surprised to find that it gives emphasis to behavior as related to jobs, work, absenteeism, employment turnover, productivity, human performance, and management.

In addition to our definition, OB has been characterized in the broad sense as a way of thinking and in a narrower sense as a body of knowledge covering a relatively specific set of core topics.

When we view OB as a way of thinking, we acknowledge that it can be systematically studied. Organizational behavior can be conceptualized as the systematic study of nonrandom cause and effect phenomena. It also directs one's thinking toward viewing behavior in a performance-related context, that is, as it leads to effectiveness or success in achieving organizationally desirable outcomes.

There is increasing agreement as to the components or topics that comprise the subject area of OB. While there continues to be considerable debate as to the relative importance of each, there appears to be general agreement that OB includes the core topics of motivation, leader behavior and power, interpersonal communication, group structure and process, learning, attitude development and perception, interpersonal change, and conflict.

IS OB WORTH STUDYING?

So far, we have only *assumed* that there is value in being able to explain and predict behavior in an organizational setting. Therefore, we need to consider some specific reasons why the study of OB is deserving of your attention and effort.

Many people are interested in learning about OB for the sake of curiosity alone. They seek to understand behavior. They have no intention of ever applying their knowledge; rather they merely seek an answer to why people behave the way they do in organizations with which they are familiar.

Beyond this understanding lies a desire to be able to predict what others will do. You may want to develop your skills to make valid predictions; that is, if X, then Y. The study of OB will develop this predictive skill as it relates to behavior within organizations.

Probably the most popular reason for studying OB is that the reader is

FIGURE 1–1

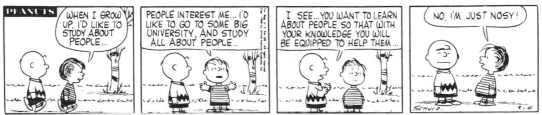

Source: Copyright 1960 by United Feature Syndicate, Inc. With permission.

interested in pursuing a career in management and wants to learn how to pre-dict behavior and apply it in some meaningful way to make organizations more effective. Having good "people skills"—which include the ability to understand your employees and to use this knowledge to get them to work efficiently and effectively for you—is a vital requirement if you are going to succeed as a man-ager.

Our final reason for studying OB may not be very exciting, but it is prag-matic—it may be a requirement for a particular degree or certificate you are seeking. In other words, you may be a captive in a required course and learning OB in your opinion may offer no obvious end that has value to you. In that case, the studying of OB is only a means toward that end. Hopefully, one of our first three reasons holds more relevance to *you*.

CONTRIBUTING DISCIPLINES TO THE OB FIELD

Organizational behavior is applied behavioral science, and as a result is built upon contributions from a number of behavioral disciplines. The predominant areas are psychology, sociology, social psychology, anthropology, and political science. As we shall learn, contributions of the psychologists have been mainly at the individual or micro level of analysis, while the latter disciplines have con-tributed to our understanding of macro concepts—group processes and organi-zation. Figure 1–2 overviews the contributions made toward a distinct field of study: Organizational Behavior.

Psychology

Psychology is the science that seeks to measure, explain, and sometimes change the behavior of humans and other animals. Psychologists concern themselves with studying and attempting to understand *individual* behavior. Those who have contributed and continue to add to the knowledge of OB are learning theorists, personality theorists, counseling psychologists, and, most importantly, organizational psychologists.

Early organizational psychologists concerned themselves with problems of fatigue, boredom, and any other factor relevant to working conditions that could impede efficient work performance. More recently, their contributions have been expanded to include learning, perception, personality, training, leadership effectiveness, needs and motivational forces, job satisfaction, performance ap-praisals, attitude measurement, and general shaping of behavior among organi-zational members to facilitate repetition of desirable behaviors.

Sociology

Whereas psychologists focus their attention on the individual, sociologists study the social system in which individuals fill their roles; that is, sociology studies

FIGURE 1–2 Toward an OB Discipline

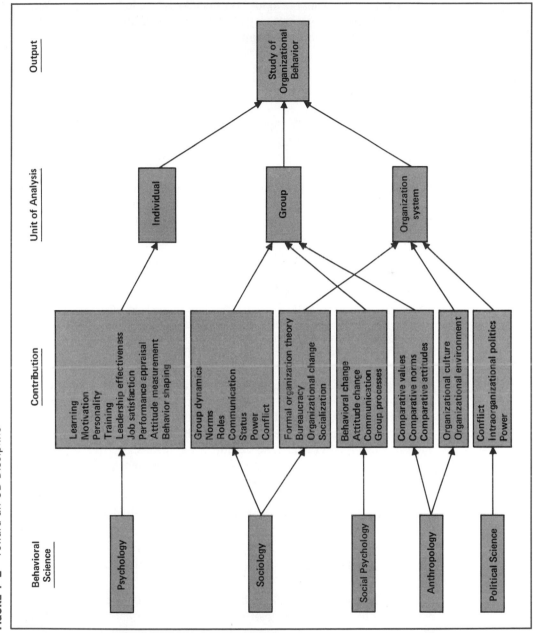

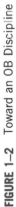

people in relation to their fellow human beings. Specifically, sociologists have made their greatest contribution to OB through their study of group behavior in organizations, particularly formal and complex organizations. Areas within OB that have received valuable input from sociologists include group dynamics, the socialization process, formal organization theory and structure, bureaucracy, communications, status, power, and conflict.

Social Psychology

A relatively new field in its own right, social psychology examines interpersonal behavior. While psychology and sociology attempt to explain individual and group behavior respectively, social psychology seeks to explain how and why individuals behave as they do in group activities. One of the major areas receiving considerable investigation by social psychologists has been *change*—how to implement it and how to reduce barriers to its acceptance. Additionally, we find social psychologists making significant contributions in measuring, understanding, and changing attitudes, communication patterns, and the ways in which group activities can satisfy individual needs.

Anthropology

Anthropologists study societies, particularly primitive ones, to learn about human beings and their activities. Recognition that how we behave is a function of our culture, for example, dramatizes the contribution social anthropologists have made to OB. Differences in fundamental values, attitudes, and norms of acceptable behavior affect the way people act and explain to a considerable degree differences in behavior between, for example, Americans and East Indians, New Englanders and Southerners, or urbanites and those who were raised and have spent all their lives in rural or farm communities.

Our individual value systems—that is, our priorities and sense of right and wrong—will affect our attitudes and behavior on the job. Additionally, the work that anthropologists have done with animals, especially in the ape family, has been valuable in drawing generalizations about individual and group behavior.

Political Science

Although frequently overlooked, the contributions of political scientists are significant to the understanding of behavior in organizations. Political scientists study the behavior of individuals and groups within a political environment. Specific topics of concern to political scientists include structuring of conflict, allocation of power, and how people manipulate power for individual self-interest.

ARE "OB" AND "MANAGEMENT" SYNONYMOUS TERMS?

Many academics, practitioners, and students confuse the subject matter in OB and that in management or administration. While there is some overlap, management and OB have different means and ends.

Organizational behavior, as noted previously, is concerned with how people, individually and in groups, act in organizations. Management is concerned with the optimum attainment of organizational goals. However, since these goals are unattainable without human input, OB is a significant subset or segment of management.

The subject of OB is intended to support the knowledge necessary to be a manager. The understanding of individual and group behavior is important for what it can contribute toward the education and development of one's managerial talents. When managers perform managerial functions—planning, organizing, leading, and controlling—they need to know how their actions will impact on people. Since managers work with and get things done through other people, an understanding of people is critical to being a successful manager. But, of course, since managers also work with physical inputs (e.g., equipment, inventories) and financial inputs, a manager requires knowledge of subjects that go beyond human behavior to include, but are not limited to: accounting, finance, marketing, production systems, purchasing, forecasting, strategy and policy formation, economics, computer science, and decision making.

THERE ARE FEW ABSOLUTES IN OB

Nearly two centuries ago, the German philosopher Georg Hegel stated that thinking develops out of conflict. He argued that for every positive thesis there exists an antithesis or counterposition that negates the thesis. He believed that the conflict between these two positions produces a synthesis that does justice to the substance of both the thesis and antithesis and yet is superior to both. While Karl Marx used Hegel's dialectic to formulate a theory of revolution, this same dialectic is also the fundamental basis upon which education is built.

The objective of education is to develop one's ability to think, reason, and understand. Education seeks to cultivate an inquiring mind with the capacity to think independently, to express thoughts clearly and logically, and to exercise good judgment. Educated individuals should be less dogmatic and more appreciative of differences than the uneducated. They should be open to changing their minds as facts or conditions change. There is considerable truth to the statement that "consistency requires you to be as ignorant today as you were a year ago."

Certainly what is true for education as a whole is also true for education in organizational behavior. Simple and universal principles are avoided because there exist no simple and universal truths or principles that consistently explain organizational behavior. Instead, OB concepts are founded on situational or contingency conditions; that is, if *X*, then *Y*, but only under conditions specified in *Z* (the contingency variables). Based on understanding of human behavior, the science of OB has developed by using general concepts and altering their application to the particular situation. So, for example, OB scholars would avoid stating that effective leaders should always seek the ideas of their subordinates before making a decision. Rather, we shall find that in some situations a participative style is clearly superior, but in other situations an autocratic decision style is more effective. In other words, the effectiveness of a particular leadership style is *contingent* upon the situation in which it is utilized.

Contingency conditions, however, represent only part of the reason that OB should not be approached from a single viewpoint. Another reason for appreciating a multiview approach to OB is that conflicting positions are inevitable due to the different value systems among OB researchers, teachers, students, and practitioners.

An individual's value system—namely, one's beliefs of what is right or wrong—influences one's perceptions, attitudes, and behavior. If, for example, you believe that intelligence is predominantly determined by heredity, the way you look at the learning and training of employees will differ from that of someone who considers intelligence to be basically determined by the environment and experiences to which one is exposed.

Given that education is concerned with developing reasoning skills rather than dogmatic answers, that issues are rarely black or white, and that how we view anything is dependent on our beliefs in what is right or wrong, it seems logical (1) to approach OB from a contingency approach and (2) to stimulate the reader's reasoning abilities by presenting opposing positions on key topic issues within OB. This book will attempt to do both.

As you proceed through this volume, you will be constantly reminded of the contingency elements in OB. Specific efforts have been made to isolate those critical situational characteristics that are influential in determining whether certain types of management actions are likely to succeed or fail. Additionally, at the end of each chapter you will find a section entitled "Point-Counterpoint."

THE VALUE OF DIALOGUE ON OB ISSUES

Bertrand Russell said, "What is wanted is not the will to believe but the wish to find out, which is the exact opposite." The Point-Counterpoint sections following each chapter are included to reinforce the view that, within the field of OB, there is much intellectual debate and that learning is facilitated more by developing an inquiring mind than by "selling" a certain belief system. For example, at the conclusion of the chapter on leadership, you will find an article that views leadership as playing an important role in an organization attaining its goals. The following article, on the other hand, proposes that there is little evidence to support the view that leadership is important in determining organizational outcomes.

The exercise is meant to demonstrate that you will rarely find universally "right" answers to issues—and that differences of opinion can also surround the interpretation and importance of research. Each of the Point-Counterpoint arguments has valid points. What is right or wrong, good or bad, is based on what you think is important and not important; on what you see and what really exists.

It is hoped that the Point-Counterpoint dialogues will develop your intellectual capabilities, reasoning skills, and ability to appreciate differences, will help you to examine your own assumptions about human behavior, and will demonstrate how differences in values, perceptions, and role requirements among OB writers have resulted in considerably different positions on the same topics. Just as abortion is seen considerably differently by femininists and Catholic priests, OB topics like conflict, power, leadership, and organization design have their liberal and conservative proponents.

More specifically, by reviewing two sides of an issue you are forced to assess the underlying values of the writers and the assumptions they base their positions upon; you will have to appraise the quality of their logic and evaluate the degree to which the conclusions drawn by each author align with the assumptions made and the facts and evidence presented to defend his or her position. Just as one can develop one's intellectual and reasoning abilities through debate, the adversary relationship in the Point-Counterpoint section should assist you in developing your intellectual and reasoning abilities and applying them successfully to OB issues.

FOR DISCUSSION

1. Contrast an intuitive approach to studying behavior with a systematic approach. Is intuition always inaccurate?

2. What does the phrase "behavior is caused" mean?

3. Define organizational behavior. How does this compare with management?

4. What is an organization? Is the family unit an organization?

5. Give four reasons for studying OB.

6. What are areas where psychology has contributed to OB? Sociology? Social psychology? Anthropology? Political science? Can you think of other academic disciplines that may have contributed to OB?

7. What is the Hegelian dialectic? What relevance does it have to education? To OB?

8. "The best way to view OB is through a contingency approach." Build an argument to support this statement.

9. "Since behavior is generally predictable, there is no need to formally study OB." Why is this statement wrong?

10. Some authors have defined the purpose of OB as being "to explain, predict, and control behavior." Do you agree or disagree? Discuss.

FOR FURTHER READING

FLIPPO, E. B., "The Underutilization of Behavioral Science by Management," in *Contemporary Management*, ed. J. W. McGuire, pp. 36–41. Englewood Cliffs, N.J.: Prentice-Hall, 1974. Considers the contribution of behavioral scientists to more effective managerial practices.

KARMEL, B., *Point and Counterpoint in Organizational Behavior* (Hinsdale, Ill.: Dryden Press, 1980). Presents four pairs of debates using the point-counterpoint format.

LAWLER, E. E. III, "Adaptive Experiments: An Approach to Organizational Behavioral Research," *Academy of Management Review,* October 1977, pp. 576–85. Looks at how research designs can be adapted to assess the relative effectiveness of different management practices and organization designs.

LIPPERT, F. G., "Toward Flexibility in Application of Behavioral Science Research," *Academy of Management Journal,* June 1971, pp. 195–201. Practitioners tend toward a superficial evaluation of behavioral science research. There are no panaceas that are useful under all circumstances.

SCHEIN, E. H., "Behavioral Sciences for Management," in *Contemporary Management,* ed. J. W. McGuire, pp. 15–32. Englewood Cliffs, N.J.: Prentice-Hall, 1974. The behavioral sciences have a potential relevance to the three basic resources that managers process: (1) money or financial resources, (2) people or human resources, and (3) information of various kinds

VAN DEN BERGHE, P. L., "Sociobiology: A New Paradigm for the Behavioral Sciences?" *Social Sciences Quarterly*, September 1978, pp. 326–32. Reviews the contention of sociobiologists that human organization is reducible to the three principles of kin selection, reciprocity, and coercion.

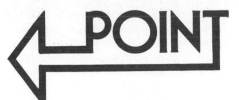

STRAUSS ET AL.

Organizational behavior is a social science

Adapted from Organizational Behavior, Research and Issues *by George Strauss, Raymond E. Miles, Charles C. Snow, and Arnold S. Tannenbaum, eds.*© *1976, 1974 by Industrial Relations Research Association. Reprinted by permission of the publisher, Wadsworth Publishing Company, Inc., Belmont, California 94002.*

Defining any academic field is difficult, but Organizational Behavior (OB) may be more difficult to define than most. As a new field, it has yet to stake out its jurisdiction definitively. Further, as an applied field, it draws very heavily on more basic fields, making it difficult to distinguish between what is rightfully OB's and what belongs to the parent discipline.

OB represents a combination of at least parts of two older fields in business schools. Human Relations and Management, but, as just mentioned, it also includes liberal elements of other disciplines, especially of psychology and sociology. Political science, economics (at least those elements dealing with decision making and information economics), anthropology, and psychiatry have also had some (probably too little) influence on the development of OB. In addition, an increasingly substantial contribution is being made by a younger generation of scholars who have received their training in business schools under the rubric of Organizational Behavior itself (or some related term).

As an academic discipline, most of what is called OB is taught in business schools and thus is focused primarily on profit-making organizations. But OB people are also interested in government, schools, hospitals, social agencies, and the like. In fact, much of the most interesting research has been done in these areas, and OB courses (though not necessarily under the title OB) are increasingly being taught in schools of education, public administration, public health, hospital administration, social work, and even forestry. It seems increasingly clear that OB principles apply (or do not apply) equally well in the nonprofit as well as in the profit sector, under socialism as well as capitalism. And they most certainly apply to unions.

OB is an applied area, but some of the best OB research is not directly applicable. Seventeen years ago, in the Industrial Relations Research Association's last review of this subject, Wilensky argued that "not everything done by the social scientist can or should help the practitioner . . . the social scientist's job is basically different from the executive's job . . . much of what he comes up with is of only limited use to the practitioner."[1] Some progress has been made since 1957 in developing management applications; nevertheless Wilensky's warning still has much validity: in general, OB research is not designed to provide solutions for specific management problems.

[1] Harold L. Wilensky, "Human Relations in the Work Place: An Appraisal of Some Recent Research," in *Research in Industrial Human Relations,* ed. C. M. Arensberg et al. (New York: Harper & Brothers, 1957), pp. 27–35.

True, much of what passes as OB "research" is mere description of management practices and sometimes consists of normative descriptions not based on empirical data. However, the best research goes beyond this and is designed to develop theories or models which in turn can help scholars and practitioners understand behavior in organizations and therefore predict and even modify behavior.

Let us be a bit more specific as to OB's value to the practitioner. Untutored, the typical person draws inferences from his own immediate experience, and, on the basis of this experience, he develops "models" that consciously or unconsciously affect his perceptions of events and how he reacts to them. To take an example: If, on the basis of early experience (or folk wisdom picked up from others), a manager concludes that workers are generally lazy and seek to shun responsibility, he is likely to supervise his own subordinates closely, thereby alienating many of them, and thus to induce them to in fact evade responsibilities. Under these circumstances, the manager's original hypothesis is confirmed.

For the practitioner who is a victim of this (and related) counterproductive cycle, OB may possibly offer three kinds of services:

1. Like any other science, OB is concerned with the relationships among organizational phenomena. On the basis of these observed relationships, theories (or models) can be developed and tested. Tested theories may, in turn, help the practitioner to understand the impact of his own current behaviors by telling him, "If you do X, there is considerable likelihood that Y will occur." As Kurt Lewin, one of the most influential of the early contributors to this field, was fond of saying, "There is nothing so practical as a good theory."

2. From the systematic study of behavior (in both real organizations and laboratory-based simulated organizations), OB research can suggest a broader range of possible behaviors to the practitioner than he had previously considered—as well as the implications of each. Combined with good theory, an expanded repertoire of managerial behaviors can significantly extend the action alternatives most practitioners possess.

3. Finally, by expanding the practitioner's range of alternative behaviors and by placing these within frameworks that provide some basis for estimating the possible impact of each form of behavior, OB research may help the practitioner make informed evaluations of future behaviors and their likely outcomes.

COUNTER POINT

WILSON

Sociobiology: studying behavior from a biological basis

Sociobiology is defined as the systematic study of the biological basis of all social behavior. For the present it focuses on animal societies, their population structure, castes, and communication, together with all of the physiology underlying the social adaptations. But the discipline is also concerned with the social behavior of early man and the adaptive features of organization in the more primitive contemporary human societies. Sociology, the study of human societies at all levels of complexity, still stands apart from sociobiology because of its largely structuralist and nongenetic approach. It attempts to explain human behavior primarily by empirical description of the outermost phenotypes and by unaided intuition, without reference to evolutionary explanations in the true genetic sense. It is most successful, in the way descriptive taxonomy and ecology have been most successful, when it provides a detailed description of particular phenomena and demonstrates first-order correlations with features of the environment. Taxonomy and ecology, however, have been reshaped entirely during the past forty years by integration into neo-Darwinist evolutionary theory—the "Modern Synthesis," as it is often called—in which each phenomenon is weighed for its adaptive significance and then related to the basic principles of population genetics. It may not be too much to say that sociology and the other social sciences, as well as the humanities, are the last branches of biology waiting to be included in the Modern Synthesis. One of the functions of sociobiology, then, is to reformulate the foundations of the social sciences in a way that draws these subjects into the Modern Synthesis. Whether the social sciences can be truly biologicized in this fashion remains to be seen.

It is part of the conventional wisdom that virtually all cultural variation is phenotypic rather than genetic in origin. This view has gained support from the ease with which certain aspects of culture can be altered in the space of a single generation, too quickly to be evolutionary in nature. The extreme orthodox view of environmentalism holds that in effect there is no genetic variance in the transmission of culture. Although the genes have given away most of their sovereignty, they maintain a certain amount of influence in at least the behavioral qualities that underlie variations between cultures. Moderately high heritability has been documented in introversion-extroversion measures, personal tempo, psychomotor and sports activities, neuroticism, dominance, depression, and the tendency toward certain forms of mental illness such as schizophrenia. Even a small portion of this variance invested in population differences might predispose societies toward cultural differences. At the very least, we should try to measure this amount. It is not valid to point to the absence of a behavioral trait in one or a few societies as conclusive evidence that the trait is environmentally induced and has no genetic disposition in man. The very opposite could be true.

In short, there is a need for a discipline of anthropological genetics. In the interval before we acquire it, it should be possible to characterize the human biogram by two indirect methods. First, models can be constructed from the most elementary rules of human behavior. Insofar as they can be tested, the rules will characterize the biogram in much the same way the ethograms drawn by zoologists identify the "typical" behavioral repertoires of animal species. The rules can be legitimately compared with the ethograms of other primate species. Variation in the rules among human cultures, however slight, might provide clues to underlying genetic differences, particularly when it is correlated with variation in behavioral traits known to be heritable.

The other indirect approach to anthropological genetics is through phylogenetic analysis. By comparing man with other primate species, it might be possible to identify basic primate traits that lie beneath the surface and help to determine the configuration of man's higher social behavior. This approach has been taken with great style and vigor in a series of popular books by Konrad Lorenz (*On Aggression*), Robert Ardrey (*The Social Contract*), Desmond Morris (*The Naked Ape*), and Lionel Tiger and Robin Fox (*The Imperial Animal*). Their efforts were salutary in calling attention to man's status as a biological species adapted to particular environments.

Let me now turn, in a very guarded context, to postulating a future scenario for sociobiology as it applies to human behavior.

When mankind has achieved an ecological steady state, probably by the end of the twenty-first century, the internalization of social evolution will be nearly complete. About this time biology should be at its peak, with the social sciences maturing rapidly. Some historians of science will take issue with this projection, arguing that the accelerating pace of discoveries in these fields implies a more rapid development. But historical precedents have misled us before: The subjects we are talking about are more difficult than physics or chemistry by at least two orders of magnitude.

Consider the prospects for sociology. There have been attempts at system building but, as in psychology, they were premature and came to little. Much of what passes for theory in sociology today is really labeling of phenomena and concepts. Process is difficult to analyze because the fundamental units are elusive, perhaps nonexistent. Syntheses commonly consist of the tedious cross-referencing of differing sets of definitions and metaphors erected by the more imaginative thinkers.

With an increase in the richness of descriptions and experiments, sociology is drawing closer each day to cultural anthropology, social psychology, and economics, and will soon merge with them. These disciplines are fundamental to sociology *sensu lato* and are most likely to yield its first phenomenological laws. In fact, some viable qualitative laws probably already exist. They include tested statements about the following relationships: the positive correlation between and within cultures of war and combative sports, resulting in the elimination of the hydraulic model of aggressive drive; precise but still specialized models of promotion and opportunity within professional guilds; and, far from least, the most general models of economics.

The transition from purely phenomenological to fundamental theory in sociology must await a full, neuronal explanation of the human brain. Only when the machinery can be torn down on paper at the level of the cell and put together again will the properties of emotion and ethical judgment come clear. Simulations can then be employed to estimate the full range of behavioral responses and the precision of their homeostatic controls. Stress will be evaluated in terms of the neurophysiological perturbations and their relaxation times. Cognition will be translated into circuitry. Learning and creativeness will be defined as the alteration of specific portions of the cognitive machinery regulated by input from the emotive centers. Having cannibalized psychology, the new neurobiology will yield an enduring set of first principles for sociology.

CHAPTER 2
Models: Toward Explaining and Predicting Behavior

AFTER STUDYING THIS CHAPTER, YOU SHOULD BE ABLE TO

Define and explain the following key terms and concepts:

Absenteeism
Causality
Dependent variables
Effectiveness
Efficiency
Independent variables

Job satisfaction
Models
Moderating variables
Productivity
Turnover

Understand:

The value of models to students of OB
The limitations of models
The types of models
The three universal components in a model
The three levels of analysis in OB

> A model is like an academic coat rack—something on which to hang theories.
>
> —S.P.R.

When confronted with the task of expressing complex things or ideas in a clear manner, we often resort to models. They help us to simplify, but in a way that minimizes the loss of accuracy and understanding. Models are used in a number of professions—by aircraft designers, economic forecasters, managers, and, as we'll show, even by textbook writers. Let us consider some examples of the use of models.

The Concorde supersonic jet is a complex physical structure composed of tons of aluminum, titanium, carpeting, and electronic equipment; however, if you know nothing about the Concorde, to describe it as an airplane that seats 160 people and can cruise at 1,200 miles per hour fails to convey an accurate picture of the aircraft. If, on the other hand, you were shown a 1:20 scale replica of the Concorde, the accuracy of your understanding of what the plane looks like would be improved.

Of course, a miniature replica of a Concorde cannot give you the sense of what it might be like breezing along 60,000 feet above the Atlantic Ocean at 1,200 miles per hour. Why not? Because the miniature is a model, built to demonstrate what a Concorde looks like. This model does not attempt, for example, to simulate the sound, feel, or interior roominess of the plane. Since our miniature is a model, it is an *abstraction of reality—a simplified representation of some real-world phenomena.* In this case, it attempts to represent the physical appearance of the Concorde.

The American economy is forecast by means of computers that have been programmed with input on such diverse parts of our society as tax rates and capital-goods spending in the steel industry. The data inputs are fed through a complex equation, and the result is an estimate of a future national product. The complex equation is a highly simplified abstraction of the American economy. It is also a mathematical model.

An organization chart—that pyramidal form hanging on the walls of personnel departments throughout the world—is also a model, portraying the formal pattern of authority relationships. It is used by managers to represent graphically the organization's hierarchy. But it, too, is a simplification. Most of us are aware that decision influence within an organization is not always shown by its organization chart. In reality, there are informal processes that, even though not shown on the chart, are important influences on decision patterns. For example, one should not assume that all those in an organization who have similar titles, and who are at the same level in the formal organization structure, are equally influential. Who knows who, who owes who, and who has the "clout" are not depicted on organization charts.

Models are a useful tool for writers in their effort to clarify complex topics. Your author believes that a good model is particularly valuable in simplifying the very complex field of OB. It can be useful in structuring the many diverse topics within OB into an integrative whole. We shall develop an OB model later in this chapter that will help you to put together the contents of this book and assist you in explaining and predicting real-life behavior in organizations. We shall approach the development of an OB model not as an end in itself, but rather as a means to the end of better understanding behavior in organization. First, however, we need to consider a typology of models—that is, the various types of models that are available to us—and then discuss the components that make up any model.

CLASSIFICATION OF MODELS

Models can be classified by a number of approaches. For example, they may be subjective or objective, static or dynamic, physical or abstract, normative or descriptive. This short listing is quite incomplete but demonstrates that models can be viewed in a number of ways. Briefly, let us review each of these classifications and show how they can relate to organizational behavior.

Subjective versus Objective Models

We carry around a number of models in our heads. These are intuitive views of how things operate. These models are subjective if they are primitive, that is, lacking in formal methods. Subjective models, for instance, are frequently the base from which decision makers in organizations appraise the behavior of job applicants in employment interviews. If the interviewer believes, based on intuition, that applicants who are aggressive and self-confident are better job performers than passive and self-doubting applicants, then a subjective model is being used.

In contrast, most formal models are objective. They substitute systematic analysis for intuition. Organizational behavior models seek objectivity and hopefully assist managers and would-be managers to replace their subjective views of behavior in the organization with formal and systematic thinking.

Static versus Dynamic Models

Models that are developed to deal with changes over time and that recognize the complexities of the environment are dynamic. Those that assume stability and maintenance of the status quo are static. In developing models of an organization and the behavior of its personnel, we must think in dynamic terms. Any other approach cannot accurately be predictive; that is, it is difficult to generalize about what will happen in the future from static models.

Physical versus Abstract Models

A mannequin in a retail store is a physical model. The accountant's model of a balance sheet—Assets = Liabilities + Owner's Equity—is abstract. Each is a simplification of reality, yet they are clearly different. The former is tangible and concrete. Examples include model planes, ships, and buildings. Abstract models are intangible and symbolic. The predominant form that abstract models take is mathematical.

In organizational behavior, we rarely deal with physical models. These are more the domain of engineers and architects. Abstract models, however, are popular for expressing OB concepts. When we say, for instance, that Performance = Motivation × Ability, we are expressing a complex relationship in a simple but abstract model.

Normative versus Descriptive Models

One of the most important distinctions that can be made between models is to classify them as either normative or descriptive. The former states what should be; the latter describes what is.

Normative models determine actions that produce an optimal solution. For the most part, management theory is composed of normative models—they attempt to present what managers *should* do. Management textbooks, for example, traditionally develop a theoretical structure for understanding the optimum functioning of managers.

In contrast, descriptive models are functioning properly when they accurately describe the activity they represent. They picture what is really going on. Valid descriptive models—ones that accurately portray what is taking place and that can explain different behaviors in varying situations or by different people—become the province of OB, since OB is concerned with real, not idealized behavior in organizations.

The above classifications present the most popular types of models. It is important to note, though, that these classes should not be considered as singular labels. Most models can be described using several of the labels presented. A model can, for example, be objective, dynamic, abstract, and normative—all at the same time.

COMPONENTS OF A MODEL

All of the models previously discussed have certain elements in common. No matter what type of model we are talking about, if it *is* a model then it will contain three universal components. These common components are an objective, variables, and relationships.

Objective

The formulation of a model begins with determining what it is that we want the model to do. Is the model attempting to predict turnover, explain motivation, select the best job applicant, ascertain the most effective leadership style, or explain why productivity within a certain department has dropped off dramatically? Once the objective is known, the key variables that may affect this objective can be identified, their order classified, and relationships defined.

Variables

General characteristics that can be measured and that change in either amplitude and/or intensity are called variables. These are critical or key elements that affect the objective we have stated. In behavior modeling, the discussion usually centers around three types of variables: dependent, independent, and moderating.

Dependent Variables. A dependent variable is a response that is affected by an independent variable. In behavioral research, popular dependent behaviors are productivity, absenteeism, and turnover. However, attitudes, such as job satisfaction, are also frequently used as dependent variables.

Independent Variables. Independent variables affect the dependent variable. "An *independent variable* is the *presumed* cause of the *dependent variable,* the *presumed effect.*"[1]

In experimental usage, the experimenter manipulates the independent variable, and then measures changes in the dependent variable. If we use worker output per hour as a dependent variable, and leadership style as the independent variable, we look for how changes in leadership style will affect worker productivity. "Whenever we state that, 'If X, then Y,' whenever we have an implication, X implies Y, we have an independent variable (X) and a dependent variable (Y)."[2]

Popular independent variables studied by OB researchers include intelligence, personality, attitudes, experience, motivation, reinforcement patterns, leadership style, reward allocations, selection methods, and organization design. By specifying the amplitude or intensity of an independent variable—for example, identifying close, moderate, and loose supervision—we can measure different levels in a dependent variable—for example, absenteeism. In this specific case, we would have three levels of the independent variable.

1. F. Kerlinger, *Foundations of Behavioral Research* (New York: Holt, Rinehart & Winston, 1965), p. 39.

2. Ibid.

Moderating Variables. Moderating variables abate the effects of the independent variable on the dependent variable. They increase complexity by saying: If X (independent variable), then Y (dependent variable) will occur, but only under conditions Z (moderating variable). To translate this into a real-life example, we might say that if we increase the amount of direct supervision in the work area (X), then there will be a change in worker productivity (Y), but this effect will be moderated by the complexity of the tasks being performed (Z).

Our discussion of variables should not be interpreted to mean that certain variable characteristics are always dependent, always independent, or always moderating. Whether a characteristic is treated as a dependent, independent, or moderating variable depends on the objective of the model. Job satisfaction, for example, would be an independent variable if the objective is to ascertain how different levels of satisfaction influence turnover. However, if the objective is to determine the impact of various pay schedules on job satisfaction, job satisfaction would become a dependent variable.

Relationships

What is the relationship among variables in our model? What is the *cause* and what is the *effect?*

Any conclusion regarding causality—that is, implying presumed cause and effect—can be highly dangerous. We must guard against assuming that a causal relation exists when only a correlation has been observed. To demonstrate, consider the following fact: Married men and women live longer than their unmarried counterparts. This statement is true, corroborated by a wealth of statistical data. Is it correct to conclude, however, that marriage causes longer life? The answer is a qualified ''No.'' Evidence suggests that people who are unlikely to live longer are also unlikely to marry or stay married, and that since most people consider marriage desirable, those who do not marry are considered odd, which puts them under social pressures and stress that can wear them down physically and reduce their life expectancy. In other words, it is one thing to determine a relationship between marriage and longevity but another to attribute causality.

Similarly, statistics clearly show that college graduates earn substantially more money during their working lives than do individuals who have not attended college. It's tempting to conclude that the college experience *caused* the higher earnings. While higher educational institutions might wish this to be true, the statistical correlation does not prove causation. It could just as easily be argued that individuals who are bright and ambitious are more likely than their less bright, less ambitious peers to choose to go to college, and that these brighter and more ambitious types would probably earn more than their peers, regardless of whether they went to college or not. The college experience, therefore, may have little, in fact, to do with the higher earnings.

We are concerned with relationships, specifically causality, for two reasons: (1) Researchers in OB use models, and can be guilty of concluding a causal relation from a correlation; and (2) a general OB model, which purports to explain and predict, implies causation between its independent and dependent variables. Let us briefly expand on each of these points.

The field of OB is building upon a base of empirical research—from studies of how people actually behave in controlled laboratory experiments and from field data gathered in real organizations. If researchers are sloppy in developing their research designs, any conclusions from such research becomes highly questionable. If researchers use unreliable measurement tools, inappropriate statistical tests, or draw incorrect conclusions from their data, our ability to make accurate statements about behavior becomes limited. Assume, for example, we employ a worker named Joan who is absent a lot. If Joan is married, with two children, and if we know that women with children have higher absenteeism than single women, can we attribute Joan's high absenteeism to her marital and child-rearing responsibilities? There may be a relationship, but the family responsibilities may not be *causing* her absenteeism.

Our other reason for being concerned with causality is that a general OB model implies that the independent variables directly cause changes in the dependent variables. In the model that we shall be using in this book, we shall articulate both types of variables and draw conclusions based on their implied relationship.

Summary

At this point, it may be helpful to summarize and synthesize. You may be asking, Who cares about causality? So what? What have models, objectives, variables, relationships, and causality got to do with understanding organizational behavior? Ah, but there is method in this madness!

The answer is really quite simple: OB is a complex field and an OB model can help us to attain our objective—to explain and predict the way people behave in organizations. Our OB model will be our road map through the vast OB maze (and through the approximately 600 pages of this book). Since, like all models, it consists of an objective, variables, and relationships, it is important to understand these concepts in order to understand the organizational behavior that is represented by the model.

VARIABLES IN OUR OB MODEL

We have stated the objective of an OB model: to explain and predict the way people behave in organizations. Our model makes many simplified assumptions and explicitly excludes moderating variables (they will be added as we go along), but it should help you to understand the key components of OB.

Our model begins by analyzing individual behavior. Using the knowledge gained at the individual level, we move on to a more complex topic, the group. Finally, we add a third level of complexity, the formal organization structural system, to arrive at our final destination: an understanding of organizational behavior. Figure 2–1 presents a skeleton on which we will construct our OB mod-

FIGURE 2–1 Basic OB Model, Stage 1

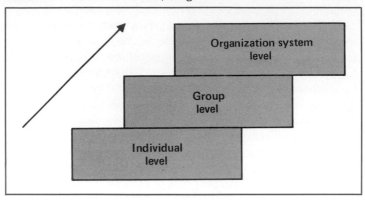

el. It proposes that there are three levels of analysis in OB, and that as we move from the individual level through to the organizational systems level, we add systematically to our understanding of behavior in organizations. The three basic levels are analogous to building blocks—each level is constructed upon the previous level. Group concepts grow out of the foundation laid in the individual section; we overlay structural constraints on the individual and group in order to arrive at organizational behavior.

The Dependent Variables

What are the key dependent variables in OB? Scholars tend to emphasize productivity, absenteeism, turnover, and job satisfaction. We shall use these four as the critical determinants of an organization's effectiveness.

Scholars have chosen these dependent variables because they are concerned with organizational effectiveness. Three behaviors appear important to defining effectiveness: membership, attendance, and productivity. Further, while job satisfaction is an attitude rather than a behavior, it is of concern because many scholars and practitioners believe that, from a socially responsible point of view, satisfaction is an important and relevant outcome. Other variables such as return on investment, growth in revenues, or market share are equally legitimate outcomes—these are frequently used by managers—but the four dependent variables we have chosen are the ones most studied by OB researchers.

Productivity. An organization is productive if it achieves its goals and does so by transferring inputs to outputs at the lowest cost. As such, productivity implies a concern for both effectiveness and efficiency.

A hospital, for example, is *effective* when it successfully meets the needs of its clientele. It is *efficient* when it can do this at a low cost. If a hospital manages to achieve higher output from its present staff by reducing the average number of days a patient is confined to a bed or by increasing the number of staff-patient contacts per day, we can say the hospital has gained productive efficiency. Similarly, a school may be effective when a certain percentage of students achieve a specified score on standardized achievement tests. The school can improve its efficiency if these higher test scores can be secured by a smaller teaching and support staff. A business firm is effective when it attains its sales or market share goals, but its productivity also depends on achieving these goals efficiently. Measures of such efficiency may include return on investment, profit per dollar of sales, and output per hour of labor.

We can also look at productivity from the perspective of the individual employee. Take the cases of Mike and Al, who are both long-distance truckers. If Mike is supposed to haul his fully loaded rig from New York to its destination in Los Angeles in sixty-eight hours or less, he is effective if he makes the 3,000 mile trip within this time period. But measures of productivity must take into account the costs incurred in reaching the goal. That is where efficiency comes in. Let us assume that Mike made the New York to Los Angeles run in sixty-seven hours and averaged seven miles per gallon. Al, on the other hand, made the trip in sixty-seven hours also but averaged nine miles per gallon. Both Mike and Al were effective—they accomplished their goal—but Al was more efficient than Mike because he consumed less gas and therefore achieved his goal at a lower cost.

In summary, one of OB's major concerns is productivity. We want to know what factors will influence the effectiveness and efficiency of individuals, of groups, and of the overall organization.

Absenteeism. The annual cost of absenteeism to U.S. organizations has been estimated at a staggering $26.4 billion.[3] It is difficult for an organization to operate smoothly and to attain its objectives if employees fail to report to their jobs. The work flow is disrupted and often important decisions must be delayed. In organizations that rely heavily upon assembly-line technology, absenteeism can be considerably more than a disruption—it can result in a drastic reduction in quality of output or, in some cases, can bring about a complete shutdown of the production facility. Examples abound, for instance, of the problems that the major U.S. automobile manufacturers have with alarmingly large increases in absences on Mondays and Fridays, especially in summer months and at the onset of the hunting and fishing seasons. Certainly, levels of absenteeism beyond the normal range have a direct impact on an organization's effectiveness and efficiency.

Turnover. A high rate of turnover in an organization means increased recruiting, selection, and training costs. It can also mean a disruption in the efficient running of an organization when knowledgeable and experienced personnel leave and replacements must be found and prepared to assume positions of responsibility. All organizations, of course, have some turnover. An organization that has no turnover probably suffers from a lack of new and fresh ideas. If the right people are leaving the organization—the marginal and submarginal em-

3. Richard M. Steers and Susan R. Rhodes, "Major Influences on Employee Attendance: A Process Model," *Journal of Applied Psychology*, August 1978, p. 391.

ployees—then turnover is functional to the operation of the organization. But when turnover is excessive or when it is confined to the superior performers, it can be a major disruptive factor, hindering the organization's effectiveness.

Job Satisfaction. The belief that satisfied employees are more productive than dissatisfied employees has been a basic tenet among managers for years. While the evidence questions this assumed causal relationship, it can be argued that a wealthy nation should not only be concerned with the quantity of life but also with improving its quality. Consistent with this view, an employee's satisfaction with his or her job (defined as the difference between the amount of rewards workers receive and the amount they believe they should receive) can be used as a reasonable substitute for the quality of work life.

Those scholars and practitioners with strong humanistic values argue that satisfaction should be a legitimate objective of an organization. Not only is satisfaction negatively related to absenteeism and turnover but, they argue, organizations have a responsibility that goes beyond dollars and cents to provide employees with jobs that are challenging and intrinsically rewarding. Therefore, although job satisfaction represents an attitude rather than a behavior, OB researchers typically consider job satisfaction an important dependent variable.

The Independent Variables

What are the major determinants of productivity, absenteeism, turnover, and job satisfaction? Our answer to that question brings us to the independent variables. Consistent with our belief that organizational behavior can best be understood when viewed essentially as a set of increasingly complex building blocks, the base or first level of our model lies in understanding individual behavior.

Values and Attitudes. Individuals enter organizations with preconceived ideas about what is right or wrong, or good or bad, and with other notions that influence the way they think and behave. Since these values and attitudes are held by individuals prior to joining an organization, they are the first step in understanding individual behavior. Values and attitudes will be discussed in the next chapter.

Personality. An individual's personality is also generally well established long before he or she enters the work force. Personalities can change, but they generally remain stable over time. So, as with values and attitudes, we shall treat personality as something people bring with them when they join an organization. An understanding of personality will tell us "how a person affects others, how he understands and views himself, and his pattern of inner and outer measurable traits."[4] This is the subject matter of Chapter 4.

4. Floyd L. Ruch and Phillip G. Zimbardo, *Psychology and Life,* 8th ed. (Glenview, Ill.: Scott, Foresman, 1971).

Perception. What we see is not reality, but rather our perception of reality. Yet, it is this perception that will influence our behavior. For example, whether or not your boss is prejudiced is irrelevant—if you *perceive* him to be, you will act as if he is! Since how we see the world will be a major influence on our behavior, the topic of perception deserves our attention. This subject is the topic of Chapter 5.

Motivation. The preceding variables, when linked with external stimuli, influence the amount of effort an individual exerts on his or her job. From a managerial perspective, motivation may be one of the most important subjects to master toward predicting our dependent variables. We shall discuss motivation in Chapter 6.

Learning. As managers, we seek to influence behavior. In this role, we attempt to change individual behavior, hopefully in ways that will improve the organization's effectiveness. To effect changes in behavior we need to know how people have learned their current behaviors. Chapter 7 presents basic principles in learning and the learning process, discusses classical and operant conditioning, and considers schedules of reinforcement.

Figure 2–2 describes the individual level, with its key components.

The behavior of people in groups is something more than the sum total of each individual acting in his or her own way. The complexity of our model is increased when we acknowledge that people's behavior when they are in groups is different from their behavior when they are alone. Therefore, the next step in the development of an understanding of OB is the study of group behavior.

Roles, Norms, and Status. Chapter 8 lays the foundation for an understanding of group behavior by presenting the concepts of roles, norms, and status. This chapter discusses how individuals in groups are influenced by the patterns

FIGURE 2–2   The Individual Level in the OB Model

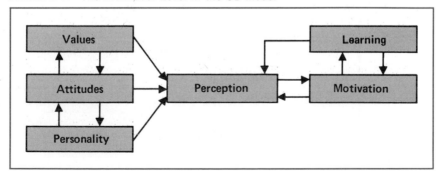

of behavior they are expected to exhibit, what the group considers to be acceptable standards of behavior, and the status hierarchy established by the group.

Group Dynamics. In Chapter 9, we present a group behavior model that builds upon the concepts of roles, norms, and status. This chapter also devotes attention to problems with group decision making.

Communication. Transmission of information becomes an issue when we move from the individual level of analysis to the group level. In order for a group to function, communication must take place. The communication process, networks, and the structuring of communication are discussed in Chapter 10.

Leadership. A group without a leader is but an uncontrolled mob. If a group is to have direction, it needs leadership. The subject of leadership—particularly the effectiveness of different leadership styles—is presented in Chapter 11.

Power. The ability to influence members of a group is a key factor in the group's behavior. This ability to influence, which we call power, is the topic of Chapter 12. In this chapter we shall try to explain how one acquires power and the effectiveness of various types of power in achieving compliance.

Conflict. The final topic in our discussion of groups is conflict. Conflict arises within the group when individual goals are incompatible with one another or with the group goals. The conflict process and the impact of conflict on organizational effectiveness are discussed in Chapter 13.

Figure 2–3 describes the concepts critical to the understanding of group behavior.

Organizational behavior reaches its highest level of sophistication when we add formal structure to our previous knowledge of individual and group behavior. Just as groups are more than the sum of their individual members, organiza-

FIGURE 2–3 The Group Level in the OB Model

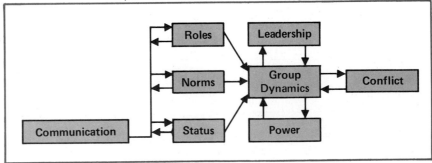

FIGURE 2–4 The Organization Systems Level in the OB Model

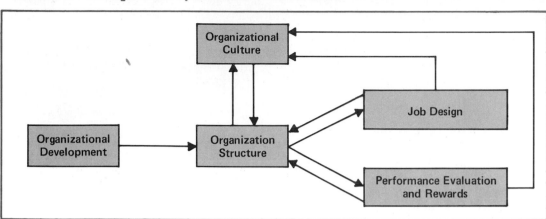

tions are not necessarily merely the summation of the behavior of a number of groups. The structural design of the formal organization and the systems used for evaluation, reward, and bringing about change must be added to our model to determine the impact that structure and organization-wide change processes have on behavior.

Organization Structure. Organizations divide the work that needs to be done into pieces and allocates these pieces among their work force; they also create job descriptions, rules, and other regulations to guide their employees; and they develop authority hierarchies that define where decisions will be made. These actions, in combination, form an organization's structure and this structure limits and regulates employee behavior in certain ways. The effect of various structural variables on performance and satisfaction will be discussed in Chapter 14.

Job Design. In Chapter 15, we shall demonstrate that the way management chooses to design individual jobs will influence behavior. Jobs can be made simple or complex, repetitive or unique, narrow or wide in scope, and interdependent or independent, to name a few of the choices open to management. The impact of these choices on employee performance and satisfaction will be discussed under the topic of job design.

Performance Evaluation and Reward Systems. The behavior of people in organizations is strongly influenced by how and on what criteria they are evaluated. Similarly, the amount and type of rewards that employees receive for their work will influence their behavior. Performance appraisals and their link to reward allocation is the subject of Chapter 16.

Organizational Culture. Each organization has its own personality made up of stable and enduring characteristics that constitute the organization's culture.

FIGURE 2–5 Basic OB Model, Stage II

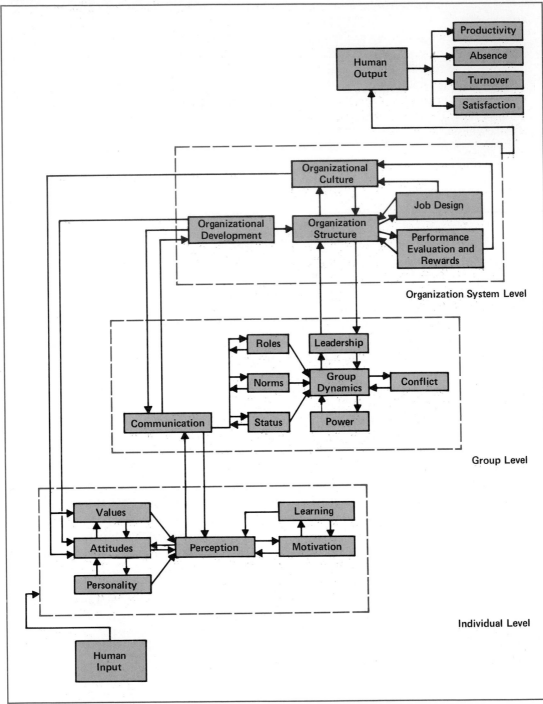

What organizational culture is, how organizations create their cultures, and the impact of culture on employee behavior will be discussed in Chapter 17.

Organizational Development. If an organization's structure can influence employee behavior, it seems logical to conclude that some behavioral outcomes may not be the ones that are desired. Are there ways to correct such states? In Chapter 18, we shall review major techniques available for initiating and facilitating changes in both structural and human processes in organizations, and the resultant impact these methods have on changing behavior.

Figure 2–4 describes the organization systems level components.

TOWARD A CONTINGENCY OB MODEL

Our final model is shown in Figure 2–5. It portrays the four key dependent variables and a large number of independent variables that research suggests have varying impact on the former. Of course, the model does not do justice to the complexity of the OB subject matter. But for the purpose of helping to explain and predict behavior, it should prove valuable.

As we noted previously, our model does not explicitly identify moderating variables because of the tremendous complexity that would be involved in such a diagram. Rather, as you advance through this book, we shall introduce important moderating variables that will improve the explanatory linkage between the independent and dependent variables. Thus, the book will follow a contingency approach—identifying independent variables, isolating moderating variables, and attempting to explain why in certain situations A causes B, yet in other situations A causes C.

You should also note that Figure 2–5 includes linkages between the three levels that were not mentioned in the previous discussion of independent variables. For instance, formal authority is linked to leadership. This is meant to convey the fact that authority and leadership are related—management exerts its influence on group behavior through leadership. Similarly, communication is the means by which individuals transmit information; thus it is the link between individual and group behavior. Communication is also central to organizational development efforts to bring about change. Finally, Figure 2–5 conveys the fact that even though an individual's values and attitudes tend to be substantially set prior to joining an organization, they can be modified by changes in organizational culture or through organizational development techniques.

FOR DISCUSSION

1. Define a model and detail several examples to illustrate your definition.

2. Identify five types of models and discuss their relevance to OB.

3. Differentiate between normative and descriptive models. Which is most appropriate for use in OB?

4. Describe three types of variables. Explain their relationship.

5. What does "causality" have to do with studying OB?

6. What are the three levels of analysis in our OB model? Are they related? If so, how?

7. If job satisfaction is not a behavior, why is it considered as an important dependent variable?

8. What are "effectiveness" and "efficiency," and how are they related to organizational behavior?

9. What are the four dependent variables in the OB model? Why have they been chosen over, for instance, percent return on investment?

10. Why are individual, group, and organization systems level behaviors each described as increasingly more complex?

FOR FURTHER READING

LORSCH, J. W., "Making Behavioral Science More Useful," *Harvard Business Review,* March–April 1979, pp. 171–80. Discusses the advantages of using a contingency view in studying behavior in organizations.

MEALIEA, L. W., and D. LEE, "An Alternative to Macro-Micro Contingency Theories: An Integrative Model," *Academy of Management Review,* July 1979, pp. 333–45. Valid contingency theories must integrate both macro (size, technology, environment) and micro (employee behavior) dimensions.

MOBERG, D. J., and J. L. KOCH, "A Critical Appraisal of Integrated Treatments of Contingency Findings," *Academy of Management Journal,* March 1975, pp. 109–24. Raises a number of questions about the theoretical nature of aggregative models of situational approaches to organization and management.

PINDER, C. C., and L. F. MOORE, "The Resurrection of Taxonomy to Aid the Development of Middle Range Theories of Organizational Behavior," *Administrative Science Quarterly,* March 1979, pp. 99–118. Argues that we should move away from systems or general models toward middle-range theories that explain a lot within a more narrow framework.

SHEPARD, J. M., and J. G. HOUGLAND, JR., "Contingency Theory: 'Complex Man' or 'Complex Organization'?" *Academy of Management Review,* July 1978, pp. 413–27. Compares the "individual differences" approach to contingency theory with the "organizational differences" approach and argues for an integration.

STAW, B. M., and G. R. OLDHAM, "Reconsidering Our Dependent Variables: A Critique and Empirical Study," *Academy of Management Journal,* December 1978, pp. 539–59. Reviews the prominent dependent variables, how they came to be, and the importance of determining whose perspective we are considering when defining dependent variables.

Control of human behavior

Adapted and edited from B. F. Skinner, "Some Issues Concerning the Control of Human Behavior: A Symposium," Science, *November 30, 1956, pp. 1057–60. With permission.*

Until only recently it was customary to deny the possibility of a rigorous science of human behavior by arguing, either that a lawful science was impossible because man was a free agent, or that merely statistical predictions would always leave room for personal freedom. But those who used to take this line have become most vociferous in expressing their alarm at the way these obstacles are being surmounted.

Now, the control of human behavior has always been unpopular. Any undisguised effort to control usually arouses emotional reactions. We hesitate to admit, even to ourselves, that we are engaged in control, and we may refuse to control, even when this would be helpful, for fear of criticism. Those who have explicitly avowed an interest in control have been roughly treated by history. Machiavelli is the great prototype. The control that Machiavelli analyzed and recommended, like most political control, used techniques that were aversive to the controllee. The threats and punishments of the bully, like those of the government operating on the same plan, are not designed—whatever their success—to endear themselves to those who are controlled. Even when the techniques themselves are not aversive, control is usually exercised for the selfish purposes of the controller and, hence, has indirectly punishing effects upon others.

Man's natural inclination to revolt against selfish control has been exploited to good purpose in what we call the philosophy and literature of democracy. The doctrine of the rights of man has been effective in arousing individuals to concerted action against governmental and religious tyranny. The literature that has had this effect has greatly extended the number of terms in our language that express reactions to the control of men. But the ubiquity and ease of expression of this attitude spells trouble for any science that may give birth to a powerful technology of behavior. Intelligent men and women, dominated by the humanistic philosophy of the past two centuries, cannot view with equanimity what Andrew Hacker has called "the specter of predictable man." Even the statistical or actuarial prediction of human events, such as the number of fatalities to be expected on a holiday weekend, strikes many people as uncanny and evil, while the prediction and control of individual behavior is regarded as little less than the work of the devil. I am not so much concerned here with the political or economic consequences for psychology, although research following certain channels may well suffer harmful effects. We ourselves, as intelligent men and women, and as exponents of Western thought, share these attitudes. They have already interfered with the free exercise of a scientific analysis, and their influence threatens to assume more serious proportions.

People living together in groups come to control one another with a technique that is not inappropriately called "ethical." When an individual behaves in a fashion acceptable to the group, he receives admiration, approval, affection, and many other reinforcements that increase the likelihood that he will continue to behave in that fashion. When his behavior is not acceptable, he is criticized, censured, blamed, or otherwise punished. In the first case the group calls him "good"; in the second, "bad." This practice is so thoroughly ingrained in our culture that we often fail to see that it is a technique of control. Yet we are almost always engaged in such control, even though the reinforcements and punishments are often subtle.

The practice of admiration is an important part of a culture, because behavior that is otherwise inclined to be weak can be set up and maintained with its help. The individual is especially likely to be praised, admired, or loved when he acts for the group in the face of great danger, for example, or sacrifices himself or his possessions, or submits to prolonged hardship, or suffers martyrdom. These actions are not admirable in any absolute sense, but they require admiration if they are to be strong. Similarly, we admire people who behave in original or exceptional ways, not because such behavior is itself admirable, but because we do not know how to encourage original or exceptional behavior in any other way. The group acclaims independent, unaided behavior in part because it is easier to reinforce than to help.

A similar difficulty arises from our use of punishment in the form of censure or blame. The concept of responsibility and the related concepts of foreknowledge and choice are used to justify techniques of control using punishment. Was So-and-So aware of the probable consequences of his action, and was the action deliberate? If so, we are justified in punishing him. But what does this mean? It appears to be a question concerning the efficacy of the contingent relations between behavior and punishing consequences. We punish behavior because it is objectionable to us or the group, but in a minor refinement of rather recent origin we have come to withhold punishment when it cannot be ex-

pected to have any effect. If the objectionable consequences of an act were accidental and not likely to occur again, there is no point in punishing. If the action could not have been avoided, punishment is also withheld if the individual is incapable of being changed by punishment because he is of "unsound mind." In all of these cases—different as they are—the individual is held "not responsible" and goes unpunished.

Just as we say that it is "not fair" to punish a man for something he could not help doing, so we call it "unfair" when one is rewarded beyond his due or for something he could not help doing. In other words, we also object to wasting *reinforcers* where they are not needed or will do no good. We make the same point with the words *just* and *right*. Thus we have no right to punish the irresponsible, and a man has no right to reinforcers he does not earn or deserve.

If the advent of a powerful science of behavior causes trouble, it will not be because science itself is inimical to human welfare but because older conceptions have not yielded easily or gracefully. We expect resistance to new techniques of control from those who have heavy investments in the old, but we have no reason to help them preserve a series of principles that are not ends in themselves but rather outmoded means to an end. What is needed is a new conception of human behavior that is compatible with the implications of a scientific analysis. All men control and are controlled. The question of government in the broadest possible sense is not how freedom is to be preserved but what kinds of controls are to be used and to what ends. Control must be analyzed and considered in its proper proportions. No one, I am sure, wishes to develop new master-slave relationships or bend the will of the people to despotic rulers in new ways. These are patterns of control appropriate to a world without science. They may well be the first to go when the experimental analysis of behavior comes into its own in the design of cultural practices.

COUNTER ⬦ POINT

ROGERS

Controlling behavior: proceed with caution

Adapted and edited from Carl R. Rogers, "Some Issues Concerning the Control of Human Behavior: A Symposium," Science, *November 30, 1956, pp. 1060–64. With permission.*

There are, I believe, a number of matters in connection with this important topic on which the authors, and probably a large majority of psychologists, are in agreement. These matters then are not issues as far as we are concerned, and I should like to mention them briefly in order to put them to one side.

I am sure we agree that men—as individuals and as societies—have always endeavored to understand, predict, influence, and control human behavior—their own behavior and that of others.

I believe we agree that the behavioral sciences are making and will continue to make increasingly rapid progress in the understanding of behavior, and that as a consequence the capacity to predict and to control behavior is developing with equal rapidity.

I believe we agree that to deny these advances, or to claim that man's behavior cannot be a field of science, is unrealistic. Even though this is not an issue for us, we should recognize that many intelligent men still hold strongly to the view that the actions of men are free in some sense such that scientific knowledge of man's behavior is impossible.

I believe that we are in agreement that the tremendous potential power of a science that permits the prediction and control of behavior may be misused, and that the possibility of such misuse constitutes a serious threat.

Consequently Skinner and I are in agreement that the whole question of the scientific control of human behavior is a matter with which psychologists and the general public should concern themselves.

With these several points of basic and important agreement, are there then any issues that remain on which there are differences? I believe there are. They can be stated very briefly: Who will be controlled? Who will exercise control? What type of control will be exercised? Most important of all, toward what end or what purpose, or in the pursuit of what value, will control be exercised?

Let us review very briefly the various elements that are involved in the usual concept of the control of human behavior as mediated by the behavioral sciences.

1. There must first be some sort of decision about goals. Usually desirable goals are assumed, but sometimes, as in George Orwell's book *1984*, the goal that is selected is an aggrandizement of individual power with which most of us would disagree. Thus the first step in thinking about the control of human behavior is the choice of goals, whether specific or general. It is necessary to come to terms in some way with the issue, "For what purpose?"

2. A second element is that, whether the end selected is highly specific or is a very general one such as wanting "a better world," we proceed by the methods of science to discover the means to these ends. We continue through further experimentation and investigation to discover more effective means.

3. The third aspect of such control is that as the conditions or methods are discovered by which to reach the goal, some person or some group establishes these conditions and uses these methods, having in one way or another obtained the power to do so.

4. The fourth element is the exposure of individuals to the prescribed conditions, and this leads, with a high degree of probability, to behavior that is in line with the goals desired.

5. The fifth element is that if the process I have described is put in motion then there is a continuing social organization that will continue to produce the types of behavior that have been valued.

Are there any flaws in this way of viewing the control of human behavior? I believe there are. The major flaw I see in this review of what is involved in the scientific control of human behavior is the denial, misunderstanding, or gross underestimation of the place of ends, goals, or values in their relationship to science. My point is that any endeavor in science, pure or applied, is carried on in the pursuit of a purpose or value that is subjectively chosen by persons. It is important that this choice be made explicit, since the particular value that is being sought can never be tested or evaluated, confirmed or denied, by the scientific endeavor to which it gives birth. The initial purpose or value always and necessarily lies outside the scope of the scientific effort that it sets in motion.

It is quite clear that the point of view I am expressing is in sharp contrast to the usual conception of the relationship of the behavioral sciences to the control of human behavior. In order to make this contrast even more blunt, I shall state this possibility in paragraphs parallel to those used before.

1. It is possible for us to choose to value man as a self-actualizing process of becoming—to value creativity, and the process by which knowledge becomes self-transcending.

2. We should proceed, by the methods of science, to discover the conditions that necessarily precede these processes and, through continuing experimentation, to discover better means for achieving these purposes.

3. It is possible for individuals or groups to set these conditions, with a minimum of power or control. According to present knowledge, the only authority necessary is the authority to establish certain qualities of interpersonal relationships.

4. Exposed to these conditions, present knowledge suggests, individuals will become more self-responsible, make progress in self-actualization, become more flexible, and become more creatively adaptive.

5. Thus such an initial choice would inaugurate the beginnings of a social system or subsystem in which values, knowledge, adaptive skills, and even the concept of science would be continually changing and self-transcending. The emphasis would be upon man as a process of becoming.

It is my hope that we have helped to clarify the range of choices that will lie before us and our children in regard to the behavioral sciences. We can choose to use our growing knowledge to enslave people in ways never dreamed of before, depersonalizing them, controlling them by means so carefully selected that they will perhaps never be aware of their loss of personhood. We can choose to utilize our scientific knowledge to make men happy, well behaved, and productive, as Skinner earlier suggested. Or we can assure that each person learns all the syllabus that we select and set before him, as Skinner now suggests. Or at the other end of the spectrum of choice we can choose to use the behavioral sciences in ways that will free, not control; that will bring about constructive variability, not conformity; that will develop creativity, not contentment; that will facilitate each person in his self-directive process of becoming; that will aid individuals, groups, and even the concept of science to become self-transcending in freshly adaptive ways of meeting life and its problems.

CASE 1A ⟶ Arnie Bentley—Househusband

October in southern California can be warm. It was, in fact, about ninety degrees on the Tuesday afternoon that your author first spoke with the familiar bearded face in the supermarket checkout line.

"Hi," I began. "Seems like every time I'm in this place I see you."

"Yeah," he responded, "you retired, too?"

"No, afraid not. I'm a professor over at State. I teach on Mondays and Wednesdays, and the rest of the time I research and write at home. I try to hit the market during the day to avoid the crowds."

The bearded face, who had now introduced himself as Arnie Bentley, told your author that he, too, liked to shop when most people were working.

"Are you retired?" I inquired. "Hell, you can't be thirty-five years old!"

"I'm thirty-three to be exact," began Arnie. "I graduated from State in 1971, with a degree in computer science. Worked for San Diego Gas and Electric for six years but hated it. So I retired."

Arnie's story fascinated me. How did he make ends meet? What did he do with himself every day? I really wanted to get to know more about Arnie Bentley. I asked him if I could buy him a cold soda, and the two of us spent the next couple of hours sitting in a small restaurant—Arnie doing most of the talking and me listening.

Arnie's "retirement" was, in actuality, a voluntary decision not to have a real job. Married, with two children, Arnie is far from well fixed. His wife is an elementary school teacher and earns $21,000 a year.

"When I left the gas company in 1978, I was making $24,000 a year. If I stayed I'd be probably making $32,000 now. But I'd be a nervous wreck. No, I'm perfectly convinced that making more money is not so all-important. We're now in a time where society offers new alternatives to working for a living. I'm not into the work ethic thing. So I've chosen to stay home and take care of the house. I guess you could say I'm a househusband. I see the kids off to school, cook, clean, do the laundry, shop, and maintain the house. I also do the typical husband chores like taking care of the yard and doing repairs."

When I asked Arnie how his wife felt about his life-style choice, he became quite serious. "At first Maggie was really upset. During the first six or nine months, I thought it was going to break up our marriage. But I held my ground. Maggie is a career woman. She's studying for her master's degree at night and she fully expects to be a school principal within five years. I really respect her ambition but the career thing isn't for me. I think

Maggie finally understood where I was coming from when I put it into the framework of the liberation movement. We talk a whole lot about women's lib. Well, I'm into male liberation! Just as women want to be free to choose, so do I! Women say they want to have the option of being physicians, lawyers, and construction workers, as well as housewives, teachers, or librarians. Well, I want those same options and I'm reaching for them. I've opted for a life-style that makes me happy and I don't care what others think.''

Questions

1. If Arnie had had the option at SDG&E of working a three-day week or to be on flexible work hours (which would have allowed him to arrive and leave when he wanted to as long as he put in his eight hours), do you think he might still be working? Discuss.
2. Given Arnie's choice of life-style, what do you think caused him to leave SDG&E? What could the company have done to retain someone like Arnie?
3. Could Arnie's life-style be the beginning of a new trend in North America? Explain.
4. Might Maggie approach her job differently because of Arnie's decision to be a househusband, than if Arnie were earning $32,000 a year as a computer specialist?
5. Using the model presented in Chapter 2, which variables might help explain the differences between Arnie's and Maggie's orientation toward working in an organization?

CASE 1B → "I Love My Work"

Stacey Friedman has been a literary agent with one of the largest literary agencies in New York for four years. Her job entails matching up authors and their manuscripts with book publishers. She has about two dozen established authors whom she represents in negotiations with the publishing houses. Stacey also regularly reviews manuscripts of new or less-established authors who want her firm to represent them.

"I live and breathe this job. I'm up at 5:30 in the morning and in the office by 7:00. I either skip lunch or use lunch as an excuse to meet with publishing editors, with one of my established authors, or to talk with a prospective client. I'm never out of the office before 7:30 P.M., and it's usually closer to 9:00. When I get home, I spend an hour or two lying in bed reading book manuscripts. I only wish I could find another five hours a day so I could squeeze in more things. God, I love my work."

You might be correct in calling Stacey a workaholic. She approaches her work almost compulsively. In college, she was in a sorority, played on her school's soccer team, and dated regularly. But Stacey's job is now her whole life. She told your author she hadn't been on a date in five months, although she had had several dozen offers. She had no social life, except for that which rotated around her work. Stacey even admitted that she hadn't had time to dust or run the vacuum cleaner over the rugs in her apartment in six weeks.

"But don't get the wrong impression when I say my apartment is a mess," interjected Stacey. "I don't care. Every morning I pop out of bed and just thank the Lord for having a job that makes me so happy. When I run into people who complain about their work, I just shake my head. How lucky I am! I'd rather be negotiating with an editor, making manuscript suggestions, discussing strategy with one of my authors, or reading some unknown author's first book than be cleaning the house, jogging around Central Park, or for that matter, making love with Burt Reynolds. I mean it when I say I've got a great job."

Stacey Friedman's enthusiasm appears to have had a very positive impact on her job performance. Her boss says she is the best young agent in the office. "She gives a hundred percent. But, of course, she's smart, too. Stacey has a bright future in this industry."

Questions

1. If you were to learn that Stacey made only $18,000 a year in her job, would you be surprised? Explain.
2. Since Stacey makes only $18,000, one can safely conclude that money is not her main source of motivation. What types of individual, organizational, and job-related factors might account for her high level of motivation?
3. Build a model showing the relationships among the factors that help explain Stacey's high level of performance and motivation.
4. Can you see any possible negative aspects of managing someone like Stacey?

CASE IC

Brave New World Revisited

Rick Johnson is Director of Human Resource Development for a large hamburger franchising operation. The company operates over three thousand restaurants in the United States and Canada, and plans to open another thousand units in the next four years.

One of Rick's responsibilities is to oversee the training of managers for the franchise units. For the past several years this training has been done in a separate educational center that adjoins the corporate headquarters in Richmond, Virginia. A new manager's training typically lasts two weeks and covers such diverse areas as budgeting, scheduling, supervisory skills, and equipment maintenance.

Rick has just returned from Boston, where he participated in a six-week executive development workshop. One of the topics introduced in the workshop particularly intrigued Rick. It was the subject of socializing new employees to their jobs. The instructor had pointed out that the way we introduce new employees to the values and norms of the organization can be a major determinant of the type of employee that results. For instance, organizations can process people formally or informally, singly or in groups, give them a mentor or let them fend on their own. Research evidence indicates that if it wants employees to be independent, creative, and individualistic, the organization should process them informally, individually, and provide no mentor. On the other hand, if an organization desires conforming and homogeneous employees, this is best achieved by making all new employees go through a structured and formal training program, have the employees go through the program as a group, and then assign a senior employee who is well schooled in the way things are done to guide and oversee the employee.

Rick Johnson's first response to the concept of socialization was one of repulsion. He said it smacked of manipulation and sounded like it came out of the book *Brave New World*. But as Rick thought about it more, he realized that whether management controlled it or not, new people to the organization always have to learn the ropes. They have to learn what the company considers acceptable and unacceptable practices. The new people could learn through trial and error, but that was slow and you couldn't be sure people learned things the way the company wanted it. It made sense, then, for management to structure an employee's socialization experiences so that employees turned out the way management desired.

With the above in mind, Rick has begun to restructure his firm's training of franchise managers. The program was already highly structured, but nearly a third of the program required the trainees to learn on the job in one of the company's local restaurants. During this part of the training, the management trainees spent four days just doing all the jobs that had to be done. They worked the grill, made fries, took and rang up orders, and cleaned tables. This was all done with a minimum of supervision. Trainees were encouraged to interact with hourly paid workers in the restaurant so as to learn how they did their jobs. Rick realized that these individualized experiences created opportunities for trainees to become socialized in ways other than the company wanted. Rick decided, then and there, that he was going to redesign the training so every future restaurant manager was a clone of the "ideal franchise manager."

Questions

1. Do you think it's possible to mold people's behavior? Explain.
2. What are the ethical issues in trying to manipulate employees?
3. What benefits would accrue to the franchising firm if Rick's program is successful? Can you think of any disadvantages?
4. Discuss how socialization impacts on the dependent variables discussed in Chapter 2.

CASE ID

"I'm Not Always Right, But I'm Right Most of the Time"

Frank Doherty is fifty-six years old. He dropped out of high school in the tenth grade to support his widowed mother and three younger brothers. At nineteen, he borrowed $200 from his uncle to buy a couple of used cars, which he hoped to resell at a profit. The rest is history. Today, Frank owns five new car dealerships. A recent article in *Automotive News* described Frank Doherty as the largest new car dealer in Texas, and among the top ten in the United States. It's estimated that his five dealerships sell better than 2,500 cars a month!

John Doherty, Frank's son, has been in the business with his dad for less than a year. A recent graduate of the University of Texas, John hoped to put what he learned while earning his B.S. and M.B.A. to work in the car business. But it was obvious to Frank that he and John had some definite differences of opinion on a number of issues. John told this case writer that the root of the problem is that "My dad is so damn dogmatic. He's been extremely successful. I mean, hell, it's hard to criticize someone who started with nothing and was a millionaire at age thirty. But, you gotta admit a lot of his success was due to being in the right place at the right time. It would have been pretty hard to lose money in Dallas with a Chevy dealership in the 1950s. And, getting the VW franchise in 1961 and the Datsun dealership in 1968 wasn't exactly bad timing! Sure, Dad had the foresight to see what the customer wanted, but that's part of the problem. Everything he's touched has turned to gold. He thinks he's infallible. You name the problem and he's instantly got the answer. Nothing burns me up more than his ideas on managing our staff.

"You know we've got about 120 salespeople working for us. We've got another 150 in the shop, and our office staff numbers better than 35. I mean, we're a pretty big operation. But Dad makes personnel decisions based on a bunch of his notions about people.

"For instance, he won't hire college graduates. He says college kids expect too much, too fast. He says they don't have patience and that they want to run the show right out of school. When that doesn't happen, they get frustrated and quit.

"Go out on the sales floor of any of our dealerships. Notice anything unusual? Did our salesmen all look like linebackers for the Dallas Cowboys? That's the result of another of Dad's crazy beliefs. He says the best salesmen are big. There's no use trying to argue with him. He thinks big guys are more aggressive and self-confident. And that results in more sales. As I said, you can't argue with him. All he says is 'Look at my track record.'

"In the office, Dad demands that the office manager keep a close eye on everybody. Dad says people are basically goof-offs. 'You leave them alone for a few minutes and they'll stop working and start playing.' The result is that our office looks like a Gestapo camp. Employees are always under close supervision.

"Everytime I try to talk with Dad about his attitudes, I get the same response. 'Listen John. Maybe my ideas aren't *always* right, but they're right *most* of the time. You may not agree with the way I run the dealerships, but you can't argue with the fact that it works.'"

Questions

1. Compare intuition and systematic study as they relate to Frank Doherty's view of human behavior.
2. What factors could explain the radical differences between father and son in their attitudes and approaches to dealing with people?
3. Do you think John can change his father's style of management? Discuss.
4. "Frank's right. College kids *do* expect too much! The best salesmen *are* big! People *are* basically goof-offs! It is just this type of generally valid insights that have made Frank the success that he is." Discuss.

PART II

The Individual

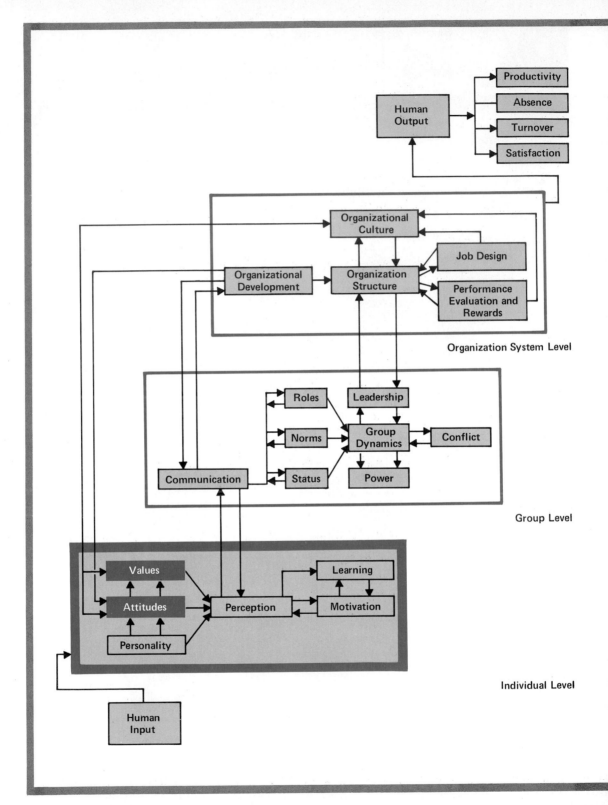

CHAPTER 3
Values and Attitudes

AFTER STUDYING THIS CHAPTER, YOU SHOULD BE ABLE TO—

Define and explain the following key terms and concepts:

Attitudes	Organizational commitment
Cognitive dissonance	Values
Job involvement	Value systems

Understand:

The source of an individual's value system
The impact of changing values
The source of an individual's attitudes
The relationship between attitudes and behavior
The role consistency plays in attitudes
How individuals reconcile inconsistencies

> When you prevent me from doing anything I want to do, that is persecution; but when I prevent you from doing anything you want to do, that is law, order and morals.
>
> —GEORGE BERNARD SHAW

It has been said that "managers, unlike parents, must work with used, not new human beings—human beings whom other people have gotten to first."[1] As such, when individuals enter an organization, they are a bit like used cars—they all have mileage on them. Some have less mileage on them than others—they have been treated carefully and have limited exposure to the realities of the elements, while others have experienced a number of rough roads and show the wear and tear of their travels. As a result of this "mileage," people enter organizations with a number of ideas of how things should be. They have preconceived notions, for example, of what constitutes a full day's work or how a boss should treat them. These notions are embedded in a value structure and a set of attitudes that have been accumulating over at least several decades. Because people enter organizations with certain "givens," we shall begin our study of OB by looking at these preconceived views in terms of the values and attitudes individuals hold when they enter the organization.

VALUES

Is capital punishment right or wrong? How about engaging in sexual relations before marriage—is it right or wrong? If a person likes power, is that good or bad? The answers to these questions are value laden. Some might argue, for example, that capital punishment is right because it is an appropriate retribution for crimes like murder or treason. However, others may argue, just as strongly, that no government has the right to take anyone's life.

Values represent basic convictions that "a specific mode of conduct or end-state of existence is personally or socially preferable to an opposite or converse mode of conduct or end-state of existence."[2] They contain a moral flavor in that they carry an individual's ideas as to what is right, good, or desirable. *Value systems* represent a prioritizing of individual values in relation to their rela-

1. Harold J. Leavitt, *Managerial Psychology,* rev. ed. (Chicago: University of Chicago Press, 1964), p. 3.
2. Milton Rokeach, *The Nature of Human Values* (New York: Free Press, 1973), p. 5.

tive importance. In other words, we all have a set of values that form a value system. This system is identified by the relative importance we assign to such values as freedom, pleasure, self-respect, honesty, obedience, equality, and so forth. We all have values and, as you will see, what we think is important influences our attitudes and our behavior.

Importance of Values

Values are important to the study of organizational behavior because they lay the foundation for the understanding of attitudes, perceptions, personality, and motivations. Individuals enter an organization with preconceived notions of what "ought" and what "ought not" to be. Of course, these notions are not value-free. On the contrary, they contain interpretations of right and wrong. Further, they imply that certain behaviors or outcomes are preferred over others. As a result, values cloud objectivity and rationality.

Values generally influence behavior. Suppose you enter an organization with the view that allocating pay on the basis of performance is right, while allocating pay on the basis of seniority is wrong or inferior. How are you going to react should you find that the organization you have just joined rewards seniority and not performance? Would your behavior be different if your values aligned with the organization's pay policies?

Sources of Our Value Systems

When we were children, why did many of our mothers tell us "you should always clean your dinner plate"? Why is it that, at least historically in our society, achievement has been considered good and being lazy has been considered bad; or that marriage is thought to be desirable and being single is not?

The answer is that, in our culture, certain values have developed over time and are continuously reinforced. Peace, cooperation, harmony, equity, and democracy are societal values that are considered desirable in our culture. These values are not fixed, but when they change they do so very slowly. It is only in the past decade, for instance, that we in North America have begun to question seriously one of our most cherished values: "Bigger is better." This conviction gave higher desirability to big cars, big homes, big incomes, and the like. It was even considered, in some circles, anti-American to question this desire to accumulate ever larger signs of achievement and success. Again, it is only very recently that we have begun to reconsider the acceptability of this notion.

The values we hold are derived from our parents, teachers, and friends, from views expressed in the media (television, radio, newspapers), and from individuals we respect and attempt to emulate—the celebrities in the entertainment, athletic, business, and political communities. Your early ideas of what is right and wrong were probably formulated from the views expressed by your parents. Think back to your early views on such topics as education, sex, and politics. For the most part, they were the same as expressed by your parents. As you grew up, and were exposed to other value systems, you may have altered a number of your values. For example, in high school, if you desired to be a member of a social club whose values included the conviction that "every person should carry a knife," there is a good probability that you changed your value system to align with members of the club, even if it meant rejecting your parents' value that "only hoodlums carry knives, and hoodlums are bad."

Interestingly, values are relatively stable and enduring. This has been explained as a result of the way in which they are originally learned.[3] As children, we are told that a certain behavior or outcome is *always* desirable or *always* undesirable. There were no gray areas. You were told, for example, that you should be honest and responsible. You were never taught to be just a little bit honest or a little bit responsible. It is this absolute or "black-or-white" learning of values that more or less assures their stability and endurance.

The process of questioning our values, of course, may result in a change. We may decide that these underlying convictions are no longer acceptable. More often, our questioning merely acts to reinforce those values we are holding.

Types of Values

At this point, we might rightfully inquire if it is possible to identify certain value "types." The most important early work in categorizing values was done by Allport and his associates.[4] They identified six types of values:

1. *Theoretical*—places high importance on the discovery of truth through a critical and rational approach
2. *Economic*—emphasizes the useful and practical
3. *Aesthetic*—places the highest value on form and harmony
4. *Social*—the highest value is given to the love of people
5. *Political*—places emphasis on acquisition of power and influence
6. *Religious*—concerned with the unity of experience and understanding of the cosmos as a whole

Allport and his associates developed a questionnaire that describes a number of different situations and asks respondents to preference rank a fixed set of answers. Based on the respondents' replies, the researchers can rank individuals in terms of the importance they give to each of the six types of values. The result is a value system for a specific individual.

Using this approach, it has been found, not surprisingly, that people in different occupations place different importance on the six value types.

Figure 3–1 shows the responses from ministers, purchasing agents, and industrial scientists. As expected, religious leaders consider religious values most important and economic values least important. Economic values, on the other hand, are of highest importance to the purchasing executives.

More recent research suggests that there is a hierarchy of levels that are

3. Ibid., p. 6.

4. Gordon W. Allport, Phillip E. Vernon, and Gardner Lindzey, *Study of Values* (Boston: Houghton Mifflin, 1951).

FIGURE 3–1 Ranking of Values by Importance among Three Groups

MINISTERS	PURCHASING EXECUTIVES	SCIENTISTS IN INDUSTRY
1. Religious	1. Economic	1. Theoretical
2. Social	2. Theoretical	2. Political
3. Aesthetic	3. Political	3. Economic
4. Political	4. Religious	4. Aesthetic
5. Theoretical	5. Aesthetic	5. Religious
6. Economic	6. Social	6. Social

Source: R. Taguiri, "Purchasing Executive: General Manager or Specialist?" *Journal of Purchasing,*
August 1967, pp. 16–21.

descriptive of personal values and life-styles. One such study identified seven levels:[5]

Level 1. *Reactive.* These individuals are unaware of themselves or others as human beings and react to basic physiological needs. Such individuals are rarely found in organizations. This is most descriptive of newborn babies.

Level 2. *Tribalistic.* These individuals are characterized by high dependence. They are strongly influenced by tradition and the power exerted by authority figures.

Level 3. *Egocentrism.* These persons believe in rugged individualism. They are aggressive and selfish. They respond primarily to power.

Level 4. *Conformity.* These individuals have a low tolerance for ambiguity, have difficulty in accepting people whose values differ from their own, and desire that others accept their values.

Level 5. *Manipulative.* These individuals are characterized by striving to achieve their goals by manipulating things and people. They are materialistic and actively seek higher status and recognition.

Level 6. *Sociocentric.* These individuals consider it more important to be liked and to get along with others than to get ahead. They are repulsed by materialism, manipulation, and conformity.

Level 7. *Existential.* These individuals have a high tolerance for ambiguity and people with differing values. They are outspoken on inflexible systems, restrictive policies, status symbols, and arbitrary use of authority.

This hierarchy has been used to analyze the problem of disparate values in organizations.[6] The research indicates that most people in today's organizations

5. Clare W. Graves, "Levels of Existence: An Open System Theory of Values," *Journal of Humanistic Psychology,* Fall 1970, pp. 131–55.

6. M. Scott Myers and Susan S. Myers, "Toward Understanding the Changing Work Ethic," *California Management Review,* Spring 1974, pp. 7–19.

operate on levels 2 through 7. But, whereas historically organizations were run by level 4 and 5 managers, there is currently a rapid movement of level 6 and 7 types into influential positions in organizations. Although probably still a minority, the number of individuals holding existential and sociocentric values is increasing. They are being heard in their fight to improve the quality rather than the material quantity of life, in their refusal to accept promotions that would require a move to another community, and in their convictions that decision making should be shared by all organizational members and not just those in managerial positions.

The seven-level categorization of values also contributes toward explaining why individuals have different attitudes and engage in varying behaviors. Tribalistic values place a high importance on acceptance of authority while existential values do not. We can, therefore, expect individuals holding these divergent values to react differently to authoritarian directions. Similarly, conformity values are consistent with achievement and Protestant ethic behavior while sociocentric values find such behavior to be undesirable. Our conclusion, then, is that values impact on behavior and, therefore, knowledge of an individual's value type should assist us in explaining and predicting his or her behavior.

The knowledge that people have different types of values has led a few of the more progressively managed organizations to initiate efforts to improve the values-job fit in order to enhance employee performance and satisfaction. Texas Instruments, for instance, has developed a program to diagnose different value types and to match properly these types with appropriate work environments within their company.

> Some individuals, for example, are classified as "tribalistic"—people who want strong, directive leadership from their boss; some are "egocentric," desiring individual responsibilities and wanting to work as loners in an entrepreneurial style; some are "sociocentric," seeking primarily the social relationships that a job provides; and some are "existential," seeking full expression of growth and self-fulfillment needs through their work, much as an artist does. Charles Hughes, director of personnel and organization development at Texas Instruments, believes that the variety of work that needs to be done in his organization is great enough to accommodate these different types of work personalities in such a manner that an individual and organizational goals are fused.[7]

Texas Instruments' efforts at matching values and work environments is obviously not widely practiced in industry. If other firms were to follow suit, they might be pleasantly surprised by the positive impact on worker productivity, attendance, resignation rates, and overall morale.

Recent Changes in Employee Values

We noted above that there is a significant increase in levels 6 and 7 types at the managerial level. Recent studies suggest that levels 6 and 7 values may becoming descriptive of employees in general. Though values are stable and enduring,

7. W. Clay Hamner and Dennis W. Organ, *Organizational Behavior: An Applied Psychological Approach* (Dallas: BPI, Inc., 1978), p. 187.

they are not rigid. More importantly, new generations can bring with them a new set of values.

Among the old work values were those implied by the following statements: (1) a woman's place is in the home, not on a paid job; (b) if a job offers economic stability, you stay with it even if it is personally unpleasant; and (c) the incentives of money and status motivate most people. The new work values put an increased importance on (a) leisure, (b) a fulfilling and meaningful paid job, and (c) control over one's activities on the job.[8]

Other studies have found age to be a major differentiator of employee values.[9] Younger workers today place a higher importance on personal freedom, short-run gratification, individualism, and openness than their parents and grandparents do. These younger workers also place less value on competition, long-term returns, and formal authority. In other words, younger employees are foresaking levels 4 and 5 values for levels 6 and 7.

What are the implications of these changes in values? Clearly, younger employees are bringing a different set of values to the work place than their older peers. This means management will need to respond to these new values if younger workers are to remain with the organization as productive members. Reliance by management on authority systems and job structures built around levels 2 through 5 values can be expected to result in reduced employee satisfaction and increased absenteeism and turnover.

ATTITUDES

Attitudes are evaluative statements—either favorable or unfavorable—concerning objects, people, or events. They reflect how one feels about something. When I say "I like my job," I am expressing my attitude about work.

Attitudes are not the same as values. Values are the broader and more encompassing concept. So attitudes are more specific than values. Values also contain a moral flavor of rightness or desirability. The statement that "discrimination is bad" reflects one's values. "I favor the implementation of an affirmative action program to recruit and develop women for managerial positions in our organization" is an attitude.

While attitudes and values are different, they are closely related. One comprehensive study took a cross section of heterogeneous value issues—including civil rights for blacks and the poor, black militancy, communism, family security, salvation, cleanliness, imaginativeness, obedience—and found values and attitudes to be significantly correlated.[10] The researcher concluded that vir-

---

8. Daniel Yankelovich, "The New Psychological Contracts at Work," *Psychology Today,* May 1978, pp. 46–50.

9. See, for instance, David J. Cherrington, Spencer J. Condie, and J. Lynn England, "Age and Work Values," *Academy of Management Journal,* September 1979, pp. 617–23.

10. Rokeach, *Human Values,* pp. 95–121.

tually any attitude will be significantly associated with some value set. The evidence allows us to say that the values people hold can explain their attitudes and, in many cases, the behaviors they engage in, but unfortunately, we cannot yet say which values underlie which attitudes and behaviors.

Sources of Attitudes

Attitudes, like values, are acquired from parents, teachers, and peer group members. In our early years, we begin modeling our attitudes after those we admire, respect, or maybe even fear. We observe the way family and friends behave and we shape our attitudes and behavior to align with theirs. People imitate the attitudes of popular individuals or those they admire and respect. If the "right thing" is to favor eating at McDonald's, you are likely to hold that attitude. If it is popular to oppose busing, you may express that view.

In contrast to values, your attitudes are less stable. Advertising messages, for example, attempt to alter your attitudes toward a certain product or service: If the people at Ford can get you to hold a favorable opinion toward their cars, that attitude may lead to a desirable behavior (for them)—the purchase of a Ford product.

In organizations, attitudes are important because they affect job behavior. If workers believe, for example, that foremen, auditors, bosses, and time and motion engineers are all in conspiracy to make the employee work harder for the same or less money, then it makes sense to try to understand how these attitudes were formed, their relationship to actual job behavior, and how they can be made more favorable. The effects of employee attitudes on job behavior will be discussed in this chapter. In Chapters 7 and 18, we will assess what can be done to make these attitudes more favorable for the organization.

Types of Attitudes

A person can have thousands of attitudes, but OB focuses our attention on a very limited number of job-related attitudes. These job-related attitudes tap positive or negative evaluations that employees hold about aspects of their work environment. Typically, there are three primary attitudes that are of concern to us: job satisfaction, job involvement, and organizational commitment.

Job satisfaction refers to an individual's general attitude toward his or her job. A person with a high level of job satisfaction holds positive attitudes toward the job, while a person who is dissatisfied with his or her job holds negative attitudes about the job. When people speak of employee attitudes, more often than not they mean job satisfaction. In fact, the two are frequently used interchangeably.

This definition of job satisfaction is clearly a very broad one. Yet this is inherent in the concept. The need to use a broad definition becomes more obvious when efforts are made to measure job satisfaction. The simplest and probably most widely used method is merely to ask individuals one question: "On the whole, are you satisfied or dissatisfied with your present job?" The Gallup Poll, for instance, has been using this question for better than thirty years.

It's possible, however, to ask people a large number of job-related questions or have them complete a standardized questionnaire. From answers to questions like "On a scale from one to five, how would you rate (a) the organization as a place to work? (b) management's interest in your welfare? and (c) the money you receive for your work?" it is possible to tap into key dimensions of job satisfaction. By combining the answers, we are able to arrive at a measure of job satisfaction.

The term "job involvement" is a more recent addition to the OB literature.[11] While there is no complete agreement over what the term means, a workable definition states that job involvement measures the degree to which a person identifies with his job, actively participates in it, and considers his performance important to his self-worth.[12] It has been assumed by OB researchers that individuals who express high involvement in their jobs are likely to be more productive, have higher satisfaction, and be less likely to resign than employees with low involvement.

The third job attitude we shall discuss is organizational commitment. This attitude expresses an individual's orientation toward the organization by tapping his or her loyalty to, identification with, and involvement in the organization.[13] Individuals who express high commitment see their identity as closely attached to that of the organization. As with job involvement, research into commitment has developed around the assumption that highly committed employees will be better performers and have lower turnover than those expressing low levels of commitment to the organization.

In summary, when we talk about job attitudes and their impact on behavior, we are referring to the positive or negative appraisals that people make about their job or organization. Job satisfaction is the most popular attitude measured in organizations, but more recently there has been increased attention given to job involvement and organizational commitment. For the most part, these attitudes are measured in order that they can be used to predict behaviors like productivity, absenteeism, and turnover.

Attitudes and Consistency

Did you ever notice how people change what they say so it doesn't contradict what they do? Perhaps a friend of yours has consistently argued that American cars are poorly built and that he'd never own anything but a foreign import. But

11. S. Rabinowitz and Douglas T. Hall, "Organizational Research on Job Involvement," *Psychological Bulletin,* March 1977, pp. 265–88.

12. S. D. Saleh and James Hosek, "Job Involvement: Concepts and Measurements," *Academy of Management Journal,* June 1976, p. 223.

13. B. Buchanan II, "Building Organizational Commitment: The Socialization of Managers in Work Situations," *Administrative Science Quarterly,* December 1974, pp. 533–46.

his dad gives him a late-model American-made car, and suddenly they're not so bad. Or, when going through sorority rush, a new freshman believes that sororities are good and that pledging a sorority is important. If she fails to make a sorority, however, notice how her attitude toward sororities changes. "I recognized that sorority life isn't all it's cracked up to be, anyway!" is not an uncommon response to an unsuccessful rush experience.

Research has generally concluded that people seek consistency among their attitudes and between their attitudes and behavior. This means that individuals seek to reconcile divergent attitudes and align their attitudes and behavior so they appear rational and consistent. When there is an inconsistency, forces are initiated to return the individual to an equilibrium state where attitudes and behavior are again consistent. This can be done by altering either the attitudes or the behavior, or by developing a rationalization for the discrepancy.

For example, a recruiter for the ABC Company, whose job it is to visit college campuses, isolate qualified job candidates, and sell them on the advantages of ABC as a place to work, would be in conflict if he personally believes the ABC Company has poor working conditions and few opportunities for new college graduates. This recruiter could, over time, find his attitudes toward the ABC Company becoming more positive. He may, in effect, brainwash himself by continually articulating the merits of working for ABC. Another alternative would be for the recruiter to become overtly negative about ABC and the opportunities within the firm for prospective candidates. The original enthusiasm that the recruiter may have shown would dwindle, probably to be replaced by open cynicism toward the company. Finally, the recruiter might acknowledge that ABC is an undesirable place to work, but as a professional recruiter his obligation is to present the positive sides of working for the company. He might further rationalize that no place is perfect to work at; therefore, his job is not to present both sides of the issue, but rather to present a "rosy" picture of the company.

Cognitive Dissonance Theory

Can we additionally assume from this consistency principle that an individual's behavior can always be predicted if we know his or her attitude on a subject? If Mr. Jones views the company's pay level as too low, will a substantial increase in his pay change his behavior; that is, make him work harder? The answer to this question is, unfortunately, more complex than merely a "Yes" or "No."

Leon Festinger, in the late 1950s, proposed the theory of cognitive dissonance.[14] This theory sought to explain the linkage between attitudes and behavior.

Dissonance means an inconsistency. Cognitive dissonance refers to any incompatibility that an individual might perceive between two or more of his attitudes, or between his behavior and his attitudes. Festinger argued that any

14. Leon Festinger, *A Theory of Cognitive Dissonance* (Stanford, Calif.: Stanford University Press, 1957).

form of inconsistency is uncomfortable and that individuals will attempt to reduce dissonance and hence the discomfort. Therefore, individuals will seek a stable state where there is a minimum of dissonance.

Of course, no individual can completely avoid dissonance. You know prejudice is wrong, but you fear the economic impact on housing prices should your neighborhood become socially mixed. Or you tell your children to brush after every meal, but *you* don't. So how do people cope? Festinger would propose that the desire to reduce dissonance would be determined by the importance of the elements creating the dissonance, the degree of influence the individual believes he or she has over the elements, and the rewards that may be involved in dissonance.

If the elements creating the dissonance are relatively unimportant, the pressure to correct this imbalance will be low. However, say a corporate manager—Mrs. Smith, who has a husband and several children—believes strongly that no company should pollute the air or water. Unfortunately, Mrs. Smith, because of the requirements of her job, is placed in the position of having to make decisions which would trade off her company's profitability against her attitudes on pollution. She knows that dumping the company's sewage into the local river (which we shall assume is legal) is in the best economic interest of her firm. What will she do? Clearly, Mrs. Smith is experiencing a high degree of cognitive dissonance. Because of the importance of the elements in this example, we cannot expect Mrs. Smith to ignore the inconsistency. There are several paths that she can follow to deal with her dilemma. She can change her behavior (stop polluting the river). Or she can reduce dissonance by concluding that the dissonant behavior is not so important after all ("I've got to make a living and, in my role as a corporate decision maker, I often have to place the good of my company above that of the environment or society"). A third alternative would be for Mrs. Smith to change her attitude ("There is nothing wrong in polluting the river"). Still another choice would be to seek out more consonant elements to outweigh the dissonant ones ("The benefits to society from our manufacturing our products more than offset the cost to society of the resulting water pollution").

The degree of influence that individuals believe they have over the elements will impact on how they will react to the dissonance. If they perceive the dissonance to be an uncontrollable result—something over which they have no choice—they are less likely to be receptive to attitude change. If, for example, the dissonance-producing behavior was required as a result of the boss's directive, the pressure to reduce dissonance would be less than if the behavior was performed voluntarily. While dissonance exists, it can be rationalized and justified.

Rewards also influence the degree to which individuals are motivated to reduce dissonance. High dissonance, when accompanied by high rewards, tends to reduce the tension inherent in the dissonance. The reward acts to reduce dissonance by increasing the consistency side of the individual's balance sheet. Since people in organizations are given some form of reward or remuneration for their services, employees often can deal with greater dissonance on their jobs than off their jobs.

These moderating factors suggest that just because individuals experience dissonance does not necessarily mean that they will directly move toward consistency, that is, toward reduction of this dissonance. If the issues underlying the dissonance are of minimal importance, if an individual perceives that the dissonance is externally imposed and is substantially uncontrollable by him, or if rewards are significant enough to offset the dissonance, the individual will not be under great tension to reduce the dissonance.

What are the organizational implications of the theory of cognitive dissonance? It can help to predict the propensity to engage in attitude and behavioral change. If individuals are required, for example, by the demands of their job, to say or do things that contradict their personal attitude, they will tend to modify their attitude in order to make it compatible with the cognition of what they have said or done. Additionally, the greater the dissonance—after it has been moderated by importance, choice, and reward factors—the greater the pressures to reduce the dissonance.

Measuring the A-B Relationship

We have maintained throughout this chapter that attitudes affect behavior. The early research work on attitudes assumed that they were causally related to behavior; that is, the attitudes people hold determine what they do. Common sense, too, suggests a relationship. Is it not logical that people watch television programs that they say they like or that employees try to avoid assignments they find distasteful?

However, in the late 1960s, this assumed relationship between attitudes and behavior (A-B) was challenged by a review of the research.[15] Based on an evaluation of a number of studies that investigated the A-B relationship, the reviewer concluded that attitudes were unrelated to behavior or, at best, only slightly related.[16] More recent research has demonstrated that there is indeed a measurable relationship if moderating contingency variables are taken into consideration.

One thing that improves our chances of finding significant A-B relationships is the use of both specific attitudes and specific behaviors.[17] It is one thing to talk about a person's attitude toward "preserving the environment" and another to speak of her attitude toward "purchasing unleaded gasoline" (which generates less air pollution in the environment). The more specific the attitude we are measuring and the more specific we are in identifying a related behavior, the greater the probability that we can show a relationship between A and B. As a case in point, researchers drew samples of drivers using unleaded and regular gas, and then asked the drivers four levels of questions ranging from items

15. A. W. Wicker, "Attitude Versus Action: The Relationship of Verbal and Overt Behavioral Responses to Attitude Objects," *Journal of Social Issues,* Autumn 1969, pp. 41–78.

16. Ibid., p. 65.

17. T. A. Heberlein and J. S. Black, "Attitudinal Specificity and the Prediction of Behavior in a Field Setting," *Journal of Personality and Social Psychology,* April 1976, pp. 474–79.

about general interest in the environment issues to a specific question about the degree of personal obligation the individual felt to buy unleaded gasoline. The A-B relationship increased from +.12 to +.59 as the questions went from the least to the most specific level.[18] That is, the more specific the question, the closer the response related to actual gasoline purchasing behavior.

Another moderator is social constraints on behavior. Discrepancies between attitudes and behavior may occur because the social pressures on the individual to behave in a certain way may hold exceptional power.[19] Group pressures, for instance, may explain why an employee who holds strong anti-union attitudes attends pro-union organizing meetings.

Of course, A and B may be at odds for other reasons. Individuals can and do hold contradictory attitudes at a given time, though as we have noted, there are pressures toward consistency. Additionally, other things besides attitudes influence behavior. But it is fair to say that, in spite of some attacks, most A-B studies yield positive results—that attitudes *do* influence behavior.[20] One of the best and most obvious confirming examples are attitude surveys taken every four years to predict presidential elections. The evidence demonstrates that, on the whole, these attitude surveys are extremely accurate predictors of voting outcomes.

An Example: Predicting Union Activity

Assume you are a senior manager at a company that is currently not unionized and you desire to keep your company nonunion.[21] It's occurred to you that one way to keep the union out would be to ensure that your employees are generally satisfied with their work environment. Two questions now arise: (1) Is it correct to assume that satisfied employees are less likely to join a union? (2) If this is true, what can you as a manager do to increase the level of employee satisfaction?

The answer to the first question lies in the A-B relationship. Research confirms that attitudes do predict union activity, as long as the attitudes are confined to aspects of work that can be expected to change as a result of unionization.[22] If employees are disgruntled over autocratic supervision, poor working conditions, or lack of job security, employee attitudes have been shown to predict at the

18. Ibid.

19. H. Schuman and M. P. Johnson, "Attitudes and Behavior," in *Annual Review of Sociology,* ed. Alex Inkeles (Palo Alto, Calif.: Annual Reviews, 1976), pp. 161–207.

20. Ibid., p. 199; and Lynn R. Kahle and Hohn J. Berman, "Attitudes Cause Behaviors: A Cross-Lagged Panel Analysis," *Journal of Personality and Social Psychology,* March 1979, pp. 315–21.

21. This position is taken for illustration purposes only. No assumption is made as to the merits or demerits of an organization being nonunionized, though there is abundant evidence that the management at a large proportion of nonunionized organizations desire to keep their nonunion status.

22. W. Clay Hamner and Frank Smith, "Work Attitudes as Predictors of Unionization Activity," *Journal of Applied Psychology,* August 1978, pp. 415–21.

group level the occurrence of unionization activity and to predict an individual's pro-union or anti-union vote.[23]

What if the employees' dissatisfaction lies with the work itself, or with some other aspect of employment that cannot be expected to be changed by unionization? Would dissatisfaction still predict union activity? The answer here appears to be negative. What we find is that this type of dissatisfaction tends to predict other behaviors. Such dissatisfaction appears to be a reasonably good predictor of absenteeism and turnover.[24]

The above findings should encourage you, as a manager, to engage in regular employee attitude surveys. Employees dissatisfied with their work are likely to be pro-union if they see the union as being able to reduce this dissatisfaction. This is consistent with our findings that say attitudes are a good predictor of future behavior when that behavior is under the control of the employee. We should also expect positive attitudes toward the job to lead to more positive outcomes. Employees who are satisfied with their working conditions can be expected to support the company in a union election. A knowledge of job attitudes, therefore, can give you information that can guide you in determining what, if any, aspects of the work situation to change if your objective is to minimize pro-union activity.

IMPLICATIONS FOR PERFORMANCE AND SATISFACTION

Attitudes and Productivity

The attitude-productivity relationship is not clear. In 1955, Brayfield and Crockett did an extensive examination of this relationship and concluded that there was minimal or no relationship between attitudes and performance.[25] Two years later, Herzberg and his associates concluded from the studies they reviewed, which in many cases differed from Brayfield and Crockett's, that there was generally a positive relationship between attitudes and productivity.[26] They were careful, however, to note that in many cases the correlations, although positive, were low. Similarly, a review in 1964 of twenty-three separate studies revealed that, in all but three cases, there was a low but positive relationship between

23. Chester Schriesheim, "Job Satisfaction, Attitudes toward Unions, and Voting in a Union Representation Election," *Journal of Applied Psychology,* October 1978, pp. 548–52.

24. Lyman Porter and Richard Steers, "Organizational, Work, and Personal Factors in Employee Turnover and Absenteeism," *Psychological Bulletin,* August 1973, pp. 151–76.

25. Arthur H. Brayfield and Walter H. Crockett, "Employee Attitudes and Employee Performance," *Psychological Bulletin,* Vol. 52 (1955), pp. 396–428.

26. Frederick Herzberg, B. Mausner, R. O. Petterson, and D. F. Capwell, *Job Attitudes: Review of Research and Opinion* (Pittsburgh: Psychological Service of Pittsburgh, 1957).

satisfaction and performance.[27] A review of the research between 1955 and 1964 supports the previously mentioned studies: It was concluded that studies of the relationship between attitudes and productivity have resulted in generally mixed findings.[28]

Recent research has been no more encouraging. Increased employee satisfaction, involvement, or commitment cannot be said to lead to higher productivity.[29] At best the relationship is unclear. Our conclusion, at least at this point in time, must be that there are no consistent findings from which we can generalize as to an individual's productivity based on his or her attitudes.

Attitudes and Withdrawal Behaviors

Early studies confirmed that employee satisfaction is inversely related to absenteeism and turnover. The greater the satisfaction expressed by the employee about his or her job, the less he or she demonstrated these withdrawal behaviors. Brayfield and Crockett found a significant but complex relationship between attitudes and both absenteeism and turnover.[30] Vroom found a consistent negative relationship between job satisfaction and turnover, but a less consistent negative relationship between satisfaction and absenteeism.[31] Other studies have found that satisfaction has a consistent impact on absenteeism, but an even more profound and consistent relationship on turnover.[32] However, the conclusion that satisfaction and absence are inversely related has come under recent attack.[33] A review of twenty-nine major studies which looked at this relationship showed that research varied dramatically with regard to methods and measures, populations used, and results reported. Attempting to correct for a number of these differences, the researchers studied 1,200 production workers and concluded that negative attitudes as expressed in the form of job dissatisfaction are unrelated to absence from work.

A recent review found a negative correlation of −.40 between satisfaction

27. Victor H. Vroom, *Work and Motivation* (New York: John Wiley, 1964).

28. Glenn P. Fournet, M. K. Distefano, Jr., and Margaret W. Pryer, "Job Satisfaction: Issues and Problems," *Personnel Psychology,* Vol. 19 (1966), pp. 165–83.

29. See, for example, Edwin A. Locke, "The Nature and Causes of Job Satisfaction," in *Handbook of Industrial and Organizational Psychology,* ed. Marvin D. Dunnette (Chicago: Rand McNally, 1976), pp. 1297–350; Richard M. Steers, "Antecedents and Outcomes of Organizational Commitment," *Administrative Science Quarterly,* March 1977, pp. 46–56; and Charles N. Greene and Robert E. Craft, Jr., "The Satisfaction-Performance Controversy—Revisited," in *Motivation and Work,* ed. Richard M. Steers and Lyman W. Porter, 2nd ed. (New York: McGraw-Hill, 1979), pp. 270–86.

30. Brayfield and Crockett, "Employee Attitudes."

31. Vroom, *Work and Motivation.*

32. Fournet, Distefano, and Pryer, "Job Satisfaction"; and Porter and Steers, "Organizational, Work, and Personal Factors."

33. Nigel Nicholson, Colin A. Brown, and J. K. Chadwick-Jones, "Absence From Work and Job Satisfaction," *Journal of Applied Psychology,* December 1976, pp. 728–37.

and employee withdrawal, leading the reviewer to the conclusion that satisfied people tend to be on the job more frequently and leave the organization less frequently than those who are dissatisfied.[34]

There is growing enthusiasm for the view that organizational commitment is a better predictor of voluntary resignations than job satisfaction.[35] If this is true, efforts to develop valid measures of organizational commitment may be of increasing importance to managers.[36]

In summary, the evidence is fairly clear that committed and satisfied employees have lower rates of both turnover and absenteeism. If we consider the two withdrawal behaviors separately, however, we can be more confident about the influence of attitudes on turnover: An individual's attitudes represent an important force on his or her decision to stay with or leave the organization. Conclusions regarding the relationship between attitudes and absenteeism must be more guarded.

Attitudes and Satisfaction

Job attitudes and job satisfaction appear to be closely connected; in fact, in many research studies these terms are used interchangeably. In studies of job attitudes, it is generally thought that the result is some measure of job satisfaction or dissatisfaction. Job satisfaction, of course, is not a behavior but rather a general feeling of contentment with the job. As a result, if attitudes are positive, job satisfaction also tends to be positive. If the individual believes that his or her job is frustrating, boring, or offers no opportunity for personal growth, we should expect satisfaction to be low. If we are interested, therefore, in having employees who are satisfied with their jobs, we should actively seek to create in them positive attitudes toward their job and the organization.

FOR DISCUSSION

1. Define values. Define attitudes. How are they similar? Different?

2. What is the source of our value system?

3. "Twenty years ago, young employees we hired were ambitious, conscientious, hard-working, and honest. Today's young workers don't have the same values." Do you agree or disagree with this manager's comments? Support your position.

34. Locke, "Nature and Causes of Job Satisfaction."

35. Lyman W. Porter, Richard M. Steers, Richard T. Mowday, and Paul V. Bulian, "Organizational Commitment, Job Satisfaction, and Turnover among Psychiatric Technicians," *Journal of Applied Psychology,* October 1974, pp. 603–9; and Peter W. Hom, Ralph Katerberg, Jr., and Charles L. Hulin, "Comparative Examination of Three Approaches to the Prediction of Turnover," *Journal of Applied Psychology,* June 1979, pp. 280–90.

36. Richard T. Mowday, Richard M. Steers, and Lyman W. Porter, "The Measurement of Organizational Commitment," *Journal of Vocational Behavior,* April 1979, pp. 224–47.

4. Values have been described as the foundation of individual behavior. On what basis do you think such a statement was made?

5. What is cognitive dissonance and how is it related to attitudes?

6. "Job candidates for a sales position are more likely to be successful if they hold egocentric values." Discuss.

7. Do you think there might be any positive and signficant relationship between the possession of certain personal values and successful career progression in organizations like E. F. Hutton & Co., the AFL-CIO, or the City of Cleveland's Police Department? Discuss.

8. What contingency factors can improve the statistical relationship between attitudes and behavior?

9. "Job satisfaction is a good predictor of productivity." Do you agree or disagree? Discuss.

10. "Job satisfaction is a good predictor of turnover." Do you agree or disagree? Discuss.

FOR FURTHER READING

COOPER, M. R., B. S. MORGAN, P. M. FOLEY, and L. B. KAPLAN, "Changing Employee Values: Deepening Discontent?" *Harvard Business Review,* January-February 1979, pp. 117–25. Survey data over twenty-five years indicates that there has been a major shift in the attitudes and values of the U.S. work force.

FISHBEIN, M., and I. AJZEN, *Belief, Attitude, Intention, and Behavior.* Reading, Mass.: Addison-Wesley, 1975. Presents a coherent and systematic conceptual framework to the diverse literature on attitudes.

IVY, T. T., V. S. HILL, and R. E. STEVENS, "Dissonance Theory: A Managerial Perspective," *Business and Society,* February 1978, pp. 17–25. Dissonance theory is shown to be especially relevant in predicting consequences of decision situations and suggesting methods by which undesirable consequences can be avoided.

KELMAN, H. C., "Attitudes Are Alive and Well and Gainfully Employed in the Sphere of Action," *American Psychologist,* May 1974, pp. 310–24. Responds to critics who question the validity and usefulness of the attitude concept.

PACKARD, V. O., *The Hidden Persuaders.* New York: David McKay, 1957. Former best seller that demonstrates how attitudes are changed by advertising and promotion.

POSNER, B. Z., and J. M. MUNSON, "The Importance of Values in Organizational Behavior," *Human Resource Management,* Fall 1979, pp. 9–14. Describes values, how they are measured, and argues that values are important to study and important for managers to know about.

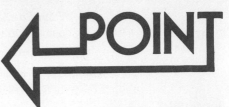

LIKERT AND KATZ

Toward achieving a high level of job satisfaction

Adapted, with permission of the publisher, from "Supervisory Practices and Organizational Structures As They Affect Employee Productivity and Morale," by Rensis Likert and Daniel Katz. Executive Personality and Job Success, AMA Personnel Series No. 120. ©1948 by American Management Associations, Inc.

One basic criterion of effective group functioning is performance, and one measure of this performance in industry is productivity. Now, we need the experience of industry in selecting operations that yield a high productivity per man-day or per man-week, and operations of a comparable nature that are lower in productivity. In this way we can take relatively marked extremes in high and low productivity at various levels of organization for comparative study. We can then go on to study what is done and how it is done, both organizationally and in managing the men; to find out what structure and what methods of working with people, what methods of managing people, yield a high level of productivity in the day-to-day situation.

A second important criterion of group functioning, we feel, is job satisfaction, morale, or whatever you wish to call it. So our research is directed toward finding out what kinds of organizational structure, what methods of working with and managing people yield a high level of job satisfaction.

In our program of research, we have been encountering one very real obstacle: It is very difficult to find industrial situations where you have

substantially equivalent measures of productivity though we have found a few.

We started first in the home office of a life insurance company. There we found a situation where there were objective measures of productivity on comparable groups doing substantially the same work. The analysis of that work, started about a year ago, is pretty well completed. We also are well along on a research study in a large public utility.

In the life insurance company, there were productivity measures in terms of cost-accounting records. We selected for study parallel sections and divisions—ones chosen had been consistently above or below average in productivity for a six-month period.

In the study of the public utility, we had a somewhat different research design. There we had no adequate measures of productivity for the various departments. After all, the electricity is on or it is off, and the plant or powerhouse is functioning, the substations are functioning, or they are not. The usual measures of productivity do not apply to substation operators or to certain other types of public utility workers. The company's thought, however, was that one very satisfactory way to proceed would be to use measures of morale.

We constructed a comprehensive written questionnaire covering the many aspects of morale on the basis of pilot studies and pretesting. This questionnaire was administered to all nonsupervisory employees, about 9,000 in number. Individual workers were not identified, but they did give the name of their work group so that work groups could be compared. A work group consisted of employees under a first-line supervisor.

On the basis of the returns of the written questionnaire we selected the forty work groups with the highest morale and the forty work groups with the lowest morale. We then went back and interviewed all the employees in the groups, about 800 in all. In addition, we interviewed all the supervisory and managerial personnel involved, from first-line supervisors, through intermediate supervisors, clear up to the president of the company. We tried to find out what they did and how they did it, in order to get some insight into what produced high and low morale.

Let us now turn to a consideration of the results of our work. With respect to productivity, we find some rather interesting facts. For example, the kind of management that puts pressure on the section heads for productivity and keeps pressing all the time to get the work out—with the supervisors and section heads, in turn, putting direct pressure on the employees—characterizes the low-production sections.

A factor that seems to characterize the high-production sections and divisions is that the supervision is more general. There is more opportunity for initiative on the part of the people below the division level and, in turn, below the section heads. This is reflected in greater job satisfaction on the part of the supervisors to whom greater responsibility is given. In fact, a major source of dissatisfaction among the supervisors in charge of low-production sections is the lack of delegation of authority so far as they are concerned. A related finding is that the high-production supervisors tend to be more employee-centered and the low-production supervisors tend to be more work-centered.

Let us turn now to some of the differences that are related to job satisfaction and morale. In our study of a public utility we found four factors relatively independent of one another that were important for morale: (1) size of the work group, (2) recency of promotion, (3) type of work, and (4) supervision.

In this company were work groups ranging in size from three to seventy people. In general the larger the work group, the lower the morale, even when other factors such as type of work were held constant. Morale was higher among the people recently promoted than among those who had made no progress in the company for some time.

As other studies have indicated, type of work is also related to morale. The blue-collar workers tended to have lower morale than white-collar workers. The more monotonous the work, the poorer the morale; the more technical, the more specialized, the more varied the work, the higher the morale.

Another factor of great importance to morale is supervision. Certain kinds of supervision produce high morale; other kinds of supervision produce low morale. In the first place, the good supervisor is one who can create a feeling of real participation on the part of his workers. Employees having good morale say, for example, that their supervisor asks their opinion and is open-minded to suggestions; that he holds discussions with them in which they are given a chance to express their own ideas, or share in reaching a decision.

All the evidence from these studies and from previous work that we have done indicates the importance of giving people a sense of real participation—not artificial or condescending, but genuine, honest-to-goodness participation, where they are respected as intelligent people who are sincerely trying to do a job.

These are some of our findings to date. They suggest that the reward-punishment type of motivation we tended to use in the past, with its emphasis on fear, in terms of traditional forms of supervision and management, is beginning to break down. The more democratic internalized type of motivation makes possible the full utilization of human resources. The dictatorial form of government organization that exists in certain parts of the world today, relying as it does upon fear and external sanctions, can never achieve the level of productivity in industry and of human happiness in the job that we can achieve within a democratic structure.

COUNTER POINT

LAWLER AND PORTER

The effect of performance on job satisfaction

Adapted and edited from Edward E. Lawler III and Lyman W. Porter, "The Effect of Performance on Job Satisfaction," Industrial Relations, October 1967, pp. 20–28. With permission.

The human relations movement with its emphasis on good interpersonal relations, job satisfaction, and the importance of informal groups provided an important initial stimulant for the study of job attitudes and their relationship to human behavior in organizations. Through the thirties and forties, many studies were carried out to determine the correlates of high and low job satisfaction. Such studies related job satisfaction to seniority, age, sex, education, occupation, and income, to mention a few. Why this great interest in job satisfaction? Undoubtedly some of it stemmed from a simple desire on the part of scientists to learn more about job satisfaction, but much of the interest in job satisfaction seems to have come about because of its presumed relationship to job performance. As Brayfield and Crockett have pointed out, a common assumption that employee satisfaction directly affects performance permeates most of the writings about the topic that appeared during this period of two decades.

It is not hard to see how the assumption that high job satisfaction leads to high performance came to be popularly accepted.

But does the available evidence support the belief that high satisfaction will lead to high performance? Since an initial study, in 1932, by Kornhauser and Sharp, more than thirty studies have considered the relationship between these two variables. Many of the earlier studies seemed to have assumed implicitly that a positive relationship existed and that it was important to demonstrate that it in fact did exist. Little attention was given to trying to understand *why* job satisfaction should lead to higher performance; instead, researchers contented themselves with routinely studying the relationship between satisfaction and performance in a number of industrial situations.

Judging from the impact of the first review of the literature on the topic, by Brayfield and Crockett, many social scientists, let alone practicing managers, were unaware that the evidence indicated how little relationship exists between satisfaction and performance. The key conclusion that emerged from the review was that "there is little evidence in the available literature that employee attitudes bear any simple—or, for that matter, appreciable—relationship to performance on the job." (The review, however, pointed out that job satisfaction did seem to be positively related, as expected, to two other kinds of employee behavior, absenteeism and turnover.)

The review had a major impact on the field of industrial psychology and helped shatter the kind of naive thinking that characterized the earlier years of the Human Relations movement.

However, before we too glibly accept the view that satisfaction and performance are unrelated, let us look carefully at the data from studies reviewed by Vroom. These studies show a median correlation of $+.14$ between satisfaction and performance. Although this correlation is not large, the consistency of the direction of the correlation is quite impressive. Twenty of the twenty-three correlations cited by Vroom are positive. By statistical tests such consistency would occur by chance less than once in a hundred times.

In summary, the evidence indicates that a low but consistent relationship exists between satisfaction and performance, but it is not at all clear *why* this relationship exists. The questions that need to be answered at this time, therefore, concern the place of job satisfaction both in theories of employee motivation and in everyday organizational practice.

There are really two bases upon which to argue that job satisfaction is important. Interestingly, both are different from the original reason for studying job satisfaction, that is, the assumed ability of satisfaction to influence performance. The first, and undoubtedly the most straightforward reason, rests on the fact that strong correlations between absenteeism and satisfaction, as well as between turnover and satisfaction, appear in the previous studies. Accordingly, job satisfaction would seem to be an important focus of organizations that wish to reduce absenteeism and turnover.

A second reason for interest in job satisfaction stems from its low but consistent *association* with job performance. Let us speculate for a moment on why this association exists. One possibility is that, as assumed by many, the satisfaction *caused* the performance. However, there is little theoretical reason for believing that satisfaction can cause performance. Vroom has pointed out that job satisfaction and job performance are caused by quite different things: " . . . job satisfaction is closely affected by the amount of rewards that people derive from their jobs . . . level of performance is closely affected by the basis of attainment of rewards. Individuals are satisfied with their jobs to the extent to which their jobs provide them with what they desire, and they perform effectively in them to the extent that effective performance leads to the attainment of what they desire."[1]

1. Victor H. Vroom, *Work and Motivation* (New York: John Wiley, 1964), p. 246.

Vroom's statement contains a hint of why, despite the fact that satisfaction and performance are caused by different things, they do bear some relationship to each other. If we assume, as seems to be reasonable in terms of motivation theory, that rewards cause satisfaction, and that in some cases performance produces rewards, then it is possible that the relationship between satisfaction and performance comes about through the action of a third variable—rewards. Briefly stated, good performance may lead to rewards, which in turn lead to satisfaction; this formulation then would say that satisfaction, rather than causing performance, as was previously assumed, is caused by it.

This model would seem to predict that because of the imperfect relationship between performance and rewards and the importance of expected equitable rewards there would be a low but positive relationship between job satisfaction and job performance. The model leads to a number of other predictions about the relationship between satisfaction and performance. If it turns out that, as this model predicts, satisfaction is dependent on performance, then it can be argued that satisfaction is an important variable from both a theoretical and a practical point of view despite its low relationship to performance. However, when satisfaction is viewed in this way, the reasons for considering it to be important are quite different from those that are proposed when satisfaction is considered to cause performance.

We have argued that it is important to consider the satisfaction level that exists in organizations. For one thing, satisfaction is important because it has the power to influence both absenteeism and turnover. In addition, in the area of job performance, we have emphasized that rather than being a cause of performance, satisfaction is caused by it. If this is true, and we have presented some evidence to support the view that it is, then it becomes appropriate to be more concerned about which people and what kind of needs are satisfied in the organization rather than about how to maximize satisfaction generally. In short, we suggest new ways of interpreting job satisfaction data.

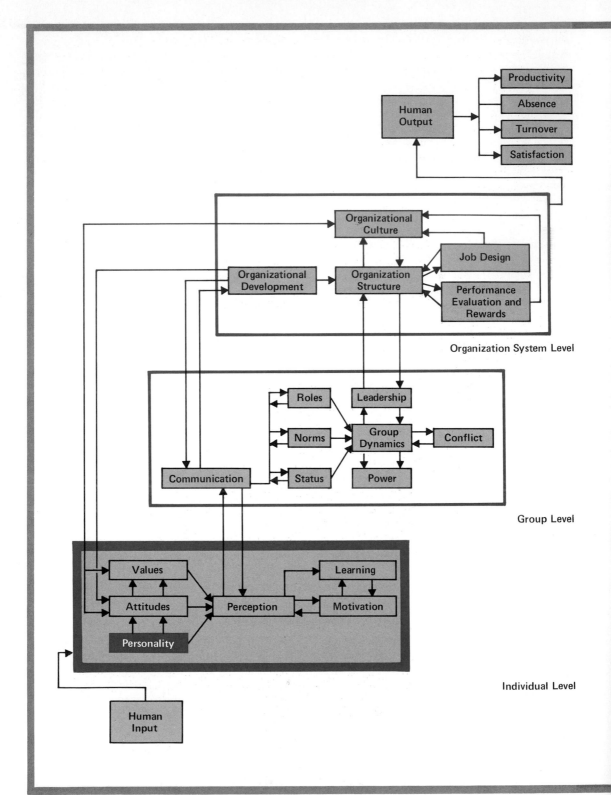

CHAPTER 4
Personality

AFTER STUDYING THIS CHAPTER, YOU SHOULD BE ABLE TO—

Define and explain the following key terms and concepts:

Anxiety	Machiavellianism
Authoritarianism	Maturation theory
Ectomorph	Mesomorph
Endomorph	*nAch*
Expressives	Personality
Extroversion	Personality traits
Instrumentals	Stress
Introversion	Type A behavior
Locus of control	Type B behavior

Understand:

The meaning of personality
The factors that determine an individual's personality
The difference between trait and type approaches
The impact of job typology on the personality—job performance
 relationship
The importance of the self-concept
The benefits and disadvantages of defensive behaviors
The sources of stress

> I ain't much, baby—but I'm all I've got.
>
> —JESS LAIR

Why are some people quiet and passive, while others are loud and aggressive? What do we know from theories of personality and personality development that can help us to explain and predict the behavior of individuals in organizations?

This chapter will attempt to answer these questions. We shall begin by defining the elusive concept of personality, looking at its determinants, and the characteristics that make up one's personality. Then we shall consider theories that propose to explain stages through which healthy individuals develop; examine a number of personality variables that have been linked to employee behavior, including defense mechanisms; assess the relationship between personality and stress; and conclude with a discussion of how the understanding of personality is relevant to explaining and predicting behavior.

WHAT IS PERSONALITY?

When we talk of personality, we do not mean that a person has charm, a pleasant attitude toward life, a smiling face, or is a finalist for "Happiest and Friendliest" in this year's Miss America contest. When psychologists talk of personality, they mean a dynamic concept describing the growth and development of a person's whole psychological system. Rather than looking at parts of the person, personality looks at some aggregate whole that is greater than the sum of the parts.

The most frequently used definition of personality was produced by Gordon Allport over forty years ago. He said personality is "the dynamic organization within the individual of those psycho-physical systems that determine his unique adjustments to his environment."[1]

Personality can be described more specifically as "how a person affects others, how he understands and views himself, and his pattern of inner and outer measurable traits."[2] In this definition, how one affects others is a function of

1. Gordon W. Allport, *Personality: A Psychological Interpretation* (New York: Holt, Rinehart & Winston, 1937), p. 48.

2. Floyd L. Ruch, *Psychology and Life,* 6th ed. (Chicago: Scott, Foresman, 1963), p. 353.

one's physical appearance and behavior. Understanding oneself refers to an awareness that each of us is a unique being with a set of attitudes and values, and that we each have a self-concept that is the result of successive interactions with the environment. Finally, the pattern of measurable traits refers to a set of characteristics that the person exhibits.

PERSONALITY DETERMINANTS

An early argument in personality research was whether an individual's personality was the result of heredity or environment. Was the personality predetermined at birth or was it the result of the individual's interaction with his or her environment? Clearly, there is no simple "black-or-white" answer. Personality appears to be a result of both influences. Additionally, there has recently been an increased interest in a third factor—the situation. Thus, an adult's personality is now generally considered to be made up of both hereditary and environmental factors, and moderated by situational conditions.

Heredity

Heredity refers to those factors that were determined at conception. Physical stature, facial attractiveness, sex, temperament, muscle composition and reflexes, energy level, and biological rhythms are characteristics that are generally considered to be either completely or substantially influenced by who your parents were, that is, by their biological, physiological, and inherent psychological makeup. The heredity approach argues that the ultimate explanation of an individual's personality is the molecular structure of the genes, located in the chromosomes. "In fact, much of the early work in personality could be subsumed under the series: Heredity is transmitted through the genes; the genes determine the hormone balance; hormone balance determines physique; and physique shapes personality."[3]

The heredity argument can be used to explain why Veronica's nose looks like her father's, or why her chin resembles her mother's. It may explain why Diane is a "gifted athlete" when both her parents were similarly gifted. More controversy would surround the conclusion, by those who advocate the heredity approach, that Michael is lethargic as a result of inheriting this characteristic from his parents.

If all personality characteristics were completely dictated by heredity, they would be fixed at birth and no amount of experience could alter them. If you were relaxed and easygoing, for example, that would be the result of your genes, and it would not be possible for you to change these characteristics. While this approach may be appealing to the bigots of the world, it is an inadequate explanation of personality.

3. Joe Kelly, *Organizational Behavior*, rev. ed. (Homewood, Ill.: Richard D. Irwin, 1974), p. 243.

Environment

Among the factors that exert pressures on our personality formation are the culture in which we are raised; our early conditioning; the norms among our family, friends, and social groups; and other influences that we experience. The environment we are exposed to plays a critical role in shaping our personalities.

For example, culture establishes the norms, attitudes, and values that are passed along from one generation to the next and create consistencies over time. An ideology that is fostered in one culture may have only moderate influence in another. For instance, we in North America have had the themes of industriousness, success, competition, independence, and Protestant ethic constantly instilled in us through books, the school system, family, and friends. North Americans, as a result, tend to be ambitious and aggressive relative to individuals raised in cultures that have emphasized getting along with others, cooperation, and the priority of family over work and career.

An interesting area of research linking environmental factors and personality has focused on the influence of birth order. It has been argued that sibling position is an important psychological variable "because it represents a microcosm of the significant social experiences of adolescence and adulthood."[4] Those who see birth order as a predictive variable propose that while personality differences between children are frequently attributed to heredity, the environment in which the children are raised is really the critical factor that creates the differences. And the environment that a firstborn child is exposed to is different from that of later-born children.

The research indicates that firstborns are more prone to schizophrenia, more susceptible to social pressure, and more dependent than the later-born.[5] The firstborn are also more likely to experience the world as more orderly, predictable, and rational than later-born children. Of course, there is much debate as to the differing characteristics of first- versus later-born children, but the evidence does indicate that firstborns of the same sex "should be more concerned with social acceptance and rejection, less likely to break the rules imposed by authority, more ambitious and hard-working, more cooperative, more prone to guilt and anxiety, and less openly aggressive."[6]

Careful consideration of the arguments favoring either heredity or environment as the primary determinant of personality forces the conclusion that both are important. Heredity sets the parameters or outer limits, but an individual's full potential will be determined by how well he or she adjusts to the demands and requirements of the environment.

4. Irving Janis, George F. Mahl, Jerome Kagan, and Robert P. Holt, *Personality: Dynamics, Development and Assessment* (New York: Harcourt, Brace & World, 1969), p. 555.

5. Jonathan R. Warren, "Birth Order and Social Behavior," *Psychological Bulletin,* Vol. 65 (1966), pp. 38–49.

6. Janis et al., *Personality,* p. 552.

Situation

A third factor, the situation, further influences the effects of heredity and environment on personality. An individual's personality, while generally stable and consistent, does change in different situations. Different demands in different situations call forth different aspects of one's personality. We should not, therefore, look at personality patterns in isolation.

While it seems only logical to suppose that situations will influence an individual's personality, a neat classification scheme that would tell us the impact of various types of situations has so far eluded us. "Apparently we are not yet close to developing a system for clarifying situations so that they might be systematically studied."[7] However, we do know that certain situations are more relevant than others in influencing personality.

> What is of interest taxonomically is that situations seem to differ substantially in the constraints they impose on behavior, with some situations—e.g. church, an employment interview—constraining many behaviors and others—e.g. a picnic in a public park—constraining relatively few.[8]

Furthermore, although certain generalizations can be made about personality, there are significant individual differences. As we shall see, the study of individual differences has come to receive greater emphasis in personality research, which originally sought out more general, universal patterns. It has been recently suggested that we return to the search for basic generalizations.

> If anatomists had proceeded in the same way as personality psychologists, we would know a great deal about minor variations in the location of the heart without ever realizing that for just about everyone everywhere it is located in the chest just slightly to the left of center. The above is not to deny the importance of individual differences; but until we know more about basic processes of personality, it is difficult to know how to fit the differences in.[9]

Valid generalizations and individual differences are equally important. In this chapter, we will look at both.

PERSONALITY CHARACTERISTICS

The early work in the structure of personality revolved around attempts to identify and label enduring characteristics that describe an individual's behavior. Popular characteristics include shy, aggressive, submissive, lazy, ambitious, loyal, or timid. These characteristics, when they are exhibited in a large number of situations, are called traits. As we shall find, the more consistent the characteristic and the more frequently it occurs in diverse situations, the more important that trait is in describing the individual.

7. Lee Sechrest, "Personality," in *Annual Review of Psychology*, Vol. 27, ed. Mark R. Rosenzweig and Lyman W. Porter (Palo Alto, Calif.: Annual Reviews, 1976), p. 10.

8. Ibid., p. 10.

9. Ibid., p. 4.

FIGURE 4–1

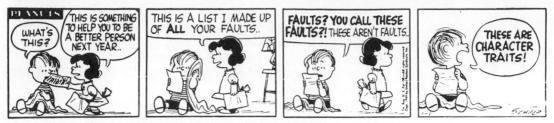

Trait Approach

Efforts to isolate traits have been hindered by the fact that there are so many of them. In one study, 17,953 individual traits were identified.[10] However, it is virtually impossible to predict behavior when such a large number of traits must be taken into account. As a result, attention has been directed toward reducing these thousands to a more manageable number—to ascertain the source of primary traits.

One researcher isolated 171 surface traits but concluded that they were superficial and lacking in descriptive power.[11] What he sought was a reduced set of traits that would identify underlying patterns. The result was the identification of sixteen personality factors, which he called source or primary traits, that are the basic underlying causes of surface traits. They are shown in Figure 4–2. These sixteen traits have been found to be generally steady and constant sources of behavior, allowing prediction of an individual's behavior in specific situations by weighing the characteristics for their situational relevance.

However, there are several problems with this approach: Terms are difficult to define, there are contradictions, and the scientific reliability of the results is open to considerable challenge.

Type Approach

An extension of the trait approach has been labeled as the type approach. Instead of looking at specific characteristics, the type approach attempts to group those qualities that go together into a single category. For example, ambition and aggression tend to be highly correlated.

Attempts to reduce the number of traits further tend to isolate introversion-extroversion and something approximating high anxiety—low anxiety as

10. G. W. Allport and H. S. Odbert, "Trait Names, A Psycholexical Study," *Psychological Monographs*, No. 47, 1936.

11. Raymond B. Cattell, "Personality Pinned Down," *Psychology Today*, July 1973, p. 40–46.

FIGURE 4–2 Sixteen Source Traits

```
 1. Reserved ..............Outgoing
 2. Less intelligent ........More intelligent
 3. Affected by feelings .....Emotionally stable
 4. Submissive ............Dominant
 5. Serious................Happy-go-lucky
 6. Expedient..............Conscientious
 7. Timid .................Venturesome
 8. Tough-minded..........Sensitive
 9. Trusting ..............Suspicious
10. Practical..............Imaginative
11. Forthright.............Shrewd
12. Self-assured ..........Apprehensive
13. Conservative ..........Experimenting
14. Group-dependent .......Self-sufficient
15. Uncontrolled ..........Controlled
16. Relaxed ..............Tense
```

the underlying interconnecting characteristics.[12] As depicted in Figure 4–3, these dimensions suggest four personality types.[13] For example, an individual with high anxiety and extroversion would be tense, excitable, unstable, warm, sociable, and dependent.

The most popular of the type approaches are Jung's work on introversion-extroversion and Sheldon's research on body typologies.

Jung. Half a century ago, Swiss psychoanalyst Carl Jung proposed that most people were predominantly either introverted or extroverted. He argued that introverts tend to be primarily oriented to the subjective world. They look inward at themselves, avoid social contacts and initiating interaction with others,

12. Raymond B. Cattell, *The Scientific Analysis of Personality* (Chicago: Aldine, 1965); and H. J. Eysenck, *The Structure of Human Personality* (London: Methuen, 1953).

13. S. R. Maddi, *Personality Theories* (Homewood, Ill.: Dorsey, 1968).

FIGURE 4–3 Four-Type Thesis

	High Anxiety	**Low Anxiety**
Extrovert	Tense, excitable, unstable, warm, sociable, and dependent	Composed, confident, trustful, adaptable, warm, sociable and dependent
Introvert	Tense, excitable, unstable, cold, and shy	Composed, confident, trustful, adaptable, calm, cold, and shy

and tend to be withdrawn and quiet and to enjoy solitude. In contrast, extroverts are primarily oriented to the outside world, friendly, enjoy interaction with others, dislike solitude, are generally aggressive, and express feelings and ideas openly.

Efforts to validate Jung's theory have shown that, as a neat dichotomy, the description of introvert-extrovert is really applicable to only the rare extremes. Most individuals tend to be *ambiverts:* that is, they alternate between introversion and extroversion.[14]

Sheldon. A development out of the heredity school of personality is the work of W. H. Sheldon, who labeled three body builds and certain personality characteristics they reflected.[15] The three types are:

1. Endomorph—fleshy and inclined toward fatness
2. Mesomorph—athletic and inclined to be muscular
3. Ectomorph—thin and inclined to be fine-boned and fragile

Sheldon's three body types and concomitant personality traits are shown in Figure 4–4.

A classification like Sheldon's has intuitive appeal. Who among us has not,

14. Robert E. Silverman, *Psychology* (New York: Appleton-Century-Crofts, 1971), p. 499.

15. William H. Sheldon, *The Varieties of Temperament* (New York: Harper & Row, 1942).

FIGURE 4–4 Sheldon's Body Types and Respective Personality Traits

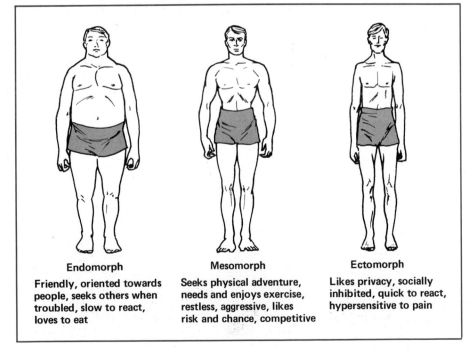

Endomorph	Mesomorph	Ectomorph
Friendly, oriented towards people, seeks others when troubled, slow to react, loves to eat	Seeks physical adventure, needs and enjoys exercise, restless, aggressive, likes risk and chance, competitive	Likes privacy, socially inhibited, quick to react, hypersensitive to pain

FIGURE 4–5 Predictive Validity of Trait or Type Approach

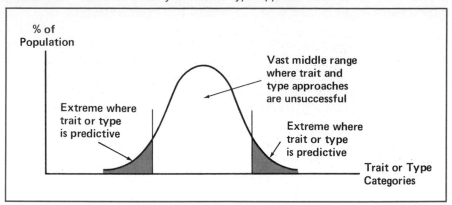

at one time or another, said something like "fat people are jolly" or "frail and sickly people tend to be smart"? Employee interviewers also fall prey to the same logic when, for instance, they operate under the assumption that tall, muscular individuals are more aggressive and hence make better salespeople. In spite of the fact that the early research by Sheldon obtained high correlations between body type and personality characteristics, later attempts to validate this research achieved low or negligible correlations. While the evidence today would question that homogeneous body types must necessarily result in homogeneous personalities, the fact is that our physical appearance, especially in the early years, does influence our self-image, which may in turn affect our personality development. For example, if you are athletic and have a muscular build, others may expect you to be aggressive, and their expectations may influence you to such a degree that you may actually become aggressive.

Summary

Neither trait nor type approaches have been highly successful in predicting behavior across a broad spectrum of situations. The reason lies in the fact that these approaches, for the most part, ignore situational contexts. The approaches are not contingency-oriented and, therefore, largely ignore the dynamic interchange that occurs in an individual's personality as a result of interaction with his or her environment.

As a result, prediction is constrained by the typologies. As noted in Figure 4–5, they tend to be so excessively broad that the classifications apply only to extreme cases—in the tails of the curve—but lack relevance in the vast middle ground. We might be able to predict some common behaviors among *extreme* extroverts or individuals who are *highly* anxious, but most people's characteristics fall in the vast middle range. As a result, we conclude that any approach to explaining personality in terms of characteristics must also consider situational variables.

TWO POPULAR
PERSONALITY DEVELOPMENT THEORIES

The issue of how personalities develop has been of major interest to psychologists for hundreds of years. Names like Sigmund Freud and Erik Erikson have become household words in psychology predominately as a result of their contention that human beings progress through stages. The healthy personality reflects the individual's successful passage through these stages, which results in successful adjustment to his or her environment. Much of the work in personality development, however, has little relevance to students of organizational behavior. In the following pages, we present two personality development theories that *are* pertinent in understanding OB. These are Chris Argyris's maturation theory and Gail Sheehy's passages theory.

Maturation Theory

Professor Chris Argyris of Harvard has postulated a maturation theory of personality development that proposes that all healthy people seek situations that offer autonomy, wide interests, treatment as an equal, and the opportunity to exhibit their ability to deal with complexity.[16] More specifically, Argyris argues that healthy individuals tend to move from immaturity to maturity:

1. From being passive to engaging in increasing activity
2. From dependence on others to independence
3. From having few ways to behave to possessing many alternatives
4. From having shallow interests to developing deeper interests
5. From having a short time perspective to having a longer time perspective
6. From being in a subordinate position to viewing oneself as equal or superordinate
7. From lack of awareness of oneself to awareness of oneself

According to Argyris, healthy people will show the behaviors of maturity while unhealthy people tend to demonstrate childlike, immature behaviors. Further, Argyris argues that most organizations tend to treat their employees like children, making them dependent, subordinate, and narrowly constrained.

Passages Theory

A more recently proposed theory postulates that individuals confront five turning points in their adult lives. Although this theory is comprehensively developed in several works,[17] the widespread success of Gail Sheehy's version in her

16. Chris Argyris, *Personality and Organization: The Conflict Between System and the Individual* (New York: Harper & Row, 1957), p. 50.

17. Roger Gould, *Transformations* (New York: Simon & Schuster, 1978); and Daniel J. Levinson, with Charlotte N. Darrow, Edward B. Klien, Maria H. Levinson, and Braxton McKee, *The Seasons of a Man's Life* (New York: Knopf, 1978).

best seller, *Passages,*[18] has resulted in the theory being typically attributed to her.

Sheehy was concerned that little had been done to document the development of personality beyond the late teenage years. As a result, she reviewed the literature, undertook extensive interviews, and concluded that adults progress through five crises:

1. *Pulling Up Roots.* This period occurs between the ages of eighteen and twenty-two, when individuals exit from home and incur physical, financial, and emotional separation from their parents. They cover their fears and uncertainty with acts of defiance and mimicked confidence. Those individuals who do not have an identity crisis at this point will have it erupt during a later transition where, Sheehy suggests, the penalties may be harder to bear.

2. *The Trying Twenties.* During the twenties, we try to grab hold of who we are and where we want to go. All things seem possible. This period is a time of opportunity, but also includes the fear (usually unfounded) that choices are irrevocable. Two forces push upon us—one is to build a firm, safe structure for the future by making strong commitments, and the other is to explore and experiment and keep flexible as to commitments.

3. *The Catch-Thirties.* Approaching the age of thirty is a time in which life commitments are made, broken or renewed. It may mean setting out on a secondary road toward a new vision or a toning down of idealistic dreams to realistic goals. Commitments are altered or must be deepened. There is change, turmoil, and often an urge to bust out of the routine.

4. *The Deadline Decade.* The ten years between the ages of thirty-five and forty-five represent a crossroad. Youth is history and we begin to see that time is running out. It is a time of both danger and opportunity. This period is characterized by a reexamination of our purposes and how we will spend our resources from now on.

5. *Renewal or Resignation.* The mid-forties bring a period of stability. It may bring staleness and result in resignation. However, for the individual who can find a purpose and direction upon which to continue building his or her life, the mid-forties may well be the best years.

What is the relationship between these five stages or crises and understanding OB? The answer is that you should expect all employees to face crises during their careers. Just as youths are notorious for undergoing identity crises during their teenage years, adults too go through stages—insecurity, opportunities presented, opportunities foregone and lost, and either the acceptance of new challenges or resignation. These crises create the opportunity for an employee to alter his or her goals, commitments, and loyalties to the organization. The infamous mid-life crisis, typically attributed to individuals in their early for-

18. Gail Sheehy, *Passages: Predictable Crises of Adult Life* (New York: Dutton, 1976), p. 13.

ties, is part of what Sheehy calls The Deadline Decade. That is, it is not unusual in fact for employees, when they reach forty, to begin to reexamine their goals and make important adjustments in their lives. Their personalities may undergo significant changes resulting in behavioral patterns quite different from those exhibited prior to their crisis. The manager who understands personality development is better able to predict these crises and recognize them as natural transitions that adults encounter.

MAJOR PERSONALITY ATTRIBUTES INFLUENCING OB

A number of specific personality attributes have been isolated as having potential for predicting behavior in organizations. The first of these attributes is related to where one perceives the locus of control in one's life. The others are achievement orientation, authoritarianism, Machiavellianism, and propensity for risk taking. In this section we shall briefly introduce these attributes and summarize what we know as to their ability to explain and predict employee behavior.

Locus of Control

Some people believe that they are masters of their own fate. Other people see themselves as pawns of fate, believing that what happens to them in their lives is due to luck or chance. The first type, who believe they control their destiny, have been labeled *internals,* while the latter, who see their life controlled by outside forces, have been called *externals.*[19]

A large amount of research comparing internals with externals has consistently shown that individuals who rate high in externality are less satisfied with their jobs, more alienated from the work setting, and less involved on their jobs than are internals.[20]

Why are externals more dissatisfied? The answer is probably because they perceive themselves as having little control over those organizational outcomes that are important to them. Internals, facing the same situation, attribute organizational outcomes to their own actions. If the situation is unattractive, they believe they have no one else to blame but themselves.

The evidence for the impact of locus of control on performance is less clear, yet it seems reasonable to hypothesize that internals should be better performers. Many of the behavior patterns that go along with the internals' per-

19. Julian B. Rotter, "Generalized Expectancies for Internal Versus External Control of Reinforcement," *Psychological Monographs,* Vol. 80, No. 609 (1966).

20. See Dennis W. Organ and Charles N. Greene, "Role Ambiguity, Locus of Control, and Work Satisfaction," *Journal of Applied Psychology,* February 1974, pp. 101–2; Terence R. Mitchell, Charles M. Smyser, and Stan E. Weed, "Locus of Control: Supervision and Work Satisfaction," *Academy of Management Journal,* September 1975, pp. 623–31; and K. E. Runyon, "Some Interactions between Personality Variables and Management Styles," *Journal of Applied Psychology,* June 1973, pp. 288–94.

spective—they search more actively for information before making a decision, are more motivated to achieve, and make a greater attempt to control their environment—are qualities that should lead to better employee performance, especially among managers.

The positive comments we have made about internals is not a complete endorsement of the internal as the ideal personality for organizational members. There is a tendency to conclude that internals are "better" than externals, and that the more internal an employee is, the better for the organization. This is not always true. We know that we live in a world in which there are forces beyond the control of the individual; therefore, very extreme internals may be overrigid, defensively overestimating their ability to control events in their life.[21] Additionally, there is evidence that imposing external strictures on the freedom to choose between job activities may produce resistance from internals resulting in poor performance.[22]

Achievement Orientation

We noted in the prior section that internals are motivated to achieve. This achievement orientation has also been singled out as a personality characteristic that varies among employees and that can be used to predict certain behaviors.

Research has centered around the need to achieve (*nAch*). People with a high need to achieve can be described as continually striving to do things better. They want to overcome obstacles, but they want to feel that their success (or failure) is due to their own actions. This means they like tasks of intermediate difficulty. If a task is very easy, it will lack challenge. High achievers receive no feeling of accomplishment from doing tasks that fail to challenge their abilities. Similarly, they avoid tasks that are so difficult that the probability of success is very low. Even if they succeed, it is more apt to be due to luck than ability. Given the high achiever's propensity for tasks where the outcome can be attributed directly to his or her efforts, the high *nAch* person looks for challenges having approximately a 50-50 chance of success.

What can we say about high achievers on the job? In jobs that provide intermediate difficulty, rapid performance feedback, and allow the employee control over his or her results, the high *nAch* individual will perform well.[23] This implies, though, that high achievers will do better in sales, professional sports, or in management than on an assembly line or in clerical tasks. That is, those individuals with a high *nAch* will not always outperform those who are low or intermediate in this characteristic. The tasks that high achievers undertake must provide the challenge, feedback, and responsibility they look for if the high *nAch* personality is to be positively related to job performance.

21. W. Clay Hamner and Dennis W. Organ, *Organizational Behavior: An Applied Psychological Approach* (Dallas: BPI, 1978), p. 182.

22. W. W. Moyer, "Effects of Loss of Freedom on Subjects with Internal or External Locus of Control," *Journal of Research in Personality,* Vol. 12 (1978), pp. 253–61.

23. John B. Miner, *Theories of Organizational Behavior* (Hinsdale, Ill.: Dryden Press, 1980), pp. 46–75.

Authoritarianism

There is evidence that there is such a thing as an authoritarian personality, but its relevance to job behavior is more speculation than fact. With that qualification, let us examine authoritarianism and consider how it might be related to employee performance.

Authoritarianism refers to a belief that there should be status and power differences among people in organizations.[24] The extremely high authoritarian personality is intellectually rigid, judgmental of others, deferential to those above and exploitative of those below, distrustful, and resistant to change. Of course, few people are extreme authoritarians, so conclusions must be guarded. It seems reasonable to postulate, however, that possessing a high authoritarian personality would be related negatively to performance where the job demanded sensitivity to the feelings of others, tact, and the ability to adapt to complex and changing situations.[25] On the other hand, where jobs are highly structured and success depends on close conformance to rules and regulations, the high authoritarian employee should perform quite well.

Machiavellianism

Closely related to authoritarianism is the characteristic of Machiavellianism (Mach), named after Niccolo Machiavelli who wrote in the sixteenth century on how to gain and manipulate power. An individual high in Machiavellianism is pragmatic, maintains emotional distance, and believes that means can justify ends. "If it works, use it" is consistent with a high Mach perspective.

A considerable amount of research has been directed toward relating high and low Mach personalities to certain behavioral outcomes.[26] High Machs manipulate more, win more, are persuaded less, and persuade others more than do low Machs.[27] Yet these high Mach outcomes are moderated by situational factors. It has been found that high Machs flourish when (1) they interact face-to-face with others rather than indirectly; (2) the situation has a minimum number of rules and regulations, thus allowing latitude for improvisation; and (3) where emotional involvement with details irrelevant to winning distracts low Machs.[28]

Should we conclude that high Machs make good employees? That answer depends on the type of job and whether you consider ethical implications in evaluating performance. In jobs that require bargaining skills (such as labor ne-

---

24. T. Adorno et al., *The Authoritarian Personality* (New York: Harper & Brothers, 1950).

25. Harrison Gough, "Personality and Personality Assessment," in *Handbook of Industrial and Organizational Psychology,* ed. Marvin D. Dunnette (Chicago: Rand McNally, 1976), p. 579.

26. R. G. Vleeming, "Machiavellianism: A Preliminary Review," *Psychological Reports,* February 1979, pp. 295–310.

27. R. Christie and R. L. Geis, *Studies in Machiavellianism* (New York: Academic Press, 1970), p. 312.

28. Ibid.

gotiation) or where there are substantial rewards for winning (as in commissioned sales), high Machs will be productive. But if means can't justify the ends, if there are *absolute* standards of behavior, or if the three situational factors noted in the previous paragraph are not in evidence, our ability to predict a high Mach's performance will be severely curtailed.

Risk Taking

People differ in their willingness to take chances. This propensity to assume or avoid risk has been shown to impact on how long it takes managers to make a decision and how much information they require before making their choice. For instance, seventy-nine managers worked on simulated personnel exercises that required them to make hiring decisions.[29] High risk-taking managers made more rapid decisions and used less information in making their choices than the low risk-taking managers. Interestingly, the decision accuracy was the same for both groups.

While it is generally correct to conclude that managers in organizations are risk aversive,[30] there are still individual differences on this dimension.[31] As a result, it makes sense to recognize these differences and even to consider aligning risk-taking propensity with specific job demands. For instance, a high risk-taking propensity may lead to more effective performance for a stock trader in a brokerage firm. This type of job demands rapid decision making. On the other hand, this personality characteristic might prove a major obstacle to accountants performing auditing activities. This latter job might be better filled by someone with a low risk-taking propensity.

PERSONALITY—JOB FIT THEORIES

In our discussion of authoritarianism, Machiavellianism, and risk taking, our conclusions were qualified to recognize that the requirements of the job moderated the relationship between possession of the personality characteristic and job performance. This concern with matching the job requirements with personality characteristics has recently received increased attention. In this section, two personality–job fit theories will be presented.

Instrumental versus Expressive Orientation

Some people see their work as a means to another end, while others desire jobs for the intrinsic satisfaction that the work itself provides. People who fall into the

29. R. N. Taylor and M. D. Dunnette, "Influence of Dogmatism, Risk-Taking Propensity, and Intelligence on Decision-Making Strategies for a Sample of Industrial Managers," *Journal of Applied Psychology*, August 1974, pp. 420–23.

30. Irving L. Janis and Leon Mann, *Decision Making: A Psychological Analysis of Conflict, Choice, and Commitment* (New York: Free Press, 1977).

31. N. Kogan and M. A. Wallach, "Group Risk Taking as a Function of Members' Anxiety and Defensiveness," *Journal of Personality*, March 1967, pp. 50–63.

first category have what is referred to as an *instrumental orientation*—they desire financial rewards from a job and the security the job provides. Those in the second category have an *expressive orientation*—they want occupational achievement and opportunities for self-fulfillment. There is evidence indicating that performance and satisfaction are higher when expressive personalities are placed in challenging jobs and instrumental personalities in nonchallenging jobs than under the opposite, incongruent personality–job fit conditions.[32]

This finding is consistent with the notion that an employee's behavior is a function of both personality and environment. To some people, work is their central life interest. For such individuals, a challenging job is required. But not all employees want a demanding job. So personality characteristics do impact on behavior, but there is evidence to suggest this impact is at least moderated to the extent that the employee perceives the job to be challenging or nonchallenging.

The Six Personality Types Model

The most researched personality–job fit theory is the six personality types model. The model states that satisfaction and the propensity to leave a job depends on the degree to which individuals successfully match their personality with a congruent occupational environment.[33]

Each one of the six personality types has a matching occupational environment. Listed below is a description of the six types and examples of congruent occupations:

Type	Occupations
1. Realistic—involves aggressive behavior, physical activities requiring skill, strength, and coordination	Forestry, farming, architecture
2. Investigative—involves activities requiring thinking, organizing, and understanding rather than feeling or emotion	Biology, mathematics, news reporting
3. Social—involves interpersonal rather than intellectual or physical activities	Foreign service, social work, clinical psychology
4. Conventional—involves rule-regulated activities and sublimation of personal needs to an organization or person of power and status	Accounting, finance, corporate management
5. Enterprising—involves verbal activities to influence others, to attain power and status	Law, public relations, small business management
6. Artistic—involves self-expression, artistic creation, or emotional activities	Art, music, writing

A Vocational Preference Inventory questionnaire has been developed which contains 160 occupational titles. Respondents indicate which of these occupations they like or dislike and these answers are used to form personality profiles. Utilizing this procedure, research strongly supports the hexagonal dia-

32. Charles A. O'Reilly, III, "Personality–Job Fit: Implications for Individual Attitudes and Performance," *Organizational Behavior and Human Performance*, February 1977, pp. 36–46.

33. John L. Holland, *Making Vocational Choices: A Theory of Careers* (Englewood Cliffs, N.J.: Prentice-Hall, 1973).

FIGURE 4–6 Hexagonal Diagram of the Relationships Among Occupational Personality Types

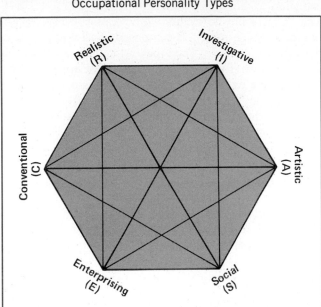

Source: From John L. Holland, *Making Vocational Choices: A Theory of Careers* (Englewood Cliffs, N.J.: Prentice-Hall 1973), p. 23. Used by permission. [This model originally appeared in J. L. Holland et al., "An Empirical Occupational Classification Derived from a Theory of Personality and Intended for Practice and Research," ACT Research Report No. 29 (Iowa City: The American College Testing Program, 1969.]

gram in Figure 4–6. This figure shows that the closer two fields or orientations are in the hexagon, the more compatible they are. Adjacent categories are quite similar, while those diagonally opposite are highly dissimilar.

What does all this mean? The theory argues that satisfaction is highest and turnover lowest where personality and occupation are in agreement. Social individuals should be in social jobs, conventional people in conventional jobs, and so forth. A realistic person in a realistic job is in a more congruent situation than a realistic person in an investigative job. A realistic person in a social job is in the most incongruent situation possible. The key points of this model are that (1) there do appear to be intrinsic differences in personality among individuals; (2) there are different types of jobs; and (3) people in job environments congruent with their personality type should be more satisfied and less likely to voluntarily resign than people in incongruent jobs.

THE SELF-CONCEPT AND DEFENSIVE BEHAVIORS

An important dimension of personality is the self-concept; that is, how one views oneself. It is generally considered from two dimensions: the "I" and the "me." Together they define, for each of us, who we are and who we are in the process of becoming. Our self-concept is important because we take it into each social situation.

The "I" is a private picture we hold of ourselves. Based on the experiences we have undergone, it is comprised of all that we have learned and accepted as part of ourselves. The "me" is the view of self as reflected in the way others behave toward us. The various ways we appear to others plus the way we think they see us makes up the "me." It is the degree of agreement that exists between the "I" and the "me" that is critical in determining behavior.

The more the "I" and the "me" agree, the more consistent and harmonious are our relationships with others. Our expected behavior will be congruent with both the way we see ourselves and the way we perceive others see us. If there is considerable divergence, the result is inconsistent expectations and increased anxiety within the individual. We are forced to reevaluate our self-concept, reduce our contacts with these "others" who are creating the discrepancy, or grow to accept the discomfort from this tension and anxiety.

Our natural response is to maintain our self-concept. This means we attempt to keep a positive view of ourselves and further try to have others accept this internal picture. The effort to maintain our self-concept, however, can result in negative outcomes, such as:

1. People respond to threats to self-concept by trying to hide those parts of themselves that they see as less than totally acceptable.
2. People pretend to be something that they are not.

FIGURE 4–7

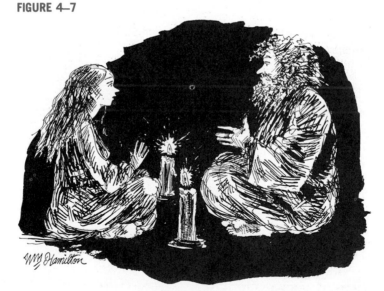

"Larry, in case we don't find enlightenment, do you think we can still get back your Pontiac dealership?"

Source: The New Yorker, July 31, 1971 Drawing by Wm. Hamilton; © 1971 The New Yorker Magazine, Inc.

3. People fall back on cautious and ritualized behavior which, for example, acts to retard new and creative ideas.

When their self-concept is threatened, one of the most natural reactions of people is to engage in some form of defensive behavior. It has been argued that "perhaps no psychological concept has more importance for administrators than psychological defense."[34] When our self-concept is attacked, our natural reaction is to protect it. Every individual will, to some extent, rely on defensive behaviors in order to maintain a stable mental health.

However, the more intense the anxiety experienced by the individual, the greater the probability that these defenses will play a significant part in his or her behavior. Perception of threats produce anxiety. These defenses do not necessarily help the individual to deal with external reality, but they increase adaptability so that internal tension can be maintained at an acceptable level.

While there are dozens of specific defensive behaviors, some of the most common include fantasy, regression, repression, compensation, identification, projection, rationalization, and reaction formation.

Fantasy. An escape from reality through daydreaming or some other form of visionary imagery is fantasizing. Employees who distort their real contribution in a committee by envisioning their comments as the critical input into a major decision are engaging in fantasy.

Regression. An individual may revert back to an earlier and less mature level of behavior when confronted with frustration. Childlike outbursts such as throwing a fit or engaging in horseplay are examples of regression.

Repression. By keeping frustration in the unconscious, we repress information threatening to the consciousness. When feelings or anxieties are excluded from the consciousness, they cannot surface to create frustration or guilt. When an employee "forgets" to tell her boss about an embarrassing situation, she is engaging in repression.

Compensation. When we exert an unusual amount of energy into one activity to make up for a deficiency in another we are exhibiting compensation behavior. This is illustrated by the individual who becomes extremely active and assumes a leadership role on the company's bowling team to compensate for his failure to advance and be promoted in his job with the company.

Identification. When a person models himself or herself after someone else by assuming the characteristics, values, attitudes or mannerisms of the other person, we refer to the behavior as identification. The new college graduate engages in identification when she patterns her behavior after the company's successful, young, female executive vice-president.

34. W. G. Bennis, E. H. Schein, F. I. Steele, and D. E. Berlew, *Interpersonal Dynamics* (Homewood, Ill.: Dorsey, 1968).

Projection. The attribution of one's own problems or motives to someone else is called projection. The employee who wants a specific promotion, is successful in obtaining it, but then proves unable to handle the new job, may insist that it was his wife who pushed him to go after the promotion. He has transferred the responsibility from his shoulders to his wife's.

Rationalization. This is the justification of inconsistent behaviors or attitudes by developing untrue but creditable explanations. "Rationalization is most obviously used to explain failures when job hunting, as in the case of the applicant for a broadcast announcer's job who explained, "They w-w-wouldn't h-hire m-me because I'm a C-C-Catholic.' "[35]

Reaction Formation. In this defense, certain actions unacceptable to the consciousness are repressed, resulting in the individual acting contrary to his or her real feelings and expressing this opposite behavior with considerable force. The individual who has developed a reputation as abrasive may be excessively friendly and cordial to reduce the anxieties created by past abrasive behavior.

Defensive behaviors are exhibited by most of us, at some time or another. Every individual must value his or her self-concept in order to maintain and develop a healthy personality. It is not surprising, therefore, that people develop protective or defensive mechanisms to ensure that health is maintained.

PERSONALITY AND STRESS

The medical profession has long been concerned about the effect of stress on health, but it is only recently that organizational researchers have begun to examine the impact of stress on worker behavior and how personality characteristics may moderate the stress-behavior relationship.

Why the recent concern with stress as an OB topic? First, stress appears to be linked to employee performance and satisfaction. So the topic is a relevant independent variable. Second, there is an implicit obligation of management to improve the quality of organizational life for employees. Because stress has been directly linked to coronary heart disease, a reduction in stress can increase both the general health and longevity of an organization's work force. Of course, this too can have performance implications.

What Is Stress?

Stress is a dynamic condition in which an individual is confronted with an opportunity, constraint, or demand related to what he or she desires and for which

35. Joe Kelly, *Organizational Behavior*, rev. ed. (Homewood, Ill.: Richard D. Irwin, 1974), p. 272.

the outcome is perceived to be both uncertain and important.[36] This is a complicated definition. Let's look at its components more closely.

Stress is not necessarily bad in and of itself. While stress is typically discussed in a negative context, it also has positive value. It is an opportunity when it offers potential gain. Consider, for example, the superior performance that an athlete or stage performer gives in "clutch" situations. Such individuals often use stress positively to rise to the occasion and perform at or near their maximum.

More typically, stress is associated with constraints and demands. The former prevent you from doing what you desire. The latter refers to the loss of something desired. So when you take a test at school or you undergo your annual performance review at work, you feel stress because you confront opportunity, constraints, and demands. A good performance review may lead to a promotion, greater responsibilities, and a higher salary. But a poor review may prevent you from getting the promotion. An extremely poor review might even result in your being fired.

Two conditions are necessary for potential stress to become actual stress.[37] There must be uncertainty over the outcome and the outcome must be important. Regardless of the conditions, it is only when there is doubt or uncertainty regarding whether the opportunity will be seized, the constraint removed, or the loss avoided that there is stress. That is, stress is highest for those individuals who perceive that they are uncertain as to whether they will win or lose and lowest for those individuals who think that winning or losing is a certainty. But importance is also critical. If winning or losing is an unimportant outcome, there is no stress. If keeping your job or earning a promotion doesn't hold any importance to you, you have no reason to feel stress over having to undergo a performance review.

Facts about Stress and Work

The research on stress has uncovered several important facts. First, stress creates some very real costs to organizations. Second, stress is additive in nature. Third, people react differently to stress situations. Each of these facts are relevant to our discussion.

Over one million Americans suffer heart attacks each year. Half of these attacks will be fatal.[38] One out of every five average, healthy, male Americans will suffer a heart attack before he reaches sixty-five years of age.[39] There is no

---

36. Adapted from Randall S. Schuler, "Definition and Conceptualization of Stress in Organizations," *Organizational Behavior and Human Performance,* April 1980, p. 189.

37. Ibid., p. 191.

38. David C. Glass, "Stress, Competition, and Heart Attacks," *Psychology Today,* December 1976, p. 54.

39. Karl Albrecht, *Stress and the Manager* (Englewood Cliffs, N.J.: Prentice-Hall, 1979), p. 33.

doubt that organizational stress is a major contributor to coronary heart disease.[40] Beyond their significance for the quality of human life, these statistics have direct implications for organizations. Stress-induced heart disease increases both short- and long-term absenteeism, and the need to replace employees due to premature retirements or death. While the linkage is less clear, stress also undoubtedly contributes to mental illness, alcoholism, drug abuse, and other work-related dysfunctional conditions and behaviors.

Stress is additive.[41] It builds up. Each new and persistent stressor adds to an individual's stress level. A single stressor, in and of itself, may seem relatively unimportant, but if it is added to an already high level of stress, it can be "the straw that breaks the camel's back." If we want to appraise the total amount of stress an individual is under, we have to sum up his or her opportunity stresses, constraint stresses, and demand stresses.

Another important fact about stress is that it does not necessarily follow from a stressor. Whether a potential stressor actually provokes a stress condition depends in large measure on the personality of the individual exposed to it. Individual differences moderate the relationship between a potential stress condition and the reaction to it.[42] Individuals react differently to common stress situations and this difference can be substantially predicted by these individuals' personality characteristics. The relevant personality constructs will be elaborated upon later in this section.

Symptoms of Stress

Stress shows itself in a number of ways. For instance, an individual who is experiencing a high level of stress may develop high blood pressure, ulcers, irritability, difficulty in making routine decisions, loss of appetite, accident-proneness, and the like. These can be subsumed under three general categories: physiological, psychological, and behavioral symptoms.[43]

Physiological Symptoms. Most of the early concern with stress was directed at physiological symptoms. This was predominately due to the fact that the topic was researched by specialists in the health and medical sciences. This research led to the conclusion that stress could create changes in metabolism, increase heart and breathing rates, increase blood pressure, bring on headaches, and induce heart attacks.

The link between stress and particular physiological symptoms is not clear.

40. See, for instance, Cary L. Cooper and Judi Marshall, "Occupational Sources of Stress: A Review of the Literature Relating to Coronary Heart Disease and Mental Ill Health," *Journal of Occupational Psychology,* Vol. 49, No. 1 (1976), pp. 11–28.

41. Hans Selye, *The Stress of Life,* rev. ed. (New York: McGraw-Hill, 1956).

42. Bernard J. Mullin and Robert L. Swinth, "Individual Differences in Perceived Stress and Performance in Response to Organizational Stressors," paper presented at the meeting of Western Academy of Management, Monterey, California, April 1981.

43. Schuler, "Definition and Conceptualization of Stress" pp. 200–5.

There are few, if any, consistent relationships.[44] This is attributed to the complexity of the symptoms and the difficulty of objectively measuring them. But of greater relevance is the fact that physiological symptoms have the least direct relevance to students of OB. Our concern is with behaviors and attitudes. Therefore, the two other symptoms of stress are more important to us.

Psychological Symptoms. Stress can cause dissatisfaction. Job-related stress can cause job-related dissatisfaction. Job dissatisfaction, in fact, is "the simplest and most obvious psychological effect" from stress.[45] But stress shows itself in other psychological states—for instance, tension, anxiety, irritability, boredom, and procrastination.

The evidence indicates that when people are placed in jobs that make multiple and conflicting demands or in which there is a lack of clarity as to the incumbent's duties, authority, and responsibilities, both stress and dissatisfaction are increased.[46] Similarly, the less control people have over the pace of their work, the greater the stress and dissatisfaction. While more research is needed to clarify the relationship, the evidence suggests that jobs that provide a low level of variety, significance, autonomy, feedback, and identity to incumbents create stress and reduce satisfaction and involvement in the job.[47]

Behavioral Symptoms. Behaviorally related stress symptoms include changes in productivity, absence, and turnover, as well as changes in eating habits, increased smoking or consumption of alcohol, rapid speech, fidgeting, and sleep disorders.

There has been a significant amount of research investigating the stress-performance relationship. Given our particular interest in factors that influence employee performance, this research is summarized in the following section.

Stress and Performance

The best-known and most thoroughly documented pattern in the stress-performance literature is the inverted-U relationship.[48] This is shown in Figure 4–8.

The logic underlying the inverted-U is that low to moderate levels of stress stimulate the body and increase its ability to react. Individuals then often per-

44. Terry A. Beehr and John E. Newman, "Job Stress, Employee Health, and Organizational Effectiveness: A Facet Analysis, Model, and Literature Review," *Personnel Psychology,* Winter 1978, pp. 665–99.

45. Ibid., p. 687.

46. Cooper and Marshall, "Occupational Sources of Stress."

47. J. Richard Hackman and Greg R. Oldham, "Development of the Job Diagnostic Survey," *Journal of Applied Psychology,* April 1975, pp. 159–70.

48. See, for instance, Joseph E. McGrath, "Stress and Behavior in Organizations," in *Handbook of Industrial and Organizational Psychology,* ed. Marvin D. Dunnette (Chicago: Rand McNally, 1976); and Robert T. Keller, "Job Stress and Employee Performance in a Manufacturing Plant," paper presented at the meeting of the National Academy of Management, San Diego, August 1981.

FIGURE 4–8 Relationship between Stress and Job Performance

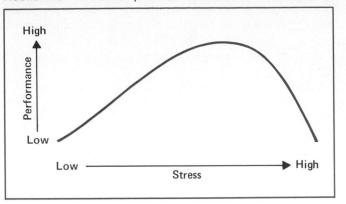

form their tasks better, more intensely, or more rapidly. But too much stress places unattainable demands or constraints on a person, which results in lower performance. This inverted-U pattern may also describe the reaction to stress over time, as well as to changes in stress intensity. That is, even moderate levels of stress can have a negative influence on performance over the long term as the continued intensity of the stress wears down the individual and saps his or her energy resources. An athlete may be able to use the positive effects of stress to obtain a higher performance during every Saturday's game in the fall season. Or a sales executive may be able to psych herself up for her presentation at the annual national meeting. But moderate levels of stress experienced continually over long periods of time—as typified by the emergency room staff in a large urban hospital—can result in lower performance. This may explain why emergency room staffs at such hospitals are frequently rotated and why it is unusual to find individuals who have spent the bulk of their career in such an environment. In effect, to do so would expose the individual to the risk of "career burnout."

The inverted-U hypothesis is moderated by at least two important contingency factors: the type of job and the personality of the individual.

Type of Job. You don't have to be an insightful behavioral scientist to hypothesize that jobs differ in such a way that a given level of stress might effect performance positively in one job and negatively in another. Casual observation would lead most of us to assume that the stress level of a scriptwriter who has to turn out a fresh half-hour comedy show every week is probably quite high. A high state of arousal is probably necessary to get a quality script. Stress stimulates a nervousness and intensity that is functional. But would that same stress level be functional for a brain surgeon? Probably not. While the brain surgeon certainly works under stress, it is of a lower level. It is more controlled. Since the surgeon is typically performing precise yet routine procedures, extremely high levels of arousal are likely to lead to a lower level of surgical performance. But this extreme arousal level may be just what is necessary for the scriptwriter to do her best work.

The evidence suggests that high stress jobs are those where incumbents have little control over their work, are under relentless time pressures, face threatening physical conditions, or have major responsibilities for financial or human resources.[49] Managers fall in this category, as do secretaries, foremen, waiters, inspectors, and clinical lab technicians. In contrast, jobs rating low on stress include farm laborer, maid, stock handler, and college professor.[50]

Probably the most widely recognized stress-inducing occupation is that of the air traffic controller.[51] At Chicago's O'Hare airport, for instance, 1,900 flights are handled each day. That equates to a takeoff or landing every twenty seconds. Each air traffic controller at O'Hare is responsible for landing a plane every two minutes while simultaneously monitoring a half dozen others on the radar screen. In such a job, there is obviously little room for error. As a result, controllers at O'Hare are allowed to work only ninety continuous minutes during peak hours. Even with these shortened time schedules, stress-induced symptoms are overwhelming. Tenure is short compared to more typical jobs. Of the 94 controllers at O'Hare in 1977, only two had been there more than ten years. Most don't last five years. Of those that made it for five years, two-thirds had either ulcers or ulcer symptoms. One study which compared over 4,000 air traffic controllers with 8,000 second-class airmen found the rate of hypertension among the controllers to be four times that of the airmen, while ulcers were more than twice as prevalent.[52]

Personality. There is an increasing amount of research to support the proposition that the effect of stress on an employee's behavior is moderated by his or her personality type. Personality traits that moderate an individual's response to stress at work include extroversion, rigidity, authoritarianism, dogmatism, locus of control, and tolerance for ambiguity.[53] The greatest interest, however, has been directed at what has come to be known as Type A and Type B personalities.[54]

The Type A personality is characterized by feeling a chronic sense of time urgency and by an *excessive* competitive drive. A Type A individual is "*aggressively* involved in a *chronic, incessant* struggle to achieve more and more in less and less time, and if required to do so, against the opposing efforts of other things or other persons."[55] In the North American culture, such characteristics tend to be highly prized and positively correlated with ambition and the success-

49. Cary L. Cooper and R. Payne, *Stress at Work* (London: John Wiley, 1978).

50. As reported in *U.S. News and World Report,* March 13, 1978, pp. 80–81.

51. See, for example, D. Martindale, "Sweaty Palms in the Control Tower," *Psychology Today,* February 1977, pp. 71–73.

52. Reported in Daniel Katz and Robert L. Kahn, *The Social Psychology of Organizations,* 2nd ed. (New York: John Wiley, 1978), p. 599.

53. These traits are reviewed in Arthur P. Brief, Randall S. Schuler, and Mary Van Sell, *Managing Job Stress* (Boston: Little, Brown, 1981), pp. 94–98.

54. Meyer Friedman and Ray H. Rosenman, *Type A Behavior and Your Heart* (New York: Knopf, 1974).

55. Ibid., p. 84.

ful acquisition of material goods. Some of the more outstanding characteristics of Type A's include:

1. Always moving, walking, and eating rapidly
2. Feelings of impatience with the rate at which most events take place
3. Striving to think or do two or more things simultaneously
4. Persistent and destructive inability to cope with leisure time
5. Obsession with numbers; success is measured in terms of how much of everything they acquire.

In contrast to the Type A personality, there is the Type B, who is exactly opposite. Type B's are "rarely harried by the desire to obtain a wildly increasing number of things or participate in an endless growing series of events in an ever decreasing amount of time."[56] Type B personalities can be identified by the following characteristics:

1. Never suffer from a sense of time urgency with its accompanying impatience
2. Feel no need to display or discuss either their achievements or accomplishments unless such exposure is demanded by the situation
3. Play for fun and relaxation, rather than to exhibit their superiority at any cost
4. Can relax without guilt

The evidence links these two distinct personality types with diverse behaviors and different performance outcomes depending on the requirements of the job.

Before we review the research findings, it is interesting to note that Type A is the predominant personality type in North America. Without knowing anything about you, it would be statistically correct for me to assume that *you* are a Type A. About 50 percent of the population are Type A, approximately 40 percent are Type B, and the remaining 10 percent are a mix of both Type A and Type B characteristics. The fact that Type A personality characteristics are associated with two to three times greater risk of heart attack than Type B characteristics[57] can additionally help to explain the wide prevalence of heart disease in North America.

Type A's operate under moderate to high levels of stress. They subject themselves to more or less continuous time pressure, creating for themselves a life of deadlines. These characteristics result in some rather specific behavioral outcomes. For example, Type A's are fast workers. This is because they emphasize quantity over quality. In managerial positions, Type A's demonstrate their competitiveness by working long hours and, not infrequently, making poor decisions because they make them too fast. Type A's are also rarely creative. Because of their concern with quantity and speed, they rely on past experiences

56. Ibid., pp. 84–85.

57. Orlando Behling and F. Douglas Holcombe, "Dealing with Employee Stress," *MSU Business Topics,* Spring 1981, p. 53.

when faced with problems. They will not allocate the time that is necessary to develop unique solutions to new problems. They rarely vary in their responses to specific challenges in their milieu; hence their behavior is easier to predict than that of Type B's.

Are Type A's or Type B's more successful in organizations? In spite of the Type A's hard work, the Type B's are the ones who appear to make it to the top. Great salesmen are usually Type A's, while senior executives are usually Type B's. Why? The answer lies in the tendency of A to trade off quality of effort for quantity.

> . . . promotion and elevation, particularly in corporate and professional organizations, usually go to those who are wise rather than to those who are merely hasty, to those who are tactful rather than to those who are hostile, and to those who are creative rather than to those who are merely agile in competitive strife.[58]

The Type A–Type B dichotomy offers us some insight into the impact of personality characteristics on the stress-performance relationship. Where high energy alone is a major determinant in job success, Type A's should be highly effective. In those jobs where originality, thought, and care are important, the Type B personality should be more successful.

IMPLICATIONS FOR PERFORMANCE AND SATISFACTION

What is the relevance of the personality literature in helping us to explain and predict behavior? The negative position is well summarized in the following statement: ". . . most research—the vast proportion of research—in personality is inconsequential, trivial, and pointless even if it is well done."[59] Part of this statement is true, but clearly it represents too extreme a position. The personality material *does* have relevance—by determining what characteristics will make for effective job performance it can aid in personnel selection; by increasing our understanding of how personality and job characteristics interact it can result in better hiring, transfer, and promotion decisions; and by providing insights into personality development it can help us to anticipate, recognize, and prevent the operationalizing of costly defenses by organizational members.

Because personality characteristics create the parameters for people's behavior, they give us a framework for predicting behavior. For example, individuals who are shy, introverted, and dislike social situations would probably make poor salespeople. Individuals who are submissive and conforming might not be effective as advertising "idea" people.

58. Friedman and Rosenman, *Type A Behavior*, p. 86.
59. Sechrest, "Personality," p. 2.

Can we predict which people would perform satisfactorily in sales, research, or assembly-line work based on their personality characteristics? The answer is a qualified "Yes." We can look at certain characteristics that tend to be related to job success, test for these traits, and use this data to make selection more effective. A person who accepts rules, conformity, and dependence and rates high on authoritarianism is likely to feel more comfortable in a structured assembly-line job, as an admittance clerk in a hospital, or as an administrator in a large public agency than as a researcher or in a job requiring a high degree of creativity. This is exactly why personality tests are used in screening job candidates—to avoid potential mismatches!

But are personality characteristics reliable predictors? This is more difficult to answer. Personality characteristics do tend to be stable, which explains why behavior patterns are generally uniform. An individual who, for example, was shy yesterday, is likely to continue to be shy today. This stability factor is a plus since any attempt to predict behavior needs consistent past data upon which to base future estimates.

> From a practical standpoint, the trait-and-type approach is most useful when the pertinent behavior patterns are absolutely consistent—that is, characteristic of a person regardless of circumstances. . . . The statement that a person has the trait of submissiveness is useful for prediction only insofar as he is submissive in all or most situations. If he is submissive only in certain circumstances, then we can predict his behavior accurately only if we know what those circumstances are.[60]

The type of work and the structure of the job represent significant situational variables that affect personality in an organizational environment. As noted above, where these variables are unstable, our ability to predict is reduced.

Another factor that reduces the predictive value of personality characteristics is inherent in the characteristics themselves: Because of the difficulty in accurately measuring each characteristic and the fact that most people possess middle-range levels of this characteristic (i.e., they are neither highly tense nor are they highly composed), personality characteristics tend to be valuable only in predicting extremes. In other words, only with individuals who demonstrate extreme levels of independence or dependence, submissiveness or dominance, self-assuredness or apprehensiveness, can we accurately predict satisfaction and behavior.

One area of recent research interest has been the relationship of personality variables to withdrawal behaviors. One review concluded that individuals who demonstrated extreme positions along certain trait continua tend to leave the organization more frequently than those in the middle range.[61] Employees

60. Richard S. Lazarus, *Personality and Adjustment* (Prentice-Hall, 1963), as cited in *Concepts and Controversy in Organizational Behavior,* 2nd ed., ed. W. R. Nord (Pacific Palisades, Cal.: Goodyear, 1976), p. 129.

61. L. W. Porter and R. M. Steers, "Organizational Work and Personal Factors in Employee Turnover and Absenteeism," *Psychological Bulletin,* August 1973, pp. 151–76.

with high levels of anxiety, achievement orientation, aggression, independence, self-confidence, and sociability are more likely to withdraw from organizations than employees with more moderate levels of these traits. However, this conclusion has come under recent attack.[62] Another researcher, using the sixteen-trait classification, found anxiety and conscientiousness to be the most important traits in explaining turnover and absenteeism.[63] In the type of jobs tested, which tended normally to have high turnover rates, high levels of anxiety and low levels of conscientiousness predicted withdrawal behaviors.

Sheehy's theory of personality development provides meaningful insights that have direct application to organizational behavior. The fact that each adult individual passes through certain critical stages suggests that certain behavior and satisfaction patterns can be predicted in employees. For example, satisfaction levels probably decline for many employees in their mid-thirties, as they begin to recognize that their dreams of fame and fortune are probably just that—dreams. They may become defensive—using projection or rationalization—in an attempt to redirect their frustration away from themselves personally. Similarly, each of the stages proposed by Sheehy should bring with them changes in the individual's personality and consequently changes in his or her work behavior.

The personality–job fit theories offer suggestions for improving worker performance by selecting individuals for jobs based on matching job characteristics with personality characteristics. Our discussion of stress also has implications for selection and placement of employees. Jobs differ in the degree of stress they create. Individuals differ in the manner in which they react to stress. Matching Type A's and Type B's with congruent jobs allows the organization to reduce the dysfunctional effects of stress and to maximize its functional benefits.

FOR DISCUSSION

1. How does *heredity* influence personality? *Environment?* The *situation?*

2. How could birth order or physical characteristics influence personality? What conclusions can one draw based on these areas of research?

3. What are traits? How many personality traits are there?

62. R. T. Mowday, L. W. Porter, and E. F. Stone, "Employee Characteristics as Predictors of Turnover among Female Clerical Employees in Two Organizations," working paper dated April 1977.

63. J. John Bernardin, "The Relationship of Personality Variables to Organizational Withdrawal," *Personnel Psychology*, Spring 1977, pp. 17–27.

4. What constrains the ability of personality traits to predict behavior?

5. What is the maturation theory? What are its implications for understanding behavior?

6. What behavioral predictions might you make if you knew an employee had (a) an external locus of control? (b) a high *nAch?* (c) a low Mach score?

7. "The type of job an employee does moderates the relationship between personality and job productivity." Do you agree or disagree with this statement? Discuss.

8. List and describe five defense mechanisms. If all people engage, at times, in defense mechanisms, what value is there in knowing about them?

9. What is the relationship between stress and performance?

10. How can our knowledge of personality help us to explain and predict behavior?

FOR FURTHER READING

ALLPORT, G. W., *Pattern and Growth in Personality.* New York: Holt, Rinehart & Winston, 1961. Surveys the most important findings from personality research and adds coordinating theory to knit together the results of this research.

BISCHOF, L. J., *Interpreting Personality Theories,* 2nd ed. New York: Harper & Row, 1970. Presents biographical background and contributions of the twenty major personality theorists.

BYRNE, D., *Introduction to Personality: Research, Theory and Applications,* 2nd ed. Englewood Cliffs, N.J.: Prentice-Hall, 1974. Clearly written text concentrating on the study of individual differences.

EPSTEIN, S., "The Stability of Behavior: On Predicting Most of the People Much of the Time," *Journal of Personality and Social Psychology,* July 1979, pp. 1097–126. A review of personality studies indicates that while personality characteristics may not permit prediction of single instances of behavior, they are effective for predicting behavior averaged over a range of situations.

HOGAN, R., C. B. DESOTO, and C. SOLANO, "Traits, Tests, and Personality Research," *American Psychologist,* April 1977, pp. 255–64. Presents five major criticisms of personality tests, reviews the evidence, and concludes that most of the criticisms are unjustified.

LICHTMAN, C. M., and R. G. HUNT, "Personality and Organization Theory: A Review of Some Conceptual Literature," *Psychological Bulletin,* October 1971, pp. 271–94. Reviews and comments on the ways different theories have dealt with, or contributed to, the structuralist versus personalistic dilemma.

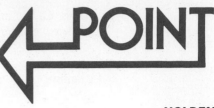

POINT

HOLDEN

Twins raised apart: some case studies

Adapted and edited from Constance Holden, "Identical Twins Reared Apart," Science, *March 1980, pp. 1323–24. ©1980 by the American Association for the Advancement of Science. With permission.*

Investigators have been bemused and occasionally astonished at similarities between long-separated twins, similarities that prevailing dogma about human behavior would ordinarily attribute to common environmental influences. How is it, for example, that two men with significantly different upbringings came to have the same authoritarian personality? Or another pair to have similar histories of endogenous depression? Or still another pair to have virtually identical patterns of headaches? Consider the following cases of identical twins being studied by Thomas Bouchard at the University of Minnesota.

The "Jim twins" were separated from birth and both coincidently named Jim by their adoptive families. Jim Springer and Jim Lewis were adopted as infants into working-class Ohio families. Reunited at the age of 39, the similarities in their lives were eerie. Both liked math and did not like spelling in school. Both had law enforcement training and worked part-time as deputy sheriffs. Both vacationed in Florida, both drove Chevrolets. Both had dogs named Toy. Both married and divorced women named Linda and had second marriages with women named Betty. They named their sons James Allan and James Alan, respectively. Both like mechanical drawing and carpentry. They have almost identical drinking and smoking patterns. Both chew their fingernails down to the nubs.

But what investigators think "astounding" is their similar medical histories. In addition to having hemorrhoids and identical pulse and blood pressure and sleep patterns, both inexplicably put on 10 pounds at the same time in their lives. What really gets the researchers is that both suffer from "mixed headache syndrome"—a combination tension headache and migraine. The onset occurred in both at the age of 18. They have these late-afternoon headaches with the same frequency and same degree of disability, and the two use the same terms to describe the pain.

The twins also have their differences. One wears his hair over his forehead, the other has it slicked back with sideburns. One expresses himself better orally, the other in writing. Although the emotional environments in which they were brought up were different, the profiles on their psychological inventories were much alike.

Another much-publicized pair are 47-year-old Oskar Stöhr and Jack Yufe. These two have the most dramatically different backgrounds of all the twins studied. Born in Trinidad of a Jewish father and a German mother, they were separated shortly after birth. The mother took Oskar back to Germany, where he was raised as a Catholic and a Nazi youth by his grandmother. Jack was raised in the Caribbean, as a Jew, by his father, and spent part of his youth on an Israeli kibbutz. The two men now lead markedly different lives: Oskar is an industrial supervisor in Germany, a devoted union man, a skier. Jack runs a retail clothing store in San Diego, is separated, and describes himself as a workaholic.

But similarities started cropping up as soon as Oskar arrived at the airport for their first meeting. Both were wearing wire-rimmed glasses and mustaches, both sported two-pocket shirts with epaulets. They share idiosyncrasies galore: they like spicy foods and sweet liqueurs, are absentminded, have a habit of falling asleep in front of the television, think it's funny to sneeze in a crowd of strangers, flush the toilet before using it, store rubber bands on their wrists, read magazines from back to front, dip buttered toast in their coffee. Oskar is domineering toward women and yells at his wife, which Jack did before he was separated. Oskar did not take all the tests because he speaks only German, but the two had very similar profiles on the Minnesota Multiphasic Personality Inventory. Although the two were raised in different cultures and speak different languages, investigator Bouchard professed himself struck by the similarities in their mannerisms, the questions they asked, their "temperament, tempo, the way they do things"—which are, granted, relatively intangible when it comes to measuring them. Bouchard also thinks the two supply "devastating" evidence against the feminist contention that children's personalities are shaped differently according to the sex of those who rear them, since Oskar was raised by women and Jack by men.

Other well-publicized twin pairs are Bridget and Dorothy, and Barbara and Daphne. Both sets are British housewives, now in their late 30's, who were separated during World War II. Bridget and Dorothy are of considerable interest because they were raised in quite different socioeconomic settings—the class difference turns out mainly to be reflected in the fact that the one raised in modest circumstances has bad teeth. Otherwise, say the investigators, they share "striking similarities in all areas," including another case of coincidence in naming children. They named their sons Richard Andrew and Andrew Richard, respectively, and their daughters Catherine Louise and Karen Louise. (Bouchard is struck by this, as the likelihood of such a coincidence would seem to be lessened by the fact that names are a joint decision of husband and wife.) On ability and IQ tests the scores of the sisters were similar, although the one raised in the lower class setting had a slightly higher score.

The other British twins, Daphne and Barbara, are fondly remembered by the investigators as the "giggle sisters." Both were great gigglers, particularly together, when they were always setting each other off. Asked if there were any gigglers in their adoptive families, both replied in the negative. The sisters also shared identical coping mechanisms in the face of stress: they ignored it. In keeping with this, both flatly avoided conflict and controversy—neither, for example, had any interest in politics. Such avoidance of conflict is "classically regarded as learned behavior," says Bouchard.

COUNTER ⟶⟵ POINT

FARBER

Twins raised apart: a review of the evidence

The literature contains references to 121 valid sets of separated twins. The following conclusions were based on a very careful analysis of this sample.

Individuals are the product of both heredity and environment. However, some things appear to be more affected by one than the other. In general, we find that physical characteristics may have substantial genetic determination. Some personality traits are more environmentally than genetically related, while others are the reverse. There is also a glaring paradox related to the personality of twins: Twins who have no contact often seem to be the most alike, despite families and cultures that sometimes seem very different.

Close analysis of the sample finds remarkable similarities, sometimes so striking as to be unnerving. Appearance, voice, gestures, and even onset of landmarks such as menstruation or menopause certainly are under a noteworthy degree of hereditary control. So also is susceptibility to symptoms and disorders ranging from menstrual complaints, to dental caries, to cardiovascular disease, to psychosis, to musculoskeletal disorders. Physical characteristics ranging from height, to weight, to menstrual symptoms are greatly alike among the twins—perhaps not surprisingly, since at least some of these traits are presumed to have significant degrees of genetic determination. However, it is a little more eerie to discover that traits such as smoking, drinking, nail biting, or gestures and mannerisms are alike despite environmental differences and lack of contact. While we find similarities among personality characteristics, investigators who have studied series of separated twins are unanimous in concluding that personality is more affected by environment than any other area of human functioning. But there are still questions to be answered.

For example, why should most of these twins laugh alike, describe symptoms in the same way, smoke similar numbers of cigarettes, choose similar creative pursuits, and sometimes even marry the same number of times? Someone will have to examine if, in fact, the similarity in mannerisms described in this sample exists in another sample, and, if it does (and I suspect it will), someone will have to fathom why twins reared in different environments should so frequently bite their nails, grimace, snicker, tap their fingers, and even have neurotic symptoms in such similar ways. That activity levels might have innate components is not hard to envision, but the suggested specificity at the level of mannerisms and nervous habits is hard to comprehend. At this point, it is reasonable to conclude that the clearest signs of genetic determination may occur in personality traits closest to neurobiological functioning—arousal, sensory patterning, tempo, units of movement, and so forth.

It is easier to conceptualize temperament as the important area to study. The similarities in characteristic mood and the similarity in the pattern of anxiety seem noteworthy. Proneness to anxiety, fearfulness, and depressive tendencies also bear similarities but probably are not worthy of interpretation in this sample, given the massive environmental traumas pervading the lives of almost all twins.

The environment, particularly family influences, shows clearly in attitudes, values, and choice of mate. The cultural or regional influences transmitted by the family and social network also are present and probably show in general personality traits ranging from emotional expressivity to drinking habits. However, since in almost every instance investigators were from the same culture, there is some control for cultural influences; there is also some obscuring of the full degree of differences that exist among Danes, Englishmen, Japanese, and Americans reared in different decades and different social milieus. Indeed, everything in these data points toward the massive and perhaps predominant influence of family and culture on attitudes and psychological traits, particularly traits increasingly removed

from direct physical involvement such as the difference between suspiciousness or indecision versus the experienced state of anxiety arousal.

There is substantial ambiguity in the data on twins. Certainly one of the more baffling is the paradox that twins with the least contact may most frequently be the most alike. Since the evidence from this sample demonstrates that twins with contact appear the most different, the differences speak eloquently to the need of each individual to be an individual—unique and clearly bounded. And, since twins evidently make themselves different as well as being made different by external forces, the pattern suggests that an approach that views the individual as an active participant in the creation of his reality is essential to understand the data. Additionally, we can infer that even though the separate environments in which twins are reared appear dissimilar to us, the twins must be making them similar or experiencing them similarly nonetheless. If true, there may be a development process and way of organizing one's perceptions that are significantly influenced by heredity.

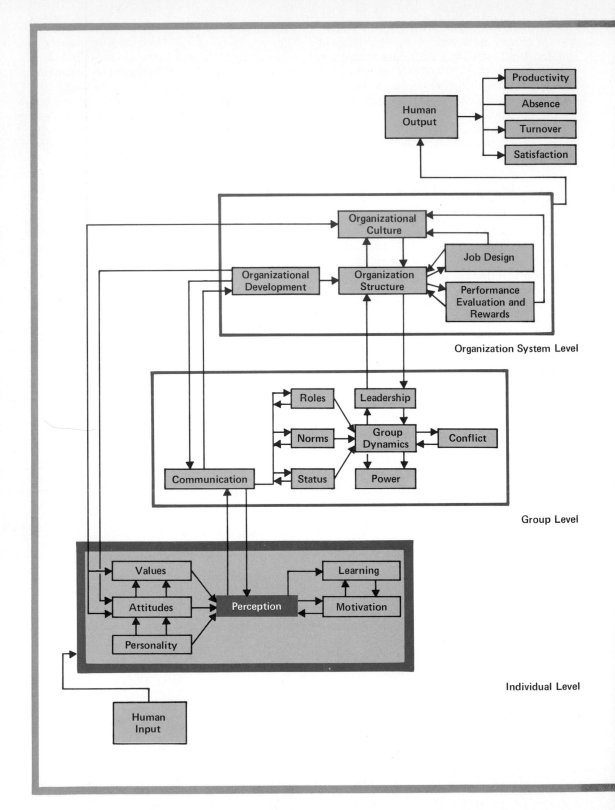

CHAPTER 5
Perception

AFTER STUDYING THIS CHAPTER, YOU SHOULD BE ABLE TO—

Define and explain the following key terms and concepts:

Assumed similarity   Perception

Attribution theory   Selective perception

Halo effect   Stereotyping

Understand:

The difference between perception and reality in determining behavior

How two people can see the same thing and interpret it differently

Why we see what we want to see

How factors residing in the perceiver shape perception

How factors in the target shape perception

How factors in the situation shape perception

Three determinants of attribution

How shortcuts can assist in or distort our judgments of others

> First umpire: "Some's balls and some's strikes and I calls 'em as they is."
>
> Second umpire: "Some's balls and some's strikes and I calls 'em as I sees 'em."
>
> Third umpire: "Some's balls and some's strikes but they ain't nothin' till I calls 'em."
>
> —HADLEY CANTRIL

Any discussion of perception begins with the realization that the way we see the outside world need not be the same as the world really is. We tend to see the world the way we want to perceive it. For supporting evidence, we need go no further than the perception of how effective a college instructor is in the classroom. It is not unusual for an instructor to be rated "excellent" by some students, and "unsatisfactory" by other students in the same class. The instructor's teaching behavior, of course, is a constant. In spite of the fact that all students see the same instructor, they perceive his or her effectiveness differently. This illustration confirms that we do not *see* reality but rather we interpret what we see and call it reality.

When distortions are low—for example, when you and I both agree that the bank robbery we just witnessed was carried out by a Caucasian male, approximately five feet, ten inches tall, 170 pounds, with dark brown hair, and wearing jeans and a light blue nylon jacket with a white patch on the right shoulder—it means that we not only saw the same thing, but that our base of interpretation was similar.

A frequently cited case of how perceptions distort reality derives from a study conducted with representatives from both management and labor.[1] Each group was given a photograph of an ordinary-looking man and asked to describe the individual in the photograph using a long list of personality characteristics. The only difference was that in half the cases the man pictured in the photograph was labeled as a plant manager and in the other half this same person was described as a union official. The results confirmed that impressions were radically different, and depended on whether the man in the photograph was seen as "union" or "management," and, of course, whether the evaluator represented "union" or "management." Management and labor representatives formed significantly different impressions, each viewing the other as less dependable and more intolerant of diverse points of view than members of their own group. Apparently, perception is like beauty in that it lies "in the eye of the beholder."

1. Mason Haire, "Role Perceptions in Labor-Management Relations: An Experimental Approach," *Industrial and Labor Relations Review,* January 1955, pp. 204–16.

As we shall find throughout this chapter, people's behavior is based on their perceptions of what reality is; therefore, the world as it is perceived is the world that is behaviorally important. Specifically, we shall define perception, discuss factors that influence perception, and introduce some unique problems that arise when we attempt to make judgments about others based on our perceptions.

WHAT IS PERCEPTION?

Perception can be defined as a process by which individuals organize and interpret their sensory impressions in order to give meaning to their environment. However, as we have noted, what one perceives can be substantially different from objective reality. It need not be, but there is often disagreement. For example, it is possible that all employees in a firm may view it as a great place to work—favorable working conditions, interesting job assignments, good pay, an understanding and responsible management—but, as most of us know, it is very unusual to find such consistencies. Any male who has attempted to get reinforcement from friends that a recently purchased necktie is good-looking understands that people see things differently.

FACTORS INFLUENCING PERCEPTION

How do we explain the fact that individuals may look at the same thing, yet perceive it differently? A number of factors operate to shape and sometimes distort perception. These factors can reside in the *perceiver,* in the object or *target* being perceived, or in the context of the *situation* in which the perception is made.

The Perceiver

When an individual looks at a target and attempts to interpret what he or she sees, that interpretation is heavily influenced by personal characteristics of the individual perceiver. Have you ever bought a new car and then suddenly noticed a large number of cars like yours on the road? It's unlikely that the number of such cars suddenly expanded. Rather, your own purchase has influenced your perception so that you are now more likely to notice them. This is an example how factors related to the perceiver influence what he or she perceives. Among the more relevant personal characteristics affecting perception are values and attitudes, personality, motives, interests, past experience, and expectations.

Values and Attitudes. In Chapter 3, we argued that values and attitudes influence behavior. They also impact on how you interpret your environment.

Sandy likes small classes because she enjoys asking a lot of questions of her teachers. Scott, on the other hand, prefers large lectures. He rarely asks questions and likes the anonymity that goes with being lost in a sea of bodies. On the first day of classes this term, Sandy and Scott find themselves walking into the university auditorium for their introductory course in psychology. They both recognize that they will be among some 800 students in this class. But given the different attitudes held by Sandy and Scott, it shouldn't surprise you to find that they interpret what they see differently. Sandy sulks, while Scott's smile does little to hide his relief in being able to blend unnoticed into the large auditorium. They both see the same thing, but they interpret it differently. A major reason is that they hold divergent attitudes concerning large classes.

Personality. An individual's personality, too, influences what he or she sees. Each person has his or her own style for organizing the environment. For instance, some people are high differentiators—they are readily able to notice differences and distinctions between objects. Other people minimize differences and tend to see their environment in relatively holistic terms.[2] Each person also has his or her own defense mechanisms. These mechanisms allow us to cope by protecting us from being deluged by external stimuli. Each of us has our own filtering system that filters in different perceptions of reality. An action by a mutual friend of ours might not threaten your self-concept, but it might mine. My defenses are up and, of course, are protecting me from perceiving things that would upset me. As a result, you and I are unlikely to perceive our friend's actions similarly.

Motives. Unsatisfied needs stimulate individuals and may exert a strong influence on their perceptions. This was dramatically demonstrated in research on hunger.[3] Individuals in the study had not eaten for varying numbers of hours. Some had eaten an hour earlier, while others had gone as long as sixteen hours without food. These subjects were shown blurred pictures, and the results indicated that the extent of hunger influenced the interpretation of the blurred pictures. Those who had not eaten for sixteen hours perceived the blurred images as pictures of food far more frequently than did those subjects who had eaten only a short time earlier.

This same phenomena has application in an organizational context, as well. It would not be surprising, for example, to find that a boss who is insecure perceives a subordinate's efforts to do an outstanding job as a threat to his own position. Personal insecurity can be transferred into the perception that others are out to "get your job," regardless of the intention of the subordinates. Likewise, people who are devious are prone to see others in the same context.

Interests. It should not surprise you that a plastic surgeon is more likely to notice an imperfect nose than is a plumber. The supervisor who has just been rep-

2. H. A. Witkin et al., *Psychological Differentiation* (New York: John Wiley, 1962).

3. David C. McClelland and J. W. Atkinson, "The Projective Expression of Needs: The Effect of Different Intensities of the Hunger Drive on Perception," *Journal of Psychology*, Vol. 25 (1948), pp. 205–22.

rimanded by her boss for the high level of lateness among her staff is more likely to notice lateness by an employee tomorrow than she was yesterday. If you are preoccupied with a personal problem, you may find it hard to be attentive in class. If you are hungry, you are more apt to notice that the person next to you in class is nibbling French fries than if you had just eaten.

The focus of one's attention appears to be influenced by his or her interests. Because our individual interests differ considerably, what one person notices in a situation can differ from what others perceive.

Past Experience. Just as interests narrow one's focus, so do one's past experiences. You perceive those things to which you can relate. However, in many instances, your past experiences will act to nullify an object's interest.

Those objects or events that have been experienced are less unusual or unique than new experiences. As a result, you are more likely to notice a machine that you have never observed before than a standard typewriter that is exactly like a thousand others you have previously seen. Similarly, you are more likely to notice the operations along an assembly line if this is the first time you have seen an assembly line. In the late 1960s and early 1970s, women and minorities in managerial positions were highly visible, if for no other reason than historically these positions were the province of white males. Now that these groups are more widely represented in the managerial ranks, we are less likely to be aware that a manager is female, black, or chicano.

Expectations. Expectations can distort your perceptions in that you will see what you expect to see. If you expect police officers to be authoritative, young people to be unambitious, personnel directors to "like people," or individuals holding public office to be "power hungry," you may perceive them this way regardless of their actual traits.

Support for the impact that expectations play in organizations was found in a study that manipulated the degree of supervision given to subordinates.[4] The experiment required a supervisor to ensure that the performance output of two subordinates was maintained at an acceptable level. In the first phase, the supervisor was given almost constant surveillance reports on the performance output of one subordinate, but only infrequent reports on the other. The experiment, therefore, required the supervisor to have greater trust in the loosely supervised subordinate. The final reports on the first phase found the two subordinates' output to be identical. In the second phase of the experiment, the supervisor was free to monitor either or both of the subjects whenever he wanted. The behavior of the supervisor in the second phase demonstrated that, in spite of the equal performance records in the first phase, the supervisor did not trust the two subordinates equally. Rather, he monitored more the subordinate who had been placed under high surveillance during the first phase. Prior expectations, based on previous levels of trust, resulted in different degrees of sur-

4. Lloyd H. Strickland, "Surveillance and Trust," *Journal of Personality*, Vol. 26 (1958), pp. 200–15.

veillance even though there was no difference in productivity to justify the different degrees of supervision.

The Target

Characteristics in the target that is being observed can affect what is perceived. Loud people are more likely to be noticed in a group than quiet ones. So, too, are extremely attractive or unattractive individuals. Motion, sounds, size, and other attributes of a target shape the way we see it.

Because targets are not looked at in isolation, the relationship of a target to its background influences perception, as does our tendency to group close things and similar things together.

Figure-Ground Perception. What we see is dependent on how we separate a figure from its general background.

What you see as you read this sentence is black letters on a white page. You do not see funny-shaped patches of black and white because you recognize these shapes and organize the blue shapes against the white background. Figure 5–1 dramatizes this effect. The figure on the left may at first look like a white vase. However, if white is taken as the background, we see two blue profiles. At first observation, the figure on the right appears to be some blue modular figures against a white background. Closer inspection will reveal the word "FLY" once the background is defined as blue.

Proximity. Objects that are close to each other will tend to be perceived together rather than separately. As a result of physical proximity or time proximity, we often put together objects or events that are unrelated. Employees in a particular department are seen as a group. If, in a department of four members, two suddenly resign, we tend to assume that their departures were related when, in

FIGURE 5–1   Figure-Ground Illustrations

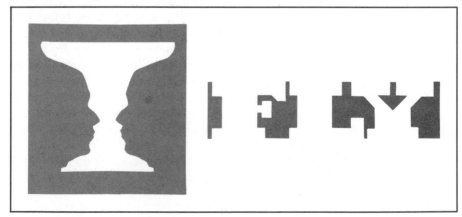

fact, they may be totally unrelated. Timing may also imply dependence when, for example, a new sales manager is assigned to a territory and, soon after, sales in that territory skyrocket. The assignment of the new sales manager and the increase in sales may not be related—the increase may be due to an introduction of a new product line or to one of many other reasons—but there is a tendency to perceive the two occurrences as related.

Similarity. Persons, objects, or events that are similar to each other also tend to be grouped together. The greater the similarity, the greater the probability that we will tend to perceive them as a common group. Women, blacks, or any other group that has clearly distinguishable characteristics in terms of features or color will tend to be perceived as alike in other, unrelated characteristics as well.

The Situation

The context in which we see objects or events is important. Elements in the surrounding environment influence our perceptions.

I may not notice a twenty-five-year-old female in an evening gown and heavy makeup at a nightclub on Saturday night. Yet that same woman, so attired for my Monday morning management class, would certainly catch my attention (and that of the rest of the class). Neither the perceiver nor the target changed between Saturday night and Monday morning, but the situation was different. Similarly, you are more likely to notice your employees goofing off if *your* boss from head office happens to be in town. Again, the situation effects your perception. The time at which an object or event is seen can influence attention, as can location, light, heat, or any number of situational factors.

PERSON PERCEPTION: MAKING JUDGMENTS ABOUT OTHERS

Thus far we have discussed perception in general terms. Objects, events, activities, and people were all used as examples of "targets" to be perceived. Now we want to narrow our focus to the perception of people. Given that we are concerned with organizational behavior, we should be specifically interested in how the general issues already presented, and additional issues unique to person perception, impact on OB.

Attribution Theory

Our perceptions of people differ from our perceptions of inanimate objects like desks, machines, or buildings because we make inferences about the actions of people that we don't make about inanimate objects. Nonliving objects are subject to the laws of nature, but they have no beliefs, motives, or intentions. People do. The result is that when we observe people, we attempt to develop explanations of why they behave in certain ways. Our perception and judgment of a person's actions, therefore, will be significantly influenced by the assumptions we make about the person's internal state.

Attribution theory has been proposed to develop explanations of how we judge people differently depending on what meaning we attribute to a given behavior.[5] Basically the theory suggests that when we observe an individual's behavior, we attempt to determine whether it was internally or externally caused. That determination, however, depends on three factors: (1) distinctiveness, (2) consensus, and (3) consistency. First, let's clarify the differences between internal and external causation, then elaborate on each of the three determining factors.

Internally caused behaviors are those that are believed to be under the personal control of the individual. Externally caused behavior is seen as resulting from outside causes; that is, the person is seen as forced into the behavior by the situation. If one of your employees were late for work, you might attribute his lateness to his partying into the wee hours of the morning and then oversleeping. This would be an internal interpretation. But if you attributed his arriving late to a major automobile accident that tied up traffic on the road that your employee regularly uses, then you are making an external attribution. As observers, we have a tendency to assume that others' behavior is internally controlled, while we tend to exaggerate the degree to which our own behavior is externally determined.[6] But this is a broad generalization. There still exists a considerable amount of deviation in attribution, depending on how we interpret the distinctiveness, consensus, and consistency of the actions.

Distinctiveness refers to how different the behavior that is being observed is from other behaviors the individual demonstrates. Is the employee who arrives late today also the source of complaints by co-workers for being a "goof-off"? What we want to know is if this behavior is unusual or not. If it is, the observer is likely to give the behavior an external attribution. If this action is not unique, it will probably be judged as internal.

If everyone who is faced with a similar situation responds in the same way, we can say the behavior shows *consensus*. Our late employee's behavior would meet this criterion if all employees who took the same route to work were also late. From an attribution perspective, if consensus is high you would be expected to give an external attribution to the employee's tardiness; whereas if other employees who took the same route made it to work on time, your conclusion as to causation would be internal.

Finally, an observer looks for *consistency* in a person's actions. Does the person respond the same way over time? Coming in ten minutes late for work is not perceived in the same way if for one employee it represents an unusual case (she hasn't been late for several months), while for another it is part of a routine

5. Harold H. Kelley, *Attribution in Social Interaction* (Morristown, N.J.: General Learning Press, 1971).

6. Walter R. Nord, ed., *Concepts and Controversy in Organizational Behavior,* 2nd ed. (Pacific Palisades, Calif.: Goodyear, 1976), p. 27.

pattern (she is regularly late two or three times a week). The more consistent the behavior, the more the observer is inclined to attribute it to internal causes.

The above explains what you have seen operating for years. All similar behaviors are not perceived similarly. We look at actions and judge them within their situational context. If you have a reputation as a good student yet blow one test in a course, the instructor is more likely to disregard the poor exam. Why? He or she will attribute the cause of this unusual performance to external conditions. It may not be your fault! But for the student who has a consistent record of being a poor performer, it is unlikely the teacher will ignore the low test score. Similarly, if everyone in class blew the test, the instructor may attribute the outcome to external causes (maybe the questions were poorly written, the room was too warm, students didn't have the prerequisites that he assumed) rather than to causes under the students' own control.

Attribution theory becomes extremely relevant when we consider how people judge others. We noted at the beginning of this section that when we observe people, in contrast to inanimate objects, we develop explanations for why they behave the way they do. These attributions, then, impact on how we interpret and judge the behavior we see. This will become clearer when we discuss how perceptions influence processes like the employment interview or performance appraisals.

Attribution theory is important because an individual's interpretations of actions will contribute to his or her behavioral responses to those actions and form a basis for the prediction of future events. We look for meaning in the behavior of others. Unfortunately, though, the reasons why people do what they do are very complex. Yet, because we still attempt to attribute causation, we end up basing our attribution on a simplification of what we see. Our ability to comprehend and store perceptual information is limited, so we reduce our observations into simple cause-and-effect sequences. As we shall demonstrate, this can bias how we judge others in organizations.

Specific Applications in Organizations

People in organizations are always judging each other. Managers must appraise their subordinates' performance. We evaluate how much effort our co-workers are putting into their jobs. When a new person joins a department, he or she is immediately "sized up" by the other department members. In many cases, these judgments have important consequences for the organization. Let us briefly look at a few of the more obvious applications.

Employment Interviews. A major input into who is hired or rejected is the employment interview. It's fair to say that few people are hired without an interview. But the evidence indicates that interviewers make perceptual judgments that are often inaccurate. Additionally, interrater agreement among interviewers is often poor; that is, different interviewers see different things in the same candidate and thus arrive at different conclusions about the applicant.

Interviewers generally draw early impressions that become very quickly entrenched. If negative information is exposed early in the interview it tends to be more heavily weighted than if that same information were conveyed later.[7] Studies indicate that most interviewers' decisions change very little after the first four or five minutes of the interview. As a result, information elicited early in the interview carries greater weight than does information elicited later, and a "good applicant" is probably characterized more by the absence of unfavorable characteristics than by the presence of favorable characteristics.

Importantly, who you think is a good candidate and who I think is one may differ markedly. Because interviews usually have so little consistent structure and interviewers vary in terms of what they consider a good candidate, judgments of the same candidate can vary widely. If the employment interview is an important input into the hiring decision, and it usually is, you should recognize that perceptual factors influence who is hired and eventually the quality of an organization's labor force.

Performance Appraisals. Although the impact of performance evaluations on behavior will be discussed fully in Chapter 16, it should be pointed out here that an employee's performance appraisal is very much dependent on the perceptual process. An employee's future is closely tied to his or her appraisal—promotions, raises, and continuation of employment are among the most obvious outcomes. The performances appraisal represents an assessment of an employee's work. While this can be objective (e.g., a salesperson is appraised on how many dollars of sales she generates in her territory), most jobs are evaluated in subjective terms. Subjective measures are easier to implement, they provide managers with greater discretion, and many jobs do not readily lend themselves to objective measures. Subjective measures are, by definition, judgmental. The evaluator forms a general impression of an employee's work. To the degree that managers use subjective measures in appraising employees, what the evaluator perceives to be "good" or "bad" employee characteristics/ behaviors will significantly influence the appraisal outcome.

Assessing Level of Effort. An individual's future in an organization is usually not dependent on performance alone. In many organizations, the level of an employee's effort is given high importance. Just as teachers frequently consider how hard you try in a course as well as how you perform on examinations, so often do managers. And assessment of an individual's effort is a subjective judgment susceptible to perceptual distortions and bias. If it is true, as some claim, that "more workers are fired for poor attitudes and lack of discipline than for lack of ability,"[8] then appraisal of an employee's effort may be a primary influence on his or her future in the organization.

7. See, for example, Edward C. Webster, *Decision Making in the Employment Interview* (Montreal: Industrial Relations Center, McGill University, 1964).

8. David Kipnis, *The Powerholders* (Chicago: University of Chicago Press, 1976).

Assessing Loyalty. Another important judgment that managers make about employees is whether they are loyal to the organization. Few organizations appreciate employees, especially those in the managerial ranks, bad-mouthing the firm. Further, in some organizations, if the word gets around that an employee is looking at other employment opportunities outside the firm, that employee may be labeled as disloyal, cutting off all future advancement opportunities. The issue is not whether organizations are right in demanding loyalty, but that many *do* and that assessment of an employee's loyalty or commitment is highly judgmental. What is perceived as loyalty by one decision maker may be seen as excessive conformity by another. An employee who questions a top management decision may be seen as disloyal by some, yet caring and concerned by others. When evaluating a person's attitude, which loyalty assessment is, we must recognize that we are again involved with person perception.

Frequently Used Shortcuts in Judging Others

One last topic we should discuss is the fact that we use a number of shortcuts when we judge others. Perceiving and interpreting what others do is burdensome. As a result, individuals develop techniques for making the task more manageable. These techniques are frequently valuable—they allow us to make accurate perceptions rapidly and provide valid data for making predictions. However, they are not foolproof. They can and do get us into trouble. An understanding of these shortcuts can be helpful toward recognizing when they can result in significant distortions.

Selectivity. Any characteristic that makes a person, object, or event stand out will increase the probability that it will be perceived. Why? Because it is impossible for us to assimilate everything we see—only certain stimuli can be taken in. This explains why you're more likely to notice cars like your own or why some people may be reprimanded by their boss for doing something that when done by another employee goes unnoticed. Since we can't observe everything going on about us, we engage in selective perception. A classic example shows how vested interests can significantly influence what problems we see.

Dearborn and Simon[9] performed a perceptual study in which twenty-three business executives read a comprehensive case describing the organization and activities of a steel company. Six of the twenty-three executives were in the sales function, five in production, four in accounting, and eight in miscellaneous functions. Each manager was asked to write down the most important problem he found in the case. Eighty-three percent of the sales executives rated sales important, while only 29 percent of the others did so. This, along with other results of the study, led the researchers to conclude that the participants perceived aspects in a situation that related specifically to the activities and goals of

9. DeWitt C. Dearborn and Herbert A. Simon, "Selective Perception: A Note on the Departmental Identifications of Executives," *Sociometry*, June 1958, pp. 140–44.

the unit to which they were attached. A group's perception of organizational activities is selectively altered to align with the vested interest they represent. In other words, where the stimuli are ambiguous, as in the steel company case, perception tends to be influenced more by an individual's base of interpretation (i.e., attitudes, interests, and background) than by the stimulus itself.

But how does selectivity work as a shortcut in judging other people? Simply, since we cannot assimilate all that we observe, we take in bits and pieces. But these bits and pieces are not chosen randomly; rather, they are selectively chosen depending on the interests, background, experience, and attitudes of the observer. Selective perception allows us to "speed read" others, but not without the risk of drawing an inaccurate picture. Because we see what we want to see, we can draw unwarranted conclusions from an ambiguous situation. If there is a rumor going around the office that your company's sales are down and that large layoffs may be coming, a routine visit by a senior executive from headquarters might be interpreted as the first step in management's identification of people to be fired, when in reality such an action may be the farthest thing from the mind of the senior executive.

Assumed Similarity. It is easy to judge others if we assume they are similar to us. Sometimes called the "like me" effect, assumed similarity means, for instance, that if you want challenge and responsibility in your job, you assume that others want the same. This assumption clouds judgments made of others.

If a person evaluates another's personality as more similar to himself than the other actually is, he distorts the other's personality to make it more like his own. When this shortcut is extensively used by a person, his observations and appraisals of others will correspond more to his own personality (as he sees it) than to the other's personality (as the other sees it).

What this means in practice is that among people who assume similarity, their perception of others is influenced more by what the observer is like than by what the person being observed is like. When observing others who actually are like them, these observers are quite accurate—not because they are more perceptive but only because they always judge people as being similar to themselves, so when they finally find one who is, they are naturally correct.

Stereotyping. When we judge someone on the basis of our perception of the group to which he or she belongs, we are using the shortcut called stereotyping. William Faulkner engaged in stereotyping in his reported conversation with Ernest Hemingway, when he said, "The rich are different from you and me." Hemingway's reply, "Yes, they have more money," indicated that other than the required difference (you need money to be rich), he refused to stereotype or generalize characteristics about people based on their wealth.

Generalizations, of course, are not without their advantages. It makes assimilating easier since it permits us to maintain consistency. It is less difficult to deal with an unmanageable number of stimuli if we use stereotypes. But the problem occurs when we inaccurately stereotype. All accountants are *not* quiet and introspective, in the same way that all salespeople are *not* aggressive and outgoing.

We are all guilty of stereotyping. If you come into your political science class on the first day to find your instructor is a female, wearing waist-length hair with a colorful headband, a tie-dyed blouse, a calf-length jean skirt, and boots, do you stereotype? If you consider such attire to be consistent with one who holds liberal political beliefs, could you not misinterpret some of her lectures? In spite of the instructor's efforts to demonstrate a neutral political stance, if you originally thought her to hold strong leftist views, you might continue to see her lectures philosophically slanted to the left only because that is what you expected from someone who dresses as she does.

In an organizational context, we frequently hear comments that represent stereotyped representations of certain groups: "Married people are more stable employees;" "Managers don't give a damn about their people, only getting the work out;" or "Union people expect something for nothing." Clearly, these phrases represent stereotypes, but if people expect these perceptions, that is what they will see, whether it represents reality or not.

Obviously, one of the problems of stereotypes is that they are so widespread, in spite of the fact that they may not contain a shred of truth, or may be irrelevant. Their being widespread may only mean that many people are making the same, inaccurate perception based on a false premise about a group. The movement of blacks and women into managerial positions has been a major source of perceptual distortion. As we noted previously, these positions were historically the sole province of white males. If white male managers expect women to be unaggressive and unable to make tough decisions or career commitments, or blacks to be lazy and irresponsible—all stereotypes that have no founding in fact—we can expect any activity on the part of women or blacks that is not aggressive, tough, ambitious, or responsible to be perceived unfavorably. Recent research finds that men view women as too emotional and unreliable to be effective managers. These perceptions are held in spite of the evidence—women are no more emotional than men on the job and, when age and type of job are held constant, male-female turnover rates are about the same.[10] Such stereotypes result in reduced promotion opportunities for women in organizations and suboptimize the organization's effectiveness when they prevent the selection of the most qualified applicant.

Halo Effect. When we draw a general impression about an individual based on a single characteristic like intelligence, sociability, or appearance, a halo effect is operating. This phenomenon frequently occurs when students appraise their classroom instructor. Students may isolate a single trait, such as enthusiasm, and

10. Francine E. Gordon and Myra H. Strober, *Bringing Women into Management* (New York: McGraw-Hill, 1975), p. 159.

allow their entire evaluation to be tainted by how they judge the instructor on this one trait. Thus, an instructor may be quiet, assured, knowledgeable, and highly qualified, but if his style lacks zeal, he will be rated lower on a number of other characteristics.

The reality of the halo effect was confirmed in a classic study where subjects were given a list of traits like intelligent, skillful, practical, industrious, determined, and warm and asked to evaluate the person to whom these traits applied.[11] Based on these traits, the person was judged to be wise, humorous, popular, and imaginative. When the same list was modified to substitute cold for warm in the trait list, a completely different set of perceptions was obtained. Clearly, the subjects were allowing a single trait to influence their overall impression of the person being judged.

The propensity for the halo effect to operate is not random. Research suggests that it is likely to be most extreme when the traits to be perceived are ambiguous or unclear in behavioral terms, when the traits have moral overtones, and when the perceiver is judging traits with which he or she has had limited experience.[12]

In organizations, the halo effect is important in understanding an individual's behavior, particularly when judgment and evaluation must be made. It is not unusual for the halo effect to occur in selection interviews or at a performance appraisal time. A stunning blonde female candidate for a secretarial position may be perceived by a male interviewer as an intelligent individual with high secretarial skills, when in fact she may be intellectually dull and poorly skilled in dictation and typing. What has happened is that a single trait—beauty—has overridden other characteristics in the interviewer's general perception about the individual. The halo effect can have a similarly distorting impact on performance evaluation, causing the full appraisal to be biased by a single trait.

IMPLICATIONS FOR PERFORMANCE AND SATISFACTION

This chapter has pointed out many ways in which perceptions can be distorted. We have noted that perception is dependent not only upon characteristics of the target being observed, but also on characteristics of the perceiver and the situation. These three factors, then, combine to structure the way we perceive and evaluate the people, events, and objects in the environment.

11. Solomon E. Asch, "Forming Impressions of Personality," *Journal of Abnormal and Social Psychology,* July 1946, pp. 258–90.

12. Jerome S. Bruner and Renato Tagiuri, "The Perception of People," in *Handbook of Social Psychology,* ed. E. Lindzey (Cambridge, Mass.: Addison-Wesley, 1954), p. 641.

Experiencing the environment is an active process in which people try to make sense out of their environment. In this active process, individuals selectively notice different aspects of the environment, appraise what they see in terms of their own experience, and evaluate what they experience in terms of their needs and values. Since people's needs and past experiences often differ markedly, so do their perceptions of the environment.[13]

Of course, our concern is more than merely describing the phenomenon of perception and making the point that what you perceive may not at all be "reality." Our concern is directed to perception as it impacts on an individual's behavior and attitudes.

Individuals behave in a given way or form certain attitudes based not on the way their external environment actually is, but rather on what they see or believe it to be. Because individuals act on their interpretations of reality rather than reality itself, it is clear that perception must be a critical determinant of our dependent variables.

An organization may spend millions of dollars to create a pleasant work environment for its employees. However, in spite of these expenditures, if an employee believes her job is lousy, she will behave accordingly. It is her perception of a situation that becomes the basis on which she behaves. The employee who perceives her supervisor as a hurdle-reducer and an aide to help her do a better job and the employee who sees the same supervisor as "big brother, closely monitoring every motion, to ensure that I keep working" will differ in their behavioral responses to their supervisor. The difference has nothing to do with the reality of the supervisor's role; the difference in behavior is due to different perceptions.

The process from reality and observation to behavioral and attitudinal outputs is summarized in Figure 5–2. Of course, the actual process happens so fast that we do not experience each of these steps. They are presented rather to allow the reader to conceptualize the process. Figure 5–2 explains why it is unlikely that two individuals will perceive "reality" in exactly the same way. It also explains that what may produce higher productivity, increased satisfaction, and higher work attendance in one individual may result in exactly the opposite outcomes for another.

Productivity

The evidence suggests that what individuals *perceive* from their work situation will influence their productivity more than will the situation itself. Whether a job is actually interesting or challenging is irrelevant. Whether a manager successfully plans and organizes the work of his subordinates and actually helps them to

13. Edward E. Lawler III and John Grant Rhode, *Information and Control in Organizations* (Pacific Palisades, Calif.: Goodyear, 1976), p. 26.

FIGURE 5–2 How Perceptions Affect Attitudes and Behavior

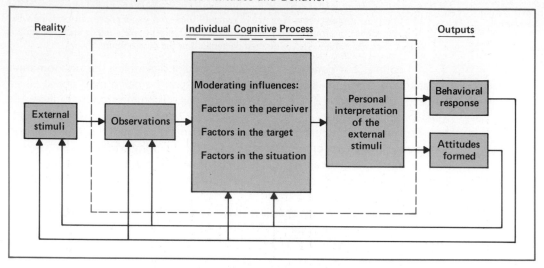

more efficiently and effectively structure their work is far less important than how his subordinates perceive his efforts. Similarly, issues like fair pay for work performed, the validity of performance appraisals, and the adequacy of the work conditions are not judged by employees in a way that assures common perceptions, nor can we be assured that individuals will interpret conditions about their job in a favorable light. Therefore, to be able to influence productivity, it is necessary to assess how workers perceive their jobs.

It is unacceptable for a sales manager to argue that "John should be selling far more of our products in his territory. His territory is a gold mine. It has unlimited potential." When John is interviewed, we find that he believes he is getting as much as possible out of his territory. Whether the salesman is right or wrong is irrelevant. The fact is that he *perceives it to be right.* If the manager hopes to improve sales in John's territory, he must first succeed in changing John's perceptions.

Absenteeism and Turnover

Like productivity, absence and turnover behavior are reactions to the individual's perceptions. Dissatisfaction with work conditions or the belief that there is a lack of promotion opportunities in the organization are judgments based on attempts to make some meaning out of one's job. Since there can be no such thing as a "bad job," only the perception that the job is bad, managers must spend time to understand how each individual interprets reality and, where there is a significant difference between what is seen and what exists, try to eliminate the distortions. Failure to deal with the differences when individuals perceive the job in negative terms will result in increased absenteeism and turnover.

Job Satisfaction

Job satisfaction is a highly subjective, general impression of the benefits that derive from the job. Clearly, this variable is critically linked to perception. If job satisfaction is to be improved, the worker's perception of the job's characteristics, supervision, and the organization as a whole must be positive.

Summary

In attempting to explain and predict behavior, reality is secondary to what is perceived. People's responses are based on their perceptions. It would be nice if they perceived reality clearly, but we have demonstrated that there are a number of influences at work that create distortions and may result in reduced levels of performance and satisfaction.

A hospital director once remarked that she was faced with a large exodus of her best nurses. When asked why, she said, "They all think they're underpaid." When asked if this was the case, she exclaimed, "Absolutely not! We have just completed a thorough area survey, and our salaries are in the upper quartile. Their complaints are unjustified. They're quitting in droves for a reason that is completely erroneous."

The director was confusing reality with perceptions. The departure of competent nurses because they viewed the hospital's salaries as too low was apparently based on a misperception. The director was right that salaries were competitive, yet the nurses are just as gone as if the hospital's salaries *were low*. The nurses' behavior was based on their *perception* of reality.

The material in this chapter would suggest that individuals be continually surveyed—through discussion, written questionnaires, or both—to ensure that employee attitudes and misperceptions are identified. Once identified, communication efforts can be made to correct them. If this feedback is not received, individuals may develop unfavorable attitudes toward their job and the organization, resulting in increased absenteeism, higher turnover, and possibly lower productivity. Further, it would suggest that managers understand how the perceptual process impacts on many key decisions that affect employees: hiring, performance appraisals, assessment of effort and loyalty, and attributing causes to specific behaviors. Perceptual errors can lead to lower employee performance, low morale, and an overall reduction in the organization's effectiveness. Managers should be well advised to pay particular attention to the shortcuts they use in judging others. These shortcuts can lead to distortions which, in turn, can lead to poor judgments and poor decisions.

FOR DISCUSSION

1. Define perception.

2. "The fact that you and I agree on what we see suggests we have similar backgrounds and experiences." Do you agree or disagree? Discuss.

3. What is attribution theory? What are its implications for explaining organizational behavior?

4. How might perceptual factors be involved when an employee receives a poor performance appraisal?

5. How does selectivity affect perception? Give an example of how selectivity can create perceptual distortion.

6. What is stereotyping? Give an example of how stereotyping can create perceptual distortion.

7. Give some positive results from using shortcuts when judging others.

8. What is the relationship between what you see and how you behave? What is the relationship between reality and how you behave?

FOR FURTHER READING

BARTLEY, S., *Perception in Everyday Life.* New York: Harper & Row, 1972. A nontechnical book that considers the operation of the perceptual systems in daily life.

KELLEY, H. H., and J. L. MICHELA. "Attribution Theory and Research" in *Annual Review of Psychology,* Vol. 31, ed. M. R. Rosenzweig and L. W. Porter, pp. 457–50. Palo Alto, Cal.: Annual Reviews, Inc., 1980. Presents several attribution "theories," illustrating both antecedents and consequences of attributions for behavior.

KEY, W. B. *Subliminal Seduction.* Englewood Cliffs, N.J.: Prentice-Hall, 1973. Argues that advertisers manipulate the media with subliminal sexual messages. Includes some eye-opening illustrations of messages that one would rarely be aware of perceiving.

MCCAULEY, C., C. L. STITT, and M. SEGAL, "Stereotyping: From Prejudice to Prediction," *Psychological Bulletin,* January 1980, pp. 195–208. Presents counterpoints to the common arguments made against stereotypes.

WEBBER, R. A., "Perceptions of Interactions between Superiors and Subordinates," *Human Relations,* June 1970, pp. 235–48. After the perceptions of thirty-four superior-subordinate pairs were analyzed, there was found to be consistent distortions in the perceptions of verbal interaction.

ZALKIND, S., and T. W. COSTELLO. "Perception: Some Recent Research and Implications for Administration," *Administrative Science Quarterly,* September 1962, pp. 218–35. Reviews the perceptual process and suggests some implications for administrative decisions and actions.

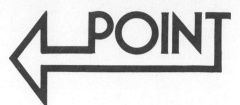

Training can improve perceptual accuracy

Adapted and edited from Bernard M. Bass, Wayne F. Cascio, J. Westbrook McPherson and Harold Tragash, "PROSPER—Training and Research for Increasing Awareness of Affirmative Action in Race Relations," Academy of Management Journal, *September 1976, pp. 353–69. With permission.*

Racially integrating the firm involves a variety of coordinated affirmative action efforts by its sponsors and its top management as well as its members at lower levels. The organization's sponsors and its top management must be convinced that for social, business, political, moral, and/or legal reasons, affirmative action is to be implemented. Policies need to be formulated which will encourage the effort. These include more objective, open recruiting, selection, and promotion policies. At all levels, managers and staff personnel need to look at their own current attitudes and behavior to examine the impediments they knowingly or unknowingly create to bar the intake and upward mobility of women, blacks, and other protected groups.

Greater realism coupled with heightened awareness may promote more effective problem solving. In turn, this should result in more effective utilization of minority group members.

This concern prompted the Xerox Corporation to sponsor the development of PROSPER—a self-guided training activity that includes before and after measurement of awareness as well as a method for stimulating awareness of racial issues.

PROSPER was intended to increase the awareness of white managers to their racial biases and how those beliefs manifest themselves in their on-the-job relationships with blacks. Furthermore, the program was designed to help white managers become sensitive to the racial stereotypes in American institutions, including industry. It was assumed that as managers become more aware of key factors that generate racial bias they would be better able to understand their own feelings and to improve their effectiveness in dealing with minorities—particularly blacks.

First the domain and dimensions of the relevant attitudes had to be determined. Several large surveys were conducted, factor analyzed, and subsequently modified in a series of trials and refactorings, finally yielding five factors of consequence: (1) the system is biased; (2) implementation of affirmative action policies is limited; (3) black employees are competent; (4) black employees need real inclusion; and (5) black employees need to build self-esteem. It was felt that these five factors would adequately profile a trainee's awareness and could serve as building blocks for the scenario and role play to follow.

The self-guided program was then constructed around the five awareness factors. The program developed was a four-hour learning experience to increase managers' awareness of racially discriminating beliefs that reduce the effective utilization of black employees. Successive pilot programs were run to refine the learning experience, to minimize cost and maximize standardization of the change approach. The entire program PROS-

PER was reduced to a single, simple work booklet, one per participant.

The exercise PROSPER was created around these five factors. After establishing an attitudinal baseline, PROSPER provided a set of in-basket memos, a role-play, and messages dealing with the five factors. Participants then retook the awareness questionnaire to see what changes, if any, had occurred. The factors provided a meaningful structure for managers to talk about their understanding and feeling about black employees.

Results with over two thousand participants show that there was a significant increase in awareness on all five factors from beginning to end of PROSPER. Merely showing up at the start of the PROSPER program was associated with a more aware position on the five factors in contrast to a group that had not yet been enrolled. Awareness was greater still at the end of PROSPER. Three to five months afterwards, awareness did decline in a sample selected for follow-up, but only about half-way back to where the larger sample was at the beginning of the administration of PROSPER.

Change in awareness, of course, does not necessarily mean behavior change. Whether a change will be accompanied by a change in behavior will depend upon the extent the organization and immediate social situation provide supports and inducements for such behavioral change, whether opportunities are available to make such changes, and whether the individual whose awareness has changed has the capability to exhibit the new behavior.

COUNTER POINT

CROW

Training may reduce perceptual accuracy

Adapted and edited from W. J. Crow, "The Effect of Training Upon Accuracy and Variability in Interpersonal Perception," Journal of Abnormal and Social Psychology, *September 1957, pp. 355–59. Copyright © 1957 by the American Psychological Association. Reprinted by permission.*

One purpose of many training programs in clinical, counseling, and personnel psychology is to increase the accuracy of the trainee's perceptions of others. The ability to "understand others" or to have "clinical intuition" is considered a basic requirement for the good practitioner. It has been difficult to evaluate the success of such training, however, because until recently there has been no way to measure, by objective tests, the subtle and complex psychological variables that are presumably detected by the practitioner.

Recent methodological improvements in the measurement of interpersonal perceptiveness have made it possible to measure the accuracy of clinical judgment in a more objective way. It is now customary to ask a person (the object) to fill out a personality questionnaire and then ask the trainee (the subject) to fill out the identical questionnaire just as he believed the object has filled it out. The measure of the subject's accuracy is the degree of correspondence between the object's actual responses and those which the subject estimated that the object had made.

Early studies using this technique for measuring interpersonal perception focused primarily upon accuracy, but attention has been called recently to the importance of other components of the interpersonal-perception situation. Cronbach has advanced a hypothesis for the relationship between accuracy and one of these components—the amount of variability in the subjects' estimations: If the subject increases the variability of his judgments from one time to another and his ability to make accurate judgments does not increase correspondingly, then he will make greater errors the second time than the first. It also follows that whenever a judgmental task is very difficult or the objects are very low in ability, subjects with little variability in their estimations will make small errors, and subjects with high variability will make large errors. Stated otherwise, accuracy and variability will be negatively correlated when the task is difficult or the subject is very inaccurate.

The purpose of the study herein reported was twofold: (a) to investigate the effects of a training program upon interpersonal perception, and (b) to test the hypothesis of the relationship between accuracy and variability in estimation.

To accomplish these purposes, interpersonal perception measures were administered at the beginning, during, and after the senior year to a class of medical students who were divided into experimental and control groups. The experimental group was instructed in physician-patient relationships and was provided with the opportunity to establish such relationships through more prolonged contact with patients than was possible for the control group. It was expected (a) that the students in the experimental group would become more accurate in interpersonal perception than students in the control group, and (b) that variability in estimation would be negatively related to accuracy of judgment.

Contrary to expectation, the group which received more training in interpersonal relations (the experimental group) did not improve in accuracy of interpersonal perception more than did the group without such special training (control group). In fact, the results support the opposite conclusion: that, as a result of their special training, the experimental group became less accurate than the control group.

The experimental group increased the variability in their estimations significantly more than did the control group. The experimental group also assumed less agreement between the way Ss [Subjects] would rate themselves and the way they "really were." These results, in conjunction with the fact that the experimental group increased in accuracy, support Cronbach's hypothesis that, if an S increases his differentiation without a corresponding increase in ability, he will make greater errors.

These results indicate that training programs devoted to increasing accuracy of interpersonal perception (as in medical education and in the training of teachers, clinical psychologists, and similar specialists) run the risk of decreasing accuracy when they increase the trainees' responsiveness to individual differences. Since very little is known about how to train people to make more accurate judgments about others, training programs frequently utilize a procedure of "exposure" and little else. The belief that placing the trainee in a position to observe others and to make judgments will produce desirable results is challenged by these findings. Such experience may lead the trainee to differentiate among people far beyond his capacity to do so accurately. In the absence of dependable measures of his accuracy, the trainee lacks knowledge of his errors and may continue inappropriate overdifferentiation long after the training has ceased.

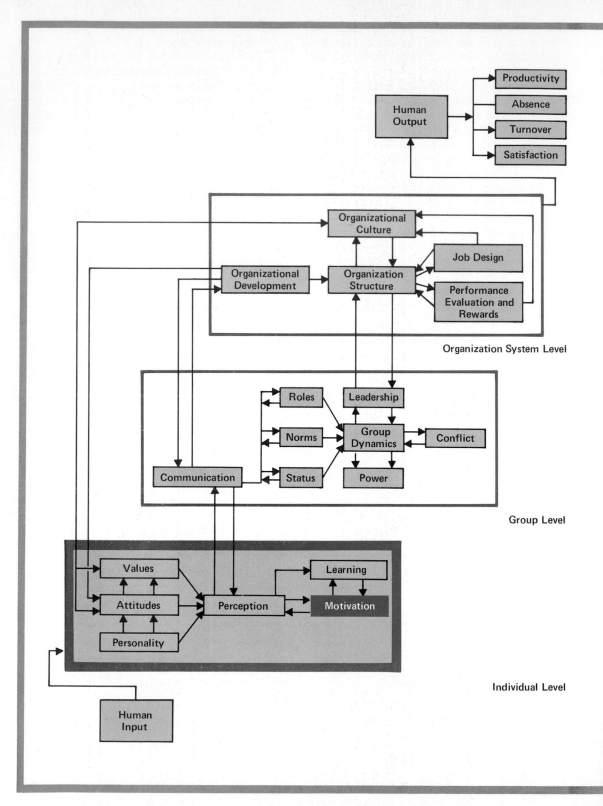

CHAPTER 6
Motivation

AFTER STUDYING THIS CHAPTER, YOU SHOULD BE ABLE TO—

Define and explain the following key terms and concepts:

Affiliation need
Cognitive evaluation theory
Equity theory
ERG theory
Expectancy theory
Extrinsic motivators
Goal-setting theory
Hierarchy of needs theory
Higher-order needs

Intrinsic motivators
Lower-order needs
Motivation
Motivation-hygiene theory
Needs
Power need
Reinforcement theory
Self-actualization

Understand:

The motivation process
The types of needs that individuals have
The priority of different needs
The difference between intrinsic and extrinsic motivators
The impact from overrewarding and underrewarding employees
The types of goals that increase performance
How reinforcers effect behavior
The key relationships in expectancy theory

> Set me anything to do as a task, and it is inconceivable the desire I
> have to do something else.
>
> —GEORGE BERNARD SHAW

In the study of individual behavior, there is probably no concept more important than motivation. A cursory look at any organization quickly suggests that some people work harder than others. An individual with outstanding abilities may consistenly be outperformed by someone with obviously inferior talents. Why do people exert different levels of effort in different activities? Why do some people appear to be "highly motivated," while others are not? These are questions we shall attempt to answer in this chapter.

WHAT IS MOTIVATION?

We might define motivation in terms of some outward behavior. People who are "motivated" exert a greater effort to perform than those who are "not motivated." However, such a definition is relative and tells us little. A more descriptive but less substantive definition would say motivation is the willingness to do something, and is conditioned by this action's ability to satisfy some need for the individual. A need, in our terminology, means some internal state that makes certain outcomes appear attractive. This motivation process can be seen in Figure 6–1.

An unsatisfied need creates tension which stimulates drives within the individual. These drives generate a search behavior to find particular goals that, if attained, will satisfy the need and lead to the reduction of tension.

Motivated employees are in a state of tension. In order to relieve this tension, they engage in activity. The greater the tension, the more activity will be needed to bring about relief. Therefore, when we see people working hard at some activity, we can conclude that they are driven by a desire to achieve some goal that they perceive as having value to them.

Figure 6–1 The Motivation Process

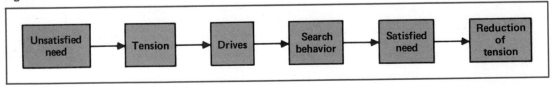

INDIVIDUAL NEEDS:
THE FOUNDATION OF MOTIVATION

Our description of the motivation process is built on the foundation of an unsatisfied need. Although needs are infrequently viewed as self-serving desires, this is in fact what they are. Therefore, an interesting way to begin our look at motivation is by looking at human beings as behaving in ways that they perceive to be in their self-interest.

Self-Interest:
The Ultimate Motivating Force

Every person, consciously or unconsciously, asks himself, "What's in it for me?" before engaging in any form of behavior. The principle that individuals are motivated by their personal self-interest underlies almost every economic theory and is contained, explicitly or implicitly, in all theories of motivation. Whether it is called self-serving behavior, need satisfaction, hedonism, or whatever, the underlying concept is the same—individuals act so as to maximize their own self-interest.

This is not to say that other people's feelings do not impinge on how we view our self-interest. Nor does it exclude the fact that many people's self-interest is to help others. St. Francis of Assisi, Joan of Arc, Albert Schweitzer, Florence Nightingale, and even the kamikaze pilots in World War II pursued their self-interest through helping others or playing out martyr roles. In each case, these individuals *believed* their behavior was in their own best interest. Whether it actually was, of course, is irrelevant—the key point is that they believed it was! People may act in ways that appear irrational—the martyr who sets himself aflame or the employee who turns in her resignation in the heat of an argument. However, their behavior is totally rational and consistent with what they believe is, at the time, in their best interest. Similarly, doing something for someone else may appear to be unselfish, but to the individual engaging in the behavior, the act satisfies some need or it would not be engaged in. While self-interest can take many forms, we can state that in most cases it takes the form of putting our personal well-being above the well-being of others.

Figure 6–2

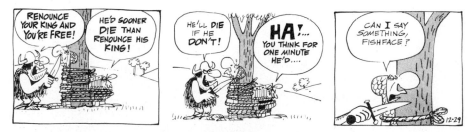

Source: By permission of Johnny Hart and Field Enterprises, Inc.

You may find the above description of self-interest underlying everyone's behavior as repulsive. Certainly, there is a strong negative connotation to the thesis. If behavior is founded on self-interest, why is it then that the concept seems so contemptible? The answer is that the lay person tends to separate self-directed behavior from other-directed behavior. When individuals directly act in their self-interest, we label the behavior as "selfish" and attribute a socially undesirable flavor to the behavior. On the other hand, as we noted above, helping someone else, being kind or thoughtful to others, working for a "cause," or trying to please another person are also examples of self-serving behavior. However, instead of being self-directed, they are other-directed. Other-directed behavior is also self-serving—self-interest is fostered through doing things for others. To illustrate, assume you enjoy having friends. We can say you have a need for affiliation. You also know that others will seek out your companionship more readily if you are friendly and pleasant to be around. So what do you do? You act other-directed! You are friendly to others and thoughtful toward their needs. Importantly, such behavior is *not* unselfish. Social people, for example, just tend to be more other-directed, since they see this as a way to achieve the ends they value. Other-directed people are not any less self-serving, but they do appear to be less selfish.

In summary, the reason the self-interest principle is often difficult for us to accept is that we tend to attribute self-interest only to behavior that is self-directed and to assume that other-directed is not self-serving; that helping others or being courteous, friendly, and agreeable to others is an end in itself. It is not! It only acts to serve some need that requires others to satisfy it.

How Many Needs Are There?

If you observed an individual's behavior for a reasonable period of time and listed reasons for his or her actions, you would be formulating a list of needs. From your efforts you might observe the need for safety, approval, independence and autonomy, achievement, respect and admiration, affection, affiliation, or basic physiological fulfillment like hunger or thirst.

Obviously, the list could be easily expanded. However, as we expanded the list we would find an increase in overlapping needs. Toward reducing ambiguity and eliminating interdependent concepts, psychologists have proposed several classification schemes.

Maslow's Hierarchy of Needs

The most widely accepted need classification scheme was proposed by Abraham Maslow over a quarter of a century ago.[1] His list of needs is conveniently short, yet covers most of the dimensions that psychologists have found to be important.

1. Abraham Maslow, *Motivation and Personality* (New York: Harper & Row, 1954).

Maslow hypothesized that within every human being there exists a hierarchy of five needs. These needs are:

1. *Physiological*—includes hunger, thirst, shelter, sex, and other bodily needs
2. *Safety*—includes security and protection from physical and emotional harm
3. *Love*—includes affection, belongingness, acceptance, and friendship
4. *Esteem*—includes internal esteem factors such as self-respect, autonomy, and achievement; and external esteem factors such as status, recognition, and attention
5. *Self-actualization*—the drive to become what one is capable of becoming; includes growth, achieving one's potential, and self-fulfillment

As each of these needs becomes substantially satisfied, the next need becomes dominant. In terms of Figure 6–3, the individual moves up the hierarchy. From the standpoint of motivation, the theory would say that although no need is ever fully gratified, a substantially satisfied need no longer motivates.

Maslow separated the five needs into higher and lower levels. Physiological and safety needs were described as lower-order, and love, esteem, and self-actualization as higher-order needs. The differentiation between the two orders

Figure 6–3 Maslow's Hierarchy of Needs

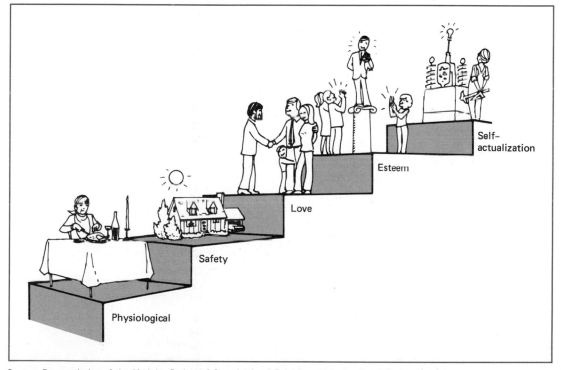

Source: By permission of the Modular Project of Organizational Behavior and Instructional Communications Centre. McGill University, Montreal, Canada

was made on the premise that higher-order needs are satisfied internally to the person, whereas lower-order needs are predominantly satisfied externally (by such things as money wages, union contracts, and tenure). In fact, the natural conclusion to be drawn from Maslow's classification is that in times of economic plenty, which has generally described the North American society since the mid-1940s, almost all permanently employed workers have had their lower-order needs substantially met.

Maslow's need theory has received wide recognition, particularly among practicing managers. This can be attributed to the theory's intuitive logic and ease of understanding. Unfortunately, however, research does not generally validate the theory. Maslow provided no empirical substantiation, and several studies that sought to validate the theory found no support.[2]

Old theories, especially ones that are intuitively logical, apparently die hard. One researcher reviewed the evidence and concluded that "although of great societal popularity, need hierarchy as a theory continues to receive little empirical support."[3] Further, the researcher stated that the "available research should certainly generate a reluctance to accept unconditionally the implication of Maslow's hierarchy."[4] Another review came to the same conclusion.[5] Little support was found for the prediction that need structures are organized along the dimensions proposed by Maslow; the prediction of a negative relationship between the level of need gratification and the activation of that need; or the prediction of a positive relationship between the level of need gratification and the activation level of the next higher need. But remember that there is a difference between finding "insufficient evidence" for a theory and labeling it "invalid." "It is clear that the available research does not support the Maslow theory to any significant degree. This does not imply that the theory is wrong, merely that it has not been supported."[6]

ERG Theory

Because of the unsuccessful efforts to support Maslow's belief that a higher need becomes an operative motivator only after the previous lower need is sat-

2. See for example, Edward E. Lawler III and J. Lloyd Suttle, "A Causal Correlational Test of the Need Hierarchy Concept," *Organizational Behavior and Human Performance,* April 1972, pp. 265–87; and Douglas T. Hall and Khalil E. Nongaim, "An Examination of Maslow's Need Hierarchy in an Organizational Setting," *Organizational Behavior and Human Performance,* February 1968, pp. 12–35.

3. Abraham K. Korman, Jeffrey H. Greenhaus, and Irwin J. Badin, "Personnel Attitudes and Motivation," in *Annual Review of Psychology,* ed. Mark R. Rosenzweig and Lyman W. Porter (Palo Alto, Calif.: Annual Reviews, 1977), p. 178.

4. Ibid. p. 179.

5. M. A. Wahba and L. G. Bridwell, "Maslow Reconsidered: A Review of Research on the Need Hierarchy Theory," *Organizational Behavior and Human Performance,* Vol. 15 (1976), pp. 212–40.

6. John B. Miner, *Theories of Organizational Behavior* (Hinsdale, Ill.: Dryden Press, 1980), p. 41.

isfied, attempts have been made to revise Maslow's thesis in order to align it more closely with the empirical research. One such approach is a modified hierarchy of three core needs proposed by Clayton Alderfer.[7]

Alderfer argues that there are three groups of core needs—existence, relatedness, and growth—hence the label: ERG theory. The existence group is concerned with providing our basic material existence requirements. They include the items that Maslow considered as physiological and safety needs. The second group of needs are those of relatedness—the desire we have for maintaining important interpersonal relationships. These social and status desires require interaction with others if they are to be satisfied, and align with Maslow's love need and the external component of Maslow's esteem classification. Finally, Alderfer isolates growth needs—an intrinsic desire for personal development. These include the intrinsic component from Maslow's esteem category and the characteristics included under self-actualization.

Whether the ERG theory has isolated the critical or important need groups is an empirical question and, at this time, the evidence is too scant to draw any definitive conclusions.[8] However, Alderfer has dealt with the overlapping problem that occurred in Maslow's hierarchy by separating the survival, social, and personal growth needs. Equally important, Alderfer has avoided the assumption that a certain group of needs—for example, the existence needs—must be substantially satisfied before another set can emerge. Variables such as education, family background, and cultural environment can alter the importance or driving force that a group of needs hold for a particular individual. The evidence demonstrating that people in other cultures rank the need categories differently—for instance, those in Spain and Japan place social needs before their physiological requirements[9]—indicates that if a need theory is going to be valid over a cross-section of the population, it must either avoid assuming that all individuals proceed through a specific sequential need hierarchy, or modify the theory to isolate the factors (i.e., age, nationality, income level, type of work performed or whatever) that differentiate individuals into homogenous need hierarchy categories. Until we have research that can differentiate these categories, it is presumptuous to say anything other than need categories exist, but movement from one category to another cannot be accurately predicted.

Achievement, Power, and Affiliation Motives

In Chapter 4, we introduced the *need to achieve* as a personality attribute. It is also one of three needs proposed by David McClelland as important in organi-

7. Clayton P. Alderfer, "An Empirical Test of a New Theory of Human Needs," *Organizational Behavior and Human Performance,* May 1969, pp. 142–75.

8. For example, the ERG theory was disconfirmed by John Rauschenberger, Neal Schmitt, and John E. Hunter, "A Test of the Need Hierarchy Concept by a Markov Model of Change in Need Strength," *Administrative Science Quarterly,* December 1980, pp. 654–70.

9. Mason Haire, Edwin E. Ghiselli, and Lyman W. Porter, "Cultural Patterns in the Role of the Manager," *Industrial Relations,* Vol. 2 (1963), pp. 95–117.

zational settings for understanding motivation.[10] These three needs are achievement, power, and affiliation. They are identified as follows:

Need for achievement—the drive to excel, to achieve in relation to a set of standards, to strive to succeed.

Need for power—the need to make others behave in a way that they would not have behaved otherwise

Need for affiliation—the desire for friendly and close interpersonal relationships

As described previously, some people who have a compelling drive to succeed are striving for personal achievement rather than the rewards of success per se. They have a desire to do something better or more efficiently than it has been done before. This drive is the achievement need (*nAch*). From research into the achievement need, McClelland found that high achievers differentiate themselves from others by their desire to do things better.[11] They seek situations where they can attain personal responsibility for finding solutions to problems, where they can receive rapid feedback on their performance so they can tell easily whether they are improving or not, and where they can set moderately challenging goals. High achievers are not gamblers; they dislike succeeding by chance. They prefer the challenge of working at a problem and accepting the personal responsibility for success or failure, rather than leaving the outcome to chance or the actions of others. Importantly, they avoid what they perceive to be very easy or very difficult tasks.

Again as noted in Chapter 4, high achievers perform best when they perceive their probability of success as being .5; that is, where they estimate that they have a 50-50 chance of success. They dislike gambling with high odds because they get no achievement satisfaction from happenstance success. Similarly, they dislike low odds (high probability of success) because then there is no challenge to their skills. They like to set goals that require stretching themselves a little. When there is an approximately equal chance of success or failure, there is the optimum opportunity to experience feelings of accomplishment and satisfaction from their efforts.

The need for power (*nPow*) is the desire to have impact, to be influential, and to control others. Individuals high in *nPow* enjoy being "in charge," strive for influence over others, prefer to be placed into competitive and status-oriented situations, and tend to be more concerned with gaining influence over others and prestige than with effective performance.

The third need isolated by McClelland is affiliation (*nAff*). This need has received the least attention of researchers. Affiliation can be viewed as a Dale Carnegie–type of need—the desire to be liked and accepted by others. Individuals with a high affiliation motive strive for friendship, prefer cooperative situations rather than competitive ones, and desire relationships involving a high degree of mutual understanding.

10. David C. McClelland, *The Achieving Society* (New York: Van Nostrand Reinhold, 1961).

11. Ibid.

McClelland's research suggests that these motives have important implications for organizational selection. For example, an individual who has a high *nAff* and a low *nPow*, and who is placed into a job requiring a strong *nPow* in order to be effective, will have the wrong motivating forces to be successful in the job. More specifically, McClelland argues that the needs for affiliation and power tend to be closely related to managerial success.[12] He says that his studies in organizations offer strong evidence that the best managers are high in their need for power and low in their need for affiliation. Another researcher concurs, adding that possession of a high power motive is a requirement for managerial effectiveness.[13] Of course, what is the cause and what is the effect is arguable. It has been suggested that a high power need may occur simply as a function of one's level in a hierarchical organization.[14] This latter argument proposes that the higher the level an individual rises to in the organization, the greater is the incumbent's power motive. As a result, powerful positions would be the stimulus to a high power motive.

Do McClelland's three need categories agree or conflict with Maslow? It appears that McClelland's research can be reconciled into Maslow's hierarchy. Achievement closely approximates Maslow's self-actualization need. Affiliation would be part of Maslow's love need. Finally, McClelland's view of power suggests that it overlaps several of Maslow's categories. For example, power can bring safety, prestige, or even the friendship of others.

Attempts to validate McClelland's research and conclusions have met with reasonable success. However, practitioners have given greatest attention to the achievement need. Given that *nAch* drives people to act on the basis of an internally induced stimulus rather than relying on externally imposed motivators, there are several implications for managers. First, since the *nAch* attributes can be taught and have been positively related to higher work performance, managers can consider having employees undergo *nAch* training to stimulate this need. Second, an understanding of the concepts behind *nAch* and the characteristics that individuals high in *nAch* seek in their jobs can assist managers in explaining and predicting employee behavior.

Needs: A Summary

We have noted that it is possible to identify hundreds, possibly even thousands of needs if we attempted to list them. Of course many overlap, so efforts have been directed toward isolating a short list of important needs that are substantially independent of each other. The most frequently cited list of needs is that identified by Maslow, though the evidence to support a five-step hierarchy has failed to appear. There do seem to be basic needs: existence and security. Then

---

12. David C. McClelland and David H. Burnham, "Power Is the Great Motivator," *Harvard Business Review,* March-April 1976, pp. 100–110.

13. John B. Miner, *Studies in Management Education* (New York: Springer, 1965).

14. D. Kipnis, "The Powerholder," in *Perspectives in Social Power,* ed. J. T. Tedeschi (Chicago: Aldine, 1974), pp. 82–123.

there are higher-order needs. But the segmentation of the higher-order needs, as done by Maslow, goes beyond the empirical research to date. The fact is, that after lower-order needs are met, it is difficult to predict with any precision which need will become most influential. Additionally, the evidence can neither support nor refute that individuals may be simultaneously motivated by several higher-order needs. As a result, in spite of the popularity of Maslow's hierarchy, Alderfer's three-need hierarchy of existence, relatedness, and growth appears to be as far as one can realistically extend the research.

Reading an Individual's Needs

It is one thing to say that if you want to understand or predict an individual's motivational level, you need to know her needs. It is something completely different to know how to read needs.

An obvious, but incorrect, manner to learn about an individual's needs and self-interest is to ask her. There are several reasons why this approach is destined for failure. Many people find it difficult to talk about such a subject. Some may not consciously know what their needs or self-interests are. Others will tell you, unintentionally, what you want to hear. They will tell you what they believe they are supposed to say. A businesswoman may tell you she wants to make a great deal of money, since she thinks that is what businesswomen are supposed to strive for. Or that same businesswoman may say she wants to create a better world for all of us to live in. Such a response is more socially desirable than admitting that she wants power or prestige. Unfortunately for those of us interested in learning about other's needs, socially desirable responses tend to overshadow true responses.

What individuals say is not a good measure of what really motivates them. What we need to do, then, is develop awareness in observing others' needs through what they say, what they don't say, and most importantly, how they behave.

Behavior is usually a stronger sign than any verbal utterance. In fact, it has been said that, "Sometimes what a person says can't be heard because his actions speak so loudly." Unfortunately, developing the skills to "read" others takes time and practice. We can point out its importance, encourage the reader to be aware of possible discrepancies between actual needs and stated needs, and suggest that efforts to develop this skill will pay handsome dividends. Additionally, we can suggest that you consider engaging in research to determine the needs of the people you want to motivate.[15]

At this point, it might also be relevant to note that you should avoid assuming that your needs are a good indicator of others' needs. The Golden Rule says, "Do unto others as you would have them do unto you." In terms of effec-

15. For approaches on researching needs, see, for example, R. J. Pellegrin and C. H. Coates, "Executives and Supervisors: Contrasting Definitions of Career Success," *Administrative Science Quarterly,* Vol. 1 (1957), pp. 506–17; Lyman W. Porter, "A Study of Perceived Need Satisfaction in Bottom and Middle Management Jobs," *Journal of Applied Psychology,* Vol. 45 (1961), pp. 1–10; and David C. McClelland, "Achievement Motivation Can Be Developed," *Harvard Business Review,* Vol. 43 (1965), pp. 6–24, 178.

tively motivating others, ignore this advice. Its basic assumption is wrong: Your needs and desires are not necessarily the same as others. People are different and to assume that what you want is what others want is certain to lead you aground in terms of understanding others and motivating them. If you need a rule to follow, try this one: "Do unto others as they would want to be done to."

EXTRINSIC VERSUS INTRINSIC MOTIVATORS

A common way to classify motivation factors is by differentiating extrinsic from intrinsic motivators. *Extrinsic motivation* refers to the value an individual receives from the environment surrounding the context of the work. Pay, supervisory relations, tenure, and compliments are illustrations of extrinsic motivators. On the other hand, *intrinsic motivation* refers to the pleasure or value associated with the content of a work task. The desire for competence, achievement, and self-actualization are basically satisfied by outcomes that individuals give themselves. If you do well on a class examination, others can bestow prestige on you through admiration and other outcomes. However, if you view the high mark on the exam as a result of hard and challenging preparation, it can give you a sense of achievement regardless of external standards imposed. Even if the exam mark was not among the highest in the class, if the subject is particularly difficult for you, the attainment of a "high C" or "low B" can be intrinsically rewarding. Athletic achievements can be viewed similarly. In spite of the fact that a four-minute mile is commonplace these days among world-class runners, if you have ordinary talents, you may get a tremendous feeling of accomplishment from breaking the six-minute barrier, even if it will not get you any medals in a track meet or many accolades from others. This feeling of achievement is an intrinsic quality that can be met only by attaining internally imposed standards.

The extrinsic-intrinsic dichotomy has been the central arena for two debates on motivation. The first questions whether the factors we traditionally call motivators are actually motivators. That is, some research has shown that work motivation only occurs from intrinsic factors and that the extrinsic factors don't motivate employees but merely placate them. This research—called the *motivation hygiene theory*—has been the subject of considerable controversy. We shall present the findings and the arguments offered by its critics. The second debate is more recent, but nearly as controversial. It surrounds the issue of whether intrinsic and extrinsic motivators are independent or additive. Specifically, do individuals who are paid to perform an interesting task attribute their behavior to external forces and does this reduce their intrinsic interest in the task itself? We shall discuss this issue under the *cognitive evaluation theory*.

Motivation-Hygiene Theory

The motivation-hygiene theory was proposed by psychologist Frederick Herzberg over twenty years ago.[16] In the belief that an individual's relation to his

16. F. Herzberg, B. Mausner, and B. Snyderman, *The Motivation to Work* (New York: John Wiley, 1959).

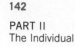

142

PART II
The Individual

work is a basic one and that his attitude to his work can very well determine his success or failure, Herzberg investigated the question, "What do people want from their jobs?" He asked people to describe, in detail, situations when they felt exceptionally good or bad about their jobs. These responses were tabulated and categorized. Factors affecting job attitudes as reported in twelve investigations conducted by Herzberg are illustrated in Figure 6–4.

From the categorized responses, Herzberg concluded that the replies people gave when they felt good about their jobs were significantly different from the replies given when they felt bad. As seen in Figure 6–4, certain characteristics tend to be consistently related to job satisfaction, and others to job dissatisfaction. Intrinsic factors, such as achievement, recognition, the work itself, responsibility, and advancement seem to be related to job satisfaction. When those questioned felt good about their work, they tended to attribute these characteristics to themselves. On the other hand, when they were dissatisfied, they

Figure 6–4 Comparison of Satisfiers and Dissatisfiers

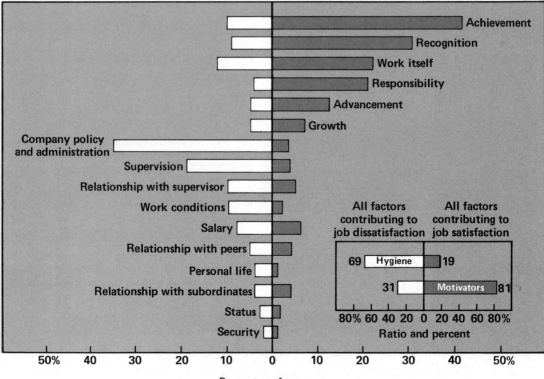

Source: Frederick Herzberg, "One More Time: How Do You Motivate Employees?" Harvard Business Review, January-February 1968, p. 57. With permission. Copyright © 1967 by the President and Fellows of Harvard College; all rights reserved.

Figure 6–5 Contrasting Views of Satisfaction-Dissatisfaction

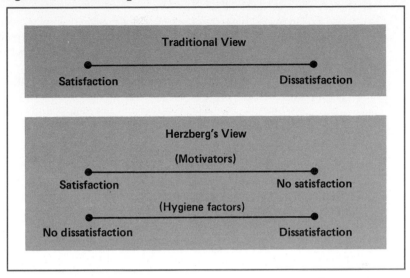

tended to cite extrinsic factors, such as company policy and administration, supervision, interpersonal relations, and working conditions.

The data suggests, says Herzberg, that the opposite of satisfaction is not dissatisfaction, as was traditionally believed. Removing dissatisfying characteristics from a job does not necessarily make the job satisfying. As illustrated in Figure 6–5, Herzberg proposes that his findings indicate the existence of a dual continuum: the opposite of "Satisfaction" is "No Satisfaction," and the opposite of "Dissatisfaction" is "No Dissatisfaction."

According to Herzberg, the factors leading to job satisfaction are separate and distinct from those that lead to job dissatisfaction. Therefore, managers who seek to eliminate factors that can create job dissatisfaction can bring about peace, but not necessarily motivation. They will be placating their work force rather than motivating them. As a result, such characteristics as company policy and administration, supervision, interpersonal relations, working conditions, and salary have been characterized by Herzberg as hygiene factors. When they are adequate, people will not be dissatisfied; however, neither will they be satisfied. If we want to motivate people on their jobs, Herzberg suggests emphasizing achievement, recognition, the work itself, responsibility, and growth. These are the characteristics that people find intrinsically rewarding.

The motivation-hygiene theory is not without its detractors. The criticisms of the theory have been based on five suggested weaknesses:

1. The procedure that Herzberg used is limited by its methodology. When things are going well, people tend to take credit themselves. Contrarily, they blame failure on the extrinsic environment.
2. The reliability of Herzberg's methodology is questioned. Since raters have to make interpretations, it is possible that they may contaminate the findings by

interpreting one response in one manner while treating another similar response differently.

3. No overall measure of satisfaction was utilized. In other words, a person may dislike part of his or her job, yet still think the job is acceptable.

4. The theory is inconsistent with previous research. The motivation-hygiene theory ignores situational variables.

5. Herzberg assumes that there is a relationship between satisfaction and productivity. But the research methodology he used looked only at satisfaction, not at productivity. To make such research relevant, one must assume a high relationship between satisfaction and productivity.[17]

Regardless of criticisms, Herzberg's theory has been widely read and few managers are unfamiliar with his recommendations. The increased popularity since the mid-1960s of vertically expanding jobs to allow workers greater responsibility in planning and controlling their work can probably be largely attributed to Herzberg's findings and recommendations.

From another perspective, Herzberg's findings appear consistent with general surveys made of workers' opinions about what they want from their job. Nationwide polls conducted by the National Opinion Research Center, for example, indicate that "more than half of the white, male work force in the United States believes that the most important characteristic of a job is that it involve work that is important and provides a sense of accomplishment."[18] Meaningful work is rated "most important" three times more frequently than "opportunities for advancement" and "high income," and seven times more frequently than the desire for "shorter work hours and much free time." In terms of preferencing order, these polls find no difference between replies of white-collar and blue-collar workers.

Cognitive Evaluation Theory

In the late 1960s, one researcher proposed that the introduction of extrinsic rewards, such as pay, for behavior that had been previously intrinsically rewarding would tend to decrease the overall level of motivation.[19] During the 1970s, this proposal—which has come to be called the cognitive evaluation theory—became the subject of much research, a large amount of which was supportive.[20]

Historically, motivation theorists had generally assumed that intrinsic and extrinsic motivators were independent—that is, the stimulation of one would not affect the other. But the cognitive evaluation theory suggests otherwise. It ar-

17. Robert J. House and Lawrence A. Wigdor, "Herzberg's Dual-Factor Theory of Job Satisfaction and Motivations: A Review of the Evidence and Criticisms," *Personnel Psychology,* Winter 1967, pp. 369–89; and Donald P. Schwab and Larry L. Cummings, "Theories of Performance and Satisfaction: A Review," *Industrial Relations,* October 1970, pp. 403–30.

18. Charles N. Weaver, "What Workers Want from Their Jobs," *Personnel,* May-June 1976, p. 49.

19. Richard deCharms, *Personal Causation: The Internal Affective Determinants of Behavior* (New York: Academic Press, 1968).

20. Edward L. Deci, *Intrinsic Motivation* (New York: Plenum, 1975).

gues that when extrinsic rewards like pay or promotions are used by organizations as payoffs for superior performance, the intrinsic rewards, which are derived from individuals doing what they like, are reduced. In other words, when extrinsic rewards are given to someone for performing an interesting task, it causes intrinsic interest in the task itself to decline.

Why would such an outcome occur? The popular explanation is that the individual experiences a loss of control over his or her own behavior so that the previous intrinsic motivation diminishes. Further, the elimination of extrinsic rewards can produce a shift—from an external to an internal explanation—in an individual's perception of causation of why he works on a task. If you're reading a novel a week because your English literature instructor requires you to, you can attribute your reading behavior to an external source. However, after the course is over, if you find yourself still reading a novel a week, your natural inclination is to say, "I must enjoy reading novels, because I'm reading one a week!"

If the cognitive evaluation theory is valid, it should have major implications for managerial practices. It has been a truism among compensation specialists for years that if pay or other extrinsic rewards are to be effective motivators, they should be made contingent on an individual's performance. But, cognitive evaluation theorists would argue, this will only tend to decrease the internal satisfaction that the individual receives from doing the job. We have substituted an external stimulus for an internal stimulus. In fact, if cognitive evaluation theory is correct, it would make sense to make an individual's pay *noncontingent* on performance in order to avoid decreasing intrinsic motivation.

We noted earlier that the cognitive evaluation theory has been supported in a number of studies.[21] Yet it has also met with attacks, specifically on the methodology used in these studies[22] and in the interpretation of the findings.[23] But where does this theory stand today? Can we say that when organizations use extrinsic motivators like pay and promotions to stimulate workers' performance that they do so at the expense of reducing intrinsic interest and motivation in the work being done? The answer is not a simple "Yes" or "No."

While further research is needed to clarify some of the current ambiguity,

21. For example, see Robert D. Pritchard, Kathleen M. Campbell, and Donald J. Campbell, "Effects of Extrinsic Financial Rewards on Intrinsic Motivation," *Journal of Applied Psychology,* February 1977, pp. 9–15; and Robert D. Pritchard and Edward L. Deci, "The Effects of Contingent and Noncontingent Rewards and Controls on Intrinsic Motivation," *Organizational Behavior and Human Performance,* Vol. 8 (1972), pp. 217–29.

22. W. E. Scott, "The Effects of Extrinsic Rewards on 'Intrinsic Motivation': A Critique," *Organizational Behavior and Human Performance,* Vol. 15 (1976), pp. 117–19; B. J. Calder and B. M. Staw, "Interaction of Intrinsic and Extrinsic Motivation: Some Methodological Notes," *Journal of Personality and Social Psychology,* Vol. 31 (1975), pp. 76–80.

23. G. R. Salancik, "Interaction Effects of Performance and Money on Self Perception of Intrinsic Motivation," *Organizational Behavior and Human Performance,* Vol. 13 (1975), pp. 339–51; Fred Luthans, Mark Martinko, and Tom Kess, "An Analysis of the Impact of Contingency Monetary Rewards on Intrinsic Motivation," *Proceedings of the Nineteenth Annual Midwest Academy of Management,* St. Louis, 1976, pp. 209–21.

the evidence does lead us to conclude that the nonadditivity of extrinsic and intrinsic rewards is a real phenomenon.[24] But its impact on employee motivation at work, in contrast to motivation in general, may be considerably less than originally thought. First, many of the studies testing the theory were done with students, not paid organizational employees. The researchers would observe what happens to a student's behavior when a reward that had been allocated is stopped. This is interesting, but it does not represent the typical work situation. In the real world, when extrinsic rewards are stopped it usually means the individual is no longer part of the organization. Second, evidence indicates that very high intrinsic motivation levels are strongly resistant to the detrimental impacts of extrinsic rewards.[25] Even when a job is inherently interesting, there still exists a powerful norm for extrinsic payment.[26] At the other extreme, on dull tasks extrinsic rewards appear to increase intrinsic motivation.[27] Therefore, the theory may have limited applicability to work organizations because most low-level jobs are not inherently satisfying enough to foster high intrinsic interest and many managerial and professional positions offer intrinsic rewards. Cognitive evaluation theory may be relevant to that set of organizational jobs which falls in between—those that are neither extremely dull nor extremely interesting.

POPULAR PROCESS THEORIES OF MOTIVATION

Let's turn our attention now to process theories of motivation. Except for a few minor exceptions, the "action" in motivation research has moved toward attempting to understand how individuals determine the amount of effort to exert. That is, what is the process by which individuals determine the choice of effort levels on a particular task? In the following pages, we shall review the four most popular theories. Each has its own emphasis. For instance, *equity theory* is specifically concerned with whether individuals perceive that rewards are being allocated fairly. *Goal-setting theory* looks at the specificity and difficulty of goals as a primary explanation of effort. *Reinforcement theory* emphasizes the pattern in which rewards are administered. *Expectancy theory* focuses on an individual's perception of the relationship of rewards to performance and the value that the individual assigns to the rewards.

24. Miner, *Theories of Organizational Behavior*, p. 157.

25. Hugh J. Arnold, "Effects of Performance Feedback and Extrinsic Reward Upon High Intrinsic Motivation," *Organizational Behavior and Human Performance*, December, 1976, pp. 275–88.

26. Barry M. Staw, "Motivation in Organizations: Toward Synthesis and Redirection," in *New Directions in Organizational Behavior*, ed. B. M. Staw and G. R. Salancik (Chicago: St. Clair, 1977), p. 76.

27. B. J. Calder and B. M. Staw, "Self-Perception of Intrinsic and Extrinsic Motivation," *Journal of Personality and Social Psychology*, April 1975, pp. 599–605.

Equity Theory

Jane Pearson graduated last year from the State University with a degree in accounting. After interviews with a number of organizations on campus, she accepted a position with one of the nation's largest public accounting firms and was assigned to their Boston office. Jane was very pleased with the offer she received: challenging work with a prestigious firm, an excellent opportunity to gain important experience, and the highest salary any accounting major at State was offered last year—$1,800 a month. But Jane was the top student in her class; she was ambitious and articulate and fully expected to receive a commensurate salary.

Twelve months have passed since Jane joined her employer. The work has proved to be as challenging and satisfying as she had hoped. Her employer is extremely pleased with her performance; in fact she recently received a $100 a month raise. However, Jane's motivational level has dropped dramatically in the past few weeks. Why? Her employer has just hired a fresh college graduate out of State University, who lacks the one-year experience Jane has gained, for $1,950 a month—$50 more than Jane now makes! It would be an understatement to describe Jane in any other terms than livid. Jane is even talking about looking for another job.

Jane's situation illustrates the role equity plays in motivation. Employees make comparisons of their job inputs and outcomes relative to those of others. We perceive what we get from a job situation (outcomes) in relation to what we put into it (inputs), and then compare our input-outcome ratio with the input-outcome ratio of relevant others. This is shown in Fig. 6-6. If we perceive our ratio to be equal to the relevant others with whom we compare ourselves, a

FIGURE 6–6 Equity Theory

RATIO COMPARISONS	PERCEPTION
$\dfrac{O}{I_A} < \dfrac{O}{I_B}$	Inequity due to being underrewarded
$\dfrac{O}{I_A} = \dfrac{O}{I_B}$	Equity
$\dfrac{O}{I_A} > \dfrac{O}{I_B}$	Inequity due to being overrewarded

Where $\dfrac{O}{I_A}$ represents the employee and

$\dfrac{O}{I_B}$ represents relevant others

state of equity is said to exist. We perceive our situation as fair—that justice prevails. If the ratios are unequal, inequity exists; that is, we tend to view ourselves as underrewarded or overrewarded. It has been proposed that an equity process takes place in which people who view any inequity as aversive will attempt to correct it.[28]

The referent than an employee selects adds to the complexity of equity theory. Evidence suggests that the reference chosen is an important variable in equity theory.[29] The three referent categories have been classified as "other," "system," and "self." The "other" category includes other individuals with similar jobs in the same organization, and also includes friends, neighbors, or professional associates. Based on information that employees receive through word of mouth, newspapers, and magazines, on such issues as executive salaries or a recent union contract, employees can compare their pay to that of others.

The "system" category considers organizational pay policies and procedures, and the administration of this system. It considers organization-wide pay policies, both implied and explicit. Precedents by the organization in terms of allocation of pay would be a major determinant in this category.

The "self" category refers to input-outcome ratios that are unique to the individual and differ from the individual's current input-outcome ratio. This category is influenced by such criteria as past jobs or commitments that must be met in terms of family role.

The choice of a particular set of referents is related to the information available about referents as well as to their perceived relevance. Based on equity theory, we might suggest that when employees envision an inequity, they may take one or more of five choices:

1. Distort either their own or others inputs or outcomes
2. Behave in some way so as to induce others to change their inputs or outcomes
3. Behave in some way so as to change their own inputs or outcomes
4. Choose a different comparison referent
5. Leave the field (quit their job)

Equity theory recognizes that individuals are concerned not only with the absolute amount of rewards they receive for their efforts; but also with the relationship of this amount to what others receive. They make judgments as to the relationship between their inputs and outcomes and the inputs and outcomes of others. Based on one's inputs, such as effort, experience, education, and competence, one compares outcomes such as salary levels, raises, recognition, and other factors. When people perceive an imbalance in their input-outcome ratio

28. J. S. Adams, "Inequity in Social Exchanges," *Advances in Experimental Social Psychology,* ed. Leonard Berkowitz (New York: Academic Press, 1965), pp. 267–300.

29. Paul S. Goodman, "An Examination of Referents Used in the Evaluation of Pay," *Organizational Behavior and Human Performance,* October 1974, pp. 170–95.

relative to others, tension is created. This tension provides the basis for motivation, as people strive for what they perceive as equity and fairness.

Specifically, the theory establishes four propositions relating to inequitable pay:

1. *Given payment by time, overrewarded employees will produce more than equitably paid employees.* Hourly and salaried employees will generate high quantity or quality of production in order to increase the input side of the ratio and bring about equity.

2. *Given payment by quantity of production, overrewarded employees will produce fewer, but higher quality units, than equitably paid employees.* Individuals paid on a piece-rate basis will increase their effort to achieve equity, which can result in greater quality or quantity. However, increases in quantity will only increase inequity since every unit produced results in further overpayment. Therefore, effort is directed toward increasing quality rather than increasing quantity.

3. *Given payment by time, underrewarded employees will produce less or poorer quality of output.* Effort will be decreased, which will bring about lower productivity or poorer-quality output than equitably paid subjects.

4. *Given payment by quantity of production, underrewarded employees will produce a large number of low-quality units in comparison with equitably paid employees.* Employees on piece-rate pay plans can bring about equity because trading off quantity of output for quality will result in an increase in rewards with little or no increase in contributions.

The above propositions have generally proven to be supported.[30] A review of the recent research tends to confirm consistently the equity thesis: Employee motivation is influenced significantly by relative rewards as well as absolute rewards. Where employees perceive inequity, they will act to correct the situation.[31] The result might be lower or higher productivity, improved or reduced quality of output, increased absenteeism, or voluntary resignation.

The above does not mean that equity theory is without problems. The theory leaves some key issues still unclear.[32] For instance, how do employees

30. Paul S. Goodman and A. Friedman, "An Examination of Adams' Theory of Inequity," *Administrative Science Quarterly,* September 1971, pp. 271–88.

31. See, for example, Michael R. Carrell, "A Longitudinal Field Assessment of Employee Perceptions of Equitable Treatment," *Organizational Behavior and Human Performance,* February 1978, pp. 108–18; Robert G. Lord and Jeffrey A. Hohenfeld, "Longitudinal Field Assessment of Equity Effects on the Performance of Major League Baseball Players," *Journal of Applied Psychology,* February 1979, pp. 19–26; and John E. Dittrich and Michael R. Carrell, "Organizational Equity Perceptions, Employee Job Satisfaction, and Departmental Absence and Turnover Rates," *Organizational Behavior and Human Performance,* August 1979, pp. 29–40.

32. Paul S. Goodman, "Social Comparison Process in Organizations," in *New Directions in Organizational Behavior,* ed. B. M. Staw and G. R. Salancik (Chicago: St. Clair, 1977), pp. 97–132.

select who is included in the "other" referent category? How do they define inputs and outcomes? How do they combine and weigh their inputs and outcomes to arrive at totals? When and how do the factors change over time? However, regardless of these problems, equity theory continues to offer us some important insights into employee motivation.

Goal-Setting Theory

Gene Broadwater, coach of the Hamilton High School cross-country team, gave his squad these last words before they approached the line for the league championship race: "Each one of you is physically ready. Now, get out there and do your best. No one can ever ask more of you than that."

You've heard the phrase a number of times yourself: "Just do your best. That's all anyone can ask for." But what does "do your best" mean? Do we ever know if we've achieved that vague goal? Would the cross-country runners have recorded faster times if Coach Broadwater had given each a specific goal to shoot for? Might you have done better in your high school English class if your parents had said, "You should strive for 85 percent or higher on all your work in English," rather than telling you to "do your best"? The research on goal-setting addresses these issues and the findings, as you will see, are impressive in terms of the impact specific and challenging goals have on performance.

In the late 1960s, it was proposed that intentions to work toward a goal are a major source of work motivation.[33] The evidence strongly supports this thesis. More to the point, we can say that specific goals increase performance and that difficult goals, when accepted, result in higher performance than easy goals.[34]

Specific hard goals produce a higher level of output than a generalized goal of "do your best." The specificity of the goal itself acts as an internal stimulus. For instance, when a trucker commits to making eighteen round-trip hauls between Baltimore and Washington, D.C., each week, this intention gives him a specific objective to reach for. We can say that, all things being equal, the trucker with a specific goal will outperform his counterpart operating with no goals or the generalized goal of "do your best."

If factors like ability and acceptance of the goals are held constant, we can also state that the more difficult the goals, the higher the level of performance. However, it's logical to assume that easier goals are more likely to be accepted. But once an employee accepts a hard task, he or she will exert a high level of effort until it is achieved, lowered, or abandoned.

If employees have the opportunity to participate in the setting of their own goals, will they try harder? The evidence is mixed regarding the superiority of

---

33. Edwin A. Locke, "Toward a Theory of Task Motivation and Incentives," *Organizational Behavior and Human Performance,* May 1968, pp. 157–89.

34. Gary P. Latham and Gary A. Yukl, "A Review of Research on the Application of Goal Setting in Organizations," *Academy of Management Journal,* December 1975, pp. 824–45.

participation over assigned goals. In some cases, participatively set goals elicit superior performance, while in other cases individuals performed best when assigned goals by their boss. But a major advantage of participation may be in increasing acceptance of the goal, itself, as a desirable one to work toward. As we noted above, resistance is greater when goals are difficult. If people participate in goal-setting, they are more likely to accept even a difficult goal than if they are arbitrarily assigned it by their boss. The reason is that individuals are more committed to choices in which they have a part. Thus, although participative goals may have no superiority over assigned goals when acceptance is taken as a given, participation does increase the probability that more difficult goals will be agreed to and acted upon.

Studies on goal-setting have demonstrated the superiority of specific and challenging goals as motivating forces. While we can't conclude that having employees participate in the goal-setting process is always desirable, participation is probably preferable to assignment when you expect resistance to accepting more difficult challenges. As an overall conclusion, therefore, we have significant evidence that intentions—as articulated in terms of goals—are a potent motivating force.

Reinforcement Theory

A counterpoint to goal-setting theory is reinforcement theory. The former is a cognitive approach, proposing that an individual's purposes direct his or her action. In reinforcement theory we have a behavioristic approach, which argues that reinforcement conditions behavior. The two are clearly at odds philosophically. Reinforcement theorists see behavior as environmentally caused. You need not be concerned, they would argue, with internal cognitive events; what controls behavior are reinforcers—any consequence which, when immediately following a response, increases the probability that the behavior will be repeated.

Reinforcement theory ignores the inner state of the individual and concentrates solely on what happens to a person when he or she takes some action. Because it does not concern itself with what initiates behavior, it is not, strictly speaking, a theory of motivation. But it does provide a powerful means of analysis of what controls behavior, and it is for this reason that it is typically considered in discussions of motivation.[35]

We shall address the reinforcement process in detail in our next chapter. There, we shall show how using reinforcers to condition behavior gives us considerable insight into how people learn. Yet we cannot ignore the fact that reinforcement has a wide following as a motivational device. In its pure form, however, reinforcement theory ignores feelings, attitudes, expectations, and other cognitive variables that are known to impact behavior. In fact, some re-

---

35. Richard M. Steers and Lyman W. Porter, *Motivation and Work Behavior*, 2nd ed. (New York: McGraw-Hill, 1979), p. 13.

searchers look at the same experiments that reinforcement theorists use to support their position and interpret the findings in a cognitive framework.[36]

Reinforcement is undoubtedly an important influence on behavior, but few scholars are prepared to argue that it is the *only* influence. The behaviors you engage in at work and the amount of effort you allocate to each task *is* effected by the consequences that follow from your behavior. If you are consistently reprimanded for outproducing your colleagues, you will likely reduce your productivity. But your lower productivity may also be explained in terms of inequity, goals, or expectancies.

Expectancy Theory: An Integrative Model

Each of the theories we have discussed so far contributes to an understanding of motivation but none has been as successful as we would like. Need theories offer insight into motivation, but have clear limitations. Motivation-hygiene and cognitive evaluation theories have been subjected to extremely critical attack, leaving little from which to generalize. Equity, goal-setting, and reinforcement theories each add to our understanding of motivation, but seem individually limited. What is necessary is a theory of motivation that considers needs, goals, perceptions, reinforcers, and the contingency aspects relevant to particular people in particular situations (i.e., individual differences like attitudes and personality). Such an integrative scheme has been formulated—it is called expectancy theory.[37] Though expectancy theory has its critics,[38] it has generally developed results that indicate that it is currently the clearest and most accurate explanation of individual motivation.

The expectancy theory argues that the strength of a tendency to act in a certain way depends on the strength of an expectation that the act will be followed by a given outcome and on the attractiveness of that outcome to the individual. It includes, therefore, three variables.[39]

1. *Attractiveness*—the importance that the individual places on the potential outcome or reward that can be achieved on the job. This considers the unsatisfied needs of the individual.
2. *Performance-reward linkage*—the degree to which the individual believes that performing at a particular level will lead to the attainment of a desired outcome.

36. Edwin A. Locke, "Latham vs. Komaki: A Tale of Two Paradigms," *Journal of Applied Psychology*, February 1980, pp. 16–23.

37. Victor H. Vroom, *Work and Motivation* (New York: John Wiley, 1964).

38. See, for example, Herbert G. Heneman III and Donald P. Schwab, "Evaluation of Research on Expectancy Theory Prediction of Employee Performance," *Psychological Bulletin*, July 1972, pp. 1–9; and Leon Reinharth and Mahmoud A. Wahba, "Expectancy Theory as a Predictor of Work Motivation, Effort Expenditure, and Job Performance," *Academy of Management Journal*, September 1975, pp. 502–37.

39. Vroom refers to these three variables as *valence, instrumentality,* and *expectancy,* respectively.

3. *Effort-performance linkage*—the perceived probability by the individual that exerting a given amount of effort will lead to performance.

While this may sound pretty complex, it really is not that difficult to visualize. Whether one has the desire to produce at any given time depends on one's particular goals and one's perception of the relative worth of performance as a path to the attainment of these goals.

Figure 6–7 is a considerable simplification of expectancy theory, but expresses its major contentions. The strength of a person's motivation to perform (effort) depends on how strongly she believes that she can achieve what she attempts. If she achieves this goal (performance), will she be adequately rewarded and, if she is rewarded by the organization, will the reward satisfy her individual goals? Let us consider the four steps inherent in the theory and then attempt to apply it.

First, what perceived outcomes does the job offer the employee? Outcomes may be positive: pay, security, companionship, trust, fringe benefits, a chance to use talent or skills, congenial relationships. On the other hand, employees may view the outcomes as negative: fatigue, boredom, frustration, anxiety, harsh supervision, threat of dismissal. Importantly, reality is not relevant here; the critical issue is what the individual employee *perceives* the outcome to be, regardless of whether or not her perceptions are accurate.

Second, how attractive do employees consider these outcomes? Are they valued positively, negatively, or neutrally? This obviously in an internal issue to the individual and considers her personal values, personality, and needs. The individual who finds a particular outcome attractive—that is, positively valued—would prefer attaining it to not attaining it. Others may find it negative and, therefore, prefer not attaining it to attaining it. Still others may be neutral.

Third, what kind of behavior must the employee produce in order to achieve these outcomes? The outcomes are not likely to have any effect on the individual employee's performance unless the employee knows, clearly and unambiguously, what she must do in order to achieve them. For example, what is "doing well" in terms of performance appraisal? What are the criteria the employee's performance will be judged on?

Fourth and last, how does the employee view her chances of doing what is asked of her? After the employee has considered her own competencies and her ability to control those variables that will determine her success, what probability does she place on successful attainment?[40]

40. This four-step discussion was adapted from K. F. Taylor, "A 'Valence-Expectancy' Approach to Work Motivation," *Personnel Practice Bulletin,* June 1974, pp. 142–48.

Figure 6–7 Simplified Expectancy Model

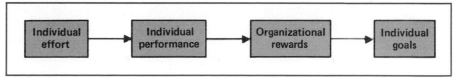

Let us use the classroom organization as an illustration of how one can use expectancy theory to explain motivation.

Most students prefer an instructor who tells them what is expected of them in the course. They want to know what the assignments and examinations will be like, when they are due or to be taken, and how much weight each carries in the final term grade. They also like to think that the amount of effort they exert in attending classes, taking notes, and studying will be reasonably related to the grade they will make in the course. If we assume that the above describes you, consider that five weeks into a class you are really enjoying (we'll call it B.A. 301), an exam is given back. You have studied hard for this exam. You have consistently made "A's" and "B's" on exams in other courses where you have expended similar effort. And the reason you work so hard is to make top grades, which you believe are important for getting a good job upon graduation. Also, you are not sure but you may want to go on to graduate school. Again, you think grades are important for getting into a good graduate school

Well, the results of that five-week exam are in. The class median was 72. Ten percent of the class scored an 85 or higher and got an "A." Your grade was 46; the minimum passing mark was 50. You're mad. You're frustrated. Even more, you're perplexed. How could you have possibly done so poorly on the exam when you usually score among the top grades in other classes by preparing as you had for this exam? Several interesting things are immediately evident in your behavior. Suddenly, you no longer are driven to attend B.A. 301 classes regularly. You find you do not study for the course either. When you do attend classes, you daydream a lot—the result is an empty notebook instead of several pages of notes. One would probably be correct in describing you as "lacking in motivation" in B.A. 301. Why did your motivational level change? You know and I know, but let's explain it in expectancy terms.

If we use Figure 6–7 to understand this situation, we might say the following: Studying and preparation in B.A. 301 (effort) is conditioned by it resulting in answering the questions on the exam correctly (performance), which will produce a high grade (reward), which you believe will lead to the security, prestige, and other benefits that accrue from obtaining a good job (individual goal).

The attractiveness of the outcome—which in this case is a good grade—is high. But what about the performance-reward linkage? Do you feel that the grade you received truly reflects your knowledge of the material? In other words, did the test fairly measure what you know? If the answer is "Yes," then this linkage is strong. If the answer is "No," then at least part of the reason for your reduced motivational level is your belief that the test was not a fair measure of your performance. If the test was of an essay type, maybe you believe the instructor's grading method was poor. Was too much weight placed on a question that you thought was trivial? Maybe the instructor does not like you and was biased in grading your paper. These are examples of perceptions that influence the performance-reward linkage and your level of motivation.

Another possible demotivating force may be the effort-performance relationship. If, after you took the exam, you believed that you could not have passed it regardless of the amount of preparation you had done, then your desire to study will drop. Possibly the instructor wrote the exam under the assumption that you had had a considerably broader background in the course's subject matter. Maybe the course had several prerequisites that you did not know about, or possibly you had the prerequisites but took them several years ago. The end result is the same: You place a low value on your effort leading to answering the exam questions correctly, and hence there is a reduction in your motivational level and you lessen your effort.

The key to expectancy theory, therefore, is the understanding of an individual's goals, and the linkage between effort and performance, between performance and rewards and, finally, between the rewards and individual goal satisfaction. As a contingency model, expectancy theory recognizes that there is no universal principle for explaining everyone's motivations. Additionally, just because we understand what needs a person seeks to satisfy does not ensure that the individual himself perceives high performance as necessarily leading to the satisfaction of these needs. If you desire to take B.A. 301 in order to meet new people and make social contacts, but the instructor organizes the class on the assumption that you want to make a good grade in the course, the instructor may be personally disappointed should you perform poorly on the exams. Unfortunately, most instructors assume that their ability to allocate grades is a potent force in motivating students. But it will only be so if students place a high importance on grades, if students know what they must do to achieve the grade desired, and if the students consider there is a high probability of their performing well should they exert a high level of effort.

Let us summarize some of the issues expectancy theory has brought forward. First, it emphasizes payoffs or rewards. As a result, we have to believe that the rewards the organization is offering align with what the employee wants. It is a theory based on self interest wherein each individual seeks to maximize her expected satisfaction: "Expectancy theory is a form of calculative, psychological *hedonism* in which the ultimate motive of every human act is asserted to be the maximization of pleasure and/or the minimization of pain."[41] Second, we have to be concerned with the attractiveness of rewards, which requires an understanding and knowledge of what value the individual puts on organizational payoffs. We shall want to reward the individual with those things she values positively. Third, expectancy theory emphasizes expected behaviors. Does the person know what is expected of her and how she will be appraised? Finally, the theory is concerned with expectations. It is irrelevant what is realistic or rational. An individual's own expectations of performance, reward, and goal satisfaction outcomes will determine her level of effort, not the objective outcomes themselves.

Does expectancy theory work? The space we have devoted to it suggests

41. Edwin A. Locke, "Personnel Attitudes and Motivation," in *Annual Review of Psychology,* ed. Mark R. Rosenzweig and Lyman W. Porter (Palo Alto, Calif.: Annual Reviews, 1975), p. 459.

that it is important, yet, as we have seen before, few theories are irrefutable, without critics, or devoid of contradictory findings. Expectancy theory is no exception.[42] Attempts to validate the theory have been complicated by methodological, criterion, and measurement problems. As a result, many published studies that purport to support or negate the theory must be viewed with caution. Importantly, most studies have failed to replicate the methodology as it was originally proposed. For example, the theory proposes to explain different levels of effort within the same person under different circumstances, but almost all replication studies have looked at different people. By correcting for this flaw, support for the validity of expectancy theory has been greatly improved.[43] Some critics suggest that the theory has only limited use, arguing that it tends to be more valid for predicting in situations where effort-performance and performance-reward linkages are clearly perceived by the individual.[44] Since few individuals perceive a high correlation between performance and rewards in their jobs, the theory tends to be idealistic. If organizations actually rewarded individuals for performance, rather than criteria such as seniority, effort, skill level, or job difficulty, then the theory's validity might be considerably greater. However, rather than invalidating expectancy theory, this criticism can be used in support of the theory and for explaining why a large segment of the work force exerts a minimal level of effort in carrying out their job responsibilities.

IMPLICATIONS FOR PERFORMANCE AND SATISFACTION

An individual's motivation, along with her skills and abilities, will be the critical determinants of individual performance. An individual's motivation also influences her satisfaction with her job and her predilections toward absenteeism or resignation.

The evidence indicates that while thousands of needs can be enumerated, they can be narrowed down to a few reasonably independent groupings. The most popular classification scheme, the need hierarchy proposed by Abraham Maslow, has generally proved weak as an explanation of motivation; ". . . .there is relatively little evidence empirically relating Maslow's model to performance, or even to psychological well-being."[45] The most accurate classification pro-

42. See footnote 38.

43. Paul M. Muchinsky, "A Comparison of Within- and Across-Subjects Analyses of the Expectancy-Valence Model for Predicting Effort," *Academy of Management Journal,* March 1977, pp. 154–58.

44. Robert J. House, H. J. Shapiro, and M. A. Wahba, "Expectancy Theory as a Predictor of Work Behavior and Attitudes: A Re-evaluation of Empirical Evidence," *Decision Sciences,* January 1974, pp. 481–506.

45. J. G. Hunt and J. W. Hill, "The New Look in Motivational Theory for Organizational Research," *Human Organization,* Summer 1969, pp. 100–109.

poses that there are three core needs—existence, relatedness, and growth. The concept of needs, regardless of the categories used to describe them, are almost universally accepted to be the base upon which the motivation process works.[46]

Existence needs of individuals in today's labor force are substantially met. The union movement and government legislation have achieved wages, hours, and working conditions for North American workers that ensure that they need pay little attention to the fear of hunger, of being without shelter, or of enduring a major hardship should they be temporarily out of work. As a result, while workers are still interested in more money and more security, particularly in times of inflation and high unemployment rates, relatedness and growth needs appear to be of increasing importance to the permanently employed.

The need to achieve has received a considerable amount of attention by psychologists. The evidence indicates that individuals who have a high need to achieve outperform low achievers. "Men with high *nAch* get more raises and are promoted more rapidly, because they keep actively seeking ways to do a better job."[47] Additionally, achievement motivation is closely related to the entrepreneurial task. As a result, those with a high need to achieve should be successful in founding and developing small businesses or in managerial positions that represent a "small business within a business," such as those who manage relatively small divisions within larger conglomerates.[48]

The best predictor of motivation and performance is expectancy theory, which builds upon many of the concepts we discussed previously; values, personality, perception, needs, equity, goals, and reinforcement. Individual motivation will be significantly determined by the probabilities a worker assigns to the following relationships: effort leading to performance, performance leading to rewards, and these rewards satisfying personal goals. It tells us that each individual has his or her own goals, and that organizations that offer uniform rewards will fail to take advantage of individual differences. Further, an individual's intrinsic motivation is stimulated where the tasks performed are perceived as challenging but not overwhelming. "Very difficult goals seem to have a positive effect on performance, only when they are accepted. Easy goals seem to have little positive effect, because even if they are achieved, individuals do not feel they have accomplished anything."[49] Importantly, where individuals perceive a weak linkage between performance and rewards, effort is reduced. The expectancy theory, when meshed with equity theory, forces us to deal not only with reality—what is—but with what individuals perceive a situation to be. Regard-

46. For an excellent article that questions the need models, see Gerald R. Salancik and Jeffrey Pfeffer, "An Examination of Need-Satisfaction Models of Job Attitudes," *Administrative Science Quarterly*, September 1977, pp. 427–56.

47. David C. McClelland, "That Urge to Achieve," *Think*, November-December, 1966, pp. 19–23.

48. John B. Miner, *Theories of Organizational Behavior*, pp. 71, 73.

49. Edward E. Lawler III and John Grant Rhode, *Information and Control in Organizations* (Pacific Palisades, Calif.: Goodyear, 1976), p. 71.

less of how closely rewards have been correlated to performance criteria, if individuals perceive this correlation to be low we can expect low performance, a decrease in job satisfaction, and an increase in turnover and absenteeism statistics.

FOR DISCUSSION

1. Define motivation. Describe the motivation process.

2. Do all people act in their self-interest? How might your answer be reconciled with traditional teachings of the church?

3. Compare and contrast Maslow's hierarchy of needs theory with (a) Alderfer's ERG theory and (b) Herzberg's motivation-hygiene theory.

4. Describe the three needs isolated by McClelland. How are they related to worker behavior?

5. "The cognitive evaluation theory is contradictory to reinforcement and expectancy theories." Do you agree or disagree? Explain.

6. "Goal-setting is part of both reinforcement and expectancy theories." Do you agree or disagree? Explain.

7. Reconcile equity and expectancy theories.

8. Reconcile reinforcement and expectancy theories.

9. Are workaholics and high achievers the same thing? Discuss.

10. Can an individual be *too* motivated, so that his or her performance declines as a result of excessive effort? Discuss.

FOR FURTHER READING

CHUNG, K. H., *Motivational Theories and Practices.* Columbus, Ohio: Grid, Inc., 1977. Reviews major theories of motivation, integrates them into a theoretical framework, and translates theory into specific motivational programs applicable to organizations.

CONNOLLY, T., "Some Conceptual and Methodological Issues in Expectancy Models of Work Performance Motivation," *Academy of Management Review,* October 1976, pp. 37–47. Reviews expectancy theory and attempts to identify weaknesses and inconsistencies in empirical studies which have sought to validate the theory.

HUNT, J. G., and J. W. HILL, "The New Look in Motivational Theory for Organizational Research," *Human Organization,* Summer 1969, pp. 100–109. Argues that the expectancy model is superior to either the Maslow or Herzberg models on both theoretical and empirical grounds.

LAWLER, E. E., III, *Motivation in Work Organizations.* Monterey, Calif.: Brooks/Cole, 1973. Reviews the literature in work motivation and satisfaction.

LOCKE, E. A., "The Ubiquity of the Technique of Goal Setting in Theories of and Approaches to Employee Motivation," *Academy of Management Review,* July 1978, pp. 594–601. Goal setting is recognized, explicitly or implicitly, by virtually every major theory of work motivation. This stems from the general recognition that rational human action is goal directed.

STEERS, R. M., and L. W. PORTER, eds. *Motivation and Work Behavior,* 2nd ed. New York: McGraw-Hill, 1979. Some of the major articles in the study of work motivation are reprinted.

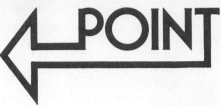

Statement of the personality-versus-organization hypothesis

Adapted and edited from George Strauss, "The Personality-Versus-Organization Theory," in Individualism and Big Business, *ed. Leonard R. Sayles (New York: McGraw-Hill, 1963), pp. 67–70. Reproduced by permission.*

Over the years, out of the contributions of individuals such as Argyris, Herzberg, Maier, Maslow, and McGregor has come a consistent view of human motivation in industry. With due regard to Chris Argyris, I would like to call it the "personality-versus-organization hypothesis."

1. Human behavior in regard to work is motivated by a hierarchy of needs, in ascending order: physical well-being, safety, social satisfaction, egoistic gratification, and self-actualization. By hierarchy is meant that a higher, less basic need does not provide motivation unless all lower, more basic needs are satisfied, and that once a basic need is satisfied, it no longer motivates.

Physical needs are the most fundamental, but once a reasonable level of physical-need satisfaction is obtained (largely through pay), individuals become relatively more concerned with other needs. First they seek to satisfy their security needs (e.g., through seniority and fringe benefits). When these, too, are reasonably satisfied, social needs (e.g., friendship and group support) take first priority. And so forth. Thus, for example, hungry men have little interest in whether or not they belong to strong social groups; relatively well-off individuals are more anxious for good human relations.

Only when most of the less pressing needs are satisfied will individuals turn to the ultimate form of satisfaction, self-actualization, which is described by Maslow as "the desire to become more and more what one is, to become everything that one is capable of becoming. . . . A musician must make music, an artist must paint, a poet must write, if he is to be ultimately happy. What a man can be, he must be."[1]

2. Healthy individuals desire to mature, to satisfy increasingly higher levels of needs; in practice, they want more and more opportunities to form strong social groups, to be independent and creative, to exercise autonomy and discretion, and to develop and express their unique personalities with freedom.

3. The organization, on the other hand, seeks to program individual behavior and reduce discretion. It demands conformity, obedience, dependence, and immature behavior. The assembly-line worker, the engineer, and the executive are all subject to strong pressures to behave in a programmed, conformist fashion. As a consequence, many individuals feel alienated from their work.

4. Subordinates react to these pressures in a number of ways, most of which are dysfunctional to the organization. Individuals may fight back through union activity, sabotage, output restriction, and other forms of rational or irrational (aggressive) behavior. Or they may withdraw and engage in regression, sublimination, childish be-

[1] A. H. Maslow, "A Theory of Human Motivation," *Psychological Review,* Vol. 40 (1943), p. 372.

havior, failure to contribute creative ideas, or to produce no more than a minimum amount of work. In any case, employees struggle not to conform (at least at first). To keep these employees in line, management must impose still more restrictions and force still more immature behavior. Thus a vicious cycle begins.

5. Management pressures often lead to excessive competition and splintering of work groups and the consequent loss of cooperation and social satisfaction. Or work groups may become even stronger, but their norms may now be anti-management, those of protecting individuals against pressures from above.

6. A subtle management, which provides high wages, liberal employee benefits, "hygienic," "decent" supervision, and not too much pressure to work, may well induce employees to think they are happy and not *dissatisfied*. But they are not (or should not be) truly *satisfied*; they are apathetic and have settled for a low level of aspiration. They do as little work as they can get away with and still hold their jobs. This unhealthy situation is wasteful both to the individual and to the organization.

7. Some differences in emphasis are found among authorities as to whether the behavior of the typical subordinate under these circumstances will be rational (reality-oriented) or irrational (frustration-oriented). In any case, organizational pressures, particularly the subjection to programmed work, may lead to serious personality disturbances and mental illness. Traditional organizational techniques thus not only prevent the organization from operating at maximum efficiency, but in terms of their impact on individual adjustments, are also very expensive to the society as a whole.

8. The only healthy solution is for management to adopt policies that promote intrinsic job satisfaction, individual development, and creativity, according to which people will willingly and voluntarily work toward organizational objectives because they enjoy their work and feel that it is important to do a good job. More specifically, management should promote job enlargement, general supervision, strong, cohesive work groups, and decentralization. In a nutshell, management should adopt what Harold Leavitt calls "power-equalization techniques."

COUNTER POINT

Strauss

Criticism of the personality-versus-organization hypothesis

Adapted and edited from George Strauss, "The Personality-Versus-Organization Theory," in Individualism and Big Business, *ed. Leonard R. Sayles (New York: McGraw-Hill, 1963). pp. 70–79. Reproduced by permission.*

The view expressed previously is, in a sense, a hypothesis as to human behavior in organizations. But it is more than a coldly objective hypothesis, it is a prescription for management behavior, and implicit in it are strong value judgments. With its strong emphasis on individual dignity, creative freedom, and self-development, this hypothesis bears all the earmarks of its academic origin.

Professors place high value on autonomy, inner direction, and the quest for maximum self-development. As much as any other group in society, their existence is work-oriented; for them, creative achievement is an end in itself and requires no further justification. Most professors are strongly convinced of the righteousness of their Protestant ethic of hard work and see little incongruity in imposing it upon the less fortunate.

And yet there are many misguided individuals (perhaps the bulk of the population) who do not share the professor's values and would not be happy in a professor's job. Further, the technical requirements of many lines of work are very different from those of academia. Academic work is best accomplished by those who adhere to academic values, but it is questionable whether these values are equally functional in other lines of work, where creativity is not required to get the job done, but only the ability to follow orders.

In the following paragraphs, I shall seek to reevaluate the personality-versus-organization hypothesis. I shall suggest, first, that it contains many debatable value judgments and, second, that it ignores what Harold Leavitt has called "organizational economics." I shall conclude that a broad range of people do not seek self-actualization on the job—and that this may be a fortunate thing, because it might be prohibitively expensive to redesign some jobs to permit self-actualization.

It seems to me that the hypothesis, as often stated, overemphasizes (1) the uniqueness of the personality-organization conflict to large-scale industry, (2) the universality of the desire to achieve self-actualization, and (3) the importance of the job (as opposed to the community or the home) as a source of need satisfaction. Too little attention is given to economic motivation.

Others are as skeptical as I am of the theory of increased alienation. In his conclusion to a survey of job-satisfaction studies, Robert Blauner questions

. . . the prevailing thesis that most workers in modern society are alienated and estranged. There is a remarkable consistence in the findings that the vast majority of workers, in virtually all occupations and industries, are moderately or highly satisfied, rather than dissatisfied with their jobs. . . . The real character of the [pre—mass production] craftsman's work has been romanticized by the prevalent tendency to idealize the past. . . .[1]

The basic hypothesis implies a strong moral judgment that people should want freedom and self-actualization; that it is somehow morally wrong for people to be lazy, unproductive, and uncreative. It seems to me that the hypothesis overemphasizes individual's desires for freedom and underemphasizes their desire for security. It can even be argued that some of the personality-versus-organization writing has a fairly antisocial, even nihilistic flavor; it seems to emphasize individual freedom and self-development as the all-important value. Yet, mature behavior does not mean freedom from all restrictions; it means successful adjustment to them.

There is an additional value judgment in the basic hypothesis that the *job* should be a primary form of need satisfaction for everyone (as it is for professors). But the central focus of many people's lives is not the job, but the home or the community. Many people find a full measure of challenge, creativity, and autonomy in raising a family, pursuing a hobby, or taking part in community affairs.

Kerr, Harbison, Dunlop, and Myers predict work, in the future, will doubtless be increasingly programmed and will provide fewer and fewer opportunities for creativity and discretion on the job. On the other hand, the hours will grow shorter, and there will be a new "bohemianism" off the job. All this suggests the irreverent notion that *perhaps* the best use of our resources is to accelerate automation, shorten the workweek just as fast as possible, forget about on-the-job satisfactions, and concentrate our energies on making leisure more meaningful.

At the same time that the hypothesis overemphasizes the job as a source of need satisfaction it also underemphasizes the role of money as a means of motivation. The hypothesis says that once employees obtain a satisfying level of economic reward, they go on to other needs and, presumably, are less concerned with money. However, the level of reward that is *satisfying* can rise rapidly over time. Further, money is a means of satisfying high needs, too—such as ego and, for some, self-actualization, e.g., the individual who (perhaps misguidedly) seeks to live his life off the job engaging in "creative" consumption. True, employees expect much better physical, psychological, and social conditions on the job today than they did fifty years ago. But they also expect more money. There is little evidence that money has ceased to be a prime motivator.

Carried to excess, anxiety and aggression are undoubtedly harmful to the organization and the individual. There is much more doubt about apathy and conformity. It is often argued that an apathetic worker who is subject to "hygienic" supervision will work only enough to avoid getting fired, that he will never exercise creativity or imagination or execute an outstanding performance. On many jobs, however, management has no use for outstanding performance. What is outstanding performance on the part of an assembly-line worker? That he works faster than the line? That he shows creativity and imagination on the job? Management wants none of these. *Adequate* performance is all that can be used on the assembly-line and probably on a growing number of other jobs in our society. Here the conformable, dependent worker may well be the best.

Considerable evidence leads to the conclusion that a relatively stable situation can exist, in which workers perform relatively routine, programmed jobs under hygienic supervision. Though these workers may not be satisfied (in the Herzberg sense), they are not actively dissatisfied; they do not feel a need for additional responsibility; and they seek meaning in life from their home and community rather than from their jobs. To be sure, these individuals are maximizing neither their productive efforts nor their possible satisfaction. But both management and employees find the situation suffices for their needs. It may well be the best we are likely to get in many situations without costly changes in such important matters as technology and child upbringing.

[1] "Work Satisfaction and Industrial Trends in Modern Society," in *Labour and Trade Unionism,* ed. Walter Galenson and Seymour Martin Lipset (New York: John Wiley, 1960), pp. 352–53.

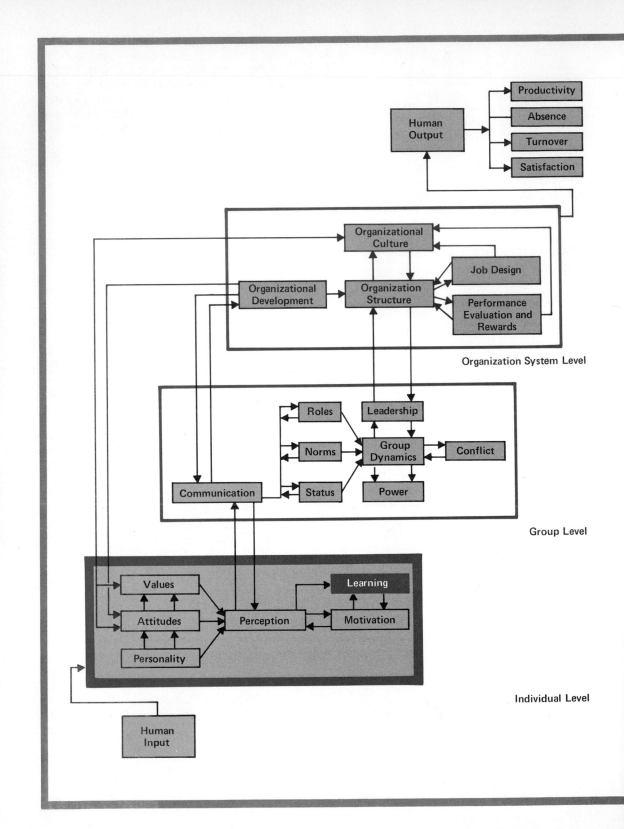

CHAPTER 7
Learning

AFTER STUDYING THIS CHAPTER, YOU SHOULD BE ABLE TO—

Define and explain the following key terms and concepts:

Classical conditioning
Conditioning
Continuous reinforcers
Fixed-interval schedule
Fixed-ratio schedule
Intermittent reinforcers
Learning
Operant conditioning

Positive reinforcement
Primary reinforcers
Punishment
Reinforcement
Secondary reinforcers
Shaping behavior
Variable-interval schedule
Variable-ratio schedule

Understand:

Why all behavior is learned
How learning theories provide insights into changing behavior
The concept of conditioning
The difference between classical and operant conditioning
The four schedules of reinforcement
The role of punishment in learning

> If you give me a dozen healthy infants and required me to select one at random, I could train him to be anything irrespective of his talents and predilection.
>
> —J.B. WATSON

The knowledge and skills that each of us possess today are something that we have acquired. You were not born with the knowledge that red lights mean stop and that Columbus discovered America in 1492, or with the skills of reading, writing, and politely turning down invitations to parties you expect to be a bore. These were acquired; that is, they have been learned. Similarly, people bring to their jobs a wealth of knowledge and skills that have been acquired in the years preceding their employment.

Certain behaviors that are desirable for employees to exhibit—being to work on time, following directions, obeying rules, doing a good job—are, for the most part, learned before we ever seek gainful employment. The fact that some people are chronically late for work, while the majority are prompt, suggests that some individuals have learned different work habits. Since most of the things people do on their job have been learned, if we want to explain and predict this behavior, we need a fundamental understanding of the concepts and processes of learning. An understanding of how people learn will also prove beneficial when we find employees behaving in ways that we consider undesirable. Why? Because change requires unlearning or extinguishing the old behaviors and re-learning new behaviors.

LEARNING AND MOTIVATION

In the previous chapter we discussed motivation. The concepts underlying motivation are also basic to understanding learning. Motivation concepts are fundamental to an understanding of learning because, without motivation, learning does not take place. There must be a stimulus, a need, and a drive to initiate learning.

In the last chapter, we also introduced reinforcement theory. This theory explained motivation from an external or environmental perspective. We could alter an individual's level of motivation by altering the consequences of his or her behavior. Reinforcement theory will be expanded upon in this chapter to show that most work-related behaviors are shaped by the environment. The way organizations manage that environment—for instance, the manner in which they pay people, the criteria they choose for giving promotions, or the frequency with which they praise a job well done—will significantly influence how employees learn and behave. There is no "looking the other way." If decision makers in organizations do not take positive action to manage their environment, it will be managed by accident. Of course, it is better that things happen by plan than by accident. Reinforcement theory offers insights into how to manage the learning process. If an employee's behavior is satisfactory, we shall want to maintain it; that is, we want to ensure that the desirable behavior is not eliminated. On the other hand, if an employee's behavior is unsatisfactory, we may want to change it.

A DEFINITION OF LEARNING

What is learning? A psychologist's definition is considerably broader than the lay person's view that "it's what we did when we went to school." In actuality, each of us is continuously going "to school." Learning is going on all the time. A generally accepted definition of learning is, therefore, *any relatively permanent change in behavior that occurs as a result of experience.* Ironically, we can say that changes in behavior indicate learning has taken place, and that learning is a change in behavior.

Obviously, the above definition suggests that we shall never see someone "learning." We can see changes, but not the learning itself. The concept is theoretical and hence not directly observable.

> You have seen people in the process of learning, you have seen people who behave in a particular way as a result of learning, and some of you (in fact, I guess the majority of you) have "learned" at some time in your life. In other words, we infer that learning has taken place if an individual behaves, reacts, responds as a result of experience in a manner different from the way he formerly behaved.[1]

Our definition has several components that deserve clarification. First, learning involves change. This may be good or bad from an organizational point of view. People can learn unfavorable behaviors—to hold prejudices or to restrict their output, for example—as well as favorable behaviors. Second, the change must be relatively permanent. Temporary changes may be only reflexive and fail to represent any learning. Therefore, this requirement rules out behavioral changes caused by fatigue or temporary adaptations. Third, our definition is concerned with behavior. Learning takes place where there is a change in actions. A change in an individual's thought process or attitudes, if accompanied by no change in behavior, would not be learning. Finally, some form of experience is necessary for learning. This may be acquired directly through observation or practice. Or, it may result from indirect experiences, such as that acquired through reading. The crucial test still remains: Does this experience result in a relatively permanent change in behavior? If the answer is "Yes," we can say that learning has taken place.

1. William McGehee, "Are We Using What We Know About Training?—Learning Theory and Training," *Personnel Psychology,* Spring 1958, p. 2.

RELEVANCE OF LEARNING TO OB

How is learning relevant to explaining and predicting behavior? A candid answer would acknowledge that it is probably of less value than some of the subjects of our previous discussions: values, attitudes, perception, and motivation. This, of course, does not mean that learning is irrelevant.

Much of the traditional literature dealing with learning is interesting to read, but the relevance of the material to the explaining and predicting of OB is marginal. On the other hand, there are topics that are important to OB. What we shall do in this chapter, therefore, is emphasize the concepts in learning that have direct impact on explaining and predicting behavior. Though learning offers important insights for those interested in "controlling" behavior, we shall downplay the control dimension and stress the descriptive aspects.

What are some key questions in OB that learning may help to provide answers to? It can help us to answer questions such as: Do we learn personality characteristics such as high achievement or anxiety? Can we change the particular values, attitudes, perceptions, personalities, or motivational levels that individuals hold?

Learning certainly has direct impact on training activities within the personnel function of an organization. It can give insights into how to best develop the talents and skills that employees will need to perform effectively. But it is the desire to change individuals that is probably of the greatest importance. The manager who undertakes to produce such changes can be likened to a teacher. He or she attempts to instruct the employee to engage in behaviors that will help the organization achieve its objectives. When individuals are late for work, sloppy, disobey directives, or engage in other types of dysfunctional behavior, the manager will attempt to teach more functional behaviors. When the employee is performing satisfactorily, the manager-teacher will need to give the employee feedback and other forms of rewards so as to maintain or strengthen these desirable behaviors.

We have already acknowledged that individuals enter an organization with a wealth of learned attitudes and behaviors. Their performance on the job is a function of their previously learned experiences. Additionally, individuals continue to learn every day on their job. Most importantly, an understanding of learning will explain why what a manager does significantly influences whether these day-to-day learning experiences will strengthen, maintain, or weaken an employee's behavior.

Learning can also be used as the prime explanation of why employers prefer to hire people with college degrees or considerable job experience, rather than individuals with only a high school education or no prior relevant experience. The employer assumes that not only have education or experience provided learning, but that learning can result in higher job performance. It is assumed that people with relevant job experience have learned more about the job, that they have acquired greater skills as a result of this learning, and that the application of these greater skills to the job will result in higher performance on the job, than if the individual had no experience. Similarly, organizations often pay more for recent graduates of four-year colleges than for individuals with four years of practical working experience. While market factors clearly influence these differences, the market rate for the college-trained applicant is usually higher because of the assumption that college better prepares an individual for the long term—that college exposure increases the potential of the individual to be more valuable to the organization.

In summary, much of the behavior we exhibit on our jobs has been learned prior to taking the job. The purpose of this chapter will be to first explain how we learned the behaviors we bring with us into the organization. From a secondary perspective, we are interested in understanding learning concepts since they provide a basis for changing the behaviors that we find unacceptable and maintaining those that are acceptable. This chapter will demonstrate that if you want to know how people are going to behave, look at how they perceive the consequences of that behavior.

CONDITIONING

Conditioning is often used as a synonym for learning, but more properly it refers to the process of acquiring a pattern of behavior. There are two main types of conditioning—*classical conditioning* and *operant conditioning*.

Classical Conditioning

Classical conditioning grew out of experiments, to teach dogs to salivate in response to the ringing of a bell, conducted by a Russian physiologist, Ivan Pavlov.

A simple surgical procedure allowed Pavlov to accurately measure the amount of saliva secreted by a dog. When Pavlov presented the dog with a piece of meat, it resulted in a noticeable increase in salivation. When Pavlov withheld the presentation of meat and merely rang a bell, the dog had no salivation. Then, Pavlov proceeded to link the meat and the ringing of the bell. After repeatedly hearing the bell before getting the food, the dog began to salivate as soon as the bell rang. After awhile, the dog would salivate merely at the sound of the bell, even if no food was offered. What had happened was that the dog had learned to respond—that is, salivate—to the bell. Let's review this experiment to introduce the key concepts in classical conditioning.

The meat was an *unconditioned stimulus;* it invariably caused the dog to react in a specific way. The reaction that took place whenever the unconditioned stimulus occurred was called the *unconditioned response* (or the noticeable increase in salivation, in this case). The bell was an artificial stimulus, or what we call the *conditioned stimulus*. While it was originally neutral, when the bell was paired with the meat (an unconditioned stimulus), it eventually produced a response when presented alone. The last key concept is the *conditioned response*. This describes the behavior of the dog salivating in reaction to the bell alone.

Using the above concepts, we can summarize classical conditioning. Essentially, learning a conditioned response involves building up an association between a conditioned stimulus and an unconditioned stimulus. Using the paired stimuli, one compelling and the other one neutral, the neutral one becomes a conditioned stimulus and, hence, takes on the properties of the unconditioned stimulus.

Classical conditioning can be used to explain why Christmas carols often bring back pleasant memories of childhood—the songs being associated with the festive Christmas spirit and initiating fond memories and feelings of euphoria. In an organizational setting, we can also see classical conditioning operating. For example, at one manufacturing plant, every time the top executives from the head office would make a visit, the plant management would clean up the administrative offices and wash the windows. This went on for years. Eventually, employees would turn on their best behavior and look prim and proper whenever the windows were cleaned—even in those occasional instances when the cleaning was not paired with the visit from the top brass. People had learned to associate the cleaning of the windows with the visit from the head office.

Classical conditioning is passive. Something happens and we react in a specific way. It is elicited in response to a specific, identifiable event. As such it can explain simple reflexive behaviors. But most behavior—particularly the complex behavior of individuals in organizations—is emitted rather than elicited. It is voluntary rather than reflexive. For example, employees choose to arrive at work on time, ask their boss for help with problems, or "goof off" when no one is watching. The learning of these behaviors is better understood by looking at operant conditioning.

Operant Conditioning

Operant conditioning argues that behavior is a function of its consequences. People learn to behave so they get something they want or avoid something they don't want. Operant behavior means voluntary or learned behavior in contrast to reflexive or unlearned behavior. The tendency to repeat such behavior is influenced as a result of the reinforcement or lack of reinforcement brought about by the consequences of the behavior. Reinforcement, therefore, strengthens a behavior and increases the likelihood that it will be repeated.

What Pavlov did for classical conditioning, noted Harvard psychologist B.F. Skinner has done for operant conditioning. Building on earlier work in the field, Skinner's research has extensively expanded our knowledge of operant conditioning. Even his staunchest critics, who represent a sizable group, admit that his operant concepts work.

Behavior is assumed to be determined from without—that is, learned—rather than from within (reflexive or unlearned). Skinner argues that by creating pleasing consequences to follow specific forms of behavior, the frequency of that behavior will increase. People will most likely engage in desired behaviors if they are positively reinforced for doing so. Rewards, for example, are most effective if they immediately follow the desired response. Additionally, behavior that is not rewarded, or is punished, is less likely to be repeated.

You see illustrations of operant conditioning everywhere. For example, any situation in which it is either explicitly stated or implicitly suggested that reinforcements are contingent on some action on your part involves the use of operant learning. Your instructor says that if you want a high grade in the course you must supply correct answers on the test. A commissioned salesperson wanting to earn a sizable income finds that it is contingent on generating high sales in her territory. Of course, the linkage can also work to teach the individual to engage in behaviors that work against the best interests of the organization. Assume your boss tells you that if you will work overtime during the next three-week busy season, you will be compensated for it at the next performance appraisal. However, when performance appraisal time comes you find that you are given no positive reinforcement for your overtime work. The next time your boss asks you to work overtime, what will you do? You will probably decline! Your behavior can be explained by operant conditioning: If a behavior fails to be positively reinforced, the probability that the behavior will be repeated declines.

SHAPING: A MANAGERIAL TOOL

Because learning takes place on the job as well as prior to it, managers will be concerned with how they can teach employees to behave in ways that most benefit the organization. When we attempt to mold individuals by guiding their learning in graduated steps, we are shaping behavior.

Consider the situation in which an employee's behavior is significantly different from that sought by management. If management only reinforced the individual when he showed desirable responses, there might be very little reinforcement taking place. In such a case, shaping offers a logical approach toward achieving the desired behavior.

We *shape* behavior by systematically reinforcing each successive step that moves the individual closer to the desired response. If an employee who has been chronically a half-hour late for work comes in only twenty minutes late, we can reinforce this improvement. Reinforcement would increase as responses more closely approximate the desired behavior.

In this section, we shall differentiate between primary and secondary reinforcers, identity methods for shaping behavior, and introduce varying schedules for applying the shaping methods.

Primary and Secondary Reinforcers

As noted previously, a reinforcer is anything that increases the strength of a behavior. A reward that accompanies or follows a behavior is the reinforcer of that behavior. All reinforcers, however, are not the same. Some are primary and others are secondary. For the most part, organizations can allocate only secondary reinforcers.

A primary reinforcer is rewarding in and of itself, and its effects are independent of past experiences. Food, water, sex, and sleep are examples of these rewards. Primary reinforcers are instinctual needs and are not learned. While important from a theoretical point of view, primary reinforcers have little relevance to understanding complex behavior in organizations.

Secondary reinforcers are conditioned needs that we have learned to value. Probably the best example of a secondary reinforcer is money—a basic reward that organizations bestow on their employees and that allows employees to obtain primary reinforcers. Other secondary reinforcers include such rewards as prestige, praise, fame, affection, attention, approval, and recognition. The effectiveness of a reinforcer depends upon the individual, his reinforcement history, and what he perceives as rewarding.

What is the importance of acknowledging two types of reinforcers? The answer is that organizationally relevant reinforcers are secondary. They must be learned through association with other reinforcers because they are not habitual or basic. Our discussion of shaping will focus on secondary reinforcers, since they are the ones that are available to managers.

Methods of Shaping Behavior

There are three ways to shape behavior: through positive reinforcement, negative reinforcement, or punishment. When a response is followed with something pleasant, it is called *positive reinforcement*. This would describe, for instance, the boss who praises an employee for a job well done. When a response is followed by the termination or withdrawal of something unpleasant, it is called *negative reinforcement*. If your college instructor asks a question and you don't know the answer, looking through your lecture notes is likely to avoid your being called on. This is a negative reinforcement because you have learned that looking busily through your notes terminates being called on by the instructor. *Punishment* is causing an unpleasant condition in an attempt to eliminate an undesirable behavior. An employee who receives a two-day suspension from work, without pay, for showing up drunk is an example of punishment.

Both positive and negative reinforcement result in learning. They strengthen a desired response and increase the probability of repetition. In the above illustrations, praise strengthens and increases the behavior of doing a good job because praise is desired. The behavior of "looking busy" is similarly strengthened and increased by it terminating the undesirable consequence of being called on by the teacher. Punishment, however, weakens behavior and tends to decrease its subsequent frequency.

Reinforcement, whether it is positive or negative, has an impressive record as a shaping tool. Our interest, therefore, is in reinforcement rather than punishment. A review of research findings on the impact of reinforcement upon behavior in organizations concluded that:

1. Some type of reinforcement is necessary to produce a change in behavior.
2. Some types of rewards are more effective for use in organizations than others.
3. The speed with which learning takes place and the lasting of its effects will be determined by the timing of reinforcement.[2]

Point 3 is extremely important and deserves considerable elaboration.

Schedules of Reinforcement

The two major types of reinforcement schedules are *continuous* and *intermittent*. A continuous schedule reinforces the desired behavior each and every time it is demonstrated. For example, in the case of someone who has historically had trouble being at work on time, every time he is *not* tardy his manager might compliment him on this desirable behavior. In an intermittent schedule, on the other hand, not every instance of the desirable behavior is reinforced, but reinforcement is given often enough to make the behavior worth repeating. This latter schedule can be compared to the workings of a gambling slot machine, which people will continue to play even when they know that it is adjusted to give a considerable return to the gambling house. The intermittent payoffs occur just often enough to reinforce the behavior of slipping in quarters and pulling the handle. Evidence indicates that the intermittent or varied form of reinforcement tends to promote more resistance to extinction or elimination than does the continuous form.[3]

An intermittent reinforcement can be of a ratio or interval type. Ratio schedules depend upon how many responses the subject makes. The individual is reinforced after giving a certain number of specific types of behavior. Interval schedules depend upon how much time has passed since the last reinforcement. With interval schedules, the individual is reinforced on the first appropriate behavior after a particular time has elapsed. A reinforcement can also be classified as fixed or variable. Intermittent techniques for administering rewards can, therefore, be placed into four categories, as shown in Figure 7–1.

2. Timothy W. Costello and Sheldon S. Zalkind, *Psychology in Administration* (Englewood Cliffs, N.J.: Prentice-Hall, 1963), p. 193.

3. Fred Luthans and Robert Kreitner, *Organizational Behavior Modification* (Glenview, Ill.: Scott, Foresman, 1975), pp. 49–52.

FIGURE 7–1 Schedules of Reinforcement

	Ratio	Interval
Fixed	Fixed–ratio	Fixed–interval
Variable	Variable–ratio	Variable–interval

Fixed-Ratio Schedule. After a fixed or constant number of responses are given, a reward is initiated. For example, a piece-rate incentive plan is a fixed-ratio schedule—the employee receives a reward based on the number of work pieces generated. If the piece rate for a zipper installer in a dressmaking factory is $5.00 a dozen, the reinforcement (money in this case) is fixed to the number of zippers sewn into garments. After every dozen is sewn in, the installer has earned another $5.00.

Fixed-Interval Schedule. When rewards are spaced at uniform time intervals, the reinforcement schedule is of the fixed-interval type. The critical variable is time, and it is held constant. This is the predominant schedule for almost all salaried workers in North America. When you get your paycheck on a weekly, semimonthly, monthly, or other predetermined time basis, you are rewarded on a fixed-interval reinforcement schedule.

Variable-Ratio Schedule. When the reward varies relative to the behavior of the individual, he or she is said to be reinforced on a variable-ratio schedule. Salespeople on commission represent examples of individuals on such a reinforcement schedule. On some occasions, they may make a sale after only two calls on potential customers. On other occasions, they might need to make twenty or more calls to secure a sale. The reward, then, is variable in relation to the number of successful calls the salesperson makes.

Variable-Interval Schedule. If rewards are distributed in time so that reinforcements are unpredictable, the schedule is of the variable-interval type. When an instructor advises her class there will be a number of pop quizzes given during the term (the exact number of which is unknown to the students), and the quizzes will account for 20 percent of the term grade, she is using such a variable-interval schedule. Similarly, a series of randomly timed unannounced visits to a company office by the corporate audit staff is an example of a variable-interval schedule.

Reinforcement Schedules and Behavior

In general, variable schedules tend to lead to higher performance than fixed schedules. For example, as noted previously, most employees in organizations are paid on fixed-interval schedules. But such a schedule does not clearly link performance and rewards. The reward is given for time spent on the job rather than for a specific response (performance). In contrast, variable-interval schedules generate high rates of response and more stable and consistent behavior because of a high correlation between performance and reward, and because of the uncertainty involved—the employee tends to be more alert since there is a surprise factor.

A summary of the effects that the various reinforcement schedules have on behavior is provided in Figure 7–2.

FIGURE 7–2 Reinforcement Schedules and Their Effects

SCHEDULE	DESCRIPTION	EFFECTS ON RESPONDING
Continuous (CRF)	Reinforcer follows every response.	1. Steady high rate of performance as long as reinforcement continues to follow every response. 2. High frequency of reinforcement may lead to early satiation. 3. Behavior weakens rapidly (undergoes extinction) when reinforcers are withheld. 4. Appropriate for newly emitted, unstable, or low-frequency responses.
Intermittent	Reinforcer does not follow every response.	1. Capable of producing high frequencies of responding. 2. Low frequency of reinforcement precludes early satiation. 3. Appropriate for stable or high-frequency responses.
Fixed-ratio (FR)	A fixed number of responses must be emitted before reinforcement occurs.	1. A fixed ratio of 1:1 (reinforcement occurs after every response) is the same as a continuous schedule. 2. Tends to produce a high rate of response which is vigorous and steady.
Variable-ratio (VR)	A varying or random number of responses must be emitted before reinforcement occurs.	1. Capable of producing a high rate of response which is vigorous, steady, and resistant to extinction.
Fixed-interval (FI)	The first response after a specific period of time has elapsed is reinforced.	1. Produces an uneven response pattern varying from a very slow, unenergetic response immediately following reinforcement to a very fast, vigorous response immediately preceding reinforcement.
Variable-interval (VI)	The first response after varying or random periods of time have elapsed is reinforced.	1. Tends to produce a high rate of response which is vigorous, steady, and resistant to extinction.

Source: From *Organizational Behavior Modification* by Fred Luthans and Robert Kreitner. Copyright © 1975 by Scott, Foresman and Company. Reprinted by permission.

IMPLICATIONS FOR PERFORMANCE
AND SATISFACTION

Any observable change in behavior is, by definition, prima facie evidence that learning has taken place. What we want to do, of course, is ascertain if learning concepts provide us with any insights that would allow us to explain and predict behavior. The evidence suggests that conditioning and shaping offer important tools for explaining levels of productivity, absenteeism rates, lateness, and the quality of employees' workmanship. These concepts also can be valuable for giving insight into how undesirable work behaviors can be modified.

Let us begin our analysis of the impact of learning on behavior by looking at the subject of superstition. Even rational and educated people who accept the logical approach of the scientific method find themselves occasionally guided by superstition. We can demonstrate that one of the causes for superstitious behavior is accidental response contingencies.

You attended a movie the night before you got an "A" on an examination. If you believe that somehow the seeing of the movie and the "A" grade were related in a causal fashion, you may believe you should go to movies before every class exam. A salesman wears his "lucky shoes" when he attempts to close his largest sale because "they" worked before—that is, the wearing of a specific pair of shoes apparently resulted in a favorable outcome. If he makes the sale, the wearing of these shoes will be further reinforced and repeated. If repeated often enough, it will eventually be reinforced again by another large sale. The end result will be the superstitious belief in a learned behavior: Particular shoes produce big sales.

Our discussion of superstition is meant to demonstrate that conditioning patterns and schedules will influence how people behave on their job. Specifically, let us look at reinforcement schedules and some examples of how positive reinforcement has been used to increase worker productivity and reduce absenteeism and tardiness.

Continuous reinforcement is initially used with weak responses or responses roughly approximating the desired productive responses. Positive reinforcement for satisfactory work is experienced, perhaps for many of the hard-core unemployables for the first time. As the work responses grow stronger and more accurate, the reinforcement is switched to a variable-ratio basis in order to facilitate stable performance and high rates of responding.[4]

Administering reward under a fixed-ratio schedule tends to produce a high rate of response which is characterized as vigorous and steady. The person soon determines that reinforcement is based on a number of responses and performs the responses as quickly as possible in order to receive the reward.[5]

Behavior resulting from a fixed-interval method of reinforcing is quite different from that exhibited by a fixed-ratio. Whereas under fixed-ratio there is a steady, vigorous response pattern, under fixed-interval there is an uneven pattern that varies from a very slow, unenergetic response immediately following reinforcement to a very fast, vigorous response immediately

4. Ibid., p. 55.

5. Fred Luthans, *Organizational Behavior,* 2nd ed. (New York: McGraw-Hill, 1977), p. 298.

preceding reinforcement. This type of behavior pattern can be explained by the fact that the person figures out that another reward will not immediately follow the last one. Therefore, the person may as well relax a little until it is time to be rewarded again.[6]

Both variable-ratio and variable-interval schedules tend to produce stable, vigorous behavior. The behavior under variable schedules is similar to that produced by a fixed-ratio schedule. Under the variable schedules, the person has no idea when reward is coming, so the behavior tends to be steady and strong.[7]

What is the role of punishment in learning? The evidence suggests that reinforcement is a more effective tool. "The punished behavior tends to be only temporarily suppressed rather than permanently changed, and the punished person tends to get anxious or 'up-tight' and resentful of the punisher."[8] Even though punishment eliminates undesired behavior more quickly than negative reinforcement does, its effect is only temporary and may later produce unpleasant side effects such as lower morale and higher absenteeism or turnover.

One of the most frequently cited organizational success stories in the use of positive reinforcement has been at Emery Air Freight.[9] Emery reports that over a three-year period, $2 million was saved in three divisions by identifying performance-related behaviors and strengthening them with positive reinforcement.

In one area, Emery sought to have freight containers used for shipments whenever possible because of specific economic savings. When employees were queried as to the percentage of shipments containerized, the standard reply was "90 percent." An analysis by Emery found, however, that the container utilization rate was only 45 percent. In order to encourage employees to use containers, Emery established a program of feedback and positive reinforcements. Each packer kept a checklist of his daily packings, both containerized and noncontainerized. At the end of each day, he computed his container utilization rate. Almost unbelievably, container utilization jumped to more than 90 percent on the first day of the program and held to that level.

Applications of positive reinforcement have also been reported by such organizations as Addressograph-Multigraph, Collins Foods International, and Dayton Hudson department stores.[10] Addressograph-Multigraph held a series of meetings between management and employees to discuss mutual needs and problems and propose solutions. At these meetings, management set standards for job performance and outlined how they were to be met, and employees identified their needs and provided a list of reinforcers to management that would help them to achieve the standards. For instance, these meetings identified that what clerk typists wanted most was a sense of belonging, a sense of

6. Ibid., p. 298.

7. Ibid., p. 299.

8. Ibid., p. 301.

9. E.J. Feeney, "At Emery Air Freight: Positive Reinforcement Boosts Performance," *Organizational Dynamics*, Winter 1973, pp. 41–50.

10. "Productivity Gains from a Pat on the Back," *Business Week*, January 23, 1978, pp. 56–62.

accomplishment, and a sense of teamwork. In return, management asked for a quicker filing on reports with fewer errors.

At Collins Foods, a reinforcement program was introduced for clerical employees in the accounting department. Supervisors and employees first met to review the department's actual performance in such areas as billing error rates. Based on this data, improvement goals were established. Employees were praised for reports containing fewer errors than the norm, and results were charted on a regular basis. Significant results were achieved; for example, the error rate in accounts payable fell from more than 8 percent to less than 0.2 percent.

Dayton Hudson experimented with reinforcement in the men's department of one of its stores. The goal was to increase the average sale from $19 to $25. Employees were taught how to make extra sales and were congratulated by supervisors each time a sale went above $19. Within two months, department sales averaged $23.

There are also impressive reports of positive reinforcement being used to cut employee absenteeism and tardiness. One researcher tells how a hardware chain established an employee lottery with monthly prizes awarded, and an additional separate larger lottery held twice a year.[11] The top monthly prize was a $25 appliance; the big prize in the larger drawing was a color television set. A monthly prize was allocated for every twenty-five employees, and each store had its own monthly lottery. The catch was that only employees who had perfect attendance and no tardiness in the prior month were eligible to participate in each month's lottery.

The impact of the lottery on employee behavior was impressive. In the first year of the program, absenteeism and tardiness were reduced to approximately one quarter of their previous rate and sick payments were reduced by 62 percent.

A similar lottery program was implemented by an electronics manufacturer in one of its plants.[12] The result: a 30.6 percent decrease in company sick-leave expenses that translated into a $3,100 savings. This savings was achieved at a total program cost of only $110.

Many organizations' personnel policies ignore the impact that positive reinforcement can have on expensive benefits such as sick pay. For the most part, rather than rewarding people for being on the job, reinforcement—in this case, money—rewards absenteeism. In organizations where employees are allowed, say, ten days' sick leave with pay each year, it is not surprising that the vast majority of them consume their full allotment of gratis days. If behavior is truly a function of its consequences, our personnel practices should be adjusted to pay employees something every day for being at work and to omit pay during absent periods. This concept was applied at a Mexican division of a large U.S. cor-

11. Walter Nord, "Improving Attendance Through Rewards," *Personnel Administration,* November-December 1970, pp. 37–41.

12. Jerry A. Wallin and Ronald D. Johnson, "The Positive Reinforcement Approach to Controlling Employee Absenteeism," *Personnel Journal,* August 1976, pp. 390–92.

poration in order to deal with chronic tardiness. Workers were given a small cash bonus, equal to approximately 3 percent of their basic daily wage, for each day they reported to work on or before the designated starting time. The result was a clearly lower level of worker tardiness. By altering the consequences, the researchers similarly altered the behavior.[13]

The telephone company has also experimented with positive reinforcement as a technique for reducing absence.[14] In one unit, thirty-eight operators averaged an 11 percent absentee rate in spite of a company-based attendance recognition plan. The problem was that this plan was calculated on the group's monthly attendance performance. Operators felt that if they missed a day early in the month there was little motivation to seek perfection through the rest of the month, since their individual and group record was already tarnished. To deal with this demotivating factor in the plan, attendance records were changed to a weekly basis. Supervisors were also encouraged to give positive vocal comment on operators' attendance records. These changes resulted in a drop in the group's absentee rate from 11 to 6.5 percent within several weeks. When this program was expanded to over 1,000 operators, absenteeism dropped from 7.5 to 4.5 percent in a three-month period.

FOR DISCUSSION

1. How do we know if someone has "learned" something?

2. Learning theory can be used to *explain* behavior and to *control* behavior. Distinguish between the two objectives. Can you think of any ethical or moral arguments why managers should not seek control over others' behavior? How valid do you think these arguments are?

3. What is the difference between classical and operant conditioning? Give examples of each.

4. What is the difference between positive and negative reinforcement?

5. What do we mean by "shaping" behavior?

6. Contrast primary with secondary reinforcers. Is one more relevant in the study of OB? If so, which? Why?

7. Identify, discuss, and give examples of four reinforcement schedules.

8. What have you "learned" in this chapter that could help you to explain the behavior of students in a classroom given (a) the instructor gives only one test—a final examination at the end of the course? (b) the instructor gives four exams during the term, all of which are announced on the first day of class? (c) the student's grade is based on the results of numerous exams, none of which are announced by the instructor ahead of time?

13. J.A. Hermann, A.I. de Montes, B. Dominguez, F. Montes, and B.L. Hopkins, "Effects of Bonuses for Punctuality on the Tardiness of Industrial Workers," *Journal of Applied Behavioral Analysis*, Winter 1973, pp. 563–70.

14. "Where Skinner's Theories Work," *Business Week*, December 2, 1972, p. 54.

HILGARD, E. R., and G. H. BOWER, *Theories of Learning,* 4th ed. Englewood Cliffs, N.J.: Prentice-Hall, 1975. Reviews theories of learning expounded by major schools of thought and associated with major intellectual figures to provide an understanding of modern learning theory, its historical context, and background.

JABLONSKY, S. F., and D. L. DEVRIES, "Operant Conditioning Principles Extrapolated to the Theory of Management," *Organizational Behavior and Human Performance,* April 1972, pp. 340–58. Presents a predictive model of individual behavior based on both operant conditioning and management literatures.

MINER, J. B., "Behavior Modification and Operant Learning," in *Theories of Organizational Behavior.* Hinsdale, Ill: Dryden Press, 1980, pp. 201–30. Reviews the evidence on behavior modification and its relevance to management practice.

MAWHINNEY, T. C., "Operant Terms and Concepts in the Description of Individual Work Behavior: Some Problems of Interpretation, Application, and Evaluation," *Journal of Applied Psychology,* December 1975, pp. 704–12. Good review of the applicability of operant conditioning to organizational behavior.

SCHNEIER, C. E., "Behavior Modification in Management: A Review and Critique," *Academy of Management Journal,* September 1974, pp. 528–48. Reviews studies explaining operant principles, organizational research testing these principles, and work done to date regarding applications of behavior modification in organizations.

SKINNER, B. F., *Beyond Freedom and Dignity.* New York: Knopf, 1971. A technology of behavior begins by destroying the assumption of man as a free and autonomous being.

LOCKE

The myths of behavior mod in organizations

Adapted and edited from Edwin A. Locke, "The Myths of Behavior Mod in Organizations," Academy of Management Review, *October 1977, pp. 543–53. With permission.*

Behaviorism asserts that human behavior can be understood without reference to states or actions of consciousness. Its basic premises are:

1. Determinism: With respect to their choices, beliefs, and actions individuals are ruled by forces beyond their control (according to behaviorism, these forces are environmental). Individuals are totally devoid of volition.

2. Epiphenomenalism: People's minds have no causal efficacy; their thoughts are mere by-products of environmental conditioning and affect neither their other thoughts nor their observable actions.

3. Rejection of introspection as a scientific method. It is unscientific, and its results (the identification of people's mental contents and processes) are irrelevant to understanding their actions.

The major theoretical concept in Skinner's version of behaviorism, the one most often applied to industry, is that of reinforcement. Behavior, Skinner argues, is controlled by its consequences. A reinforcer is some consequence which follows a response and makes similar responses more likely in the future. To change the probability of a given response, one merely modifies either the contingency between the response and the reinforcer or the reinforcer itself. The concept of reinforcement is, by design, devoid of any theoretical base, e.g., the experiences of pleasure and pain. The term is defined by its effects on behavior and only by these effects. Reinforcements modify responses automatically, independent of the organism's values, beliefs or mental processes, i.e., independent of consciousness.

While this theory of behavior may be appealing in its simplicity, the facts of human behavior do not correspond to it. All behavior is not controlled by reinforcements given to an acting organism. People can learn a new response by seeing other people get reinforced for that response; this is called "vicarious reinforcement." People sometimes learn by imitating others who are not reinforced for their actions; this is called "vicarious learning." Some behaviorists now acknowledge that people can control their own thoughts and actions by "talking to themselves," i.e., thinking. This is called "self-reinforcement" or "self-instruction." These last two concepts flatly contradict the assumption of determinism.

Recent experiments and reviews of the learning literature have further undermined the behaviorist position. Not only do an individual's values, knowledge, and intentions have a profound effect on behavior, but even the simplest forms of learning may not occur in the absence of conscious awareness on the part of the learner.

One thesis to be explored here is that "behavior mod" applications to industry do not actually rest on behaviorist premises—they do not ignore the employee's consciousness and/or assume it to be irrelevant to the employee's behavior.

If true, this thesis would mean that, since organizational changes do not automatically condition the employee's response, attention must be paid to what the employee *thinks* about such changes. Are they wanted? Are they understood? What are they expected to lead to, etc.?

A second issue concerns the originality of the techniques used by behavior mod practitioners in industry. Because the concept of reinforcement is defined solely by its consequences, if an alleged reinforcer does not reinforce, it is not a reinforcer. If it does, it is. Since the concept of reinforcement itself has no content (no defining characteristics independent of its effects on behavior), how are behavior modifiers to know what to use as reinforcers? In practice, behaviorists must use rewards and incentives which they observe people already acting to gain and/or keep; they must cash in on what they already know or believe people value or need. Thus, when it comes to the choice of reinforcers, behavior mod can offer nothing new. A second thesis is that the actual techniques used by behavior modifiers in industry to "reinforce" behavior are no different from the rewards and incentives already used by nonbehaviorist practitioners in this field or related fields. If this thesis is true, then the claims of originality by behavior mod practitioners are spurious.

Behavior mod advocates might reply that even if the particular reinforcers they use are not new, they do have something original to offer the practicing manager, namely, the idea of contingency. While the contingency idea is emphasized strongly in behaviorism, it is certainly not new. It has been used, if inconsistently, for centuries by animal trainers, parents, diplomats, and employers. Furthermore the principle does not work unless the individual is aware of the contingency. Finally, the principle is of limited usefulness in real-life work situations where the manager cannot control everything that happens to subordinates.

The conclusion is inescapable that behavior mod in industry is neither new or behavioristic. The specific techniques employed by behavior mod advocates have long been used in industry and other fields. What the behaviorists call reinforcers do not condition behavior automatically, but affect action through and in conjunction with the individual's mental contents and processes (integrations, goals, expectancies, etc.). While operant conditioning principles avoid the necessity of dealing with phenomena which are not directly observable, such as the minds of others, for this very reason they lack the capacity to explain human action.

The typical behaviorist response to arguments like the foregoing is, in effect, "Who cares why the procedures work, so long as they work?" This is the kind of pragmatic answer one might expect from primitive witch doctors who are challenged to explain their "cures." One has the right to expect more from a modern-day scientist.

Unless one knows why and how something "works," one does not know *when* it will work or even *that* it will work in a given circumstance. Many things which behaviorists do to change behavior, do, in fact, change it. But many of them do not, and most behaviorists do not have the slightest idea what accounts for these inconsistencies. Post hoc speculations about past conditioning or improper scheduling of the reinforcements do not solve this problem.

As several writers have pointed out, there are numerous contextual assumptions which are untrue, nonuniversal, or inappropriate in most applied settings, which behaviorists make when applying their techniques. Examples are the assumptions that individuals are basically passive responders to external stimulation; and that when subjects are being exposed to reinforcers, they will not think about what is happening, talk to anyone else about it, focus on the long-term implications, or consider their own goals.

There is a common element in the above assumptions, a premise which underlies and unites all of the behaviorist theories of human behavior and of management. It is the premise that *humans do not possess a conceptual faculty*. While Skinner does not openly deny that people have minds, he does assert that the environment is the ultimate cause of all thinking and action. *But if mind is an epiphenomenon, then, for all practical purposes, it does not exist.*

Since people can choose to think (a fact which can be validated by introspection), the behaviorist view of human nature is false. Thus the claim that behaviorism, taken literally, can serve as a valid guide to understanding and modifying human behavior in organizations is a myth.

COUNTER POINT

GRAY

The myths of the myths about behavior mod in organizations

Adapted and edited from Jerry L. Gray, "The Myths of the Myths About Behavior Mod in Organizations; A reply to Locke's Criticisms of Behavior Modification," Academy of Management Review, *January 1979, pp. 121–29. With permission.*

Locke makes some sweeping criticisms of behavior modification theory applied to organizations. Aside from his apparent bias toward cognitive theories of human behavior, his criticisms are unjustified due to Locke's incorrect interpretations of behavior modification as well as logical inconsistencies in his arguments.

Specifically, I have noted seven different (but related) contentions by Locke which are either erroneous in their interpretation, or are logically inconsistent with the premises he establishes. His contentions are:

1. Individuals are not given credit for "thinking" in behavior mod (the "deterministic" viewpoint),

2. Behavior modification has no scientific base,

3. Self-reinforcement or vicarious learning is inconsistent with the principles of behavior mod,

4. Studies which show that individuals "think" are evidence that behavior mod is wrong,

5. The principles involved in behavior mod are not new,

6. Behavior modification does not work unless the individual is aware of the contingencies,

7. Behavior mod does not work if the manager does not have control over all the contingencies.

While I believe that behavior modification does have some theoretical and practical problems associated with it, Locke's extreme bias toward cognitive explanations of behavior prevent him from seeing any of behavior modification's positive aspects and, in some cases, he interprets data to suit his own preconceived models.

1. *Individuals are not given credit for thinking in behavior modification.* The origin of Locke's error in interpretation here is obvious if one examines his citations in the article. Locke's definition of "behaviorism" is correctly stated and attributed to Skinner; however, his *interpretation* of the definition is clearly his own, as indicated by the citation of his own work. It is true that behavior can be *understood* without reference to states or actions of consciousness, but this does not mean that individuals are incapable of thinking or consciously working through their choices of action, a point of view which Locke incorrectly attributes to the behaviorist philosophy.

The operant conditioning model allows for individual choice of action within the reinforcements available. Given any stimulus, the individual has the choice to *engage* in any number of different behaviors, depending upon how he perceives the situation. The individual can choose not to engage in a behavior that is likely to be reinforced or to experiment with other behaviors to learn of their reinforcing consequences. In either case, the individual is free to "think" about the outcomes and act accordingly.

What Locke is probably objecting to is *not being able to control the reinforcements,* rather than the individual not being able to control (i.e., think through) his actions or assist in designing the system. But this is akin to the person who was just caught speeding complaining that he cannot decide whether or not the policeman should give him a ticket! Organizations are no different; some people control the rewards and punishments over others (they are usually called managers).

2. *Behavior modification has no scientific base.* First, Locke's contention regarding the independent properties of reinforcement is clearly wrong. Moreover, the reinforcements are not automatic (in operant conditioning). Second, the fact that behavior mod is based upon experiences of pleasure and pain does not in itself mean that it is devoid of a theoretical base. On the contrary, these experiences are very observable events, although it is this very point with which Locke takes issue, i.e., observing an event and defining it in terms of its consequences. Perhaps the most useful criterion for the theory test is its ability to predict behavior. Although space limitations prohibit a comprehensive review of the literature comparing behavior mod with other "theories," it is proposed here that there is considerable evidence (laboratory and field studies) to suggest that behavior modification is a far better predictor of behavior than other theories.

3. *Self-reinforcement or vicarious learning is inconsistent with the principles of behavior mod.* Locke contends that vicarious reinforcement, vicarious learning, and self-reinforcement concepts that have received considerable support in the cognitive process literature, contradict the assumptions of determinism. Again, it must be pointed out that Locke is referring to his own definition of determinism, one which effectively defines away any other explanation of behavior. Using the interpretation posed earlier, it should be clear that self-reinforcement, vicarious learning, and vicarious reinforcement are merely derivations of reinforcement theory.

4. *Studies which show that individuals*

"think" are evidence that behavior mod is wrong. Locke states that practitioners of behavior mod (behavioral psychotherapists) also violate the main premises of behavior mod by assuming that: (a) patients are conscious, (b) they can think, (c) they can introspect, and (d) they can control the actions of their own minds and bodies.

Of course, the root of Locke's criticism here is again in his definition of behaviorism which, as previously noted, is erroneous.

Operant conditioning and the correct system of applying contingencies *must* make the basic assumptions that employees can think, they can introspect, and they have control over their own actions. To the extent that these conditions do apply, the company merely defines the system through which the employees can benefit by engaging in those behaviors which will result in reinforcement.

5. *The principles involved in behavior mod are not new.* While I would certainly agree with Locke's statement here, it would have to go under the "who cares?" category. If Locke were trying to integrate this "old" theory with some recent findings then his comment might have relevance. However, the flavor of his writing suggests that "if-it's-not-created-recently-then-it's-no-good" syndrome.

Behavior mod has added an entirely new dimension to the practice of management. As a body of knowledge, it systematically specifies which managerial behaviors are appropriate under what conditions. Just because people have used reinforcement principles in the past does *not* mean that there is no originality (or value) in a systematic analysis which partially describes the necessary and sufficient conditions for behavior change.

6. *Behavior modification does not work unless the individual is aware of the contingencies.* While this statement is certainly correct, one wonders why Locke offers it as a criticism of behavior mod. Is he advocating that we *not* let people know how the reward system works? One cannot imagine *any* system working well if the contingencies are vague or inconsistent. In fact, probably one of the greatest contributions of behavior mod is its emphasis on management's responsibility to let employees know what types of

behavior are desirable and what the rewards are so that the employees can make rational decisions.

7. *Behavior mod does not work if the manager does not have control over all the contingencies.* Again, Locke's statement is correct, but it can hardly be called a criticism—a limitation, perhaps, but not a criticism. Locke's implication is that this limitation is not characteristic of the cognitive approaches. Yet we know that any manager's influence is limited by the degree to which he controls reinforcements for his subordinates.

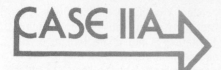

Business Is Good at Consolidated— Check It Out!

Consolidated Printers is not a household name, yet they are the largest firm in their industry. For thirty-seven years, they have specialized in making checks. When you sit down to pay your monthly bills, odds are that you write your payments on checks printed by Consolidated.

The check-printing business has proven recession-proof. For Consolidated, sales have increased in each and every one of its thirty-seven years. Located in the small beach community of Seaside, about 100 miles north of Los Angeles, the company dominates the $200 million a year check-printing industry. Recent estimates indicate that Consolidated controls better than 70 percent of the market. However, because Consolidated is a family-held company, exact figures are not available. What is known is that Randall Phillips and his children, who own Consolidated, are extremely wealthy. The Phillips Foundation, for instance, regularly distributes several million dollars a year for charitable purposes. It is also well known in Seaside that the company has been investing large sums of surplus funds in land and venture capital investments.

Consolidated Printers is the dominant employer in Seaside. Though nonunion, its employees are well paid. Hourly wages range from a low of $8.24 an hour, to as high as $15.40 for some of the skilled engravers and machine engineers. But because of recent high demand for checks, most employees have been working overtime. Last month, for instance, the *average* production worker grossed more than $2,700. Randall Phillips, in a recent interview in the *Seaside Sentinel,* commented that ''Consolidated people don't lack for motivation. They're currently the highest-paid employees in the county. But it's going to get better. Within sixty days, we will be putting into place a new productivity incentive plan which will allow selected employees to earn sizable annual bonuses based on a sophisticated productivity formula that has been developed by our cost accounting staff. All in all, the future is bright for Consolidated Printing and we expect to share this good fortune with our employees who make it all possible.''

It came as quite a shock to Mr. Phillips when he received a letter from a group of a half-dozen anonymous employees, in which they outlined a long list of grievances. Among their complaints were the following:

''We're sick of all this overtime. You and the other honchos in the administrative offices might like working nights and Saturdays, but we enjoy being with our families and friends, and having time to kick back and live a little.

''The new bonus plan is a sham. None of us can figure out how it works. As usual, it will be those people that kiss up to management that'll benefit. Stop manipulating us. We have no intention of working harder for something we don't have any chance of getting.

"How can you talk as if we're one big happy family and at the same time be preparing to throw us all out of work? It's common knowledge in town that the company has bought land in the Phoenix area and everyone says that you're going to close this plant and move the company to Arizona. Why should we give a damn about Consolidated Printers when you're abandoning us?"

Questions

1. From the standpoint of employee perceptions, what is happening here?
2. Judging by what you know about the need hierarchy theory, why are these half-dozen employees unhappy?
3. What role does expectancy theory play in this case?
4. What might the company have done to prevent these negative reactions?

CASE IIB

Money Isn't Everything, I Guess!

Mike Brady has been with the National Broadcasting Company in New York for six years. After graduating from college, he joined NBC in the programming department and has risen to the position of assistant director for daytime programming. Twenty-eight years old and single, Mike appears to enjoy his job and has consistently received good performance appraisals by his bosses. But about six months ago, the programming offices were abuzz with the rumor that Mike would be leaving NBC. It appears the source of this rumor was Mike's current boss, Linda Lawrence.

You see, Mike Brady is the grandson of J.D. Brady, the founder and owner of the Brady Oil Company. The elder Brady, who died about a year ago, left an estate valued at over $300 million. It included oil properties, a 50,000-acre ranch, property holdings in ten states, and assorted other assets. While Mike was never close to J.D.—Mike's mother and father divorced when he was a baby, both of his parents remarried, and he was raised by his mother and stepdad in very middle-class surroundings—his grandfather apparently had not forgotten him. As one of J.D.'s five grandchildren, he was awarded 8 percent of the estate by his grandfather's will, or what would amount to more than $15 million after taxes.

Apparently, when Linda read in the newspaper that Mike was inheriting the millions from his grandfather's estate, she just assumed that Mike would be leaving his job. After all, his salary at NBC was less than $38,000 a year. And he was young, handsome, single, and well-educated. As a multimillionaire, with the world at his feet, you couldn't expect Mike to continue working at a regular job, with regular hours, and three weeks of vacation a year. At least, that's what Linda thought.

But the months have passed and Mike appears as committed to his job as ever. The money he inherited has been invested and is supervised by a professional investment firm. Mike, however, continues to show up for work early, often works late when necessary, and appears to be totally unaffected by his new wealth. One of his close friends commented that Mike told him he had no intention of leaving his job. "I really like my work. Just because I came into some money doesn't change anything. What am I supposed to do? Become a jet-setter and spend my time commuting between homes in Paris, London, New York, and Beverly Hills? Come on, that's not for me. My grandfather worked hard for what he got. I don't know any idle rich. Both my real dad and stepdad went to work every day. I was brought up to value hard work and thrift. I guess that's the way I'll always be."

Linda Lawrence was puzzled. She knew if she inherited $15 million, she couldn't turn in her resignation fast enough.

Questions

1. If you inherited $15 million, would it change *your* life? Would you work? At what?
2. From a motivation viewpoint, can you explain Mike's behavior?
3. How do Mike's values influence his behavior?
4. How can the principles of operant conditioning be used to explain Mike's behavior?
5. Based on what you know about personality, examine potential reasons for the difference in Mike and Linda's attitudes toward work.
6. What percent of the male work force do you think would say they would continue to work if they got enough money to live comfortably for the rest of their life? Explain.

The Green Bay Legend

Vince Lombardi is a legend in football. He single-handedly turned the Green Bay Packers from a mediocre pro team in the mid-1950s into a football dynasty in the 1960s. It was generally agreed that there were half a dozen other pro coaches who knew as much strategically and tactically as Lombardi, but what set him apart and made his team winners was his ability to motivate his players. He was able to get the extra 10 percent which other coaches couldn't. How did he get that extra 10 percent?

For one thing, he used participation. He'd put in a new play on a given morning, have his players practice it all afternoon, and come by the rooms of players he respected that night and ask, "Well, what do you think? Will it work?"

He also was excellent at figuring out what would motivate each individual player. Some guys needed to be driven, some needed a friendly pat on the rear, while others needed to be just left alone.

One player told how, after playing an excellent game, he had been totally ignored by Lombardi. Not a kind word, not anything. At workouts on the following Tuesday and Wednesday, Lombardi chewed him up and down. The player couldn't understand it. He so desperately wanted recognition from his coach. After Wednesday's practice, in the locker room, as the players were leaving for their cars, Lombardi singled out this player, walked up to him, hit him on the rear, and said, "I just want you to know that you're the best damn offensive tackle in pro football." The player remarked how that one sentence inspired him for months.

Frank Gifford, the premier receiver, said about Lombardi, "I was always trying to please him. When we played a game, I couldn't care less about the headlines on Monday. All I wanted was to be able to walk into the meeting Tuesday morning and have Vinny give me that big grin and pat me on the fanny and let me know that I was doing what he wanted me to do. A lot of our guys felt that way. We had guys who would run through a stadium wall for him—and then maybe cuss him in the next breath. . . ."

Lombardi knew how to challenge his teams. After his team broke a two-game winning streak, Lombardi walked into the locker room to find the players laughing and clowning around. Lombardi didn't think anything was funny. "Nobody wants to pay the price," he said. "I'm the only one here that's willing to pay the price. You guys don't care. You don't want to win."

The team was stunned. Nobody knew what to do, but the silence was broken when one player stood up and said, "My God, I want to win," and then somebody else said, "Yeah, I want to win," and pretty soon there were forty guys standing, all shouting, "I want to win." Lombardi had succeeded in making them ashamed and angry.

All-Pro defensive lineman Willie Davis gave an example of how Lombardi could make you feel important and, by doing so, get you around to his way of thinking.

> I guess maybe my worst days in football were the days I tried to negotiate my contracts with the old man. I'd get myself all worked up before I went in to see him. I'd drive up from my home in Chicago, and all the way, I'd keep building up my anger, telling myself I was going to draw a hard line and get just as much money as I deserved.
>
> One year, I walked into his office feeling cocky, you know, 'Roll out the cash, Jack, I got no time for small change.' All he had to do was say one harsh word, and I was really going to let him have it. I never got a word in. Soon as he saw me, he jumped up and began hugging me and patting me and telling me, 'Willie, Willie, Willie, it's so great to see you. You're the best trade I ever made. You're a leader. We couldn't have won without you, Willie. You had a beautiful year. And, Willie, I need your help. You see, I've got this budget problem. . . .'
>
> He got me so off balance, I started feeling sorry for him. He had me thinking, 'Yeah, he's right, he's gotta save some money for the Kramers and the Greggs and the Jordans,' and the next thing I knew, I was saying, 'Yes, sir, that's fine with me,' and I ended up signing for about half what I was going to demand. When I got out of that office and started driving back to Chicago, I was so mad at myself, I was about to drive off the highway.

Questions

1. Analyze Lombardi's motivational style by using cognitive evaluation theory, equity theory, and goal-setting theory.
2. What motivation theory best describes Lombardi's approach to motivating his players? Explain.
3. Could Lombardi's approach be used in industry? Explain.

Adapted from Jerry Kramer and Dick Schaap, *Lombardi: Winning Is the Only Thing* (New York: World Publishing, 1970).

CASE IID → The Right Woman in the Wrong Job

Alix Maher described herself as humanistic. She was politically liberal, and believed socialism could rectify many ills in American society. But Alix needed to eat, and so she chose a teaching career in elementary education. In her mid-thirties, after nearly ten years of teaching, she decided to quit. When asked why, she told this casewriter that inflation demanded that she get a job that paid more money. The salary she was making as a teacher was not enough to allow her to keep her head above water. After nearly sixty days of job searching, she obtained a position with the telephone company.

After six weeks of training and three months on the job, Alix spoke candidly about how things were going.

"First, let me say that I took this job because the pay was very good and everyone told me the phone company is a good place to work. I should also tell you that I'm basically shy and unaggressive so when I interviewed for this job I really tried hard to come across as strong and confident. I guess it worked 'cause I got the job.

"I know right now, I'm not going to make it on this job. The demands on me and the things I have to do go against what I believe in. Let me tell you what I mean.

"I'm called a problem solver. If a commercial firm is having a communications problem, I come in and solve it. If that was all that the job required, I'd do very well. I've got a good mind and I like solving problems. But you really are expected to push the more sophisticated telephone systems. The job, then, is really sales. My bosses don't judge me on how well I solve customer problems. They judge me on how much upgraded telephone equipment I've convinced the customer he needs.

"I guess my dilemma boils down to this. In a large number of cases, I think I can solve the customer's problem with no additional telephone equipment. I listen to the customer, I study his operation, and I try to come up with a solution that will be effective and at the lowest cost possible. This often can be done with little or no new equipment. So, I feel good because I've satisfied my customer's needs. But, that doesn't make my employer happy. The telephone company wants to sell more telephone equipment. We meet every Monday morning to review the problems we faced last week, and how we solved them by advising the purchase of more sophisticated communications equipment. I don't understand why we've got to push the sales of new and expensive equipment. The telephone company is huge. Its profits are enormous. Why do they need to make more money? Why can't they just service the needs of their customers without trying to sell them something?"

Questions

1. Analyze the discrepancy between Alix and the demands of her job by using (a) the hierarchy of values and (b) the six personality types model.
2. Given what you know about personality and learning, could Alix learn to do the job she is expected to do? Why or why not?

3. What could the telephone company have done to avoid this problem with Alix?
4. Based on your knowledge of cognitive dissonance, what can you expect Alix to do? Why?

EXERCISE IIA

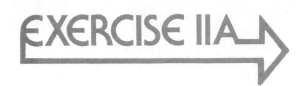

Value Assessment

Directions. Read each statement in turn then circle both the *number and letter* appearing next to either Yes or No that best indicate your feeling of like or dislike for the activity described. *Be sure to answer each question.* A sample response is a follows:

"Enjoy eating ice cream"	(2A) Yes	2A No

1. Meet new people and get acquainted with them.	5D Yes	5D No
2. Take a carload of children for an outing.	6D Yes	6D No
3. Serve as a companion to an elderly person.	7D Yes	7D No
4. Like to be with people despite their physical deformities.	8D Yes	8D No
5. Work with a group to help the unemployed.	9D Yes	9D No
6. Work with labor and management to help solve their conflicts.	10D Yes	10D No
7. Go with friends to a movie.	4D Yes	4D No
8. Help distribute food at a picnic.	3D Yes	3D No
9. Play checkers with members of your family.	2D Yes	2D No
10. Make a phone call for movie reservations.	1D Yes	1D No
11. Collect specimens of small animals for a zoo or museum.	5A Yes	5A No
12. Do algebra problems.	6A Yes	6A No
13. Develop an international language.	7A Yes	7A No
14. Do an experiment with the muscle and nerve of a frog.	8A Yes	8A No
15. Study the various methods used in scientific investigations.	9A Yes	9A No
16. Do research on the relation of brainwaves to thinking.	10A Yes	10A No
17. Visit a research laboratory in which small animals are being tested in a maze.	4A Yes	4A No
18. Plan the defense and offense you are to use before a tennis game.	3A Yes	3A No

19. Read the biography of Louis Pasteur.	2A	Yes	2A	No
20. See moving pictures in which scientists are heroes.	1A	Yes	1A	No
21. Judge entries in a photo contest.	5C	Yes	5C	No
22. Sketch action scenes on a drawing pad.	6C	Yes	6C	No
23. Participate in a summer theater group.	7C	Yes	7C	No
24. Compare the treatment of a classical work as given by two fine musicians.	8C	Yes	8C	No
25. Mold a statue in clay.	9C	Yes	9C	No
26. Be a ballet dancer.	10C	Yes	10C	No
27. Be a sign painter.	4C	Yes	4C	No
28. Plant flowers and shrubbery around a home.	3C	Yes	3C	No
29. Listen to jive and jazz records.	2C	Yes	2C	No
30. Play the jukebox.	1C	Yes	1C	No
31. Lead a round-table discussion.	5B	Yes	5B	No
32. Be chairman of an organizing committee.	6B	Yes	6B	No
33. Buy a run-down business and make it grow.	7B	Yes	7B	No
34. Borrow money in order to put over a business deal.	8B	Yes	8B	No
35. Run for political office.	9B	Yes	9B	No
36. Own and operate a bank.	10B	Yes	10B	No
37. Be a bank teller.	4B	Yes	4B	No
38. Take a course in Business English.	3B	Yes	3B	No
39. Major in commercial subjects in school.	2B	Yes	2B	No
40. Collect lunch money at the end of a school cafeteria line.	1B	Yes	1B	No
41. Send a letter of condolence to a neighbor.	5D	Yes	5D	No
42. Help people to be comfortable when traveling.	6D	Yes	6D	No
43. Belong to several social agencies.	7D	Yes	7D	No
44. Treat wounds to help people get well.	8D	Yes	8D	No
45. Help an agency locate living places for evicted families.	9D	Yes	9D	No
46. Be a medical missionary to a foreign country.	10D	Yes	10D	No
47. Attend a dance.	4D	Yes	4D	No
48. Dine with classmates in the school cafeteria.	3D	Yes	3D	No
49. Play checkers.	2D	Yes	2D	No
50. Ride in a bus to San Francisco or a neighboring city.	1D	Yes	1D	No
51. Be a laboratory technician.	5A	Yes	5A	No
52. Be a scientific farmer.	6A	Yes	6A	No
53. Develop new kinds of flowers in a small greenhouse.	7A	Yes	7A	No
54. Solve knotty legal problems.	8A	Yes	8A	No
55. Develop improved procedures in a scientific experiment.	9A	Yes	9A	No
56. Develop new mathematical formulas for research.	10A	Yes	10A	No
57. Look at the displays on astronomy in an observatory exhibit.	4A	Yes	4A	No
58. Visit the fossil display at a museum.	3A	Yes	3A	No

59.	Keep a chemical storeroom or physical laboratory.	2A	Yes	2A	No	
60.	Sell scientific books.	1A	Yes	1A	No	
61.	Judge window displays in a contest.	5C	Yes	5C	No	
62.	Collect rare and old recordings.	6C	Yes	6C	No	
63.	Be an interior decorator.	7C	Yes	7C	No	
64.	Make a comparative study of architecture.	8C	Yes	8C	No	
65.	Write a new arrangement for a musical theme.	9C	Yes	9C	No	
66.	Paint a mural.	10C	Yes	10C	No	
67.	Visit a flower show.	4C	Yes	4C	No	
68.	Make and trim household accessories like lamp shades, etc.	3C	Yes	3C	No	
69.	Dance to a fast number.	2C	Yes	2C	No	
70.	Paint the kitchen with colors of your choice.	1C	Yes	1C	No	
71.	Install improved office procedures in a big business.	5B	Yes	5B	No	
72.	Plan business and commercial investments.	6B	Yes	6B	No	
73.	Be an active member of a political group.	7B	Yes	7B	No	
74.	Address a political convention.	8B	Yes	8B	No	
75.	Operate a race track.	9B	Yes	9B	No	
76.	Become a U.S. Senator.	10B	Yes	10B	No	
77.	Purchase supplies for a picnic.	4B	Yes	4B	No	
78.	Live in a large city rather than a small town.	3B	Yes	3B	No	
79.	Work at an information desk.	2B	Yes	2B	No	
80.	Be a private secretary.	1B	Yes	1B	No	

Turn to page 532 for scoring directions and key.

Source: J. Shorr, "The Development of a Test to Measure Intensity of Values," *Journal of Educational Psychology*, vol. 44 (1953), pp. 266–74.

EXERCISE IIB →

Attitude Measure of Women as Managers

Instructions	*Rating Scale*
The following items are an attempt to assess the attitudes people have about women in business. The best answer to each statement is your *personal opinion*. The statements cover many different and opposing points of view; you may	1 = Strongly Disagree 2 = Disagree 3 = Slightly Disagree 4 = Neither Disagree nor Agree 5 = Slightly Agree

find yourself agreeing strongly with some of the   6 = Agree
statements, disagreeing just as strongly with   7 = Strongly Agree
others, and perhaps uncertain about others.
Whether you agree or disagree with any
statement; you can be sure that many people
feel the same way you do.

Using the numbers from 1 to 7 on the rating scale on the upper right, mark
your personal opinion about each statement in the blank that immediately
precedes it. Remember, give your *personal opinion* according to how much you
agree or disagree with each item. Please respond to all 21 items.

___ 1. It is less desirable for women than men to have a job that requires
responsibility.

___ 2. Women have the objectivity required to evaluate business situations
properly.

___ 3. Challenging work is more important to men than it is to women.

___ 4. Men and women should be given equal opportunity for participation in
management training programs.

___ 5. Women have the capability to acquire the necessary skills to be
successful managers.

___ 6. On the average, women managers are less capable of contributing to an
organization's overall goals than are men.

___ 7. It is not acceptable for women to assume leadership roles as often as
men.

___ 8. The business community should someday accept women in key
managerial positions.

___ 9. Society should regard work by female managers as valuable as work by
male managers.

___10. It is acceptable for women to compete with men for top executive
positions.

___11. The possibility of pregnancy does not make women less desirable
employees than men.

___12. Women would no more allow their emotions to influence their
managerial behavior than would men

___13. Problems associated with menstruation should not make women less
desirable than men as employees.

___14. To be a successful executive, a woman does not have to sacrifice some
of her femininity.

___15. On the average, a woman who stays at home all the time with her
children is a better mother than a woman who works outside the home
at least half time.

___16. Women are less capable of learning mathematical and mechanical skills
than are men.

___17. Women are not ambitious enough to be successful in the business world.

___18. Women cannot be assertive in business situations that demand it.

___19. Women possess the self-confidence required of a good leader.

___20. Women are not competitive enough to be successful in the business world.

___21. Women cannot be aggressive in business situations that demand it.

Turn to page 533 for scoring directions and key.

Source: James R. Terborg, Lawrence H. Peters, Daniel R. Ilgen, and Frank Smith, "Organizational and Personal Correlates of Attitudes Toward Women as Managers," *Academy of Management Journal,* March 1977, p. 93. With permission.

EXERCISE IIC →

Needs Test

Indicate how important each of the following are in the job you would like to get. Write the numbers 1, 2, 3, 4, or 5 on the line after each item.

1 = Not Important
2 = Slightly Important
3 = Moderately Important
4 = Very Important
5 = Extremely Important

1. Cooperative relations with my co-workers.___
2. Developing new skills and knowledge at work.___
3. Good pay for my work.___
4. Being accepted by others.___
5. Opportunity for independent thought and action.___
6. Frequent raises in pay.___
7. Opportunity to develop close friendships at work.___
8. A sense of self-esteem.___
9. A complete fringe benefit program.___
10. Openness and honesty with my co-workers.___
11. Opportunities for personal growth and development.___
12. A sense of security from bodily harm.___

Turn to page 533 for scoring directions and key.

Source: Adapted from Clayton P. Alderfer, *Existence, Relatedness, and Growth: Human Needs in Organizational Settings* Copyright © 1972 by The Free Press, a Division of Macmillan Publishing Co., Inc.

PART III

The Group

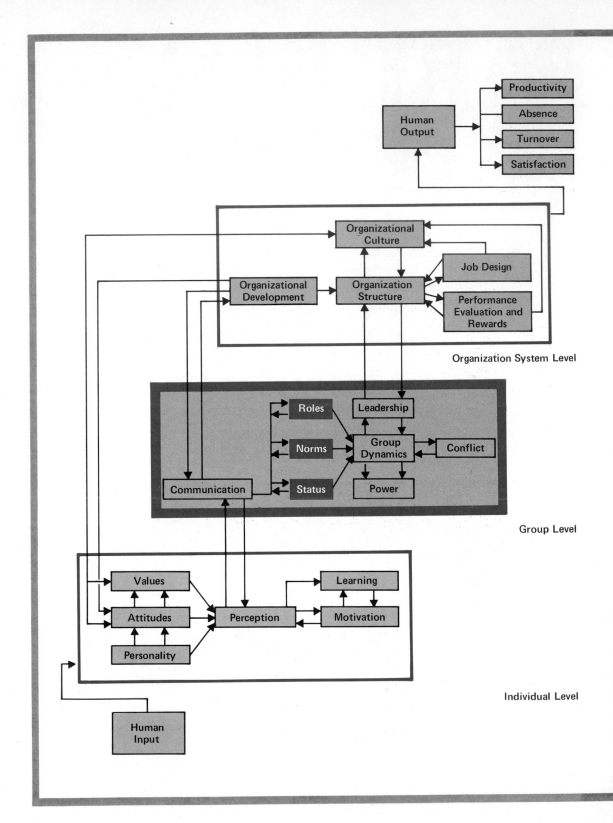

Human
Output

Productivity

Absence

Turnover

Satisfaction

Organizational
Culture

Organizational
Development

Organization
Structure

Job Design

Performance
Evaluation and
Rewards

Organization System Level

Roles

Leadership

Norms

Group
Dynamics

Conflict

Communication

Status

Power

Group Level

Values

Learning

Attitudes

Perception

Motivation

Personality

Individual Level

Human
Input

CHAPTER 8
Foundations of Group Behavior

AFTER STUDYING THIS CHAPTER, YOU SHOULD BE ABLE TO—

Define and explain the following key terms and concepts:

Command group
Conformity
Formal group
Friendship group
Group
Informal group
Interest group
Norms
Psychological contract

Role
Role conflict
Role expectations
Role identity
Role perception
Status
Status equity
Status hierarchy
Task group

Understand:

The difference between formal and informal groups
Why people join groups
How role requirements change in different situations
How norms exert influence on an individual's behavior
The importance of the Hawthorne studies to the understanding of behavior
The need for status
The sources of status

One Supreme Court Justice to another: "This daily metamorphosis never fails to amaze me. Around the house I'm a perfect idiot. I come to court, put on a black robe, and, by God, I'm IT!"

—M. HANDELSMAN

Groups are a relatively new way of looking at organizational behavior. Fifty years ago it was acceptable to say that organizations were composed of individuals and leave it at that. It was not really until the 1930s and 1940s that comtemporary ideas about groups came along: awareness that the behavior of individuals in groups is something more than the sum total of each acting in his or her own way. In other words, when individuals are in groups they act differently from when they are alone. Today, we recognize the vital role an understanding of groups plays in explaining the larger phenomena of organizational behavior.

DEFINING AND CLASSIFYING GROUPS

A group is defined as two or more individuals, interacting and interdependent, who come together to achieve particular objectives. Groups can be either formal or informal. By formal, we mean defined by the organization's structure, with designated work assignments establishing tasks and work groups. In formal groups, the behaviors that one should engage in are stipulated by and directed toward organizational goals. In contrast, informal groups are alliances that are neither structured nor organizationally determined. These groups are natural formations in the work environment, which appear in response to the need for social contact.

It is possible to further subclassify groups as command, task, interest, or friendship groups.[1] Command and task groups are dictated by the formal organization, whereas interest and friendship groups are informal alliances.

The *command group* is determined by the organization chart. It is composed of the subordinates who report directly to a given manager. An elementary school principal and her twelve teachers form a command group, as do the director of postal audits and his five inspectors.

Task groups, also organizationally determined, represent those working

1. Leonard R. Sayles, "Work Group Behavior and the Larger Organization," in *Research in Industrial Relations,* ed. Conrad Arensburg et al. (New York: Harper & Row, 1957), pp. 131–45.

together to complete a job task. However, a task group's boundaries are not limited to its immediate hierarchial superior. It can cross command relationships. For instance, if a college student is accused of a campus crime, it may require communication and coordination between the Dean of Academic Affairs, the Dean of Students, the Registrar, the Director of Security, and the student's advisor. Such a formation would constitute a task group. It should be noted that all command groups are also task groups, but because task groups can cut across the organization, the reverse need not be true.

People who may or may not be aligned into common command or task groups may affiliate to attain a specific objective with which each is concerned. This is an *interest group*. Employees who band together to have their vacation schedule altered, to support a peer who has been fired, or to seek increased fringe benefits represent the formation of a united body to further their common interest.

Groups often develop because the individual members have one or more common characteristics. We call these formations *friendship groups*. Social allegiances, which frequently extend outside the work situation, can be based on similar age, support for "Big Red" Nebraska football, having attended the same college, or the holding of similar political views, to name just a few such characteristics.

Informal groups provide a very important service by satisfying their members' social needs. Because of interactions that result from the close proximity of work stations or task interactions, we find workers playing golf together, riding to and from work together, lunching together, and spending their breaks around the water cooler together. We must recognize that these types of interactions among individuals, even though informal, deeply affect their behavior and performance.

WHY DO PEOPLE JOIN GROUPS?

There is no single reason why individuals join groups. Since most people belong to a number of groups, it is obvious that different groups provide different benefits to their members. The most popular reasons for joining a group are related to our needs for security, identity, affiliation, power, and engaging in common tasks.

Security

"There's strength in numbers." By joining a group, we can reduce the insecurity of "standing alone"—we feel stronger, have fewer self-doubts, and are more resistant to threats. New employees are particularly vulnerable to a sense of isolation and turn to the group for guidance and support. However, whether we are talking about new employees or those with years on the job, we can state that few individuals like to stand alone. We get reassurances from interacting with others and being part of a group. This often explains the appeal of unions—if management creates an environment in which employees feel insecure, they are likely to turn to unionization to reduce their feelings of insecurity.

Identity, Self-Esteem, and Status

"I'm proud to be a member of the Blue Angels," commented a Navy pilot. He was acknowledging the role that a group can have in giving prestige. Group membership means "I'm somebody." It can fulfill extrinsic needs by giving an individual status and recognition. For new freshmen in college, fraternities, sororities, the gymnastics team, or the pep club represent groups in which membership may be sought in order to reinforce feelings of worth. The move from high school to college often means going from being a "wheel" to being a "nobody." Membership in one or more college groups can help to reassure us that we are important. Similarly, many employees in organizations place a high value on meeting their esteem needs and look to membership in both formal and informal groups for satisfaction of these needs.

Groups can also fulfill intrinsic needs. Our self-esteem is bolstered when we are accepted by a highly valued group. Being assigned to a task force whose purpose is to review and make recommendations for the location of the company's new corporate headquarters can fulfill one's intrinsic needs for competence and growth, as well as one's extrinsic needs for status and influence.

Affiliation

"I'm independently wealthy, but I wouldn't give up my job. Why? Because I really like the people I work with!" This quote, from a $25,000-a-year purchasing agent who inherited several million dollars' worth of real estate, verifies that groups can fulfill our social needs. People enjoy the regular interaction that comes with group membership. For many people, these on-the-job interactions are their primary source for fulfilling their need for affiliation. For almost all people, work groups significantly contribute to fulfilling their need for friendships and social relations.

Power

"I tried for two years to get the plant management to increase the number of female restrooms on the production floor to the same number as the men have. It was like talking to a wall. But I got about fifteen other women who were production employees together and we jointly presented our demands to management. The construction crews were in here adding female restrooms within ten days!"

This episode demonstrates that one of the appealing aspects of groups is that they represent power. What often cannot be achieved individually becomes possible through group action. Of course, this power may not be sought only to make demands on others. It may be desired merely as a countermeasure. In order to protect themselves from unreasonable demands by management, individuals may align with others.

Informal groups additionally provide opportunities for individuals to exercise power over others. For individuals who desire to influence others, groups can offer power without a formal position of authority in the organization. As a group leader, you may be able to make requests of group members and obtain compliance without any of the responsibilities that traditionally go with formal managerial positions. So, for people with a high power need, groups can be a vehicle for fulfillment.

Group Goals

"I'm part of a three-person team studying how we can cut our company's transportation costs. They've been going up at over 30 percent a year for several years now so the corporate controller assigned representatives from cost accounting, shipping, and marketing to study the problem and make recommendations."

This task group was created to achieve a goal that would be considerably more difficult if pursued by a single person. There are times when it takes more than one person to accomplish a particular task—there is a need to pool talents, knowledge, or power in order to get a job completed. In such instances, management will rely on the use of a formal group.

KEY GROUP CONCEPTS

The foundation for explaining and predicting group behavior can be found in three concepts—roles, norms, and status. We have all heard these words before. They may even be a standard part of your vocabulary. But if you expect to be able to analyze groups, you are going to have to feel comfortable with these concepts and understand thoroughly the theory that underlies them. This chapter seeks to achieve that end.

Roles

Shakespeare said, "All the world's a stage, and all the men and women merely players." Using the same metaphor, all group members are actors, each playing a *role*. By this term, we mean a set of expected behavior patterns attributed to someone occupying a given position in a social unit. The understanding of role behavior would be dramatically simplified if each of us chose one role and "played it out" regularly and consistently. Unfortunately, we are required to play a number of diverse roles, both on and off our jobs. As we shall see, one of the tasks in understanding behavior is grasping the role that a person is currently playing.

For example, on his job, Bill Patterson is a plant manager with Electrical

Industries, a large electrical equipment manufacturer in Phoenix. He has a number of roles that he fulfills on that job—for instance, Electrical Industries employee, member of middle management, electrical engineer, and the primary company spokesman in the community. Off the job, Bill Patterson finds himself in still more roles: husband, father, Catholic, Rotarian, tennis player, member of the Thunderbird Country Club, and president of his homeowner's association. Many of these roles are compatible, while some create conflicts. For instance, how does his religious involvement influence his managerial decisions regarding layoffs, expense account padding, or providing accurate information to government agencies? A recent offer of promotion requires Bill to relocate, yet his family very much wants to stay in Phoenix. Can the role demands of his job be reconciled with the demands of husband and father roles?

The issue should be clear: Like Bill Patterson, we all are required to play a number of roles, and our behavior varies with the role we are playing. Bill's behavior when he attends church on Sunday morning is different from his behavior on the golf course later that same day. You, too, act differently in the role of student than you do when you play husband or wife, or boyfriend or girlfriend. In fact, I personally find it humorous to think of the student role and how it totally fails to simulate the managerial environment that we like to think we, in academia, are preparing students for. We want to prepare students to be articulate decision makers. Yet, look at most testing procedures. It will be indeed the rare boss who calls you into his office, invites you to sit down, requests that you take out a piece of paper, asks you half-a-dozen questions, and tells you to write up these answers and turn them in in fifty minutes. Is it surprising, then, that many students have a difficult time moving out of the role of student (passive, note-taking regurgitator) to the role of employee in a real organization?

Role Identity. There are certain attitudes and actual behaviors consistent with a role and they create the role identity. People have the ability to shift roles rapidly when they recognize that the situation and its demands clearly require major changes. For instance, when union stewards were promoted to foremen positions, it was found that their attitudes changed from pro-union to pro-management within a few months of their promotion. When these promotions had to later be rescinded because of economic difficulties in the firm, it was found that the demoted foremen had once again adopted their pro-union attitudes.[2]

When the situation is more vague and the role one is to play less clear, people often revert to old role identities. An investigation of high school reunions verified this view.[3] At the reunions studied, even though participants had been away from high school and their peers for five, ten, or twenty or more years, they reverted back to their old roles. The "ins" replayed their former roles, as did the "outs." Even though entirely new criteria were being used in

2. S. Lieberman, "The Effects of Changes in Roles on the Attitudes of Role Occupants," *Human Relations,* November 1956, pp. 385–402.

3. Ralph Keyes, *Is There Life After High School?* (New York: Warner Books, 1976).

the real world for success, the former "jocks," student officers, and the cheer-leaders acted as "ins" and the others expected them to. In spite of the fact that some of the former losers were now winners by society's standards, they found it very difficult to deal with the winner's role when placed in an environment in which they had always been losers. With the role requirements ill-defined, identities became clouded, and individuals reverted back to old patterns of behavior.

Role Perception. One's view of how one is supposed to act in a given situation is a role perception. Based on an interpretation of how we believe we are supposed to behave, we engage in certain types of behavior.

Where do we get these perceptions? One author suggests that we all learn roles from such media as movies, books, and television, and from friends.[4] If this is true, we might propose that many policemen may have formed their role identities from their perception of *Serpico* or "Starsky and Hutch"; law students may learn their roles from *The Paper Chase;* or journalists may be emulating their favorite character on "Lou Grant." Of course, the primary reason apprenticeship programs exist in many trades and professions is to allow individuals to watch an "expert" so they can learn to act as they are supposed to.

Role Expectations. Role expectations are defined as how others believe you should act in a given situation. How you behave is determined, to a large part, by the role defined in the context in which you are acting. The role of a U.S. senator is viewed as having propriety and dignity, whereas a football coach is seen as aggressive, dynamic, and inspiring to his players. In the same context, we might be surprised to learn that the neighborhood priest moonlights during the week as a bartender. Why? Because our role expectations of priests and bartenders tend to be considerably different. When role expectations are concentrated into generalized categories, we have role stereotypes. As illustrated in Figure 8–1, we have created a stereotype when we assume that individuals who wear jeans, beads, macrame belts, and long hair must be unemployed and have rejected established institutions and values.

Television's Archie Bunker holds a number of role stereotypes. He perceives all blacks as lazy, women as subservient, college students as anti-American, welfare recipients as chislers, and so on. Many of the "All in the Family" and "Archie Bunker's Place" story lines are built around Archie's stereotypes and the weakness of these stereotypes to predict behavior.

During the last several decades we have seen a major change in the general population's role stereotypes of females. In the 1950s, a woman's role was to stay home, take care of the house, raise children, and generally care for her husband. Today, most of us no longer hold this stereotype. Boys *can* play with Barbie Dolls and girls *can* play with G.I. Joes. Girls can aspire to be doctors, lawyers, and astronauts as well as the more traditional activities of nurse, school

4. Joe Kelly, *Organizational Behavior: An Existential Systems Approach,* rev. ed. (Homewood, Ill.: Irwin-Dorsey, 1974), p. 323.

FIGURE 8–1
DOONESBURY

by Garry Trudeau

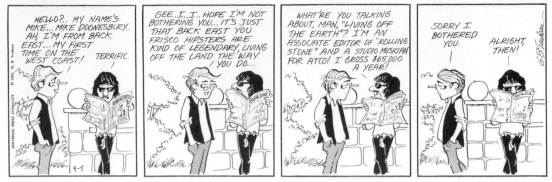

Source: G.B. Trudeau, Call Me When You Find America (New York: Bantam, 1973).

teacher, secretary, or housewife. In other words, many of us have changed our role expectations of women and, similarly, many women carry new role perceptions.

In the workplace, it can be helpful to look at the topic of role expectations through the perspective of the *psychological contract.* There is an unwritten agreement that exists between employees and their employer. This psychological contract sets out mutual expectations—what management expects from workers and vice versa.[5] In effect, this contract defines the behavioral expectations that go with every role. Management is expected to treat employees justly, provide acceptable working conditions, clearly communicate what is a fair day's work, and give feedback on how well the employee is doing. Employees are expected to respond by demonstrating a good attitude, following directions, and showing loyalty to the organization.

What happens when role expectations as implied in the psychological contract are not met? If management is derelict in keeping up its part of the bargain, we can expect negative repercussions on employee performance and satisfaction. When employees fail to live up to expectations, the result is usually some form of disciplinary action up to and including firing.

The psychological contract should be recognized as a "powerful determiner of behavior in organizations."[6] It points out the importance of communicating accurately role expectations. In Chapter 17, we shall discuss how organizations socialize employees in order to get them to play out their roles in the way management desires.

5. See, for example, John P. Kotter, "The Psychological Contract," *California Management Review,* Spring 1973, pp. 91–99.

6. Edgar H. Schein, *Organizational Psychology,* 3rd ed. (Englewood Cliffs, N.J.: Prentice-Hall, 1980), p. 24.

Role Conflict. When an individual is confronted by divergent role expectations, the result is role conflict. It exists when an individual finds that compliance with one role requirement may make more difficult the compliance with another. At the extreme it would include situations where two or more role expectations are mutually contradictory.

Many believe that the topic of role conflict is the most critical role concept in attempting to explain behavior. This, for example, is one of the classic problems of college presidents, a fact which became highly evident in the late 1960s. The college president is forced to reconcile diverse role expectations by faculty, students, board members, alumni, and other administrators. The behavior expectations that are perceived as acceptable by one group are often totally in disagreement with the expectations of other groups.[7]

Our previous discussion of the many roles Bill Patterson had to deal with included several role conflicts—for instance, Bill's attempt to reconcile the expectations placed on him as head of his family and as an executive with Electrical Industries. The former emphasizes stability and concern for the desire of his wife and children, as you will remember, to remain in Phoenix. Electrical Industries, on the other hand, expects its employees to be responsive to the needs and requirements of the company. Although it might be in Bill's financial and career interests to accept a relocation, the conflict comes down to choosing between family and career role expectations.

The issue of ethics in business demonstrates a well-publicized area of role conflict among corporate executives. A recent study found that 57 percent of *Harvard Business Review* readers had experienced the dilemma of having to choose between what was profitable for their firms and what was ethical.[8]

All of us have faced and will continue to face role conflicts. The critical issue, from our standpoint, is how conflicts, imposed by divergent expectations within the organization, impact on behavior. Certainly they increase internal tension and frustration. There are a number of behavioral responses one may engage in. For example, one can give a formalized bureaucratic response. The conflict is then resolved by relying on the rules, regulations, and procedures that govern organizational activities. For example, a worker faced with the conflicting requirements imposed by the corporate controller's office and his own plant manager, decides in favor of his immediate boss—the plant manager. Similarly, many college professors create a formal environment in class by calling their students "Mr." and "Ms.," and expecting to be called "Professor"—in order to avoid allowing friendships to interfere with the objective requirements of the professorial role. Other behavioral responses may include withdrawal, stalling, negotiation or, as we found in our discussion of dissonance in Chapter 3, redefining the facts or the situation to make them appear congruent.

7. Stephen P. Robbins, *Positional Authority of Selected College and University Presidents as Perceived by Their Interacting Publics,* doctoral dissertation, University of Arizona, 1971.

8. Steven N. Brenner and Earl A. Molander, "Is the Ethics of Business Changing?" *Harvard Business Review,* January-February 1977, pp. 57–71.

The Good Student Game. How roles pervade us and how well we understand them is demonstrated in the "Good Student Game." You should be able to see some of your own role playing through this description.

The game begins when its organizer announces to a group of twelve to twenty innocents: "I want to lead you in a learning game. Whoever plays must observe a small set of rules and roles. These create an artificial stage. Within it, let's try to have a real discussion of how people act out their parts in the classroom game called " 'good student.' "

. . . The first rule assumes that everyone's a "good student"—independent, critical, with his own unique viewpoint.

"So, I'm always free to ask any of you to express a view that differs from one just given. You can extend it or contradict it. The second rule assumes that a 'good student' is in command of the material and can make connections between its parts. So I can call on anyone to explain the connection between any two points other people have previously made." (The organizer, of course, need have no idea whether points are in fact connectable: that's not his problem. He doesn't mention this, but goes on to ask for volunteers to play three standard "good student" roles.) "One way to present yourself as a 'good student' is to display your command of the material. Another is to brown-nose, to agree with the teacher. But you can also win points by creative disagreement. . . . So we'll want a Yes Man. When I ask—about anything—*Is that right, Mr. Yes?* he replies, *Yes, that is right,* and then explains why. Likewise, we'll want a No Man, whose job is to answer, when asked, *No, that is wrong,* and then explain why. Is all this clear?"

"Are the rest of us supposed to play roles?"

"No. No one else should try to act a role. Everyone is free to respond as himself. Even the people who play Mr. Yes (and) Mr. No . . . should respond as themselves except when I call on them specifically in role. Let's try to keep the discussion as real and substantive as we can."

"Very well, how do 'good students' project themselves?"

"They come to class on time."

"They hand in their homework."

"Yes, yes, some others."

"Eye contact with the teacher is very important, so is volunteering information."

"Seeing him after class to talk about something."

"What about the way people look? *You*—how do you look when you've just been asked a question you can't answer but you don't want the teacher to know?"

"I sit up straight and wrinkle my forehead, searching, maybe he'll speak first."

"And you?"

"I lean forward a little and look earnest, and try to talk about something else."

"And you. . . ?"

Soon the discussion reveals that the choices of where to sit, of posture, dress and expression, of complaisant or sarcastic attitude, are rich elements in a variety of ways of projecting oneself to teacher and class as a "good student." The organizer leads the group on, to recognize complete strategies:

"What might go with sitting in the back row and looking out the window to project a particular 'good student' image?"

"Missing a lot of classes but seeing the professor in his office, maybe not during regular hours."

"Being casual with your homework but sparkling on the final."

"You—what's the connection between the last two answers?"

"Both ways the student shows he knows what's important."

"Very good. This strategy will work with every teacher, is that right, Mr. No?"

"No, that's wrong."

"Because?"

"Because some teachers are uptight about petty detail."

"In other words, what's important is what *they* think is important. So it's clear different strategies work with different teachers and different classes. Now who can say why? What besides skill determines whether a projection of yourself as 'good student' will be successful?"

"If it helps the teacher play his own role well, if it complements his role."

"Is that right, Mr. Yes?"

"Yes that's right, because then it satisfies his image of himself, it *feeds* his ego."

"Then does the image or role of a 'good student' necessarily resemble the image of the 'good teacher' he's facing?"

"No."

"Give an example—anyone."

"The class freak and the scholarly professor who translates the freak's occasional insights so the rest of the dull class can understand them."

"That'll do."

. . . the players, led by the organizer, comment on their own performance:

"How long do you think it takes to figure out what a teacher expects from you—which 'good student' roles will work with him?"

"Maybe like three weeks."

"Anyone think the time is shorter? You do—how short?"

"Oh, you can tell where most teachers are at in the first day or so."

"How? Tell *him* why it doesn't take three weeks."

"The way the teacher talks about midterms and homework, how he's dressed, whether he wants to bullshit a bit or get right down to the subject—things like that."

"You—did that explanation make sense? Do you see why three weeks is too long?"

"Yes, I can see that the sizing-up starts right at the beginning, like whether the teacher asks the class questions about themselves."

"What is there in what he just said that presents *him* as a 'good student'?"

"He admits his mistake."

"Anyone have a better answer?"

"He not only admits it, he shows he's learned by adding something new."

"Right on! Now go back. When I asked five of you how you looked when trying not to show you didn't know the answer to a question, everyone gave a different answer, which showed you're individuals—that's very good. But everyone answered in words. No one demonstrated the look itself, even though you know how many words a picture's worth. Why didn't you?"

"You wanted us to answer in words."

"How do you know? As a matter of fact, I was hoping someone wouldn't."

"I think it's because you're articulate."

"Why is *that* a 'good student' response?"

"He was uncertain and afraid you'd tell him he was wrong, so he took care to qualify it."

"Right. But I think he is right. How *does* my being articulate work?"

"What do you mean?"

"I mean the other side of the 'good student' game is the 'good teacher' game. In what ways have I been presenting myself as a 'good teacher' here?"

"Well, first, you stand at the front and you're always moving, so we have to focus on you. Second, you look people in the eye—that's how you call on them to speak, too. Third, you keep trying to probe deeper for answers. Fourth. . . ."

"Stop. Anyone—how is *he* projecting himself as a 'good student'?"

"I'm *not* playing 'good student'."

"I don't think you are trying to. Someone else answer."

"He volunteered."

"Something less trivial."

"He said, *first, second, third.*"

"Right! How is that a presentation of a 'good student'?"

"It shows an orderly mind."

"Do you *always* say 'first, second, third'?"

"No."

"Why did you say it here? How did I cue that response?"

"*You* speak like that, even though you don't say the numbers."

"In what way was *that* presentation as 'good student'?"

"He gave you a sharp answer, even though it might have displeased you personally."

"How do you know that strategy's a good one to choose with me?"

"Because you wear your hair long."[9]

The presentation of the "Good Student Game" was meant to show how we read student and teacher roles. But it also demonstrated the impact that position plays in determining role. Because the teacher or organizer can stand in front of the room while students sit in neat rows and columns, he finds himself taking on certain behavior patterns. Had one of the students taken the position in front of the class, his role too would have been affected. Let us briefly look at the increasing body of literature that suggests the role played is influenced by spatial factors.

Spatial Influences on Role. Research evidence indicates that the way individuals position themselves within a group; that is, the spatial arrangement that they voluntarily develop, is far from random.

> In discussion groups, it has been suggested that the more autocratic leader sits at the head of the table . . . the more democratic leader tends to sit in the middle of the group.

> It would be wrong to conclude that mere location is the critical factor in determining the role which an individual will take up. It seems much more plausible to believe that dominant individuals select locations for reasons of tradition, or because this choice advertises the role they are going to take up.[10]

9. Excerpted from Michael Rossman, "Is That Right, Mr. Yes?" *Change*, January-February, 1970, pp. 7–10. With permission.

10. Kelly, *Organizational Behavior*, p. 537.

Spatial factors can also determine who within a group will be chosen or accepted for a leadership role. When one wants to take on the role of adversary or to emphasize superior-subordinate relationships, it is natural to place a barrier between himself and others (such as a desk) to identify a we-they distinction.

This may more readily be illustrated by comparing a traditional classroom situation, where the instructor stands in front of the class before a podium, with the students clearly established in neat rows and columns, and a less structured situation with the chairs geographically dispersed about in a circle and the instructor taking one of the seats in the circle. The latter positioning can be expected to increase group interaction, reduce the feeling of superior-subordinate interaction, and place the instructor on a more equal footing with the students.

The importance of spatial arrangements was found in a study of faculty offices at a small, coeducational liberal arts college.[11] Two groups were identified: faculty whose office arrangements had desks between themselves and their students (db) and those who did not have a desk between the students and themselves (dnb). The researcher found that senior faculty members were significantly more likely to use the db design. Seventy-three percent of the senior faculty used the db design, compared with only 47 percent of the younger faculty. Of particular interest was the finding that dnb instructors were rated more positively on overall student ratings of the courses they taught and of themselves as instructors. Again, studies such as this suggest the interrelationship between spatial factors and the roles individuals play. In some cases, spatial factors influence role, and in other cases role influences spatial factors.

Norms

In North America, no one looks twice at the twenty-year-old male holding hands with a twenty-year-old female. However, in many communities, two adult females holding hands might attract attention. And two adult males holding hands is almost sure to attract awkward glances. Why? Norms!!

All groups have established norms, that is, acceptable standards of behavior that are shared by the group's members. Norms tell members what they ought or ought not to do under certain circumstances. From an individual's standpoint, they tell what is expected of you in certain situations. When agreed to and accepted by the group, norms act as a means of influencing the behavior of group members with a minimum of external controls. Norms differ among groups, communities, and societies, but they all have them.

Formalized norms are written up in organizational manuals, setting out rules and procedures for employees to follow. By far, the majority of norms are informal. You do not need someone to tell you that throwing paper airplanes or engaging in prolonged bull sessions at the water cooler are unacceptable behaviors when the "big boss from New York" is touring the office. Similarly, we all know that when we are in an employment interview discussing what we did

11. Richard L. Sweigenhaft, "Personal Space in the Faculty Office: Desk Placement and the Student-Faculty Interaction," *Journal of Applied Psychology*, August 1976, pp. 529–32.

not like about our previous job, there are certain things we should not talk about (difficulty in getting along with co-workers or our supervisor), while it is very appropriate to talk about other things (inadequate opportunities for advancement, or unimportant and meaningless work). Evidence suggests that even high school students recognize that in such interviews certain answers are more socially desirable than others.[12]

We have seen how students understand role playing in the classroom in their ability to identify and agree on role characteristics of a "good student." Of course, students also quickly assimilate classroom norms. Depending upon the environment created by the instructor, the norms may support unequivocal acceptance of the material suggested by the instructor, or, at the other extreme, students may be expected to question and challenge the instructor on any point that is unclear. For example, in most classroom situations, the norms dictate that one not engage in loud, boisterous discussion that makes it impossible to hear the lecturer, nor humiliate the instructor by pushing him or her "too far," even if one has obviously located a weakness in something the instructor has said. Should some in the classroom group behave in such a way as to violate these norms, we can expect pressure to be applied against the deviant members so as to bring their behavior into conformity with group standards.

The Hawthorne Studies. It is generally agreed among behavioral scientists that full-scale appreciation of the importance norms play in influencing worker behavior did not occur until the early 1930s. This enlightenment grew out of a study undertaken at Western Electric Company's Hawthorne Works in Chicago between 1927 and 1932.[13] Conducted under the direction of Harvard psychologist Elton Mayo, the Hawthorne studies concluded that a worker's behavior and sentiments were closely related, that group influences were significant in affecting individual behavior, that group standards were highly effective in establishing individual worker output, and that money was less a factor in determining worker output than group standards, sentiments, and security. Let us briefly review the Hawthorne investigations and demonstrate the importance of these findings in explaining group behavior.

The Hawthorne researchers began by examining the relation between the physical environment and productivity. Illumination, temperature, and other working conditions were selected to represent this physical environment. The researchers' initial findings contradicted their anticipated results.

They began with illumination experiments with various groups of workers. The researchers manipulated the intensity of illumination upward and downward, while at the same time noting changes in group output. Results varied, but one thing was clear: In no case was the increase or decrease in output in

12. Anne Harlan, Jeffrey Kerr, and Steven Kerr, "Preference for Motivator and Hygiene Factors in a Hypothetical Interview Situation: Further Findings and Some Implications for the Employment Interview," *Personnel Psychology,* Winter 1977, pp. 557–66.

13. Much of this description was adapted from "The Hawthorne Studies: A Synopsis," reported in *Man and Work in Society,* ed. E. L. Cass and F. G. Zimmer, (New York: Van Nostrand Reinhold, 1975), pp. 278–306.

proportion to the increase or decrease in illumination. So the researchers introduced a control group: An experimental group was presented with varying intensity of illumination, while the controlled unit worked under a constant illumination intensity. Again, the results were bewildering to the Hawthorne researchers. As the light level was increased in the experimental unit, output rose for each group. But to the surprise of the researchers, as the light level was dropped in the experimental group, productivity continued to increase in both. In fact, a productivity decrease was observed in the experimental group only when the light intensity had been reduced to that of moonlight. Mayo and his associates concluded that illumination intensity was only a minor influence among the many influences that affected an employee's productivity, but they could not explain the behavior they had witnessed.

As a follow-up to the illumination experiments, the researchers began a second set of experiments in the relay-assembly test room at Western Electric. A small group of women were isolated away from the main work group so their behavior could be more carefully observed. They went about their job of assembling small telephone relays in a room laid out similar to their normal department. The only difference was the placement in the room of a research assistant who acted as an observer—keeping records of output, rejects, working conditions, and a daily log sheet describing everything that happened. Over a two-and-a-half-year period, this small group's output increased steadily as did its morale. The number of personal absences and those due to sickness were approximately one-third of those recorded by women in the regular production department. What became evident was that this group's performance was significantly influenced by its status of being a "special" group. The women in the test room thought being in the experimental group was fun, that they were in sort of an elite group, and that management was concerned with their interest by engaging in such experimentation.

A third experiment in the bank wiring observation room was similar in design to the experiment in the relay test room, except male workers were used. Additionally, a sophisticated wage incentive plan was introduced on the assumption that individual workers will maximize their productivity when they see that it is directly related to economic rewards. The most important finding coming out of this experiment was that employees did not individually maximize their outputs. Rather, their output became controlled by a group norm that determined what was a proper day's work. Output was not only being restricted, but individual workers were giving erroneous reports. The total for a week would check with the total week's output, but the daily reports showed a steady, level output regardless of actual daily production. What was going on?

Interviews determined that the group was operating well below its capability and was leveling output in order to protect itself. Members were afraid that if they significantly increased their output the unit incentive rate would be cut, the expected daily output would be increased, layoffs might occur, or that slower men would be reprimanded. So the group established its idea of a fair output—neither too much nor too little. They helped each other out to ensure that their reports were nearly level.

The norms that the group established included a number of "don'ts." *Don't* be a rate-buster, turning out too much work. *Don't* be a chisler, turning out too little work. *Don't* be a squealer on any of your peers.

How did the group enforce these norms? Their methods were neither gentle nor subtle. They included sarcasm, name-calling, ridicule, and even physical punches to the upper arm of members who violated the group's norms. Members would also ostracize individuals whose behavior was against the group's interest.

The Hawthorne studies made an important contribution to our understanding of group behavior—particularly the significant place that norms have in determining individual work behavior.

Social Desirability and Conformity. Groups create within themselves an environment that places members under great pressure to conform to the group's norms. As noted previously, what these norms are depends on the group and its purposes. However, most groups tend to advocate both behavior and attitudes that are socially desirable. In other words, norms set by groups in organizations are influenced by a larger set of standards established at the societal level.

Do you agree with the following statements?

Minorities should receive equal opportunities in organizations.

Conflict is bad in any organization.

Businessmen should act socially responsible.

Political behavior in organizations should be eliminated.

Individuals should be rewarded on the basis of merit.

It is wrong to covet power.

Most of us would agree with all six—they reflect "apple pie and flag" responses. We have been conditioned to say and do the "right thing." Of course, you may say one thing and do something else. Nevertheless, socially desirable attitudes and behaviors are important determinants of group norms.

The impact that group pressures for conformity can have on an individual member's judgment and attitudes was demonstrated in the now-classic studies by Solomon E. Asch.[14] Asch made up groups of seven or eight people, who sat in a classroom and were asked to compare two cards held by the experimenter. One card had one line, the other had three lines of varying length. As shown in Figure 8–2, one of the lines on the three-line card was identical to the line on the one-line card. Also, as shown in Figure 8–2, the difference in line length was quite obvious; under ordinary conditions, subjects made fewer than 1 percent errors. The object was to announce aloud which of the three lines matched the single line. But what happens if all the members in the group begin to give incorrect answers? Will the pressures to conform result in the unsuspecting subject (USS) altering his or her answer to align with the others? That was what Asch

14. Solomon E. Asch, "Effects of Group Pressure Upon the Modification and Distortion of Judgments," in *Groups, Leadership and Men,* ed. Harold Guetzkow (Pittsburgh: Carnegie Press, 1951), pp. 177–90.

FIGURE 8–2 Examples of Cards Used in Asch Study

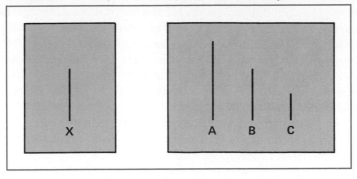

wanted to know. So he arranged the group so only the USS was unaware that the experiment was "fixed." The seating was prearranged: The USS was placed so as to be the last to announce his or her decision.

The experiment began with several sets of matching exercises. All the subjects gave the right answers. On the third set, however, the first subject would give an obviously wrong answer—for example, saying "C" in Figure 8–2. The next subject gave the same wrong answer, and so did the others until it got to the unknowing subject. He knew "B" was the same as "X," yet everyone had said "C." The decision confronting the USS is this: Do you state a perception publicly that differs from the preannounced position of the others? Or, do you give an answer that you strongly believe is incorrect in order to have your response agree with the other group members?

The results obtained by Asch demonstrated that over many experiments and many trials, subjects conformed in about 35 percent of the trials; that is, the subjects gave answers that they knew were wrong but that were consistent with the replies of other group members.

What can we conclude from this study? The results suggest that there are group norms that press us toward conformity. We desire to be one of the group and avoid being visibly different. We can generalize further to say that when an individual's opinion of objective data differs significantly from that of others in his group, he feels extensive pressure to align his opinions to conform with that of the others.

Summary. Our discussion has clarified that groups establish norms that control members by channeling their behavior. Based on these norms, group members conform. They learn that certain types of behavior are approved and others are not. The group uses its reward mechanisms to reinforce those behaviors that conform with its norms and to extinguish those that do not.

Status

While teaching a college course on adolescence a few years ago, the instructor asked the class to list things that contributed to status when they were in high school. The list was long, including such activities as being a "jock," being able to cut class without getting caught, and dating a cheerleader. Then the instructor asked the students to list things that didn't contribute to status. Again, it was easy for the students to create a long list—getting straight "A's," having your mother drive you to school, and so forth. Finally, the students were asked to develop a third list—those things that didn't matter one way or the other. There was a long silence. Finally, a young female in the back row volunteered, "In high school, nothing didn't matter."[15]

Status permeates far beyond the walls of high school. It would not be incorrect to rephrase the above quotation to read, "In the status hierarchy of life, nothing doesn't matter." In spite of the fact that most of us are quick to declare how unimportant status is, most of us are greatly concerned with acquiring status symbols. Fortunately, or unfortunately, depending on your predilections, we live in a class-structured society. In spite of attempts to make our world more egalitarian, we have made little movement toward a classless society. As far back as scientists have been able to trace human groupings, we have had chiefs and Indians, noblemen and peasants, the haves and the have-nots. This continues to be the case today. Even the smallest group will develop roles, rights, and rituals to differentiate its members. Status is an important factor in understanding behavior because it is a significant motivator and has major behavioral consequences when individuals perceive a disparity between what they perceive their status to be and what others perceive it to be.

Status is a prestige grading, position, or rank within a group. It may be formally imposed by a group, that is, organizationally imposed, through titles or amenities. This is the status that goes with being crowned "the heavyweight champion of the world," or being elected "most congenial." We are all familiar with the trappings that are associated with high organizational status—large offices with thick carpeting on the floor and an adjoining bathroom with a shower, impressive titles, high pay and fringe benefits, preferred work schedules, and so on. Whether management acknowledges the existence of a status hierarchy, organizations are filled with amenities that are not uniformly available to everyone and, hence, carry status value.

More often, we deal with status in an informal sense. Status may be informally acquired by such characteristics as education, age, sex, skill, or experience. Anything can have status value if others in the group evaluate it as such. But just because status is informal does not mean that it is less important or that there is less agreement on who has it or who does not. This was supported when individuals were asked to rank the status of their high school classmates a number of years following graduation.[16] The respondents were able to place former classmates into a status hierarchy and the rankings were almost identical. We can and do place people into status categories and there appears to be high agreement among members as to who is high, low, and in the middle.

15. Keyes, *Is There Life After High School?*
16. Ibid.

In his classic restaurant study, William F. Whyte demonstrated the importance of status.[17] Whyte proposed that people work more smoothly if high-status personnel customarily originate action for lower-status personnel. He found a number of instances where, when those of lower status were initiating action, this created a conflict between formal and informal status systems. For example, he cited one instance in which waitresses passed their customers' orders on to countermen—and thus low-status servers were initiating action for high-status cooks. By the simple addition of an aluminum spindle to which the order could be hooked, a buffer was created, thus allowing the countermen to initiate action on orders when they felt ready.

Whyte also noted that in the kitchen, supply men secured food supplies from the chefs. This was, in effect, a case of low-skilled employees initiating action upon the high-skilled. Conflict was stimulated when several supply men explicitly and implicitly urged the chefs to "get a move on." However, Whyte observed that one supply man had little trouble. He gave the chef the order and asked that the chef call him when it was ready, thus reversing the initiating process. In Whyte's analysis, he suggested several changes in procedures, which aligned interactions more closely with the accepted status hierarchy and resulted in substantial improvements in worker relations and effectiveness.

A more recent illustration of the status hierarchy can be seen on the "Tonight Show," hosted by Johnny Carson. Certainly being on the show has status, but there is a hierarchy of clearly preferable treatment a guest can receive.

The lowest position in the hierarchy is the comedian or singer who comes on late in the show, does a routine, and then disappears during a commercial. The next step up is being invited by Johnny to sit down and banter with the host. But not all those who sit down are of equal status and this is readily demonstrated by whether they stay or depart after their interview. The high-status guests—Bob Hope and Burt Reynolds, for example—get up and leave. The implication is that they have other, more important things to do. The "lesser stars" sit on the couch for the remainder of the show.

The status hierarchy on the "Tonight Show" doesn't stop with the time one spends on the couch. Being a guest host obviously carries higher status than merely being an interviewee. In the industry, it is generally agreed that when an entertainer reaches the guest host spot on the Carson show, he or she has made it—high status has been achieved. Of course, greater status still goes to those who guest for a whole week rather than merely filling in on Monday nights!

Sources of Status. Status is given by the group and, as such, is a value perception. It varies by time and place. It may mean being Catholic, Protestant, white, black, Puerto Rican, young, old, male, female, an "Ivy Leaguer," or a third-generation resident in the community, or possessing some physical characteristic. Among professional wrestlers, high weight is valued and therefore possesses

17. William F. Whyte, "The Social Structure of the Restaurant," *American Journal of Sociology,* January 1954, pp. 302–8.

status. Among professional jockeys or members of Weight Watchers, low weight carries status. In Montreal, speaking English with a French accent has a different status connotation than it does in Houston. Being able to dunk a basketball means a lot among a group of young boys putting together a basketball team in New York City, but nothing to a group of young boys fishing off the Atlantic City pier. Whether what you have, know, or can do has status depends on who is doing the evaluating.

Among most middle-class North Americans, certain things appear to have universal status: being the author of a best-selling book, being interviewed by Johnny Carson on the "Tonight Show," having dinner at the White House. Why is it, though, that some things tend to have universal status recognition while others are highly localized? The answer appears to lie in the scarceness of the activity and its visibility. Johnny Carson will interview fewer than a thousand people on his show this year and more than 10 million people will be in attendance by way of their television sets. In contrast, there will be about twenty thousand young men this year who will be captains of their high school football team and the extent of visibility each receives will be highly restricted. So Jack Winthrop, captain of the Burlington (Vermont) High School football team, has high status in northern Vermont and is unknown throughout the rest of the world. On the other hand, Dr. Jonas Salk, of polio vaccine fame, attracts the admiration of most of the Western world.

In many groups, vocabulary alone is a prime determinant of group acceptance and status. Speech that is frequently spotted with certain phrases can suggest that a person is "in," a member of a certain status element. For example, the human potential movement has its own vocabulary that identifies its members:

"I'm into _____" (Select from one of the following: est, TM, T.A.).
"I know where it's at."
"What are you getting?"
"I'm confronting my hostility."
"I can really relate to that."
"Is that your Child speaking?"
"I really need stroking."

Basically, organizations give status through one of four ways: through organizational association—"I'm with the FBI"; occupation—"He's a Supreme Court Justice"; organizational level—"He holds the position of executive director"; or salary—"I make a hundred thousand dollars a year." Additionally, status may be a personal attribute valued by others, such as: age, education, sex, race, religion, physical appearance, communicative skills, experience, or competence. Figure 8–3 lists some examples of items that can carry high status in organizations. Obvious ones include large offices, thick carpeting on the floor, impressive titles, and high pay. For example, one oil company's regional executives got the four prestige corner offices on the "executive" floor of the firm's

FIGURE 8–3 Examples of What May Connote Formal Status

Titles
Director
Manager
Chief
Head
Senior

Relationships
Work for an important individual
Job requires you to work with high-ranking organizational members
Work in a critical group or on an important assignment

Pay and Fringe Benefits
Expense account
Liberal travel opportunities
Reserved parking space with your name on it
Company-paid car
Key to executive washroom

Work Schedule
Day work rather than evening or shift
Freedom from punching a time clock
Freedom to come and go as one pleases

Office Amenities
Large office
Large desk with high-back chair
Windows with attractive view
Private secretary to screen visitors

building. Though the offices are of equal size, the quality of the views are unequal and are allocated by rank. The better views go to those with higher status.

Illustrations abound of status trappings in industry. Bank of America executives know that they have made it when they are given stationery with the bank's logo in gold rather than black ink. At Ford Motor Company, low-level executives' perks are limited to little more than an outside parking space. Middle-management positions come with larger offices, windows, plants, an intercom system, and a secretary. Senior executives get an office with a private lavatory, signed Christmas cards from the chairman, an indoor parking space, and their company cars washed and gassed on request.[18] Western Electric, the manufacturing and supply arm of the Bell System, has its complement of status symbols that relate to rank. As junior managers move up through the company, they typically first have a black Touch-Tone telephone. They then progressively move up to a colored Touch-Tone phone, a Touch-Tone desk set with a "hands free" device, a Touch-Tone model with a set of insertable programmed

18. "Top-Dollar Jobs," *Time*, June 2, 1980, p. 60.

cards that dial the desired number; an electronic preset dialing system requiring only the touch of one button to dial a specific number; and—for the president and executive vice-presidents—a Picturephone.[19]

Even workloads have status connotations. Among college professors, a frequent measure of prestige is teaching load. Paradoxically, the status of teachers among their peers is directly related to how little they teach! Four or five courses a week are viewed as a lot of work and is considered low status. Three is more than competitive and suggests that the teacher is being given some release time to engage in research. Two courses is better yet. Teaching only one course a semester is very infrequent and hence carries very high status. Of course, the eminent status position is reserved for the "teacher" who has succeeded in achieving the ultimate—no teaching load!

Status Equity. It is important for group members to believe that the status hierarchy is equitable. When inequity is perceived, it creates disequilibrium resulting in various types of corrective behavior.

The concept of equity presented in Chapter 6 applies to status. Individuals expect rewards to be proportionate to costs incurred. If Sally and Betty are the two finalists for the head nurse position in a hospital, and it is clear that Sally has more seniority and better preparation for assuming the promotion, Betty will view the selection of Sally to be equitable. However, if Betty is chosen because she is the daughter-in-law of the hospital director, Sally will believe there is an injustice.

The trappings that go with formal positions are also important elements in maintaining equity. If we believe there is an inequity between the perceived ranking of an individual and the status accouterments he or she is given by the organization, we are experiencing status incongruence. Some examples of incongruence are the supervisor earning less than her subordinates, the more desirable office location being held by a lower-ranking individual, or paid country club membership being provided by the company for division managers but not for vice-presidents. Employees expect the things an individual has and receives to be congruent with his or her status.

In spite of our acknowledgement that groups generally agree within themselves on status criteria and hence tend to rank individuals fairly closely, individuals can find themselves in a conflict situation when they move between groups whose status criteria are different or where groups are formed of individuals with heterogeneous backgrounds. Businessmen may use income, total wealth, or size of the companies they run as determinants. Government bureaucrats might use the size of their agencies. Academics may use the number of grants received or articles published. Blue-collar workers may use years of seniority, job assignments, or bowling scores. Where groups are made up of heterogeneous individuals or where heterogeneous groups are forced to be interdependent, there is a

19. Stephen P. Robbins, *Personnel: The Management of Human Resources* (Englewood Cliffs, N.J.: Prentice-Hall, 1978), p. 294.

potential for status differences to initiate conflict as the group attempts to reconcile and align the differing hierarchies.

CLOTHING AND THE KEY GROUP CONCEPTS

The clothes you wear—whether you are male or female—are an identifying costume that is an important ingredient in determining how others perceive you and behave toward you. What you wear can define your social role, your status level, and specify behavioral norms that you are expected to demonstrate.

It is not just chance that finds young medical interns wearing their white coats when they go down the street for lunch. What better way can they quickly communicate to others that they are doctors? Similarly, foremen wear white shirts to identify themselves as different. One plant superintendent recently remarked, "If one day everyone, foremen and operatives alike, arrived all wearing white shirts, I expect the next day foremen would be wearing arm bands or hats or something to distinguish themselves from the masses."

Your clothes on the job are your *uniform*. It need not be overalls or a traditional work uniform—whatever you wear to work identifies your status, group membership, and legitimacy. And, those who fail to wear the appropriate uniform for the role they play create ambiguity in role expectations. Consider the story told by a young male college professor (Leonard Bickman) at Smith College who preferred to dress casually although the expectations of his students' parents aligned with a "tie and jacket" appearance.

> . . . After being introduced to "Dad" as Len Bickman, one father asked me how I liked it at Amherst. I hesitated a few seconds, uncertain of his meaning, and replied that I did not teach at Amherst but at Smith. It was then *Dad's* turn to be confused. My clothes had led him to believe that I was a student, i.e., a low status person. Although he apologized, I could not help but feel that he was angry with me for disrupting his system for categorizing people.[20]

A more detailed account of how clothes influence behavior has been offered by clothing consultant, John Molloy.[21] Based on data secured from thousands of interviews, Molloy argues that what you wear is not important for the influence the clothes will have on you, but for the impact of your attire on other's attitudes and behavior toward you. Although the quality of his research may be dubious, his basic argument is plausible.

For example, Molloy suggests that men never wear short-sleeve shirts, always wear suits, and avoid black raincoats. Short-sleeve shirts are viewed as symbols of the lower-middle class, as are sport jackets. Molloy proposes that men are more likely to be believed, respected, and obeyed if they wear a suit. Of course, the color of the suit must be chosen to align with the image they wish

---

20. Leonard Bickman, "Clothes Make the Person," *Psychology Today*, April 1974, pp. 49–51.

21. John T. Molloy, *Dress for Success* (New York: Warner Books, 1975); and *The Women's Dress for Success Book* (New York: Warner Books, 1977).

to convey. The darker the suit, the more authority it transmits. Dark blue and dark gray solids and pinstripes give you credibility with the upper-middle class, but only the former gets high credibility ratings with the lower-middle class. If a male wants to be liked, Molloy recommends light grays, light-blue solids, and medium-range business plaids. Women, too, should wear suits. He finds that the perfect businesswoman's uniform is a highly tailored, dark-colored, skirted suit.

Molloy even proposes that a male's raincoat is not just a raincoat. The color chosen has a major impact on how people perceive the wearer. Beige raincoats are generally worn by members of the upper-middle class and black ones by members of the lower-middle class. Thus, if a man wants to be treated as a "somebody," Molloy states that he should never wear a black raincoat.

IMPLICATIONS FOR PERFORMANCE AND SATISFACTION

Roles, norms, and status have a significant impact on group behavior. Let us review the influence of each.

Roles

How is it relevant to understand group behavior to know that a woman, for example, has to reconcile her roles of mother, Methodist, Democrat, councilwoman, and warden of the Michigan State Penitentiary for Women? Knowledge of the role that a person is attempting to enact can make it easier for us to deal with the person, for we have insight into her expected behavior patterns. Additionally, knowledge of a job incumbent's role makes it easier for others to work with her, for she should behave in ways consistent with others' expectations. In other words, when a person plays out her role as it is supposed to be played, it improves the ability of others to predict the behavior of the role incumbent. We can predict an individual's behavior in new encounters by superimposing the role requirements of the situation upon her. We can, for example, expect a person to become more authoritarian when she moves from her role of wife to that of law enforcement officer.

Knowledge of an incumbent's role perception and others' expectations can also be beneficial in predicting role conflict and possibly explaining the behavior of the individual experiencing the conflict.

Norms

Norms control group member behavior by establishing standards of right or wrong. If we know the norms of a given group, it can help us to explain the attitudes and behaviors of its members. Where norms support high output, we can expect individual performance to be markedly higher than where group norms aim to restrict output. Similarly, acceptable standards of absence will be dictated by the group norms. Given the inverse correlation between satisfaction and turnover, it would also be reasonable to assume that if the group's norms reinforce complaining and consistent outward demonstration of job dissatisfaction, the propensity for members to terminate employment may be greater. On the other hand, members may enjoy this bitching and it may not affect turnover rates. To illustrate, it is not unusual for union members to play the role of "abused and exploited worker." The group may establish such a role stereotype as part of the norm. In such cases, it may have no real influence on satisfaction or quit rates.

Status

Status inequities create frustrations and can adversely influence productivity, satisfaction, and willingness to remain with an organization. There appears to be a strong correlation between the prestige of an occupation and members' satisfaction with their job.

> The prestige of an occupation depends on the amount of skill the job calls for, the degree of specialized education and training it requires, the level of responsibility and autonomy involved in work performance, and the income which it brings. All these factors have a direct relationship to satisfaction and at the same time are linked to status.[22]

"The higher the status of occupation, the more satisfied are persons who engage in it."[23] In North America, professionals have the highest occupational prestige and they also have the highest level of work satisfaction. Among 3,000 workers in sixteen industries polled, higher satisfaction scores were recorded by professional and white-collar occupations such as university professors, mathematicians, physicists, chemists, lawyers, and school superintendents. In contrast, significantly lower scores were made by skilled tradesmen and blue-collar workers.[24]

Other values of status should not be overlooked: Status provides motivation through the provision of organizational incentives, and status can be an effective indirect power base. Those individuals whom group members perceive as having status increase their ability to influence other members of the group.

22. David J. Lawless, *Effective Management: Social Psychological Approach* (Englewood Cliffs, N.J.: Prentice-Hall, 1972), p. 252.

23. Reported by Robert L. Kahn in "The Work Module," *Psychology Today*, February 1973, p. 39.

24. Ibid.

FOR DISCUSSION

1. Compare and contrast command, task, interest, and friendship groups.

2. What might motivate you to join a group?

3. Identify five roles you play. What behaviors do they require? Are any of these roles in conflict? If so, in what way? How do you resolve these conflicts?

4. What is the relationship between where you sit in relation to others and the role you are playing?

5. What is the relationship between the psychological contract and role expectations?

6. "The imposition of group norms is enforced via management authority rather than by group acceptance." Do you agree or disagree? Discuss.

7. Describe the Hawthorne studies. What is the importance of this research to understanding group behavior?

8. In the work environment, how is the status of an individual member determined?

9. How does the concept of status influence organizational effectiveness?

10. What is the "appropriate uniform" for (a) a female principal of a junior high school? (b) a female telephone lineman? (c) a male executive secretary? (d) a female banker? (e) a bartender in a swank New York City nightclub? (f) a star basketball player? (g) the President of the United States? and (h) your course instructor?

FOR FURTHER READING

BERGER, J., S. J. ROSENHOLTZ, and M. ZELDITCH, "Status Organizing Processes," in *Annual Review of Sociology,* Vol. 6, ed. A. Inkeles. pp. 479–508. Palo Alto, Calif.: Annual Reviews, 1980. Reviews theory and research on characteristics around which evaluations and beliefs about people come to be organized.

FRANKE, R. H., and J. D. KAUL, "The Hawthorne Experiments: First Statistical Interpretation," *American Sociological Review,* October 1978, pp. 623–43. The first statistical interpretation of the major Hawthorne experiments failed to support the assumption by the early researchers that unmeasured changes in the human relations of workers caused output changes.

HUNT, J. G., "Status Congruence: An Important Organization Function," *Personnel Administration,* January-February 1969, pp. 19–24. Reviews evidence concerning the effects of status congruence on group behavior and explores some of the managerial implications of the findings.

KATZ, D., and R. L. KAHN, *The Social Psychology of Organizations,* 2nd ed., chap. 7. New York: John Wiley, 1978. Excellent but sophisticated appraisal of roles. Offers a particularly good treatment of role expectations.

RIZZO, J. R., R. J. HOUSE, and S. I. LIRTZMAN, "Role Conflict and Ambiguity in Complex Organizations," *Administrative Science Quarterly,* June 1970, pp. 150–63. Role conflict and role ambiguity are negatively related to need fulfillment; and weakly, but positively, related to anxiety and propensity to leave the organization.

ROY, D. F., "Banana Time: Job Satisfaction and Informal Interaction," *Human Organization,* Vol. 18, No. 4 (1960), pp. 158–68. Fascinating account of how a small group of machine operators kept from "going nuts" in a situation of monotonous work activity by talking, fooling around, and game playing.

Suppose we took groups seriously

Adapted from Harold J. Leavitt, Man and Work in Society, ed. Eugene Louis Cass and Frederick G. Zimmer. ©1975 by Western Electric Company, Inc. Reprinted by permission of Van Nostrand Reinhold, a division of Litton Educational Publishing, Inc.

This is mostly a fantasy, but not a utopian fantasy. It tries to spin out some of the things that might happen if we really took small groups seriously; if, that is, we really used groups, rather than individuals, as the basic building blocks for an organization. The fantasy comes in proposing to start with groups, not add them in; to design organizations from scratch around small groups, rather than around individuals.

Why would groups be more interesting than individuals as basic design units around which to build organizations? What are the prominent characteristics of small groups? Why are they interesting? Here are several answers:

First, small groups seem to be good for people. They can satisfy important membership needs. They can provide a moderately wide range of activities for individual members. They can provide support in times of stress and crisis. They are settings in which people can learn not only cognitively but empirically to be reasonably trusting and helpful to one another. Second, groups seem to be good problem-finding tools. They seem to be useful in promoting innovation and creativity. Third, in a wide variety of decision situations, they make better decisions than individuals do. Fourth, they are great tools for implementation. They gain commitment from their members so that group decisions are likely to be willingly carried out. Fifth, they can control and discipline individual members in ways that are often extremely difficult through impersonal quasi-legal disciplinary systems. Sixth, as organizations grow large, small groups appear to be useful mechanisms for fending off many of the negative effects of large size. They help to prevent communication lines from growing too long, the hierarchy from growing too steep, and the individual from getting lost in the crowd.

There is a seventh, but altogether different, kind of argument for taking groups seriously. Groups are natural phenomena, and facts of organizational life. They can be created but their spontaneous development cannot be prevented. The problem is not shall groups exist or not, but shall groups be planned or not?

An architect can design a beautiful building that either blends smoothly with its environment or contrasts starkly with it. But organization designers may not have the same choice. If we design an organization that is structurally dissonant with its environment, it is conceivable that the environment will change to adjust to the organization. It seems much more likely, however, that the environment will reject the organization. If designing organizations around groups represents a sharp counterpoint to environmental trends maybe we should abort the idea.

Our environment, one can argue, is certainly highly individualized. But one can also make a less solid argument in the other direction; an argument that American society is going groupy rather than individual this year. Or at least that it is going groupy as well as individual. The evidence is sloppy at best. One can reinterpret the student revolution and the growth of antiestablishment feelings at least in part as a reaction to the decline of those institutions that most satisfied social membership needs. One can argue that the decline of the church, of the village, and of the extended family is leaving behind a vacuum of unsatisfied membership and belongingness motives. Certainly popular critics of American society have laid a great deal of emphasis on the loneliness and anomie that seem to have resulted not only from materialism but from the emphasis on individualism. It seems possible to argue that, in so far as there has been any significant change in the work ethic in America, the change has been toward a desire for work that is socially as well as egoistically fulfilling, and that satisfies human needs for belongingness and affiliation as well as needs for achievement.

In effect, the usual interpretation of Abraham Maslow's need hierarchy may be wrong. Usually the esteem and self-actualization levels of motivation are emphasized. Perhaps the level that is becoming operant most rapidly is neither of those, but the social-love-membership level.

Just what does it mean to design organizations around groups? Operationally, how is that different from designing organizations around individuals? One approach to an answer is simply to take the things that organizations do with individuals and try them out with groups. The idea is to raise the level from the atom to the molecule, and *select* groups rather than individuals, *train* groups rather than individuals, *pay* groups rather than individuals, *promote* groups rather than individuals, *design jobs* for groups rather than for individuals, *fire* groups rather than individuals, and so on down the list of activities that organizations have traditionally carried on in order to use human beings in their organizations.

Groups in organizations are not an invention of behavioral types. They are a natural phenomenon of organizations. Organizations develop informal groups, like it or not. It is both possible and sensible to describe most large organizations as collections of groups in interaction with one another; bargaining with one another, forming coalitions with one another, cooperating and competing with one another. It is possible and sensible too to treat the decisions that emerge from large organizations as a resultant of the interplay of forces among groups within the organization, and not just the resultant of rational analysis.

On the down side, small face-to-face groups are great tools for disciplining and controlling their members. Control of individual behavior is also a major problem of large complex organizations. This problem has driven many organizations into elaborate bureaucratic quasi-legal sets of rules, ranging from job evaluation schemes to performance evaluations to incentive systems; all individually based, all terribly complex, all creating problems of distributive justice. Any organizational design that might eliminate much of the legalistic superstructure therefore begins to look highly desirable.

Management should consider building organizations using a material now understood very well and with properties that look very promising, the small group. Until recently, at least, the human group has been primarily used for patching and mending organizations that were originally built of other materials.

The major unanswered questions in my mind are not in the understanding of groups, nor in the potential utility of the group as a building block. The more difficult to answer question is whether or not the approaching era is one in which Americans would willingly work in such apparently contra-individualistic units. I think we are.

COUNTER POINT

Where groups were taken seriously

Adapted from Richard E. Walton, Man and Work in Society, *ed. Eugene Louis Cass and Frederick G. Zimmer. © 1975 by Western Electric Company, Inc. Reprinted by permission of Van Nostrand Reinhold. Updated from "Stonewalling Plant Democracy,"* Business Week, *March 28, 1977, pp. 78–82.*

In January 1971, General Foods Corp. opened a dog food plant in Topeka, Kansas, designed around work groups. Self-managing work teams assumed collective responsibility for large segments of the production process. These teams performed many of the functions normally reserved for management—they made job assignments, scheduled coffee breaks, interviewed job applicants and made the hiring decisions, and even decided pay raises.

Teams had from seven to fourteen members. They were large enough to embrace a set of interrelated tasks and small enough to allow effective face-to-face meetings for decision making and coordination. An attempt was made to design every set of tasks in a way that would include functions requiring higher human abilities and responsibilities, such as planning, diagnosing mechanical problems, and liaison work. The aim was to make all sets of tasks equally challenging although each set would comprise unique skill demands. Consistent with this aim was a single job classification for all operators, with pay increases geared to mastering an increasing number of jobs, first within the team and then in the total plant. Because there were no limits on how many team members could qualify for higher pay brackets, employees were encouraged to teach each other. Within several years nearly half of the employees had earned the top rate for mastering all of the jobs in the plant.

In lieu of a "foreman" whose responsibilities typically are to plan, direct, and control subordinates, a "team leader" position was created with the responsibility for facilitating team development and decision making. Operators were provided information and decision rules that enabled them to make production decisions ordinarily made by higher levels of supervision. Management refrained from specifying in advance any plant rules. Rather, rules have evolved over time from collective experience.

Differential status symbols that characterize traditional work organizations were minimized—for example, by a single office-plant entrance and a common decor throughout offices, cafeteria and locker room. The physical layout was designed to facilitate rather than discourage the congregating of workers during working hours. These ad hoc gatherings not only afforded enjoyable exchanges but also provided opportunities to coordinate work and to learn about other jobs.

A half-dozen years after the plant was open, it was difficult to determine if the group concept was working. After the initial euphoria, a time when General Foods encouraged publicity about the Topeka plant, the company refused to let reporters inside the plant. Reports of problems were surfacing, although the plant's performance was not questioned. For instance, the plant's unit costs are 5 percent less than under a traditional factory system, while turnover and lost-time accident statistics are highly favorable. What has been noticed are a slight drop in quality, a build-up of problems because of fewer team meetings, and increased competition because of jealousy between teams and team leaders.

One of the more obvious problem areas is pay.

The system was established for team members to vote on pay raises for their fellow employees, but that proved difficult. One worker commented that "You work with somebody for five years and get to be pretty good friends. It's a little tough to decide on pay raises." As a result, although workers still discuss one another's raises, it has been reported that the real decisions are made by management.

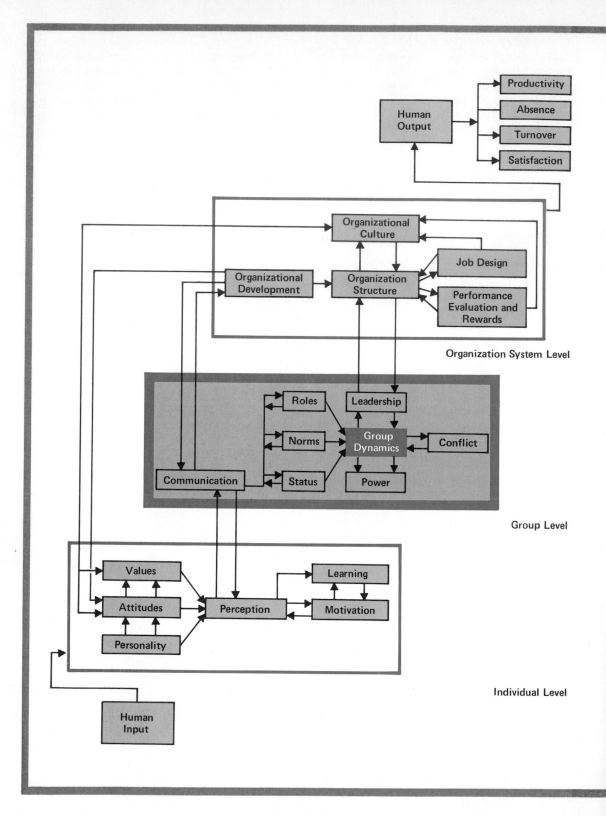

CHAPTER 9
Group Dynamics

AFTER STUDYING THIS CHAPTER, YOU SHOULD BE ABLE TO—

Define and explain the following key terms and concepts:

Activities

Cohesiveness

Delphi Technique

Emergent behavior

Groupthink

Human relations specialist

Interaction analysis

Interactions

Nominal Group Technique

Required behavior

Ringelmann effect

Risky-shift phenomenon

Sentiments

Sociogram

Sociometry

Task specialist

Understand:

Two methods for analyzing group structure and interactions

The group-behavior model

The benefits and disadvantages of group decision making

How groupthink can reduce group effectiveness

How the risky-shift phenomenon can reduce group effectiveness

The benefits and disadvantages of cohesive groups

> To get something done, a committee should consist of no more than three people, two of them absent.
>
> —LAURENCE J. PETER

In the previous chapter, group behavior was described in a relatively static state. In this chapter, we shall look at the dynamic interacting factors in groups. We begin by introducing several methods that you can use to analyze group behavior, then proceed to develop a group-behavior model, identify the key contingency variables that effect group behavior, discuss characteristics of group decision making, and assess the value of group cohesiveness.

METHODS OF GROUP ANALYSIS

Before we present our model to assist you in explaining and predicting group behavior, let's answer the question, How would I go about analyzing a group?

Honesty requires the admission that there are no easy methods by which to analyze group relationships. There are, however, two techniques that, although somewhat difficult to implement, can assist you in identifying the existence of informal groups, their leaders, conflicts, and the degree to which members are attracted to each other. These techniques are *sociometry* and *interaction analysis*.

Sociometry

One way to look at the structure of a group is through the use of sociometry, which is a preference analysis based on who members like and dislike in their group. The techniques in sociometry are not new—they date back over three decades.[1] But they are effective for depicting group interaction.

Sociometry developed from the belief that interactions in a group are based on people's feelings of like and dislike toward each other. The method involves asking group members whom they like or dislike, or whom they wish to work with or not to work with. From this data, collected by interviews, it is possible to develop attractiveness and interaction rankings and patterns that can be

---

1. J. L. Moreno, "Contributions of Sociometry to Research Methodology in Sociology," *American Sociological Review,* June 1947, pp. 287–92.

depicted in a tabular of graphic format. The latter, an example of which is shown in Figure 9–1, is by far the most popular way to show sociometric results.

In Figure 9–1, we see a simple sociogram based upon the preferred choices of attraction and rejection reported by eight social service workers, labeled as A through H. The preferences show the direction of attraction or rejection; for example, D is attracted to B, A and B are mutually attracted, and F rejects H. This sociogram shows several interesting things. A, B, and C appear to be a cohesive clique, each indicating attraction to the other. B assumes leadership characteristics: A, C, D, E, and G all are attracted to him. E and F are attracted to each other, but neither are popular. Additionally, H can be described as an isolate. He is not a preferred choice of any of the other service workers.

Sociometry provides a means for us to identify attractions, repulsions, and the direction of preferences between group members. It allows us to pick out the stars, the isolates, the powerful individuals, and other groupings. It can also be used for determining job assignments so as to further performance. For example, in one study on a Chicago construction project, some carpenters and bricklayers were allowed to self-select work partner teams, while others were assigned to teams randomly.[2] Job satisfaction was significantly higher among the teams that were self-chosen; and they also had significantly lower turnover, labor costs, and material costs. The self-selecting teams even had a small but positive advantage over the randomly chosen teams in productivity.

A final point about sociometry: It should be viewed as a method for measuring a dynamic, ever-changing preference pattern. Preferences change as group members change and can fluctuate over a range of goals. For example, in a New York training school for girls, different pairings were preferred depending

2. R. Van Zelst, "Sociometrically Selected Work Teams Increase Production," *Personnel Psychology,* Autumn 1952, pp. 175–85.

FIGURE 9–1   Sociogram

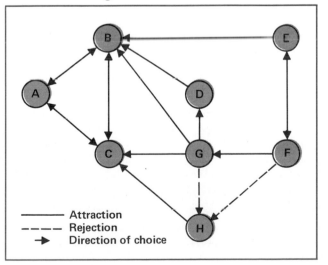

upon whether the girls were expressing their choice for a roommate or a work-mate.[3] This finding strikes home when you think of your personal first choice with whom to play tennis, attend the ballet, listen to a lecture by Art Buchwald, or go drinking at the local pub. Your preference probably changes depending on the activity, and the same idea operates with sociometric analysis.

Interaction Analysis

Another approach for analyzing interaction patterns among members of a group is interaction analysis, as proposed by R.F. Bales.[4] Interaction analysis requires one to observe individual interactions and tabulate the number of discussions taking place between individuals, noting who initiates these discussions and who addresses discussion to the entire group. Bales proposed that every observable group interaction could be placed into one of twelve categories. The first six embrace socioemotional factors: showing disagreement or agreement, tension or tension release, solidarity or antagonism. The second six are task-oriented: giving or asking for suggestions, opinions, information. Utilizing his interaction analyses, Bales found that there is a significant difference in the roles played by the two people who do the most talking within the group. One is the idea person, who takes on the role of the group's task specialist. This person's communications fall into the categories of giving suggestions, opinions, and information. He or she says things like: "Do it this way," "You work on that project," "That's the wrong way to go about it." The other role is the human-relations specialist—the best-liked member of the group, who makes friendly, encouraging, and supportive comments. This person might say things like: "Way to go," "This is a great group," "Let me help you with that problem." The human-relations specialist initiates more interactions that fall into the categories showing agreement, solidarity, and tension release.

While the two roles can be played by one person, Bales concluded that groups function more effectively when these roles are played by two separate members. This allows one to emphasize getting the job done, while the other emphasizes the social aspects of the situation, keeping the group running smoothly. The task specialist concentrates on the group's performance and the human-relations specialist keeps satisfaction high.

As noted at the beginning of this section, the effective application of group analysis is not easy. Sociometry is particularly difficult because of the cumbersomeness of asking people whom they like or dislike, and then ensuring that this data is kept current. Although observation and category demarcation in interaction analysis is also difficult, direct observation is less obtrusive than interviewing. Additionally, video-tape equipment now makes interaction analysis a more viable alternative for observing and analyzing group behavior.

3. J. L. Moreno, ed., *The Sociometry Reader* (New York: Free Press, 1960).

4. R. F. Bales, *Interaction-Process Analysis: A Method for the Study of Small Groups* (Reading, Mass.: Addison-Wesley, 1950).

GROUP-BEHAVIOR MODEL

George Homans developed a model—an adaptation of which is shown in Figure 9–2—to describe work-group behavior.[5] Even though it is more than three decades old, the model continues to have considerable value for explaining group behavior. Basically, it attempts to identify the outputs of group effort: Tasks are accomplished, intrinsic satisfactions are received, and/or personal growth is experienced. It considers those factors outside of the group itself, personalities of members, the formal requirements of the group, and the actual behaviors that emerge. The model proposes that there is a chain of influences whereby background and individual personal factors impact on the formal system to produce actual behaviors, which in turn produce the outcomes of group behavior. However, before we can discuss the model in detail, we need to define five of its most critical components: activities, interaction, sentiments, required behavior, and emergent behavior.

Defining the Key Components

Activities are the physical movements that individuals make that can be observed by others. They include things like running, sitting, writing, and operating a machine.

Interaction refers to the verbal and nonverbal communication and contacts that actually take place between people. It occurs when two or more people in some way affect each other through interpersonal behavior. Students

5. George C. Homans, *The Human Group* (New York: Harcourt Brace Jovanovich, 1950).

FIGURE 9–2 Group Behavior Model

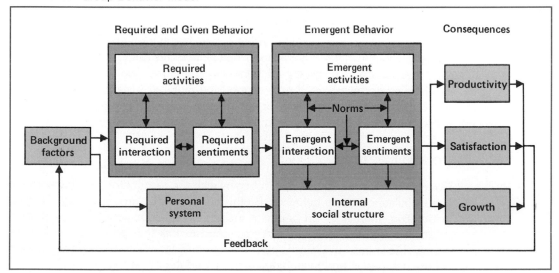

discussing an upcoming class examination, a quarterback calling signals in the huddle, and an employee waving at an acquaintance on the other side of the office are all examples of people interacting together. When we observe and analyze interaction, we look for *frequency* with which interaction occurs, the *duration* or length of the interaction, and finally the *order* of the interaction—who does the initiating. Frequency, duration, and order of interaction give us insight into the importance of the interaction, and the relative status of those who are interacting.

Sentiments are the values, attitudes, and beliefs within a person. They include all the positive and negative feelings that group members hold about each other. Because feelings are often not directly observable, they must be inferred from the activities and interactions that express them. The student who fails to talk in class, in spite of 30 percent of his grade being based on class participation, holds certain sentiments toward class discussion. If the student does not express these views, the instructor must infer what sentiments are involved. In analyzing sentiments, we look at the *number* of people who share them, how *intense* their feelings are, and the *degree* of conviction they have. Prejudice towards a certain individual, for example, may be narrowly or widely shared, mildly or strongly felt, flexible or entrenched.

Required behavior refers to the activities, interactions, and sentiments that are defined by the group's formal leaders and assigned to the members as their specified roles. Individuals are required to perform these behaviors if they are to maintain their standing within the group. For example, the accounts payable clerk must tally the invoices that are received daily, stamp them in, alphabetize and merge them with purchase orders, prepare the payment vouchers, forward them to the treasurer's office for disbursement, and talk with suppliers and the purchasing agent if discrepancies occur. Failure to engage in these required behaviors would disrupt the operation of the formal system.

Emergent behavior refers to behavior that is not required; it is in addition to what is required. Our accounts payable clerk, for example, has social needs that will be met through the group. He or she may tease new members, discuss plans for an upcoming vacation, throw paper clips at a co-worker several desks away, or agree with the other accounts payable clerks not to process more than forty vouchers a day. Emergent behavior, therefore, relates to the personal needs of group members. It may support the required system by making work more interesting and satisfying, or it can be detrimental when it interferes with the formal system's efficiency and effectiveness.

Background Factors

Now let us return to Figure 9–2. It begins with the recognition that background factors influence group behavior. By this we mean that groups do not function in isolation. Influences on behavior include, in addition to the group setting, those things, places, people, processes, and events that go on outside of the group. The more obvious of these background factors are the organizational culture, job design and technology utilized, and the reward system.

Organizational culture is a term that captures the internal atmosphere or personality of the organization. How things are supposed to be done, what is appropriate attire, or whether it's acceptable to question the boss's decision are determined by an organization's culture. Since work groups are part of the larger organization, the culture of the larger system sets parameters for the behavior of members who are part of the subsystems. The way that things are generally done in the overall organization will be a major determinant of the ways things will be done in groups within the organization.

Job design and technology refer to the means the group uses to achieve its objectives; that is, how it turns inputs into outputs. Formal authority patterns, the sequencing of work flows, standardized methods and procedures, the layout of facilities, and the actual materials, tools, and equipment that group members use are all part of job design and technology. How do these factors influence group behavior? By defining constraints on what social interactions and emergent behaviors are possible. Certainly it's easier to talk with your friend if her work station is only five feet from yours, there are no physical barriers separating the two of you, supervision is infrequent, and the noise level is very low. In contrast, it would be more difficult to interact if there is considerable physical separation, walled barriers, close supervision, high noise levels, or high-speed conveyor belts that cannot be left unattended. Because job design and technology are a major influence on who is likely to, must, or cannot interact with whom, and on when interaction can take place, they both cause and limit activities, interactions, and sentiments.

The organization's formal *reward system* influences group members by identifying which behaviors will be rewarded and which will not. The ways in which pay is allocated, recognition and praise are given, and promotions are determined are issues that group members will be concerned about. But they also will be influenced by the informal rewards that the group itself can offer. The group's ability to give or withhold support, for example, is a powerful influence on its members' behavior. The end result is that the combination of formal and informal rewards clarify which activities, interactions, and sentiments pay off and which do not.

The background factors we have described are not the only ones that influence group behavior. We could also consider economic factors, the external status hierarchy, government legislation, and the like. However, culture, technology, and rewards are probably the three most important. The key point to be made is that background factors form the "givens" that influence observed behavior.

Personal System

The personal system box in Figure 9–2 acknowledges that the personal characteristics of individuals influence the behavior that emerges from the required system. Just as culture, technology, and rewards define and limit group behavior, so do the past experiences that people bring with them when they enter a group. As we discussed in Part 2, people bring to organizations a given set of values, certain attitudes, and established personality characteristics. The same obviously holds true when they enter groups. What individuals have learned from their prior experiences becomes a factor in determining the behavior that will emerge in the group. As we shall see, the personal system interacts with the formal (required) system to influence the informal (emergent) system.

Required and Emergent Behavior

The required behaviors, while distinct in our discussion, are actually highly intertwined and mutually dependent. For instance, assume Barbara is a co-worker of yours and you frequently have to confer with her in the completion of your work assignments. You see Barbara at her desk, you walk over to her, you sit down, talk with her a bit, and agree to continue your discussion later in the afternoon. You have certain sentiments toward Barbara, implied by your going over to her desk. Going to the desk was an activity. Her asking you to "sit down" is an activity and interaction. It also confirms the good feelings you have about her. Your decision to continue your talk initiates the sentiment-activity-interaction chain. The point should be clear: The three concepts are closely linked.

Careful analysis of the required and personal systems can aid the observer in attempting to predict emergent behavior. For example, more frequent than usual interaction, and more favorable sentiments, can be expected to emerge between members whose given sentiments are similar. High status derived from the external social system is apt to be related, initially at least, to emergent interpersonal sentiment and rank in the internal social structure. Further, emergent interaction is more likely between members who are required to interact, between those whose jobs place them near each other, and so forth. Emergent behavior is likely to be related to the demands of the technology, including such conditions as heat, noise, and lighting, as well as the degree of repetitiveness and mechanical pacing required by the job. The extent to which certain sentiments are required, such as identification with the total process or willingness to innovate or take responsibility, will have more or less obvious influence on emergent sentiments, activity and interaction.

Homans hypothesized that interaction and interpersonal sentiment are closely related; that, in the absence of contrary influences, favorable sentiments emerge between members who interact frequently and frequent interaction emerges between members who like each other. Unfavorable sentiments are directed against members who do not share or who violate the norms generally accepted in the group. Furthermore, these unfavorable sentiments frequently lead to the emergence of further activities that have the function of punishing the violators of the norm and that, in turn, may well lead to further defensive or aggressive activities by the violators.

The quantity and quality of interaction between the two members—say, A and B—is related not only to the sentiment between them, but also to the extent to which A perceives B's activities as violating the norms of the group. However, if these efforts fail, and B persists in violating the norm, he or she will be the recipient of increasingly unfavorable sentiments and consequently decreasing interaction.

Summary

The Homans model argues that certain background factors combine with the required activities, interactions, and sentiments that the work group faces, plus the personal characteristics of the group members, to create both a formal and informal internal system. This, in turn, will determine the group's productivity, its level of satisfaction, and its ability to develop, change, and innovate. These outcomes—productivity, satisfaction, and growth—may or may not be supportive of the required system. Sometimes work groups invent improved methods, informally help one another, and do other things to bolster the required system. At other times, their emergent behavior may actually be in conflict with the required tasks defined by management and result in reduced productivity. Either way, the Homan's model offers you insight into group behavior and can assist you in explaining and predicting certain group consequences.

CONTINGENCY VARIABLES
THAT AFFECT GROUP BEHAVIOR

The Homans group-behavior model has given us some general insights into the working of groups. Now, we want to look at a few of the more important contingency variables that will further improve our ability to explain and predict group behavior. Among these variables are the sex and personal characteristics of members, the number of members in the group, and the degree of heterogeneity among members.

Sex of Members

The evidence has consistently shown males as more aggressive, self-assertive, and fearless than females. Women, on the other hand, are more likely to be compassionate, sympathetic, and emotional than men. Most importantly, these individual characteristics are demonstrated in groups. That is, males are generally more aggressive than females and they behave more aggressively in groups.[6]

Sex differences in group behavior have also been observed in regard to conformity behavior.[7] The evidence has shown that men are usually more influencial in groups than women are, and that women conform more than men in group situations. However, more recent investigations suggest that these re-

---

6. Marvin E. Shaw, *Contemporary Topics in Social Psychology* (Morristown, N.J.: General Learning Press, 1976), pp. 348–49.

7. Ibid.

sults may be due to the type of task studied. Researchers historically looked at tasks that were traditionally identified as male tasks. Not surprisingly, then, males had greater influence. When the task was not clearly male-related, the sex differences were eliminated.

One must carefully qualify the research on sex differences. Many differences are unquestionably the result of sex-related roles imposed upon men and women by our culture. Given that most of the studies that found sex differences were conducted prior to equal rights legislation and the women's movement, these differences may no longer be applicable.

Personality Characteristics of Members

There has been a great deal of research on the relationship between personality traits and group attitudes and behavior. The general conclusion is that attributes that tend to have a positive connotation in our culture tend to be positively related to group productivity, morale, and cohesiveness. These include traits such as sociability, self-reliance, and independence. In contrast, negatively evaluated characteristics such as authoritarianism, dominance, and unconventionality tend to be negatively related to the dependent variables.[8]

Is any one personality characteristic a good predictor of group behavior? The answer is "No." The magnitude of the effect of any *single* characteristic is small, but taken *together* the consequences for group behavior is of major significance. We can conclude, therefore, that personality characteristics of group members play an important part in determining behavior in groups.

Number of Members

Does the size of a group affect the group's overall behavior? The answer to this question is a definite "Yes," but the effect depends on what dependent variables you look at.[9] The evidence indicates, for instance, that smaller groups are faster at completing tasks than larger ones. However, if the group is engaged in problem solving and you are appraising the group in terms of its ability to obtain high-quality answers, large groups consistently get better marks than their smaller counterparts. If you are interested in cohesiveness, researchers have found that it decreases as group size increases.

One of the most important findings related to the size of a group has been labeled the Ringelmann effect.[10] It directly challenges the logic that the produc-

---

8. Ibid., pp. 350–51.

9. Edwin J. Thomas and Clinton F. Fink, "Effects of Group Size," *Psychological Bulletin,* July 1963, pp. 371–84.

10. W. Moede, "Die Richtlinien der Leistungs-Psychologie," *Industrielle Psychotechnik,* Vol. 4 (1927), pp. 193–207.

tivity of the group as a whole should at least equal the sum of the productivity of each individual in that group.

A common stereotype about groups is that the sense of team spirit spurs individual effort and enhances the productivity of all. Ringelmann, a German psychology student in the late 1920s, compared the results of individual and group performance on a rope-pulling task. He expected that the group's effort would be equal to the sum of the efforts of individuals within the group. That is, three people pulling together should exert three times as much pull on the rope as one person, and eight people should exert eight times as much pull. Ringelmann's results, however, did not confirm his expectations. Groups of three people exerted a force only two-and-a-half times the average individual performance. Groups of eight collectively achieved less than four times the solo rate.

Replications of Ringelmann's research with similar tasks have generally supported his findings.[11] Increases in group size are inversely related to individual performance. More may be better in the sense that the total productivity of a group of four is greater than one or two, but the individual productivity of each group member declines.

What causes the Ringelmann effect? It may be due to a belief that others in the group are not pulling their own weight. If you see others as lazy or inept, you can reestablish equity by reducing your effort. Another explanation is the dispersion of responsibility. Because the results of the group cannot be attributed to any single person, the relationship between an individual's input and the group's output is clouded. In such situations, individuals may be tempted to become "free riders" and coast on the group's efforts. In other words, there will be a reduction in efficiency where individuals think that their contribution cannot be measured.

The implications for OB of this effect on work groups are significant. Where managers utilize collective work situations to enhance morale and teamwork, they must also provide means by which individual efforts can be identified. If this is not done, management must weigh the potential losses in productivity against any possible gains in worker satisfaction.[12]

Heterogeneity of Members

Most group activities require a variety of skills and knowledge. Given this requirement, it would be reasonable to conclude that heterogenous groups—those made up of dissimilar individuals—would be more likely to have diverse

11. Alan G. Ingham, George Levinger, James Graves, and Vaughn Peckham, "The Ringelmann Effect: Studies of Group Size and Group Performance," *Journal of Experimental Social Psychology,* July 1974, pp. 371–84; Bibb Latané, Kipling Williams, and Stephen Harkins, "Many Hands Make Light the Work: The Causes and Consequences of Social Loafing," *Journal Of Personality and Social Psychology,* November 1979, pp. 822–32.

12. Bibb Latané, Kipling Williams, and Stephen Harkins, "Social Loafing," *Psychology Today,* October 1979, p. 110.

abilities and information, and should be more effective. Research studies substantiate this conclusion.[13]

When a group is heterogeneous in terms of personality, opinions, abilities, skills, and perspectives, there is an increased probability that the group will possess the needed characteristics to effectively complete its tasks.[14] The group may be more conflict-laden and less expedient as diverse positions are introduced and assimilated, but the evidence generally supports that heterogeneous groups perform more effectively than those that are homogeneous.

CHARACTERISTICS OF GROUP DECISION MAKING

Groups are frequently used in organizations for the purpose of solving problems or making decisions. The use of decision-making groups—typically called committees—is common in almost all medium-sized and large business firms, government agencies, hospitals, schools, and other organizations.

Why are committees so pervasive in organizations? As we noted previously, groups allow the coming together of people with heterogeneous characteristics. This diversity of ideas can bring about a better dialogue and hence better comprehension of a problem and the development of more creative alternatives, all of which result in more effective group performance. Additionally, the use of committees increases the chance that those who have to accept and implement a decision will do so. If you have participated on a committee and played an active part in its deliberation, you're more likely to see that its decisions are carried out and to exert the extra effort to ensure that they work. So the popularity of committees can be attributed to their ability to develop and implement effective decisions.

The advantages of group decisions do not come without costs. Groups are vulnerable to two important phenomena that affect the group's ability to appraise alternatives and arrive at decision solutions.

The first phenomenon, called *groupthink,* is related to norms. It describes situations where group pressures for conformity deter the group from critically appraising unusual, minority, or unpopular views. Groupthink is a disease that attacks many groups and can dramatically hinder their performance. The second phenomenon we shall review is called *risky-shift.* It indicates that in appraising a given set of alternatives, decisions reached by a group in some situations are more risky than the decisions that individuals in the group reach when they are alone. Let us look at each of these phenomena in more detail.

13. See, for example, R. L. Hoffman, "Homogeneity of Member Personality and Its Effect on Group Problem Solving," *Journal of Abnormal and Social Psychology,* January 1959, pp. 27–33; and R. L. Hoffman and N. R. F. Maier, "Quality and Acceptance of Problem Solutions by Members of Homogeneous and Heterogeneous Groups," *Journal of Abnormal and Social Psychology,* March 1961, pp. 401–07.

14. Shaw, *Contemporary Topics,* p. 356.

A number of years ago your author had a peculiar experience. During a faculty meeting that he attended, a motion was placed on the floor stipulating each faculty member's responsibilities in regard to counseling students. The motion received a second, and the floor was opened for questions. There were none. After about fifteen seconds of silence, the chairman asked if he could "call for the question" (fancy terminology for permission to take the vote). No objections were voiced. When the chairman asked for those in favor, a vast majority of the thirty-two faculty members in attendance raised their hand. The motion passed and the chairman proceeded to the next item on the agenda.

Nothing in the above process seemed unusual, but the story is not over yet. About twenty minutes following the end of the meeting, a professor came roaring into my office with a petition. The petition said that the motion on counseling students had been rammed through and requested the chairman to replace the motion on the next month's agenda for discussion and a vote. When I asked this professor why he had not spoken up less than an hour earlier, he just gave me a frustrated look. He then proceeded to tell me that in talking with people after the meeting, he realized there actually had been considerable opposition to the motion. He didn't speak up, he said, because he thought he was the only one opposed. Conclusion: The faculty meeting we had attended had been attacked by the deadly groupthink "disease."

Have you ever felt like speaking up in a meeting, classroom, or informal group, but decided against it? One reason may have been shyness. On the other hand, you may have been a victim of groupthink, the phenomenon that occurs when group members become so enamoured with seeking concurrence that the norm for consensus overrides the realistic appraisal of alternative courses of action and the full expression of deviant, minority, or unpopular views. It describes a deterioration in an individual's mental efficiency, reality testing, and moral judgments as a result of group pressures.[15]

We have all seen the symptoms of the groupthink phenomenon:

1. Group members rationalize any resistance to the assumptions they have made. No matter how strong the evidence may contradict their basic assumptions, members behave so as to continually reinforce those assumptions.
2. Members apply direct pressures on those who momentarily express doubts about any of the group's shared views or who question the validity of arguments supporting the alternative favored by the majority.
3. Those members who have doubts or hold differing points of view seek to avoid deviating from what appears to be group consensus by keeping silent about misgivings and even minimizing to themselves the importance of their doubts.
4. There appears to be an illusion of unanimity. If someone does not speak, it is assumed that he or she is in full accord. In other words, abstention becomes viewed as a "Yes" vote.[16]

15. Irving L. Janis, *Victims of Groupthink* (Boston: Houghton Mifflin, 1972).
16. Ibid.

In studies of American foreign policy decisions, the above symptoms were found to prevail when government policy-making groups failed: unpreparedness at Pearl Harbor in 1941, the U.S. invasion of North Korea, the Bay of Pigs fiasco, and the escalation of the Vietnam War by introduction of bombing during the Johnson administration. Importantly, these four groupthink characteristics could not be found where group policy decisions were successful: the Cuban missile crisis and the formulation of the Marshall Plan.[17]

Three clear illustrations of the groupthink phenomenon are the reported description of high-level decision making during the Vietnam War, the period leading up to the attempted Bay of Pigs invasion of Cuba, and Richard Nixon's effort to undermine Democratic candidates during the 1972 presidential campaign.

During the Vietnam War, many of the key people in the Johnson administration were victims of groupthink. In late 1964, before the heavy bombing of North Vietnam began, it was proposed in a policy meeting that six weeks of air strikes would induce the North Vietnamese to seek peace talks. When someone inquired what would happen if that failed, the answer was that another four weeks would certainly do the trick. There were members of this group who did not accept the notion that the propensity for the North Vietnamese to talk peace was directly related to the tonnage of bombs dropped, but the group used subtle pressures to deal with dissenters. Acceptance by the group was predicted on the dissenters meeting two conditions: (1) Doubts were not to be expressed outside the policy group for fear it would aid the opposition, making it appear that the administration was not unanimous in its position; and (2) criticisms were to be kept within the limits of an acceptable deviation, which meant that it was not permissible to challenge any of the fundamental assumptions upon which the group's prior commitments had been made. As an illustration of the climate that existed in these meetings, it is said that President Johnson used to greet Bill Moyers, who had developed a reputation as a dissenter among the group, with, "Well, here comes Mr. Stop-the-Bombing."[18]

Meetings on the Bay of Pigs invasion were attended by senior advisors; officials from within the State, Defense, and Treasury Departments; the Attorney General; White House staff advisors; the Joint Chiefs of Staff; and CIA officials. Arthur Schlesinger, one of Kennedy's most respected advisors, reported that he had strong reservations about the invasion proposal, yet he failed to present his views when issues were being discussed and decisions reached. He indicated that, at the time, he felt that his dissenting opinions were not likely to influence the group away from the invasion plan and would probably have resulted in his being labeled as a "nuisance."[19]

The evidence suggests that Schlesinger was not the only member at those meetings who had doubts but restrained himself from voicing them. From var-

17. Ibid.
18. Ibid.
19. Ibid.

ious sources it was reported that Secretary of State Dean Rusk asked more critical questions of his associates than he did in the policy meetings; that Secretary of Defense Robert McNamara held assumptions about the invasion that were at odds with those the group was operating under, and that the Joint Chiefs questioned the plan's feasibility from a military standpoint. In spite of the fact that many of President Kennedy's most valued advisors and officials had serious reservations about the invasion plan, they did not raise them openly in the group for fear of being seen as "soft" by their colleagues or of receiving social disapproval.[20]

Another example of groupthink at work is the Watergate affair. During the Watergate hearings, the following encounter took place between Senator Howard Baker and Herbert Porter, a member of Richard Nixon's White House staff. Baker wanted to know how Porter found himself "in charge of or deeply involved in a dirty tricks operation of the campaign." Porter replied that he had had qualms about his behavior, but that he ". . . was not one to stand up in a meeting and say that this should be stopped . . . I kind of drifted along." When Baker asked why he had allowed himself to get into such a predicament, Porter replied, "In all honesty, because of the fear of the group pressure that would ensue, of not being a team player. . . . I felt a deep sense of loyalty to him [President Nixon] or was appealed to on that basis."[21]

Groupthink appears to be closely aligned with the conclusions Asch drew in his experiments with a lone dissenter. Individuals who hold a position that is different from the dominant majority are under pressure to suppress, withhold, or modify their true feelings and beliefs. As members of a group, we find it is more pleasant to be in agreement—to be a positive part of the group—than to be a disruptive force, even if disruption is necessary to improve the effectiveness of the group's decisions. All groups, to some degree, suffer from groupthink. It is a natural byproduct of individual desire for consensus and agreement. However, as some of the examples above indicate, it can have a significant destructive effect upon a group's performance.

The Risky-Shift Phenomenon

In comparing group decisions that have a clear dimension of risk with the individual decisions of members within the group, evidence suggests that there are differences. In some cases, the group decisions may be more conservative than the individual decision,[22] but far more often the shift is toward greater risk taking. In any given instance of group decision making, laboratory experiments indicate that there is a distinct possibility that the solution will have a higher degree

20. Ibid.

21. *The Washington Post*, June 8, 1973, p. 20, as reported in Jerry B. Harvey, "The Abilene Paradox: The Management of Agreement," *Organizational Dynamics*, Summer 1974, p. 68.

22. D. C. Barnlund, "A Comparative Study of Individual, Majority, and Group Judgment," *Journal of Abnormal and Social Psychology*, January 1959, pp. 55–60.

of risk attached to it than many of the members would have been willing to take on their own.[23] This phenomenon is called risky-shift.

The risky-shift is actually a special case of groupthink. The decision of the group reflects the type of decision-making norm that develops during the group's discussion, and this norm tends to be toward the assumption of more aggressive and risky alternatives than the individuals would reach alone.

> Caution, which the members feel privately, may not be communicated in a group setting, and there emerges the impression that other participants are more daring. Once again we have a group situation in which participation may lead to a leveling rather than a sharpening of the differences among members.[24]

What might cause the risky-shift phenomenon to occur? Four explanations have been proposed: the familiarization hypothesis, the leadership hypothesis, the risk-as-value hypothesis, and the diffusion-of-responsibility hypothesis.[25]

The *familiarization* argument is that group discussion allows individuals to become more familiar with the situations being discussed, and this increased familiarity is responsible for the observed shift toward risk. Initially, there is a "feeling out" or "go slow" period, but once individuals feel generally comfortable, they become more bold and daring. If one accepts this view, then any procedure that will increase familiarity with an issue involving risk will cause persons to assume more risk on that issue.

The *leadership* hypothesis suggests that risk takers are perceived as group leaders, and are more dominant and influential in the group discussion, and, as a result, the risky-shift can be explained in terms of the influence of risky leaders.

A third argument is the *risk-as-value* hypothesis. It assumes that moderate risk has a stronger cultural value than caution in our society, that we generally admire persons who are willing to take risks, and that group discussion motivates individuals to show that they are at least as willing as their peers to take risks. Those whose initial private positions were less risky than the group average will recognize their relative cautiousness and recommend greater risk in order to restore their self-perceptions as being relatively risky people.

The final explanation, which seems intuitively to be the most palatable, is the *diffusion-of-responsibility* position. It proposes that group decisions free the individual from accountability for the group's final choice. If the decision fails, no one individual can be held wholly responsible.

No one of the four hypotheses can fully account for the risky-shift phenomenon. Each has some credibility. However, in our search to explain and

---

23. See, for example: N. Kogan and M. A. Wallach, "Risk Taking as a Function of the Situation, the Person, and the Group," in *New Directions in Psychology*, Vol. 3 (New York: Holt, Rinehart & Winston, 1967); and M. A. Wallach, N. Kogan, and D. J. Bem, "Group Influence on Individual Risk Taking," *Journal of Abnormal and Social Psychology*, Vol. 65 (1962), pp. 75–86.

24. J. P. Campbell et al., *Managerial Behavior, Performance, and Effectiveness* (New York: McGraw-Hill, 1970), p. 433.

25. Russell D. Clark III, "Group-Induced Shift Toward Risk: A Critical Appraisal," *Psychological Bulletin*, October 1971, pp. 251–70.

predict behavior, we should be aware of the phenomenon and its implication for proposals to make organizational decision making more democratic. Although we cannot say that groups will *always* be less cautious than individuals, the evidence indicates that allowing groups rather than individuals to make decisions that contain a clear dimension of risk increases the probability that the decisions will involve a higher degree of risk.

TOWARD IMPROVED GROUP DECISION MAKING

The most common form of group decision making takes place in interacting groups. But as our discussion of groupthink demonstrated, face-to-face interacting groups often censor themselves and pressure individual members toward conformity of opinion. Two group decision-making techniques have been suggested that attempt to structure the decision process so as to reduce many of the problems inherent in the traditional interacting group. These are the *Nominal Group Technique* and the *Delphi Technique.*[26]

Nominal Group Technique

The Nominal Group Technique restricts discussion or interpersonal communication during the decision-making process; hence, the term *nominal*. Group members are all physically present, as in a traditional committee meeting, but members operate independently. Specifically, the following steps take place:

1. Members meet as a group but, before any discussion takes place, each member independently writes down his or her ideas on the problem.
2. This silent period is followed by each member presenting one idea to the group. Each member takes his or her turn, going around the table, presenting a single idea until all ideas have been presented and recorded (typically on a flip chart or chalkboard). No discussion takes place until all ideas have been recorded.
3. The group now discusses the ideas for clarity and evaluates them.
4. Each group member silently and independently rank orders the ideas. The final decision is determined by the idea with the highest aggregate ranking.

The chief advantage of the Nominal Group Technique is that it permits the group to meet formally but does not restrict independent thinking as does the interacting group.

Delphi Technique

A more complex and time-consuming alternative is the Delphi Technique. It is similar to the Nominal Group Technique except that it does not require the physical presence of the group's members. In fact, the Delphi Technique never

26. The following discussion is based on André L. Delbecq, A. H. Van deVen and D. H. Gustafson, *Group Techniques for Program Planning: A Guide to Nominal and Delphi Processes* (Glenview, Ill.: Scott, Foresman, 1975).

allows the group members to meet face-to-face. The following steps characterize the Delphi Technique:

1. The problem is identified and members are asked to provide potential solutions through a series of carefully designed questionnaires.
2. Each member anonymously and independently completes the first questionnaire.
3. Results of the first questionnaire are compiled at a central location, transcribed, and reproduced.
4. Each member receives a copy of the results.
5. After viewing the results, members are again asked for their solutions. The results typically trigger new solutions or cause changes in the original position.
6. Steps 4 and 5 are repeated as often as necessary until consensus is reached.

Like the Nominal Group Technique, the Delphi Technique insulates group members from the undue influence of others. Because it does not require the physical presence of the participants, the Delphi Technique can be used for decision making among geographically scattered groups. For instance, Sony could use the technique to query its managers in Tokyo, Brussels, Paris, London, New York, Toronto, Rio de Janeiro, and Melbourne as to the best worldwide price for one of the company's products. The cost of bringing the executives together at a central location is avoided. Of course, the Delphi Technique has its drawbacks. Because the method is extremely time-consuming, it is frequently not applicable where a speedy decision is necessary. Additionally, the method may not develop the rich array of alternatives that the interacting or Nominal Group Technique does. The ideas that might surface from the heat of face-to-face interaction may never arise.

GROUP COHESIVENESS

Intuitively, it would appear that groups in which there is a lot of internal disagreement and a lack of a cooperative spirit would be relatively less effective in completing their tasks than groups in which individuals generally agree, cooperate, and where members like each other. Research to test this intuition has focused on the concept of group cohesiveness, defined as the degree to which members are attracted to one another and share the group's goals. That is, the more that members are attracted to each other and the more that the group's goals align with their individual goals, the greater the group's cohesiveness. In the following pages, we shall review the factors that have been found to influence group cohesiveness, then look at the relationship between cohesiveness and group productivity.

Determinants of Cohesiveness

What factors determine whether group members will be attracted to one another? Cohesiveness can be affected by such factors as time spent together, the severity of initiation, group size, external threats, and previous successes.

Time Spent Together. If you rarely get an opportunity to see or interact with other people, you're unlikely to be attracted to them. The amount of time that people spend together, therefore, influences cohesiveness. As people spend more time together they become more friendly. They naturally begin to talk, respond, gesture, and engage in other interactions. These interactions typically lead to the discovery of common interests and increased attraction.[27]

The opportunity for group members to spend time together is dependent on their physical proximity. We would expect more close relationships among members who are located close to one another rather than far apart. People who live on the same block, ride the same car pool, or share a common office are more likely to become a cohesive group because the physical distance between them is minimal. For instance, among clerical workers in one organization it was found that the distance between their desks was the single most important determinant of the rate of interaction between any two of the clerks.[28]

Severity of Initiation. The more difficult it is to get into a group the more cohesive that group becomes. The hazing that fraternities typically put their pledges through is meant to screen out those who don't want to "pay the price" and to intensify the desire of those who do to become fraternity actives. But group initiation needn't be as blatant as hazing. The competition to be accepted to a good medical school results in first-year medical school classes that are highly cohesive. The common initiation rites—applications, test taking, interviews, and the long wait for a final decision—all contribute to creating this cohesiveness. Similarly, the months or often years that an apprentice trade worker must put in to developing his or her skills before being advanced to journeyman status results in union journeymen generally being a cohesive group.

Group Size. If group cohesiveness tends to increase with the time members are able to spend together, it seems logical that cohesiveness should decrease as group size increases, since it becomes more difficult for a member to interact with all the members. This is generally what the research indicates.[29] As group size expands, interaction with all members becomes more difficult, as does the ability to maintain a common goal. Not surprisingly, too, as a single group's size increases, the likelihood of cliques forming also increases. The creation of groups within groups tends to decrease overall cohesiveness.

Evidence suggests that these size-cohesiveness conclusions may be moderated by the gender of the group members.[30] In experiments comparing

27. C. Insko and M. Wilson, "Interpersonal Attraction as a Function of Social Interaction," *Journal of Personality and Social Psychology,* December 1977, pp. 903–11.

28. John T. Gullahorn, "Distance and Friendship as Factors in the Gross Interaction Matrix," *Sociometry,* February-May 1952, pp. 123–34.

29. E. J. Thomas and C. F. Fink, "Effects of Group Size," *Psychological Bulletin,* July 1963, pp. 371–84.

30. L. Libo, *Measuring Group Cohesiveness* (Ann Arbor, Mich.: Institute of Social Research, 1953).

groups of four and sixteen members, some made up of males only, some with females only, and others mixed, the small groups proved to be more cohesive than large ones as long as all the members were of the same sex. But when the groups were made up of both males and females, the larger groups were more cohesive. Members of both sexes liked the mixed groups more than the single-sex groups, and apparently the opportunity to interact with a larger set of both sexes increased cohesiveness. While it is dangerous to generalize from this study, we should nevertheless be aware of the possible moderating effect of sex on the size-cohesiveness relationship, especially nowadays as the work force becomes more equally divided between males and females.

External Threats. Most of the research supports the proposition that a group's cohesiveness will increase if the group comes under attack from external sources.[31] Management threats frequently bring together an otherwise disarrayed union. Efforts by management to unilaterally redesign even one or two jobs or to discipline one or two employees occasionally grab local headlines when the entire work force walks out in support of the abused few. These examples illustrate a cooperative phenomenon that can develop within a group when it is attacked from outside.

While a group generally moves toward greater cohesiveness when threatened by external agents, this does not occur under all conditions. If group members perceive that their group may not meet an attack well, then the group becomes less important as a source of security, and cohesiveness will not necessarily increase. Additionally, if members believe the attack is directed at the group merely because of its existence and that it will cease if the group is abandoned or broken up, there is likely to be a decrease in cohesiveness.[32]

Previous Successes. Everyone loves a winner! If a group has a history of previous successes it builds an esprit de corps that attracts and unites members. Successful firms find it easier to attract and hire new employees. The same holds true for successful research groups, well-known and prestigious universities, and winning athletic teams. When Bill Bowerman was head track coach at the University of Oregon during the 1960s, he never had trouble attracting the country's top track and field athletes to his campus. The best athletes wanted to come to Oregon because of Bowerman's highly successful program. In fact, Bowerman claims to never have initiated contact with an athlete. In contrast to track coaches at other major universities, if an athlete wanted to compete at Oregon, he had to prove his interest by taking the first step. Continuing with another university example, for those readers who harbor ambitions of attending a top-quality graduate school of business, you should recognize that the success

---

31. A. Stein, "Conflict and Cohesion: A Review of the Literature," *Journal of Conflict Resolution,* March 1976, pp. 143–72.

32. Alvin Zander, "The Psychology of Group Processes," in *Annual Review of Psychology,* Vol. 30, ed. M. R. Rosenzweig and Lyman W. Porter (Palo Alto, Calif.: Annual Reviews, 1979), p. 436.

of these schools attracts large numbers of aspiring candidates—many have twenty or more applicants for every vacancy. Again, everyone loves a winner!

Cohesiveness and Group Productivity

The previous section indicates that, generally speaking, group cohesiveness is increased when members spend time together and undergo a severe initiation, when the group size is small, when external threats exist, and when the group has a history of previous successes. But is increased cohesiveness always desirable from the point of view of management? Is it related to increased productivity?

Research has generally shown that highly cohesive groups are more effective than those with less cohesiveness,[33] but the relationship is more complex than merely allowing us to say high cohesiveness is good. First, high cohesiveness is both a cause and outcome of high productivity. Second, the relationship is moderated by the degree to which the group's attitude aligns with its formal goals or those of the larger organization of which it is a part.

Cohesiveness influences productivity and productivity influences cohesiveness. Camaraderie reduces tension and provides a supportive environment for the successful attainment of group goals. But as already noted, the successful attainment of group goals, and the members' feelings of having been a part of a successful unit, can serve to enhance the commitment of members. Basketball coaches, for example, are famous for their endearment of teamwork. They believe that if the team is going to win games, members have to learn to play together. Popular coaching phrases include, "There are no individuals on this team" and, "We win together, we lose together." The other side of this view, however, is that winning reinforces camaraderie and leads to increased cohesiveness; that is, successful performance leads to increased intermember attractiveness and sharing.

More important has been the recognition that the relationship of cohesiveness and productivity depends on the alignment of the group's attitude with its formal goals, or for work groups, those of the larger organization of which it is a part.[34] The more cohesive a group, the more its members will follow its goals. If these attitudes are favorable (i.e., high output, quality work, cooperation with individuals outside the group), a cohesive group will be more productive than a less cohesive group. But if cohesiveness is high and attitudes unfavorable, there will be decreases in productivity. If cohesiveness is low and there is support of goals, productivity increases but less than in the high cohesiveness—high support situation. Where cohesiveness is low and attitudes are not in support of the organization's goal, there seems to be no significant effect of cohesiveness upon productivity. These conclusions are summarized in Figure 9–3.

33. See, for example, L. Berkowitz, "Group Standards, Cohesiveness, and Productivity," *Human Relations*, November 1954, pp. 509–19.

34. Stanley E. Seashore, *Group Cohesiveness in the Industrial Work Group* (Ann Arbor: University of Michigan, Survey Research Center, 1954).

FIGURE 9–3   Relationship of Cohesiveness to Productivity

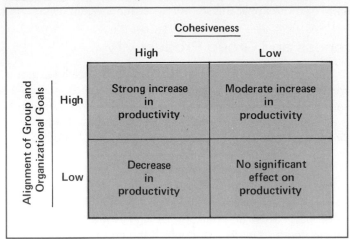

High cohesiveness tends to have a positive impact on satisfaction, and the reduction of absenteeism, tardiness, and turnover among group members. However, it may or may not affect productivity, depending on the coalignment between the group's goals and the organization's goals.

IMPLICATIONS FOR PERFORMANCE AND SATISFACTION

Sentiments, activities, and interactions within a group are important factors in explaining and predicting emergent behavior. The Homans model demonstrates the interdependence of these concepts, and how both the formal and informal systems are critical determinants of the group's productivity, its level of satisfaction, and its ability to develop, change, and innovate.

There are forces within groups that can adversely influence their decision-making effectiveness. Groupthink, if unchecked, can deter a group's creativity and its ability to change and develop innovative approaches to problems. Groups also may take greater risks in decision making than do their individual members alone. Where increased risk in decision making leads to reduced performance, the risky-shift phenomenon was shown to have an adverse impact on group outcomes. One possible solution is the use of heterogeneous groups. The evidence indicates that creating groups with individuals who have dissimilar characteristics leads to more effective decision making.

The identification of the Ringelmann effect advises management to keep in mind the negative impact on productivity as groups get larger. If large groups are used, efforts should be made to provide measures of individual performance within the group.

Cohesiveness is an important variable influencing group behavior. High cohesiveness has a positive impact on satisfaction, and the reduction of absenteeism and turnover, but its effect on productivity depends on the degree of coalignment that exists between the group's attitude or goals and the goals of the larger organization of which it is a part.

FOR DISCUSSION

1. Draw a sociometric analysis for a group with which you are familiar. Explain the patterns you have described.

2. Contrast the role of the task specialist with the role of the human-relations specialist in a group.

3. What are the key components in Homan's group behavior model? Explain the model.

4. Identify four contingency variables and discuss how they affect group behavior.

5. What is groupthink? Is the concept applicable to the family unit as well as to public or private organizations? Explain.

6. What is risky-shift? When might this phenomenon improve group effectiveness? When might it reduce effectiveness?

7. Describe the four possible causes of the risky-shift phenomenon.

8. What can management do to improve group decision-making effectiveness?

9. What factors influence the degree to which group members will be attracted to each other?

10. "High cohesiveness in a group leads to higher group productivity." Do you agree or disagree? Explain.

FOR FURTHER READING

ALDERFER, C. P., "Group and Intergroup Relations," in *Improving Life at Work*, ed. J. R. Hackman and J. L. Suttle, pp. 227–96. Santa Monica, Calif.: Goodyear, 1977. Reviews groups in social systems, small group behavior, and the dynamics of intergroup relations.

CARTWRIGHT, D., and A. ZANDER, eds., *Group Dynamics: Research and Theory*, 3rd ed. New York: Harper & Row, 1968. The classic reference for important readings in group dynamics.

"Conversation . . . with George C. Homans," *Organizational Dynamics*, Autumn 1975, pp. 34–54. In an informal dialogue, Homans candidly talks about interpersonal relationships within small groups in industry, the lessons from Hawthorne, and his views on determinism.

HOUSE, W. C., "Effects of Group Cohesiveness on Organization Performance," *Personnel Journal,* Vol. 45 (1966), pp. 28–33. Explores the relationship between group cohesiveness, morale, and productivity toward making more effective use of existing work groups.

JEWELL, L. N., and H. J. REITZ, *Group Effectiveness in Organizations.* Glenview, Ill.: Scott, Foresman, 1981. Reviews the various ways to improve group effectiveness.

STOGDILL, R. M., "Group Productivity, Drive and Cohesiveness," *Organizational Behavior and Human Performance,* August 1972, pp. 26–43. The research does not support the view that high group cohesiveness leads to high productivity; rather, group drive is the variable most consistently related to productivity.

POINT

HOLDER

Decision making by consensus

Adapted and edited from Jack J. Holder, Jr., "Decision Making by Consensus," Business Horizons, *April 1972, pp. 47–54. Copyright, 1972, by the Foundation for the School of Business at Indiana University. Reprinted by permission.*

Consensus is defined basically as agreement by all parties involved in some group decision or action; it occurs only after deliberation and discussion of pros and cons of the issues, and when all (not a majority) of the managers are in agreement. Each member of the group must be satisfied as to the ultimate course of action to be taken.

Decision making by consensus has been a common practice at Yellow Freight System, Inc., since the early 1950s, especially among the top management group of the company. The process is not a simple one. Some of the more important variables include the leader, the followers, the organizational structure, communications, leadership styles, motivation of group members, and the group itself. Many additional factors could be listed.

The various work groups at Yellow Freight extend from the top company officers to the dock foreman and his crew of dock workers. Our work groups are important to us, and as a result we are highly motivated to behave in ways consistent with the goals and values of the group in order to obtain recognition, support, security, and favorable reactions. We can conclude that management will make full use of the potential capacities of its human resources only when each person in an organization is a member of one or more effective functioning work groups that have a high degree of group loyalty, effective skills of interaction, and high performance goals.

The work group provides several advantages in the decision-making process. For example, technical knowledge and expertise may be shared; in fact, in an effective group the motivation is high to communicate accurately all relevant and important information. In addition, individual contributions make the group do a rigorous job of sifting ideas; members become experienced in effective group functioning and leadership; and group regulation of individual members can be exercised. Finally, each member is highly motivated to do his best to implement decisions and to achieve group goals. There are indications that an organization operating in a group fashion can be staffed for less than peak loads at each point.

The most important advantage of group decision making by consensus, in addition to the opportunity for knowledgeable managers to combine all their efforts to reach a decision, is that the members of the group have an ego identification with the goals. A manager's involvement in decision making in this manner makes him work hard to follow through with the decision; because he helped to make the decision he will help make it succeed.

Decision making by consensus may take more

time than decision making by majority. However, in the long run, as has been proven by Yellow Freight's past operations, the best decisions are made by consensus of all parties involved.

Decision making by consensus has been practiced at Yellow Freight since the present management assumed control of the company in the early 1950s. On important matters, the chairman of the board never took action without first discussing the decision with the president; the reverse was also true. Complete agreement was necessary before any action was taken. In later years, and after organizational changes, a new president and executive vice-president joined the chairman and honorary chairman of the board to form a decision-making group for major decisions.

The proper implementation of participative management for consensus decisions can be illustrated in some examples.

First, company officers and division managers decide jointly each year, and on a consensus basis, the goals and objectives for the company during the coming year. In a management-by-objectives process, the division managers have a voice in establishing the goals against which they will be judged.

Second, when a consensus decision is being sought regarding the opening of a new terminal, the division manager should utilize the ability of a number of people. Through his own expert ability, and with a regional and branch manager, sufficient data can be generated indicating whether customer potential is present. Since the opening of a new terminal affects the entire system, the division manager would necessarily have to work with a number of people before a decision could be made. Other managers who should be involved in this decision would include the vice-president of sales, the vice-president of operations, the president of the company, and the chairman of the board.

Third, personnel promotions and shifts at all levels of the company should definitely involve consensus decisions by the appropriate management. When a new branch manager is being selected, a regional manager should work with his division manager, who may involve the vice-presidents of sales and operations, and the president of the company. The regional manager should also look to other branch managers for their opinions and reactions to his suggestions regarding the vacancy.

Fourth, if a branch manager is making a decision to establish or terminate an agreement with an interline carrier, he should involve a number of people in this decision-making group because of their various levels of expertise. The regional manager, the salesman, and, possibly, the office manager (because of accounts receivable) should be involved. It would also be appropriate for the city dispatcher to be included.

When a new account is obtained, the branch manager should involve several people in the terminal in a participative management process. In deciding how this account is to be handled, he should involve the salesman, the operations manager, and the city dispatcher in all aspects of the new account and the procedures necessary to handle that account properly.

Any personnel shift in the terminal should involve several people related to the departments involved. For example, suppose the branch manager wants to move a dock foreman into the position of city dispatcher. The dock foreman's immediate supervisor, the present city dispatcher, the regional manager, the division manager, and other relevant individuals should be a part of the decision-making group. In case a branch manager wants to promote a shift supervisor to operations manager, the group should include city dispatch, line dispatch, office manager, regional manager, division manager, and others in the terminal.

If a consensus cannot be reached by a group, they should forego a decision at that time. Time as a prime consideration for a decision should be minimized. The group's decision not to make a specific decision on an important question may, or may not, be a consensus decision. Yellow Freight's experience has proven that when a decision cannot be reached, action should be deferred. Subsequent events will make a consensus decision easier to achieve because the action requiring a decision will have changed one way or the other.

Hasty decisions, made without a consensus, have proven unprofitable. This is true in many areas, but is especially true in matters relating to operating changes, terminal openings or closings, personnel changes and promotions, and general policy matters.

Naturally, a consensus decision cannot be reached on every administrative and day-to-day decision. The makeup of the decision-making group will vary, but should involve all those individuals immediately related to the problem area.

Once the group is formed, all must have a voice in the decision, and all must agree on the course of action to be taken. With most companies experiencing high rates of change and increased growth, it is important that we continue to make decisions by consensus.

COUNTER POINT

HAMPTON, SUMMER, AND WEBBER

Group decision making is not always better

Adapted and edited from Organizational Behavior and the Practice of Management *by David R. Hampton, Charles E. Summer, and Ross A. Webber. Copyright © 1973 by Scott, Foresman and Company. Reprinted by permission*

"A camel is a racehorse designed by a committee." So goes one of many aphorisms on the inadequacies of groups as decision makers. In spite of the fun in such complaint, however, committees continue to make decisions, because they offer advantages in breadth of experience, varied knowledge, absorption of antagonism, and mutual support.

To compare some aspects of individual versus group performance, numerous exercises have been conducted with managers and students. In Webber's research, he found five-person research groups take longer than the average of individuals working alone (50 percent longer), but over three-fourths of the groups produce better performance (an average of 30 percent better). Most groups, however, are worse than the best individual in the group.

These findings support Shaw's early contention that a group may be an advantage where being correct or avoiding mistakes is of greater importance than speed. The group does seem to improve on the performance of most people. In short:

1. The best individuals are usually better than groups as to accuracy, speed, and efficiency.
2. The average individual is faster and more efficient than most groups, but he makes more errors.
3. Groups are more accurate but slower than most individuals.

The superiority of groups over individuals, however, depends on prior experience and training. Hall's research, utilizing a "lost on the moon" exercise, presents findings very similar to Webber's results: The mean individual score for Hall was 47.5 (0 is perfect, 112 is totally wrong); the mean score for ad hoc groups was 34. In addition, Hall found that improved performance followed the reading of a one-page handout on developing group consensus—the mean score of such instructed groups was 26. Of the instructed groups, 75 percent produced group decisions that surpassed even the best individual decisions. Only 25 percent of the uninstructed groups did this.

Age and position level also seem to affect group performance on exercises. Various groups participated in Webber's research: Among others, they included high-level general executives averaging forty-seven years of age, forty-year-old middle managers, thirty-two-year old managers, and graduate and undergraduate business students about twenty-five and twenty years old respectively. The findings are distinctive. There were no significant differences in task performance among the different categories of people when they worked as individuals. *Yet, lower-level young men were more effective in utilizing group decision making than older, higher-level managers. The* difference between group performance and average individual performance decreased with increasing age and level of the group members. Younger groups improved more on individual performance. In fact, college students constituted the *only groups* that had higher group scores than their best individual. Among all the others, the best individual was better than the group.

So younger people seem to be more effective in utilizing groups for decision making than older and higher-level managers. Time and age seem to weaken the ability to work jointly with others—or perhaps the younger students came through an educational system that placed greater emphasis on group activity. The reasons why might also include less sensitivity to status, more personal flexibility, greater willingness to express opinions, and more "team spirit." Nonetheless, all age groups offered advantages and disadvantages compared to most individuals—more correct answers, fewer errors, but slower progress.

In summary, there are important differences in decision making by individuals and by groups. Groups offer advantages on certain kinds of problems when conditions are favorable—mainly on specific problems with clear-cut answers when open communication is facilitated because status and hierarchical distinctions are absent or not important. Training, experience, age, and personality also affect group effectiveness, but groups tend to make fewer errors, to be willing to take higher risks, and to improve on the performance of average individuals—but not always on that of the best group members.

Whether the advantages of group decision making justify the additional time required depends on three critical factors: (1) whether speed is essential (as when a military unit is under attack or a prospective customer is threatening to terminate negotiations); (2) whether an incorrect decision can be tolerated (as it cannot when making important defense decisions in Washington or styling decisions in Detroit); and (3) whether the organization has an exceptional individual who would be hindered by a group (as the United States had with President Lincoln, or as a few corporations have had with entrepreneurial giants).

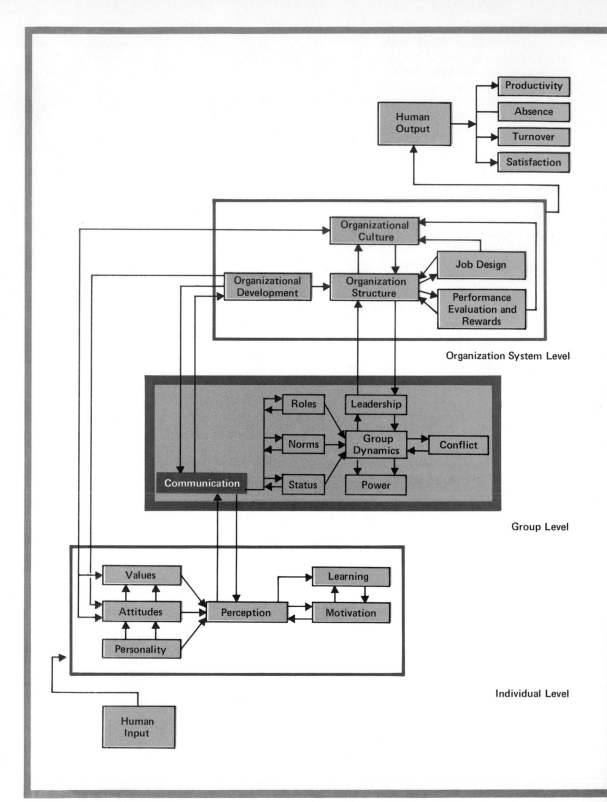

CHAPTER 10
Communication

AFTER STUDYING THIS CHAPTER, YOU SHOULD BE ABLE TO—

Define and explain the following key terms and concepts:

Channel
Communications
Communication networks
Communication process
Decoding
Encoding

Feedback loop
Grapevine
Informational cues
Jargon
Kinesics
Message

Understand:

The centrality of communication to group functioning
The process of communication
The relationship of perception to communication
The uses of language to create group identity
The benefits and disadvantages of each of five communication
   networks
Factors effecting the use of the grapevine
The difference between verbal and nonverbal communication
How physical, individual, and semantic barriers affect
   communication

> Every improvement in communication makes the bore more terrible.
> —FRANK M. COLBY

Probably the most frequently cited source of interpersonal conflict is poor communication.[1] Because we spend nearly 70 percent of our waking hours communicating—writing, reading, speaking, listening—it *seems* reasonable to conclude that one of the most inhibiting forces to successful group performance is a lack of effective communication.

No group can exist without communication: the transference of meaning among its members. It is only through transmitting meaning from one person to another that information and ideas can be conveyed. Communication, however, is more than merely imparting meaning. It must also be understood. In a group where one member speaks only German and the others do not know German, the individual speaking German will not be fully understood. Therefore, communication must include both the *transference and understanding* of meaning.

An idea, no matter how great, is useless until it is transmitted and understood by others. Perfect communication, if there were such a thing, would exist when a thought or idea were transmitted so that the mental picture perceived by the receiver was exactly the same as that envisioned by the sender. Although elementary in theory, perfect communication is never achieved in practice, for reasons we shall expand upon later.

Before making too many generalizations concerning communication and problems in communicating effectively, we should construct a model to depict and explain the components in the communication process.

COMMUNICATION-PROCESS MODEL

Before communication can take place, a purpose, expressed as a message to be conveyed, is needed. It passes between a source (the sender) and a receiver. The message is encoded (converted to symbolic form) and passed by way of some medium (channel) to the receiver, who retranslates (decodes) the mes-

---

1. See, for example, Kenneth W. Thomas and Warren H. Schmidt, "A Survey of Managerial Interests with Respect to Conflict," *Academy of Management Journal*, June 1976, p. 317.

sage initiated by the sender. The result is a transference of meaning from one person to another.[2]

Figure 10–1 depicts the communication process. This model is made up of seven parts: (1) the communication source, (2) encoding, (3) the message, (4) the channel, (5) decoding, (6) the receiver, and (7) feedback. Unfortunately, each of these components has the potential to create distortion, and therefore, impinges upon the goal of communicating perfectly.

The source initiates a message by encoding a thought. Four conditions have been described that affect the encoded message: skill, attitudes, knowledge, and the social-cultural system.

My success in communicating to you is dependent upon my writing skills; in the writing of textbooks, if the authors are without the requisite skills, their message will not reach students in the form desired. One's total communicative success includes speaking, reading, listening, and reasoning skills as well. As we discussed in Chapter 3, our attitudes influence our behavior. We hold predisposed ideas on numerous topics, and our communications are affected by these attitudes. Further, we are restricted in our communicative activity by the extent of our knowledge on the particular topic. We cannot communicate what we do not know; and should our knowledge be too extensive, it is possible that our receiver will not understand our message. Clearly, the amount of knowledge the source holds about his subject will affect the message he seeks to transfer. And finally, just as attitudes influence our behavior, so does our position in the social-cultural system in which we exist. Your beliefs and values, all part of your culture, act to influence you as a communicative source.

The message itself can cause distortion in the communicative process, regardless of the supporting apparatus used to convey it. Our message is the actual physical product from the source encoding. "When we speak, the speech is the message. When we write, the writing is the message. When we paint, the picture is the message. When we gesture, the movements of our arms, the expressions on our face are the message."[3] Our message is affected by the code or group of symbols we use to transfer meaning, the content of the message itself, and the decisions that the source makes in selecting and arranging both codes and content. Each of these three segments can act to distort the message.

The channel is the medium through which the message travels. It is selected by the source, who must determine which channel is formal and which one is

2. David K. Berlo, *The Process of Communication* (New York: Holt, Rinehart & Winston, 1960), pp. 30–32.

3. Ibid., p. 54.

FIGURE 10–1   The Communication Process

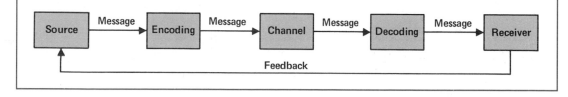

informal. Formal channels are established by the organization and transmit messages that relate to the professional activities of members. They traditionally follow the authority network within the organization. Other forms of messages, such as personal or social, follow the informal channels in the organization.

The receiver is the object to whom the message is directed. But before the message can be received, the symbols in it must be translated into a form that can be understood by the receiver. This is the decoding of the message. Just as the encoder was limited by his skills, attitudes, knowledge, and social-cultural system, so is the receiver equally restricted. Just as the source must be skillful in writing or speaking, the receiver must be skillful in reading or listening, and both must be able to reason. One's level of knowledge influences his ability to receive, just as it does his ability to send. Additionally, the receiver's predisposed attitudes and cultural background can distort the message being transferred.

The final link in the communicative process is a feedback loop. "If a communication source decodes the message that he encodes, if the message is put back into his system, we have feedback."[4] Feedback is the check on how successful we have been in transferring our messages as originally intended. It determines whether understanding has been achieved.

BARRIERS TO EFFECTIVE COMMUNICATION

It was stated previously that perfect communication is an ideal that cannot be achieved. The reason is that there are physical, individual, and semantic barriers to the transference of meaning.

Organizations, because they have formal structures, cannot help but create barriers to effective communication. The existence of excessive hierarchy creates physical distance between people. Additionally, the reliance in organizations upon having clear lines of authority in a structured hierarchy requires that formal communications follow prescribed channels through the organization. As a result, messages must frequently pass through many layers of the organization, each offering a potential for distortion. Remember the parlor game of "Telephone," where one person makes up a story that is passed around the group until it reaches the final member, who relates, in her own words, the message that she has received? Anyone who has played that game can see the distortion that can occur as information is passed between levels in an organization.

Human limitations also act as a hindrance to effective communication. Instead of listening in a rational objective manner to what is being said, we occasionally become emotionally involved. Judgments are imposed in place of rational fact appraisal. People inject their value systems into what they hear or read, and, too often, instead of decoding objectively, lose rationality—either be-

4. Ibid., p. 103.

cause they do not agree with what is being said or, if they have mentally stereo-typed the sender, by perceiving the message to be different from the way it was intended. As a result, the receiver hears what he or she expects to hear.

March and Simon reported that organizational channeling of information introduces both physical and individual barriers into material that is communi-cated.[5] They found that when information was passed between levels, it be-came altered as people interpreted "facts" differently.

The higher up an individual moves within an organization, the more he or she becomes dependent on subordinates to interpret information and direct what they perceive to be the critical data upward through the organization's hi-erarchy. For example, when information is passed through a chain of individ-uals, facts are continually interpreted. The information that finally reaches the individual at the end of the chain has been substantially filtered. What one per-son perceives as superfluous along the chain, another may view as critical. The result is a restricted flow of accurate information, distorted by the values of the communicators as to what is and is not important. Former group vice-president of General Motors, John DeLorean, has said that this filtering of communica-tions through levels at GM made it nearly impossible for senior managers to get objective information because "lower-level specialists . . . provided information in such a way that they would get the answer they wanted. I know," said De-Lorean, "I used to be down below and do it . . . now I was being presented with information that limited alternatives."[6]

Things mean different things to different people. This is particularly true with word connotations. "The meanings of words are *not* in the words; they are in us."[7] The word "flush," as an illustration, has a number of meanings. It can be a verb, noun, adverb, or adjective. Each of the following is a correct usage of the word: Your face becomes *flush* because you are angered (i.e., red in the face). Be sure to flush out the bathtub (i.e., clean with a sudden flow of water). She exhibited the first *flush* of youth (i.e., a sudden, vigorous growth). She is always *flush* with money (i.e., well-supplied or abundant). Better sit down, you're feeling *flush* (i.e., sudden feeling of great heat). The bed is *flush* to the wall (i.e., making an even or unbroken line). He took a blow *flush* to his chin (i.e., direct). He won the poker hand with a straight *flush* (i.e., cards that are all of the same suit).

Semantic problems can impede the communication that is essential for ef-fective organizational performance. A poor choice of symbols, confused mean-ing of symbols, or the ignoring of nonverbal cues could mean distorted communiques. For example, it has been reported that the differences in the

---

5. James G. March and Herbert A. Simon, *Organizations* (New York: John Wiley, 1958).

6. John DeLorean, quoted in Stephen P. Robbins, *The Administrative Process* (Engle-wood Cliffs, N.J.: Prentice-Hall, 1976), p. 404.

7. S. I. Hayakawa, *Language in Thought and Action* (New York: Harcourt Brace Jovano-vich, 1949), p. 292.

training of purchasing agents and engineers contribute to their difficulty in communicating.[8]

Background factors and group allegiance can also be distorting determinants. As we noted in Chapter 5, selectivity operates to influence what people see. Similarly, it can operate to distort communications.

The response, "I don't understand what you're saying," may result from any of the barriers noted above. Occasionally, an inadequate communication is recognized immediately: "That contradicts what you told me yesterday," or "What you're asking is not clear to me," gives rapid feedback to the sender that there is a problem. More often, there is an absence of feedback, and the sender is unaware of the ineffectiveness of the communication until later, when the behavior of the receiver indicates a lack of communication, or when the receiver states something approximating, "Oh, *that's* what you meant . . . ," or "I thought you meant. . . ."

NONVERBAL COMMUNICATION

Anyone who has ever paid a visit to a singles bar or a nightclub is aware that communication need not be verbal in order to convey a message. A glance, a stare, a smile, a frown, a provocative body movement—they all convey meaning. This example illustrates that no discussion of communication would be complete without a discussion of nonverbal messages. These include body movements, the intonations or emphasis we give to words, facial expressions, and the physical distance between the sender and receiver.

The academic study of body motions has been labeled *kinesics*. It refers to gestures, facial configurations, and other movements of the body. But it is a relatively new field and it has been subject to far more conjecture and popularizing than the research findings support. Hence, while we acknowledge the fact that body movement is an important segment of the study of communication and behavior, conclusions must be necessarily guarded. Recognizing this qualification, let us briefly consider the ways body motions convey meaning.

It has been argued that *every body movement* has a meaning and that no movement is accidental.[9] For example, through body language:

> We say, "Help me, I'm lonely. Take me, I'm available. Leave me alone, I'm depressed." And rarely do we send our messages consciously. We act out our state of being with nonverbal body language. We lift one eyebrow for disbelief. We rub our noses for puzzlement. We clasp our arms to isolate ourselves or to protect ourselves. We shrug our shoulders for indifference, wink one eye for intimacy, tap our fingers for impatience, slap our forehead for forgetfulness.[10]

8. George Strauss, "Work-Flow Frictions, Interfunctional Rivalry and Professionalism: A Case Study of Purchasing Agents," *Human Organization,* Summer 1964, pp. 136–49.

9. Ray L. Birdwhistell, *Introduction to Kinesics* (Louisville, Ky.: University of Louisville Press, 1952).

10. Julius Fast, *Body Language* (Philadelphia: M. Evans, 1970), p. 7.

While we may disagree with the specific meaning of the above movements, body language adds to and often complicates verbal communication. A body position or movement does not by itself have a precise or universal meaning, but when it is linked with spoken language, it gives fuller meaning to a sender's message.

If you read the verbatum minutes of a meeting, you could not grasp the impact of what was said in the same way you could if you had been there or saw the meeting on film. Why? There is no record of nonverbal communication. The emphasis given to words or phrases is missing. To illustrate how *intonations* can change the meaning of a message, consider the student in class who asks the instructor a question. The instructor replies, "What do you mean by that?" The student's reaction will be different depending on the tone of the instructor's response. A soft, smooth tone creates a different meaning than an intonation that is abrasive with strong emphasis placed on the last word.

The *facial expression* of the instructor in the above illustration will also convey meaning. A snarled face says something different than a smile. Facial expressions, along with intonations, can show arrogance, aggressiveness, fear, shyness, and other characteristics that would never be communicated if you read a transcript of what had been said.

The way individuals space themselves in terms of *physical distance* also has meaning. What is considered proper spacing is largely dependent on cultural norms. For example, what is "businesslike" distance in some European countries would be viewed as "intimate" in many parts of North America. If someone stands closer to you than is considered appropriate, it may indicate aggressiveness or sexual interest. If farther away than usual, it may mean disinterest or displeasure with what is being said.

It is important for the receiver to be alert to these nonverbal aspects of communication. You should look for nonverbal cues as well as listen to the literal meaning of a sender's words. You should particularly be aware of contradictions between the messages. The boss may say that she is free to talk to you about that raise you have been seeking, but you may see nonverbal signals that suggest that this is *not* the time to discuss the subject. Regardless of what is being said, an individual who frequently glances at her wristwatch is giving the message that she would prefer to terminate the conversation. We misinform others when we express one emotion verbally, such as trust, but nonverbally communicate a contradictory message that reads, "I don't have confidence in you." These contradictions often suggest that "actions speak louder (and more accurately) than words."

PERCEPTION AND THE CREATION OF MEANING

We have been looking at communication as a process subject to a number of potential distortions. A more recent approach to communication is one that emphasizes the impact of perception on the transference of meaning.[11] The central theme of this viewpoint is that meanings are not *transferred* from one person to another. Rather, receivers of the message *create* their own meanings from incoming sensory cues.[12] As we shall show, there is an increasing body of evidence that demonstrates that the way a person perceives and interprets communications will have a significant impact on his or her job satisfaction.

Think about this for a moment: "One cannot NOT communicate."[13] Every word, action, silence, or inaction carries meaning. Regardless of intention, meaning is attached to others' behaviors. So you have communicated as soon as someone has derived meaning from your actions or inactions. What does this mean in terms of interpersonal behavior? Simply, that people will create their own meanings to cues they receive from others and this interpretation is a major determinant of their satisfaction or dissatisfaction. Two areas of investigation have applied this perspective.

Applying Equity Theory to Communication

In Chapter 6, we introduced equity theory as a partial explanation of an individual's motivation. When employees perceive an inequity between their input-outcome ratio and those of relevant others, they will attempt to correct this inequity. We can look at this same concept from a communication perspective.

What is communicated is perceived and evaluated. But not all individuals are privy to all information. If your boss confides information to you that is withheld from others, that information in effect is seen as a reward. Communications, therefore, have a reward value that is subject to social comparisons. More specifically, it has been proposed that the communication process is modified as follows:[14] First, attention is paid to information to establish whether communication has actually taken place. Second, if communication has occurred, meaning must be attached in order to create a message. Third, the meaning must be evaluated in terms of importance; that is, is it relevant and does it have high saliency for the receiver? Finally, if it is relevant and has high saliency, an outcome is established. If equity exists, the message provides the receiver with a reward that serves his or her personal needs and enhances job satisfaction. Perceived inequity, on the other hand, is likely to lead to job dissatisfaction. So the fact that someone possesses information that you don't is only pertinent if you see that information as important and relevant. Then, and only then, will you compare the messages you receive with what you expect to receive in order to assess whether equity exists.

Although there is no substantive research to support the process we have

11. See, for example, W. C. Redding, *Communication within the Organization* (New York: Industrial Communications Council, 1972).

12. Paul L. Wilkens and Paul R. Timm, "Perceived Communication Inequity: A Determinant of Job Dissatisfaction," *Journal of Management*, Spring 1978, pp. 107–19.

13. Ibid., p. 108.

14. Ibid., p. 114.

described, propositions have been offered concerning four outcomes: (1) quantity of salient messages, (2) timeliness of salient messages, (3) interaction conditions, and (4) the opportunity to initiate salient messages. In terms of predicting satisfaction, the following four hypotheses are made:

1. Employees who perceive they do not receive as many salient messages as others in relation to their inputs (i.e., effort, ability, experience, education) to the group or organization will feel "less in the know" and will tend to be less satisfied on the job.

2. Employees who see themselves as the "last to know" some important information are likely to be less satisfied than ones who get this information at earlier times.

3. Employees who get a message under positive interaction conditions (e.g., the boss comes into their office and tells them) will be more satisfied than if they receive the same message under less positive conditions (e.g., it is overheard in the restroom).

4. Employees who see themselves as having fewer opportunities to initiate actions which result in the reception of important messages (e.g., opportunities to question or participate in decision making) will be more dissatisfied.[15]

Looking for Informational Cues

Another way in which perception enters into communication is related to informational cues and their impact on how people perceive their jobs. The characteristics of a job are not fixed and objective; rather, they are socially constructed realities that are defined by signals or messages that an employee receives from others. Studies demonstrate that, if these cues are manipulated (i.e., a co-worker or boss comments on the existence or absence of features such as difficulty, challenge, or autonomy in the job), employees are more satisfied with their jobs when they receive positive informational cues.[16]

It was traditionally believed that people responded to the objective characteristics of the jobs that they were doing. For instance, as we'll discuss in Chapter 15, jobs that offer employees a variety of identifiable and relevant tasks, as well as autonomy and feedback, seem to lead to more motivated, satisfied, and productive employees.[17] But attributes like variety, identity, or autonomy are not fully objective. The same job may be perceived differently by different groups. Even the same attribute may be seen as positive in one setting and negative in another. It seems reasonable to suggest, therefore, that employees may respond to both informational influences and objective characteristics.

This is just what the research indicates. In one study, investigators manipu-

15. Ibid., p. 116.

16. Charles A. O'Reilly III and David F. Caldwell, "Informational Influence as a Determinant of Perceived Task Characteristics and Job Satisfaction," *Journal of Applied Psychology,* April 1979, pp. 157–65; and Sam E. White and Terence R. Mitchell, "Job Enrichment versus Social Cues: A Comparison and Competitive Test," *Journal of Applied Psychology,* February 1979, pp. 1–9.

17. J. Richard Hackman, "Work Design," in *Improving Life at Work,* ed. J.R. Hackman and J. L. Suttle, (Santa Monica, Calif: Goodyear, 1977), pp. 96–162.

lated both the task characteristics and information cues in a simulated selection task.[18] They found that informational cues had a greater impact on job satisfaction than the objective characteristics of the task itself. Similarly, when another set of investigators manipulated task characteristics and information cues in a simulated routine clerical task, they too found that the informational cues were the dominant force determining job satisfaction.[19]

These findings underline that an employee's attitudes reflect both objective characteristics of the job or task and the informational influence of others. Moreover, the communication an employee receives from others in terms of informational cues may be a more powerful motivation force than the actual properties of the task. To generalize beyond the research, it may be that the informational cues that we get on our job from bosses, co-workers, and subordinates are as important as goal setting, equitable compensation, or intrinsically meaningful tasks in creating high motivation, high productivity, and favorable attitudes about our work.

SPECIAL GROUP LANGUAGES

Now we turn to the role that language plays in communication. Specifically, we want to show that one of the identifying characteristics of a group is its vocabulary—the language used by its members.

Specialized vocabularies are certainly prevalent among occupational groups, particularly among those occupations that take on professional status—doctors, lawyers, nurses, accountants, psychologists. But group members do not need to be certified in order to develop a *jargon* that means little to those individuals outside the occupation. Stevedores, electricians, actors, government bureaucrats, prostitutes, and members of street gangs all have a language with which they can communicate among themselves.

Occupation represents only one criterion upon which a jargon can be based. Age, race, nationality, religion, and economic background are a few of the many criteria that influence whether you use certain words or phrases, or even if you understand what is being said. For instance, U.S. residents might be bewildered if a friend asked them to help move the chesterfield. Canadians wouldn't bat an eye; they would know their friend was referring to a large couch. If someone had spent the past twenty-five years on a deserted island, isolated from the outside world, you can imagine their confusion when confronted with jargon-laden phrases such as "He's uptight"; "I wish he'd get off my case"; "It's the feeling she's going with"; and "Do you want to get it on?"

Most of us, even though we like to think we are reasonably intelligent, would have some difficulty understanding the following paragraph. The writer is

18. O'Reilly and Caldwell, "Informational Influence."
19. White and Mitchell, "Job Enrichment versus Social Cues."

FIGURE 10–2

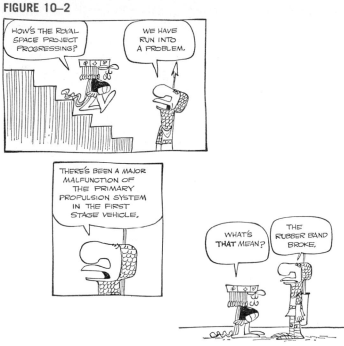

Source: Johnny Hart, *The Wondrous Wizard of Id*.

analyzing a letter written by four distinguished retired naval officers to the President on the issue of United States control of the Panama Canal Zone:

> It is reasonable to reflect that the tyrannization of the military by the commander-in-chief brings on sycophancy. That, therefore, one should not jump to conclusions based on what the men who hold their offices at the pleasure of the President are saying about the Panama Canal. But after all, if it were so obvious that the four retired admirals were correct, and that their counterparts in office are incorrect in assuring us that we do not need more in the Panama area than the treaty is in fact giving us, then our chiefs of staff are being charged with preferring their positions over the safety of the United States. One is reluctant to come to that conclusion.[20]

Where did this quote come from? From an academic journal? No—from William Buckley's daily newspaper column. Certainly, eloquence like Buckley's is impressive, but it limits his ability to transfer his ideas to others. By his use of language, he has condensed his audience to a select group of individuals whom he is trying to influence. By his language alone, Buckley assures himself that he will have a restricted audience. In contrast, a U.S. presidential candidate who spoke like Buckley would have a very difficult time getting elected since the majority of the American populace would either be unable to understand what he

20. *Burlington (Vt.) Free Press*, September 7, 1977.

FIGURE 10–3 Test Your Ability To Understand Black Street Language

What is:
1. Bad?
2. A crib?
3. Fat-mouthing?
4. A fox?
5. A grey-boy?
6. Hanging?
7. Humbuggin?
8. A jackleg?
9. Later?
10. A Mack man?
11. A natural?
12. An oreo?
13. Racking?
14. A splib?
15. Stepping?

ANSWERS: (1) Good, strong, or brave. (2) Where one lives; place of domicile. (3) Talking too much. (4) A pretty girl. (5) A white male. (6) Doing nothing. (7) Fighting. (8) An amateur. (9) Goodbye. (10) A pimp. (11) An Afro haircut. (12) A black person who thinks or acts like a white. (13) Studying. (14) A black person. (15) Dancing.

Source: Adapted from Thomas Kochman, " 'Rapping' in the Black Ghetto," *TransAction*, February 1969, pp. 26–34; *Rappin' and Stylin' Out: Communication in Urban Black America*, ed. Thomas Kochman (Urbana: University of Illinois Press, 1972); and William Safire, "Getting Down," *New York Times Magazine*, January 18, 1981, pp. 6, 8.

or she was saying or unwilling to listen with the intensity necessary to bring about understanding.

To demonstrate how effective jargon can be for group members, try the short quiz in Figure 10–3. If you are a black who was raised in an urban environment, it should not be too difficult to get a score of 10 or more right. If you are not a member of this group, a score of 3 or 4 right is quite good.

Group jargon is effective for identifying group members, allocating status to those who can communicate with the language, and for improving understanding among members. It can also facilitate keeping others on the outside who do not understand the language and creating charisma for those (group members) who do. Physicians do this when they use terms like "congenital" (existing from birth) or "arteriosclerosis" (hardening of the arteries). Social scientists can refer to "antecedent conditions," "beta weights," "single zero-order correlations," and "unstandardized regression coefficients," knowing that those in the group to whom their message is directed will know their meaning.

COMMUNICATION NETWORKS

The channels by which information flows are critical once we move beyond groups of two or three individuals. The way a group structures itself will determine the ease and availability with which members can transmit information.

Most studies of communication networks have taken place in groups created in a laboratory setting. As a result, the research conclusions tend to be constrained by the artificial setting and limited to small groups. Five common networks are shown in Figure 10–4; these are the chain, all-channel, wheel,

"Y," and circle. For our discussion purposes, let us think in an organizational context, and assume that the organization has only five members. We can then translate the networks in Figure 10–4 into their organizational equivalent.

The Five Common Networks

The chain would represent a five-level hierarchy where communications cannot move laterally, only upward and downward. In a formal organization, this type of network would be found in direct-line authority relations with no deviations. For example, the payroll clerk reports to the payroll supervisor, who in turn reports to the general accounting manager, who reports to the plant controller, who reports to the plant manager. These five individuals would represent a chain network.

If we turn the "Y" network upside down, we can see two subordinates reporting to a supervisor, with two levels of hierarchy still above the supervisor. This is, in effect, a four-level hierarchy.

If we look at the wheel diagram in Figure 10–4 as if we were standing above the network, it becomes obvious that the wheel represents a supervisor with four subordinates. However, there is no interaction between the subordinates. All communications are channeled through the supervisor.

The circle network allows members to interact with adjoining members, but no further. It would represent a three-level hierarchy in which there is communication between superiors and subordinates, and cross communication at the lowest level.

Finally, the all-channel network allows each of the subjects to communicate freely with the other four. Of the networks discussed, it is the least structured. While it is like the circle, in some respects, the all-channel network has no central position. However, there are no restrictions; all members are equal. This network is best illustrated by a committee, where no one member either formally or informally assumes a dominant or take-charge position. All members are free to share their viewpoints.

FIGURE 10–4 Common Communication Networks

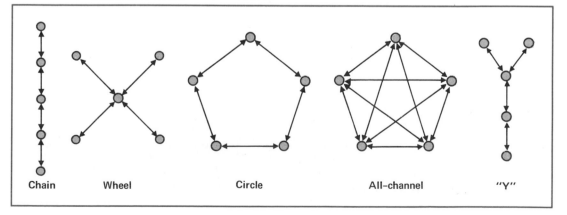

Chain   Wheel   Circle   All–channel   "Y"

The Five Networks and Group Effectiveness

Certain communication networks foster speed of decision making. Some are more effective in ensuring that directions are followed and for control purposes. Others have demonstrated success in maintaining high levels of morale. No single network will be best for all group efforts; rather, the network used should reflect the goals of the group.[21]

Laboratory experiments have found that the circle is considerably slower than either the chain or the wheel for transmitting information among all members, and that the circle rates poorest in accuracy of communication flows. As a result, the wheel and chain are rated as the most effective in terms of high job performance. However, morale is significantly higher in the circle, and, for complex problems, the circle and all-channel networks are faster and more effective. The "Y" shares advantages and disadvantages of the wheel and chain. It is fast, generates high performance, but with lower satisfaction.

The Informal Group Communication Network

The previous discussion of networks emphasized formal communication patterns, but the formal system is not the only communication system in a group or organization. Let us, therefore, now turn our attention to the informal system—where information flows along the well-known grapevine and rumors can flourish.

A classic study of the grapevine was reported thirty years ago.[22] The researcher investigated the communication pattern among sixty-seven managerial personnel in a small manufacturing firm. The basic approach used was to learn from each communication recipient how he first received a given piece of information and then trace it back to its source. It was found that, while the grapevine was an important source of information, only 10 percent of the executives acted as liaison individuals, that is, passed the information on to more than one other person. For example, when one executive decided to resign to enter the insurance business, 81 percent of the executives knew about it, but only 11 percent transmitted this information on to others.

Two other conclusions from this study are also worth noting. Information on events of general interest tended to flow between the major functional groups (i.e., production, sales) rather than within them. Also, no evidence surfaced to suggest that any one group consistently acted as liaisons; rather, different types of information passed through different liaison persons.

21. Alex Bavelas and Dermot Barrett, "An Experimental Approach to Organizational Communication," *Personnel*, March 1951, pp. 370–71.

22. Keith Davis, "Management Communication and the Grapevine," *Harvard Business Review*, September-October 1953, pp. 43–49.

An attempt to replicate this study among employees in a small state government office also found that only 10 percent act as liaison individuals.[23] This is interesting since the replication contained a wider spectrum of employees—including rank and file as well as managerial personnel. However, the flow of information in the government office took place within rather than between functional groups. It was proposed that this discrepancy might be due to comparing an executive-only sample against one which also included rank-and-file workers. Managers, for example, might feel greater pressure to stay informed and thus cultivate others outside their immediate functional group. Also, in contrast to the findings of the original study, the replication found that a consistent group of individuals acted as liaisons by transmitting information in the government office.

Is the information that flows along the grapevine accurate? The evidence indicates that about 75 percent of what is carried is accurate.[24] But what conditions foster an active grapevine? What gets the rumor mill rolling?

It is frequently assumed that rumors start because they make titillating gossip. Such is rarely the case. Rumors emerge as a response to situations that are *important* to us, where there is *ambiguity*, and under conditions that arouse *anxiety*.[25] Work situations frequently contain these three elements, which explains why rumors flourish in organizations. The secrecy and competition that typically prevail in large organizations—around such issues as the appointment of new bosses, the relocation of offices, and the realignment of work assignments—create conditions that encourage and sustain rumors on the grapevine. A rumor will persist either until the wants and expectations creating the uncertainty underlying the rumor are fulfilled, or until the anxiety is reduced.

What can we conclude from the above discussion? Certainly the grapevine is an important part of any group or organization's communication network and well worth understanding. It identifies for managers those confusing issues that employees consider important and anxiety-creating. It acts, therefore, as both a filter and a feedback mechanism, picking up the issues that employees consider relevant. For employees, the grapevine is particularly valuable for translating formal communications into their group's own jargon. Maybe more importantly, again from a managerial perspective, it seems possible to analyze grapevine information and to predict its flow, given that only a small set of individuals (around 10 percent) actively pass on information to more than one other person. By assessing which liaison individuals will consider a given piece of information to be relevant, we can improve our ability to explain and predict the pattern of the grapevine.

23. Harold Sutton and Lyman W. Porter, "A Study of the Grapevine in a Governmental Organization," *Personnel Psychology*, Summer 1968, pp. 223–30.

24. Keith Davis, cited in Roy Rowan, "Where Did *That* Rumor Come From?" *Fortune*, August 13, 1979, p. 134.

25. Ralph L. Rosnow and Gary Alan Fine, *Rumor and Gossip: The Social Psychology of Hearsay* (New York: Elsevier, 1976).

IMPLICATIONS FOR PERFORMANCE
AND SATISFACTION

Communication is a concept that embraces a number of the topics previously discussed. Perception, motivation, roles, and norms are subjects that are intimately related to the communication process and determinants of the effectiveness with which meaning is transmitted.

Take the topic of perception. We know that people react to their perceptions rather than reality. Job satisfaction, for instance, appears to be significantly influenced by an individual's judgments of equity or inequity in the receipt and evaluation of salient messages and by whether or not she receives positive or negative social cues about her job. This perceptual focus can be expanded further. If individuals perceive that a communication is threatening, they will behave accordingly, regardless of the sender's intent. The resulting behavior might be increased defensiveness, less compliance with directions, lower output, decreased job satisfaction, or an increase in the search for alternative employment opportunities.

A study of nearly 700 public utility employees confirms the importance of perception in communication.[26] It was found that processes that were seen to maximize important aspects and minimize unimportant aspects in communications were significantly correlated with the employees' satisfaction with work, satisfaction with supervision, and satisfaction with co-workers. However, processes that were seen as selectively withholding information were found to be negatively correlated with satisfaction. The problem, of course, is that what may be perceived as screening out unimportant information in one case may be perceived as the selective withholding of relevant information in another case.

We cited how different networks influence satisfaction and performance. The evidence suggests that job satisfaction is highest in the circle and all-channel networks, where democracy was most simulated. These networks also proved to generate more effective performance in the solution of complex problems. Where high performance requires close supervision and tight controls, the wheel was found to be most effective.

Findings in the chapter further suggest that the goal of perfect communication is unattainable. Yet, there is evidence that demonstrates a positive relationship between effective communication (which includes factors such as perceived trust, perceived accuracy, desire for interaction, top management receptiveness, and upward information requirements) and worker productivity.[27] Choosing the correct channel, clarifying jargon, and utilizing feedback may, therefore, make

---

26. Paul M. Muchinsky, "Organizational Communication: Relationships to Organizational Climate and Job Satisfaction," *Academy of Management Journal,* December 1977, pp. 592–607.

27. Susan A. Hellweg and Steven L. Phillips, "Communication and Productivity in Organizations: A State-of-the-Art Review," in *Proceedings of the 40th Annual Academy of Management Conference,* Detroit, Michigan, 1980, pp. 188–92.

for more effective communication, but candidness requires the admission that the human factor generates distortions that can never be fully eliminated. The communication process represents an exchange of messages, but the outcome is meanings that may or may not approximate those that the sender intended. Whatever the sender's expectations, the decoded message in the mind of the receiver represents his or her reality. And it is this "reality" that will determine performance, along with the individual's level of motivation and his or her degree of satisfaction. The issue of motivation is critical, so we should briefly review how communication is central in assessing an individual's degree of motivation.

You will remember from expectancy theory that the degree of effort an individual exerts depends on his or her perception of the effort-performance, performance-reward, and reward-goal satisfaction linkages. If individuals are not given the data necessary to make the perceived probability of these linkages high, motivation will be less than it could be. If rewards are not made clear, if the criteria for determining and measuring performance are ambiguous, or if individuals are not relatively certain that their effort will lead to satisfactory performance, then effort will be reduced. So communication plays a significant role in determining the level of motivation.

The messages that a person receives will be used as a base from which decisions will be made. People require information. Where this is withheld, perceived to be withheld, insufficient, transmitted so as to be ambiguous or threatening, satisfaction may be low and turnover high. Interestingly, the rapid growth in the participation school of organizational behavior[28] can be directly attributed to this issue. Participation was proposed as a solution based on the belief that individuals wanted to know about and influence the decisions that affected them. It was proposed that individuals who participated in decisions were more knowledgeable and more motivated to carry them out, that is, the popular contention was that people would not sabotage the decisions in which they themselves had participated.

FOR DISCUSSION

1. "Communication is the transference of meaning among group members." Discuss this definition and indicate what is missing from this definition to ensure that communications are effective.

28. The participation school is a loose label used to describe those individuals in the 1950s and 1960s who advocated that the solution to the "people problem" in organizations was to get them to participate in decisions that affected them. Names frequently associated with this school include Chris Argyris, Warren Bennis, Rensis Likert, and Douglas McGregor.

2. Describe the communication process, identifying its key components. Give an example of how this process operates with both oral and written messages.

3. What is the importance of the statement that "people will create their own meanings to cues they receive from others"?

4. "Ineffective communication is the fault of the sender." Do you agree or disagree? Discuss.

5. Describe the advantages and disadvantages of each of these networks: (a) all-channel, (b) chain, (c) circle, (d) wheel, and (e) "Y."

6. For each of the above networks, indicate the conditions under which it will be most effective.

7. What is jargon? What value does it have for improving communication? How can it stymie communication?

8. "Rumors start because something makes titillating gossip." Do you agree or disagree? Discuss.

FOR FURTHER READING

GUETZKOW, H., and H. A. SIMON, "The Impact of Certain Communication Nets Upon Organization and Performance in Task-Oriented Groups," *Management Science,* Vol. 1 (1955), pp. 233–50. Networks analyzed did not create differences among the groups with respect to the time needed for handling the operating task when an optimal organization was used. These same nets did introduce important differences in the organizing difficulties encountered.

HALL, J., "Communication Revisited," *California Management Review,* Spring 1973, pp. 56–67. More often than not, the communication dilemmas cited by people are not communication problems at all, but rather symptoms of difficulties at more basic and fundamental levels of organizational life.

HANEY, W. V., *Communication and Organizational Behavior,* 3rd ed. Homewood, Ill.: Richard D. Irwin, 1973. The classic reference on the subject of communication and its relationship to organizational behavior.

JOHNSON, B. M., *Communication: The Process of Organizing.* Boston: Allyn & Bacon, 1977. Argues that all organizations are created through communication. The book is about how people communicate to organize cooperative activities.

McCASKEY, M. B., "The Hidden Messages Managers Send," *Harvard Business Review,* November-December 1979, pp. 135–48. Managers convey messages about themselves in three ways: through their metaphors, office settings, and body language.

ROBERTS, K. H., C. A. O'REILLY III, G. E. BRETTON, and L. W. PORTER, "Organizational Theory and Organizational Communication: A Communication Failure?" *Human Relations,* May 1974, pp. 501–24. Brings together the theoretical views of organizations to suggest one perspective from which future organizational communication research might be considered.

POINT

ROGERS

Barriers and gateways
to communication

Adapted and edited from Carl R. Rogers in Carl R. Rogers and F.J. Roethlisberger, "Barriers and Gateways to Communication," Harvard Business Review, August 1952, pp. 46–50. Copyright © 1952 by the President and Fellows of Harvard College; all rights reserved.

I should like to propose, as a hypothesis for consideration, that the major barrier to mutual interpersonal communication is our very natural tendency to judge, to evaluate, to approve (or disapprove) the statement of the other person or the other group. Let me illustrate my meaning with some very simple examples. Suppose someone, commenting on this discussion, makes the statement, "I didn't like what that man said." What will you respond? Almost invariably your reply will be either approval or disapproval of the attitude expressed. Either you respond, "I didn't either; I thought it was terrible," or else you tend to reply, "Oh I thought it was really good." In other words, the primary reaction is to evaluate it from *your* point of view, your own frame of reference.

Or take another example. Suppose I say with some feeling, "I think the Republicans are behaving in ways that show a lot of good sound sense these days." What is the response that arises in your mind? The overwhelming likelihood is that it will be evaluative. In other words, you will find yourself agreeing, or disagreeing or making some judgment about me such as "He must be a conservative," or "He seems solid in his thinking." Or let us take an illustration from the international scene. Russia says vehemently, "The treaty with Japan is a war plot on the part of the United States." We rise as one person to say, "That's a lie!"

This last illustration brings in another element connected with my hypothesis. Although the tendency to make evaluations is common in almost all interchange of language, it is very much heightened in those situations where feelings and emotions are deeply involved. So the stronger our feelings, the more likely it is that there will be no mutual element in the communication. There will be just two ideas, two feelings, two judgments, missing each other in psychological space.

I am sure you recognize this from your own experience. When you have not been emotionally involved yourself and have listened to a heated discussion, you often go away thinking, "Well, they actually weren't talking about the same thing." And they were not. Each was making a judgment, an evaluation, from his own frame of reference. There was really nothing that could be called communication in any genuine sense. This tendency to react to any emotionally meaningful statement by forming an evaluation of it from our own point of view is, I repeat, the major barrier to interpersonal communication.

Is there any way of solving this problem, of avoiding this barrier? I feel that we are making exciting progress toward this goal, and I should like to present it as simply as I can. Real communication occurs, and this evaluative tendency is avoided, when we listen with understanding. What does this mean? It means to see the expressed idea and attitudes from the other person's point of view, to sense how it feels to him, to achieve his frame of reference in regard to the thing he is talking about.

Stated so briefly, this may sound absurdly simple, but it is not. It is an approach that we have found extremely potent in the field of psychotherapy. It is the most effective agent we know for altering the basic personality structure of an individual and for improving his relationships and his communications with others. If I can listen to what he can tell me, if I can understand how it seems to him, if I can see its personal meaning for him, if I can sense the emotional flavor that it has for him, then I will be releasing potent forces of change in him.

To summarize, I have said that our research and experience to date would make it appear that breakdowns in communication, and the evaluative tendency which is the major barrier to communication, can be avoided. The solution is provided by creating a situation in which each of the different parties comes to understand the other from the *other's* point of view. This has been achieved in practice, even when feelings run high, by the influence of a person who is willing to understand each point of view empathically, and who thus acts as a catalyst to precipitate further understanding.

This procedure has important characteristics. It can be initiated by one party, without waiting for the other to be ready. It can even be initiated by a neutral third person, provided he can gain a minimum of cooperation from one of the parties.

This procedure can deal with the insincerities, the defensive exaggerations, the lies, the "false fronts" that characterize almost every failure in communication. These defensive distortions drop away with astonishing speed as people find that the only intent is to understand, not to judge.

This approach leads steadily and rapidly toward the discovery of the truth, toward a realistic appraisal of the objective barriers to communication. The dropping of some defensiveness by one party leads to further dropping of defensiveness by the other party, and truth is thus approached.

This procedure gradually achieves mutual communication. Mutual communication tends to be pointed toward solving a problem rather than toward attacking a person or group. It leads to a situation in which I see how the problem appears to you as well as to me, and you see how it appears to me as well as to you. Thus accurately and realistically defined, the problem is almost certain to yield to intelligent attacks; or if it is in part insoluble, it will be comfortably accepted as such.

COUNTER POINT

KURSH

The benefits
of poor communication

Adapted and edited from Charlotte Olmsted Kursh, "The Benefits of Poor Communication," The Psychoanalytic Review, *Summer-Fall 1971, pp. 189–208. Through the courtesy of the editors and the publisher, National Psychological Association for Psychoanalysis, New York, N.Y.*

In this day and age one of the most popular forms of piety has to do with communication, somewhat narrowly defined. An ailment called "lack of communication" has taken the place of original sin as an explanation for the ills of the world, while "better communication" is trotted out on every occasion as a universal panacea.

Yet some of the basic assumptions underlying these popular views deserve more examination than they have had. One is the way in which poor communication resembles original sin: Both tend to get tangled up with control of the situation. Although if one defines communication as mutual understanding, this does not imply control for either party and certainly not for both, the equation of good communication with control appears in the assumption that better communication will necessarily reduce strife and conflict. Each individual's definition of better communication, like his definition of virtuous conduct, becomes that of having the other party accept his views—which would reduce conflict at that party's expense. As long as both feel this way the stroll can continue indefinitely, but strictly speaking has very little to do with communication difficulties per se. A better understanding of the situation might serve only to underline the differences rather than to resolve them. Indeed, many of the techniques thought of as poor communication were apparently developed with the aim of bypassing or avoiding confrontation, and some of them continue to be reasonably successful in this aim.

Another assumption that grows from this view is that when a conflict has gone on for a long time and shows every sign of continuing, lack of communication must be one of the basic problems. Usually if the situation is examined more carefully, plenty of communication will be found to be going on; the problem is again one of equating communication with agreement.

Still a third assumption, somewhat related but less squarely based on the equation of communication with controls, is that *it is always in the interest of at least one of the parties to an interaction and often of both to attain maximum clarity as measured by some more or less objective standard.* Aside from the difficulty of setting up this standard—whose standard? and doesn't this give *him* control of the situation?—there are some sequences, and perhaps many of them, in which it is to the interests of both parties to leave the situation as fuzzy, amorphous, and undefined as possible. This is notably true in culturally or personally sensitive and taboo areas involving prejudices, preconceptions, etc., but it can, for similar reasons, also be true when the area is merely a new one that could be seriously distorted by using old definitions and old solutions.

A final assumption is that poor communication is primarily a matter of *faulty techniques* of speaking, writing, listening, or reading, that improvements in technique can be learned and in every case will improve the quality of social life. While it is usually recognized that these "faulty techniques" were learned in a situation where they were probably more or less functional, the possibility is hardly considered that they might still be functional, or what that function might be.

Let us begin with the relatively simple case of the conscious lie. Although there is grudging agreement that a lie can be a benefit to the liar at least temporarily, it is usually considered to be damaging, if not fatally so, both to the lied-to and to the communication system as a whole. Lies do have a number of effects on the system aside from their immediate benefits to the liar, but by no means all of them are as negative as is sometimes assumed.

When the butler says, or used to say: "Mrs. Jones is not at home," her physical presence on the property was not germane to the issue and both the butler and the visitor understood the statement to mean: "We don't want any visitors right now, or at any rate don't want you as a visitor. Go away quietly without making a fuss." It can hardly be classified as a lie any longer, regardless of its truth or falsity as a report on the physical presence of Mrs. Jones. No deception was either intended or achieved, but a face-saving formula had evolved for coding a request that worded differently might have been offensive in that particular society.

Although a society in which no one's statements can ever be taken uncritically at face value has a communication system that can be tiresomely intricate for the decoder, at least it helps to develop an altogether healthy scepticism. A society in which all reports were as honest as the reporter could make them might well engender a dangerous credulity and a tendency to equate the known good faith of the reporter with the correctness and the adequacy of his report. Authority can be, though honest, as misleading as a conscious liar—but one is far less likely to spot the mistakes if one has not learned to doubt the good intentions.

Meaningless speech and the pseudocommunicational event are what most people seem to mean by poor communication. In neither case is the problem primarily one of *faulty techniques;* they both take considerable skill to deploy effectively.

Indeed, even if group therapy techniques and other measures aimed at "better communication" were entirely successful, one suspects that the conflict of interests between listener and speaker would soon resurrect all the old problems under a new guise. For what is the purpose of "good communication"? Listeners desire more explicit information from speakers in order to construct more effective speech themselves, and the effectiveness of speech is judged not by the information it imparts but by the extent to which the implicit commands and requests of the speaker are obeyed. The realistic and sensible victim who has had his own communications used against him once or twice understandably retreats into the comparatively safe, if sometimes obscure and thorny, thickets of "poor communication." There is a real basic problem in that the exercise of power is incompatible with good communication, but good communication unrelated to any action or exercise of power is useless.

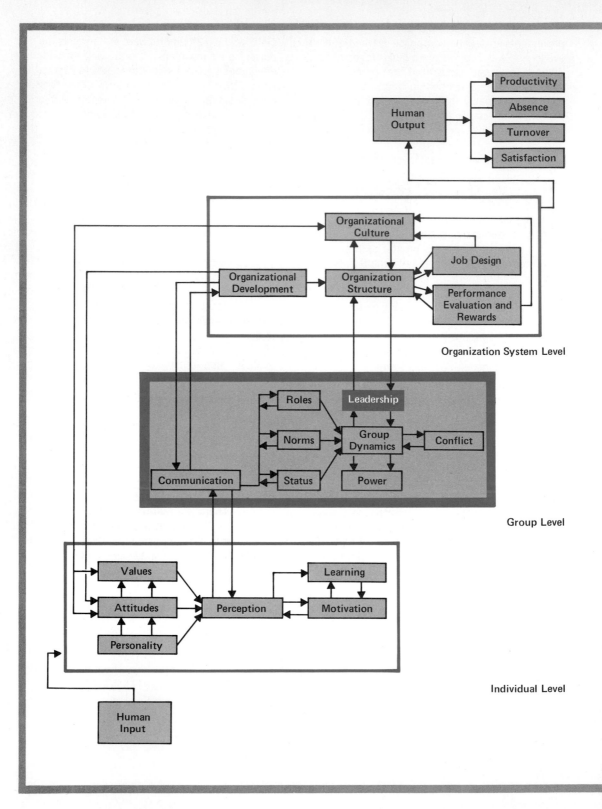

CHAPTER 11
Leadership

AFTER STUDYING THIS CHAPTER, YOU SHOULD BE ABLE TO—

Define and explain the following key terms and concepts:

Autocratic leaders	Initiating structure
Behavioral theories	Leader
Consideration	Leader-participation model
Democratic leaders	LPC
Employee-oriented leaders	Managerial grid
Fiedler contingency model	Production-oriented leaders
House path-goal model	Trait theories

Understand:

The nature of leadership
The conclusions of trait theories
The limitations of behavioral theories
The difference between initiating structure and consideration
Why no leadership style is ideal in all situations
The strengths and limitations in current contingency theories

> If anything goes bad, then I did it. If anything goes semi-good, then we did it. If anything goes real good, then you did it. That's all it takes to get people to win football games for you.
>
> —COACH PAUL "BEAR" BRYANT

It has been accepted as a truism that good leadership is essential to business, to government, and to the countless groups and organizations that shape the way we live, work, and play.[1] If leadership is such an important factor, the critical issue is: What makes a great leader? The tempting answer to give is: Great followers! While there is some truth to this response, the issue is far more complex.

WHAT IS LEADERSHIP?

Leadership is the ability to influence a group toward the achievement of goals. The source of this influence may be formal, such as that provided by the possession of managerial rank in an organization. Since management positions come with some degree of formally designated authority, an individual may assume a leadership role as a result of the position he or she holds in the organization. But not all leaders are managers nor, for that matter, are all managers leaders. Just because an organization provides its managers with certain rights is no assurance that they will be able to effectively lead. We find that nonsanctioned leadership, that is, the ability to influence that arises outside of the formal structure of the organization, is as important or more important than formal influence. In other words, leaders can emerge from within a group as well as being formally appointed.

TRANSITION IN LEADERSHIP THEORIES

The leadership literature is voluminous, and much of it is confusing and contradictory. In order to make our way through this "forest," we shall consider three basic approaches to explaining what makes an effective leader. The first sought

1. Fred E. Fiedler, "Style or Circumstance: The Leadership Enigma," *Psychology Today,* March 1969, p. 39.

to find universal personality traits that leaders had to some greater degree than nonleaders. The second approach tried to explain leadership in terms of the behavior that a person engaged in. Both of these approaches have been described as "false starts," based on their erroneous and oversimplified conception of leadership.[2] Most recently, we have looked to contingency models to explain the inadequacies of previous leadership theories in reconciling and bringing together the diversity of research findings. In this chapter, we shall present the contributions and limitations of each of the three approaches and conclude by attempting to ascertain the value of the leadership literature in explaining and predicting behavior.

TRAIT THEORIES

If one were to describe a leader based on the general connotations presented in today's media, one might list qualities such as intelligence, charisma, decisiveness, enthusiasm, strength, bravery, integrity, self-confidence, and so on—possibly eliciting the conclusion that effective leaders must be one part Boy Scout and two parts Jesus Christ. The search for characteristics such as those listed that would differentiate leaders from nonleaders occupied the early psychologists who studied leadership.

Is it possible to isolate one or more personality traits in individuals we generally acknowledge as leaders—Adolph Hitler, Susan B. Anthony, Joe "Bananas" Bonnano, Cezar Chavez, Martin Luther King, Jr., Joan of Arc, Mahatma Gandhi—that nonleaders do not possess? We may agree that these individuals meet our definition of a leader, but they represent individuals with utterly different characteristics. If the concept of traits were to be proved valid, there had to be found specific characteristics that all leaders possess.

Research efforts at isolating these traits resulted in a number of dead ends. If the search was to identify a set of traits that would always differentiate leaders from followers and effective from ineffective leaders, the search failed. Perhaps it was a bit optimistic to believe that there could be consistent and unique personality traits that would apply across the board to all effective leaders no matter whether they were in charge of the Hell's Angels, the Mormon Tabernacle Choir, the American Cancer Society, the Ku Klux Klan, or the Congress of Racial Equality.

If, however, the search was to identify traits that were consistently associated with leadership, the results can be interpreted in a more impressive light. For example, intelligence, dominance, self-confidence, high energy level, and task-relevant knowledge are five traits that show consistently positive correla-

---

2. Victor H. Vroom, "The Search for a Theory of Leadership," in *Contemporary Management: Issues and Viewpoints,* ed. Joseph W. McGuire (Englewood Cliffs, N.J.: Prentice-Hall, 1974), p. 396.

tions with leadership.[3] But "positive correlations" should not be interpreted to mean "definitive predictors." The correlations between these traits and leadership have generally been in the range of +.25 to +.35[4]—interesting results, but not earth-shattering!

The above results represent the conclusions based on seventy years of trait research. These modest correlations coupled with the inherent limitations of the trait approach—which ignores the needs of followers, generally fails to clarify the relative importance of various traits, and ignores situational factors—naturally led researchers in other directions. Although there has been some resurgent interest in traits during the past decade, a major movement away from traits began as early as the 1940s. Leadership research from the late 1940s through the mid-1960s emphasized the preferred behavioral styles that leaders demonstrated.

BEHAVIORAL THEORIES

The inability to strike "gold" in the trait mines led researchers to look at the behaviors that specific leaders exhibited. They wondered if there was something unique in the way that effective leaders behave. For example, do they tend to be more democratic than autocratic?

Not only, it was hoped, would the behavioral approach provide more definitive answers about the nature of leadership but, if successful, it would have practical implications quite different from those of the trait approach. If trait research had been successful, it would have provided a basis for *selecting* the "right" person to assume formal positions in groups and organizations requiring leadership. In contrast, if behavioral studies were to turn up critical behavioral determinants of leadership, we could *train* people to be leaders. The difference between trait and behavioral theories, in terms of application, lies in their underlying assumptions. If trait theories were valid, then leaders are basically born: You either have it or you do not. On the other hand, if there were specific behaviors that identified leaders, then we could teach leadership—we could design programs that implanted these behavioral patterns in individuals who desired to be effective leaders. This was surely a more exciting avenue for it would mean that the supply of leaders could be expanded. If training worked, we could have an infinite supply of effective leaders.

There were a number of studies that looked at behavioral styles. We shall briefly review the two most popular studied: the Ohio State group and the University of Michigan group. Then we shall see how the concepts that these studies developed could be used to create a grid for looking at and appraising leadership styles.

3. Ralph M. Stogdill, *Handbook of Leadership: A Survey of Theory and Research* (New York: Free Press, 1974).

4. Ibid.

Ohio State Studies

The most comprehensive and replicated of the behavioral theories resulted from research that began at Ohio State University in the late 1940s.[5] These studies sought to identify independent dimensions of leader behavior. Beginning with over a thousand dimensions, they eventually narrowed the list into two categories that substantially accounted for most of the leadership behavior described by subordinates. They called these two dimensions initiating structure and consideration.

Initiating structure refers to the extent to which a leader is likely to define and structure his or her role and those of subordinates in the search for goal attainment. It includes behavior that attempts to organize work, work relationships, and goals. The leader characterized as high in initiating structure could be described in terms such as: assigns group members to particular tasks; expects workers to maintain definite standards of performance; and emphasizes the meeting of deadlines.

Consideration is described as the extent to which a person is likely to have job relationships that are characterized by mutual trust, respect for subordinates' ideas, and regard for their feelings. He shows concern for his followers' comfort, well-being, status, and satisfaction. A leader high in consideration could be described as one who helps subordinates with personal problems, is friendly and approachable, and treats all subordinates as equals.

Extensive research, based on these definitions, found that leaders high in initiating structure *and* consideration (a "high-high" leader) tended to achieve high subordinate performance and satisfaction more frequently than those who rated low on either consideration, initiating structure, or both. However, the "high-high" style did not *always* result in positive consequences. For example, leader behavior characterized as high on initiating structure led to greater rates of grievances, absenteeism, and turnover and lower levels of job satisfaction for workers performing routine tasks. Other studies found that high consideration was negatively related to performance ratings of the leader by his superior. In conclusion, the Ohio State studies suggested that the "high-high" style generally resulted in positive outcomes, but enough exceptions were found to indicate that situational factors needed to be integrated into the theory.

University of Michigan Studies

Leadership studies undertaken at the University of Michigan's Survey Research Center, at about the same time as those being done at Ohio State, had similar

5. Ralph M. Stogdill and Alvin E. Coons, eds., *Leader Behavior: Its Description and Measurement,* Research Monograph No. 88 (Columbus: Ohio State University, Bureau of Business Research, 1951). For an updated literature review of the Ohio State research, see Steven Kerr, Chester A. Schriesheim, Charles J. Murphy, and Ralph M. Stogdill, "Toward a Contingency Theory of Leadership Based Upon the Consideration and Initiating Structure Literature," *Organizational Behavior and Human Performance,* August 1974, pp. 62–82.

research objectives: to locate behavioral characteristics of leaders that appeared to be related to measures of performance *effectiveness.*

The Michigan group also came up with two dimensions of leadership behavior which they labeled *employee-oriented* and *production-oriented.*[6] Leaders who were employee-oriented were described as emphasizing interpersonal relations; they took a personal interest in the needs of their subordinates and accepted individual differences among members. The production-oriented leaders, in contrast, tended to emphasize the technical or task aspects of the job—their main concern was in accomplishing their group's tasks and the group members were a means to that end.

The conclusions arrived at by the Michigan researchers strongly favored the leaders who were employee-oriented in their behavior. Employee-oriented leaders were associated with higher group productivity and higher job satisfaction. Production-oriented leaders tended to be associated with low group productivity and lower worker satisfaction.

The Managerial Grid

A graphic portrayal of a two-dimensional view of leadership style has been developed by Blake and Mouton.[7] They propose a managerial grid based on the styles of "concern for people" and "concern for production," which essentially represent the Ohio State dimensions of consideration and initiating structure or the Michigan dimensions of employee-oriented and production-oriented.

The grid, depicted in Figure 11–1, has nine possible positions along each axis, creating eighty-one different positions in which the leader's style may fall. The grid does not show results produced, but rather the dominating factors in a leader's thinking in regard to getting results.

Based on the findings from the research Blake and Mouton conducted, they concluded that managers perform best under a 9,9 style, as contrasted, for example, with a 9,1 (task-oriented) or the 1,9 (country-club type) leader. Unfortunately, the grid offers a better framework for conceptualizing leadership style than for presenting any tangible new information in clarifying the leadership quandary since there is little substantive evidence to support the conclusion that a 9,9 style is most effective in all situations.

Summary of Behavioral Theories

We have described the most popular and important of the attempts to explain leadership in terms of the behavior exhibited by the leader. There were other

6. R. Kahn and D. Katz, "Leadership Practices in Relation to Productivity and Morale," in *Group Dynamics: Research and Theory,* 2nd ed., ed. D. Cartwright and A. Zander (Elmsford, N.Y.: Row, Paterson), 1960.

7. Robert R. Blake and Jane S. Mouton, *The Managerial Grid* (Houston: Gulf Publishing, 1964).

FIGURE 11–1 The Managerial Grid

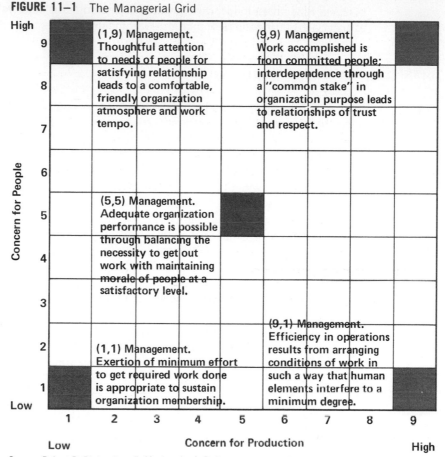

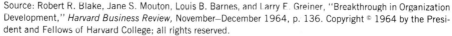

Source: Robert R. Blake, Jane S. Mouton, Louis B. Barnes, and Larry F. Greiner, "Breakthrough in Organization Development," *Harvard Business Review,* November–December 1964, p. 136. Copyright © 1964 by the President and Fellows of Harvard College; all rights reserved.

efforts,[8] but they faced the same problem that confronted the Ohio State and Michigan findings: They had very little success in identifying consistent relationships between patterns of leadership behavior and group performance. General statements could not be made because results would vary over different ranges of circumstances. What was missing was consideration of the situational factors that influence success or failure. For example, it seems unlikely that Martin Luther King, Jr., would have been a great leader of his people at the turn of the century, yet he was in the 1950s and 1960s. Would Ralph Nader have risen to lead a consumer activist group had he been born in 1834 rather than 1934, or

8. See, for example, the three styles—autocratic, participative, and laissez-faire—proposed by Kurt Lewin and Ronald Lippitt, "An Experimental Approach to the Study of Autocracy and Democracy: A Preliminary Note," *Sociometry,* No. 1, 1938, pp. 292–380; or the more recent 3-D Theory proposed by William J. Reddin, *Managerial Effectiveness* (New York: McGraw-Hill, 1970).

in Costa Rica rather than Connecticut? It seems quite unlikely, yet the behavioral approaches we have described could not clarify these situational factors.

CONTINGENCY THEORIES

It became increasingly clear to those who were studying the leadership phenomenon that the predicting of leadership success was more complex than isolating a few traits or preferable behaviors. The failure to obtain consistent results led to a new focus on situational influences. The relationship between leadership style and effectiveness suggested that under condition a, style x would be appropriate, while style y would be more suitable for condition b, and style z for condition c. But what were the condtiions a, b, c, and so forth? It was one thing to say that leadership effectiveness was dependent on the situation, and another to be able to isolate those situational conditions.

There has been no shortage of studies attempting to isolate critical situational factors that affect leadership effectiveness. One author, in reviewing the literature, found that the task being performed (i.e., complexity, type, technology, size of the project) was a significant moderating variable, but additionally uncovered studies that isolated situational factors such as style of the leader's immediate supervisor, group norms, span of management, external threat and stress, time demands, and organizational climate.[9]

Several approaches to isolating key situational variables have proven more successful than others and, as a result, have gained wider recognition. We shall consider four of these: the autocratic-democratic continuum; and the Fiedler, the path-goal, and the Vroom-Yetton models.

Autocratic-Democratic Continuum Model

If autocratic and democratic behavior were viewed only as two extreme positions, this model would be correctly labeled as a behavioral theory. However, they are merely two of many positions along a continuum. At one extreme the leader makes the decision, tells his subordinates, and expects them to carry out that decision. At the other extreme, the leader fully shares his decision-making power with his subordinates, allowing each member of the group to carry an equal voice—one person, one vote. Between these two extremes fall a number of leadership styles, with the style selected dependent upon forces in the leader himself, his operating group, and the situation. Although this represents a contingency theory, we shall find, upon investigating other contingency approaches, that it is quite primitive.

As depicted in Figure 11–2, there is a relationship between the degree of authority used and the amount of freedom available to subordinates in reaching decisions. This continuum is seen as a zero-sum game; as one gains, the other

9. Jeffrey C. Barrow, "The Variables of Leadership: A Review and Conceptual Framework," *Academy of Management Review,* April 1977, pp. 231–51.

FIGURE 11-2 Leadership–Behavior Continuum

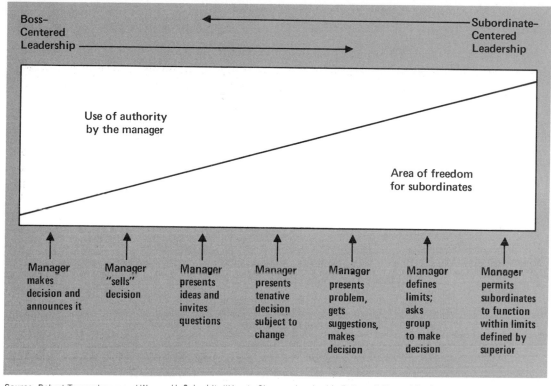

loses, and vice versa.[10] However, much of the research using this model has been concentrated on the extreme positions.

After reviewing eleven separate studies, Filley, House, and Kerr found seven to demonstrate that participative leadership has positive effects upon productivity while there were no significant effects in the other four. Although only three of the eleven investigations reported on participative leadership's effect on subordinate satisfaction, all showed positive results.[11]

Hamner and Organ reached a similar conclusion when they reviewed the research:

> Generally speaking, we find that participative leadership is associated with greater satisfaction on the part of subordinates than is nonparticipative leadership; or, at worst, that participation does not lower satisfaction. We cannot summarize so easily the findings with respect to pro-

10. Robert Tannenbaum and Warren H. Schmidt, "How to Choose a Leadership Pattern," *Harvard Business Review*, March–April 1958, pp. 95–101.

11. Alan C. Filley, Robert J. House, and Steven Kerr, *Managerial Process and Organizational Behavior*, 2nd ed. (Glenview, Ill.: Scott, Foresman, 1976), p. 223.

ductivity. Some studies find participative groups to be more productive; some find nonparticipative groups to be more effective; and quite a few studies show no appreciable differences in productivity between autocratically versus democratically managed work groups.[12]

The previous suggests a clear link between participation or the democratic style of leadership and satisfaction, but the relationship of this style to productivity is less apparent. The research can be interpreted as saying that people like democracy, but that it will not necessarily result in higher productivity.

A contingency approach would recognize that neither the democratic nor autocratic extreme is effective in all situations. The following models more comprehensively appraise these situational characteristics.

Fiedler Model

The first comprehensive contingency model for leadership was developed by Fred Fiedler.[13] His model proposes that effective group performance depends upon the proper match between the leader's style of interacting with his or her subordinates and the degree to which the situation gives control and influence to the leader. Fiedler developed an instrument, which he called the least-preferred co-worker (LPC) questionnaire, that purports to measure whether a person is task- or relationship-oriented. Further, he isolated three situational criteria—leader-member relations, task structure, and position power—that he believes can be manipulated so as to create the proper match with the behavioral orientation of the leader. In a sense, the Fiedler model is an outgrowth of trait theory, since the LPC questionnaire is a simple psychological test. However, Fiedler goes significantly beyond trait and behavioral approaches by attempting to isolate situations, relating his personality measure to his situational classification, and then predicting leadership effectiveness as a function of the two.

The above description of the Fiedler model can appear somewhat abstract. Let us now look at the model in more pragmatic detail.

Fiedler's LPC questionnaire contains sixteen bipolar adjectives (such as pleasant-unpleasant, efficient-inefficient). The questionnaire asks the respondent to: "Think of all the co-workers you have ever had. Now describe, using the bipolar-adjective scale, one person you are least able to work with." Fiedler proposes that, based on the answer, he can determine the leadership orientation of the respondent. If the least-preferred worker is viewed in relatively favorable terms, Fiedler suggests, the respondent can be said to be primarily interested in good personal relations with his co-worker; he is what may be generalized as relationship-oriented. Contrarily, if the least-preferred co-worker is

---

12. W. Clay Hamner and Dennis W. Organ, *Organizational Behavior: An Applied Psychological Approach* (Dallas: Business Publications, 1978), pp. 396–97.

13. Fred E. Fiedler, *A Theory of Leadership Effectiveness* (New York: McGraw-Hill, 1967).

seen in relatively unfavorable terms, the respondent is primarily interested in performing well, or is task-oriented.

As we noted, the three contingency dimensions that Fiedler considers are leader-member relations, task structure, and position power. They are defined as follows:

1. *Leader-member relations*—the degree of confidence, trust, and respect subordinates have in their leader
2. *Task structure*—the degree to which the job assignments are procedurized (i.e., structured or unstructured)
3. *Position power*—the degree of influence a leader has over power variables such as hiring, firing, discipline, promotion, and salary increases

Fiedler states that the more positive the leader-member relations, the more highly structured the job activity, and the greater the position power, the greater the leader's influence. For example, a very favorable situation—that is, where the three variables are positive—might involve a payroll manager who is well respected and whose subordinates have confidence in her, in a job that provides considerable freedom for her to reward and punish her subordinates, where the activities to be done (i.e., wage computation, check writing, report filing) are specific and clear. On the other hand, an unfavorable situation might be the disliked chairman of a voluntary United Fund-raising team.

Fiedler's study of over 1,200 groups resulted in the graph shown in Figure 11–3. Eight categories result from mixing the three contingency variables. These categories are as follows:

Category	Leader-Member Relations	Task Structure	Position Power
I	Good	High	Strong
II	Good	High	Weak
III	Good	Low	Strong
IV	Good	Low	Weak
V	Poor	High	Strong
VI	Poor	High	Weak
VII	Poor	Low	Strong
VIII	Poor	Low	Weak

Basically, Fiedler says the shape of the curve in Figure 11–3 implies that task-oriented leaders tend to perform better in situations that are very favorable to them, and also in situations that are very unfavorable. These are the right and left sides of the curve, which fall below the dotted line. So, Fiedler would predict that when faced with a category I, II, III, or VIII situation, task-oriented leaders perform better. Relationship-oriented leaders, however, perform better in moderately favorable situations, that is, in categories IV through VII.

One should not surmise that Fiedler has closed all the gaps and put to rest

FIGURE 11–3 Findings from Fiedler Model

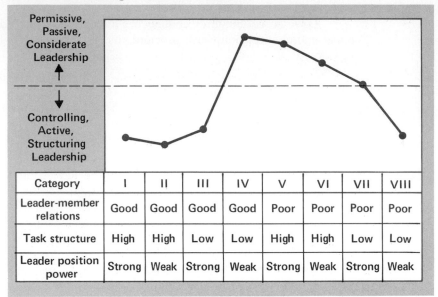

Category	I	II	III	IV	V	VI	VII	VIII
Leader-member relations	Good	Good	Good	Good	Poor	Poor	Poor	Poor
Task structure	High	High	Low	Low	High	High	Low	Low
Leader position power	Strong	Weak	Strong	Weak	Strong	Weak	Strong	Weak

Source: Adapted from Fred E. Fiedler, "The Effects of Leadership Training and Experience: A Contingency Model Interpretation," *Administrative Science Quarterly*, December 1972, p. 455. With permission.

all the questions underlying leadership effectiveness. Continued research strongly confirms that the Fiedler model predicts categories I and IV with relatively high consistency. Predictions for categories V and VIII are confirming, but at a more moderate level. Most pertinent, the model's predictions appear irrelevant to categories II, III, VI, and VII.[14]

The ability of the model to predict in several categories may mean that Fiedler has made some important insights into leadership. On the other hand, the model has a number of weaknesses.[15] First, the contingency variables are complex and difficult to assess. It's often difficult in practice to determine how good the leader-member relations are, how structured the task is, and how much position power the leader has. Second, the model gives little attention to the characteristics of the subordinates. Third, no attention is given to varying technical competencies of the leader or the subordinates. The model assumes that both the leader and subordinates have adequate technical competence. Fourth, the correlations Fiedler presents in defense of the model are relatively weak. Though generally in the right direction, they are often low and statistically nonsignificant. Finally, the LPC instrument is open to question. The logic under-

14. John B. Miner, *Theories of Organizational Behavior* (Hinsdale, Ill.: Dryden Press, 1980), pp. 307–9.

15. Edgar H. Schein, *Organizational Psychology,* 3rd ed. (Englewood Cliffs, N.J.: Prentice-Hall, 1980), pp. 116–17.

lying the LPC is not well understood and studies have shown that respondent's LPC scores are not stable.[16]

In spite of these criticisms, the Fiedler model continues to be a dominant input in the development of a contingency explanation of leadership effectiveness. Its greatest contribution may be in the direction it has taken leadership research, rather than in any definitive answers that it provides.

Path-Goal Model

Robert House, of the University of Toronto, has proposed a contingency model for leadership that integrates the expectancy model of motivation with the Ohio State leadership research.[17] The model considers the effort-performance and performance-goal satisfaction linkages, and the leadership dimensions of initiating structure and consideration. The model describes the leader as responsible for:

> . . . increasing the number and kinds of personal payoffs to the subordinates for work-goal attainment and making paths to these payoffs easier to travel by clarifying the paths, reducing roadblocks and pitfalls, and increasing the opportunities for personal satisfaction en route.[18]

Since the theory is described in terms of path clarification, need satisfaction, and goal attainment, it is referred to as the path-goal model of leadership. That is, initiating structure acts to "clarify the path" and consideration makes the path "easier to travel."

You will remember that the Ohio State group concluded that effective leaders would score high on both initiating structure and consideration. Yet, there were exceptions. What House has done, therefore, is to reconcile the apparent contradictions in the findings of the Ohio State group. The "high-high" leader is not always the most effective, so House asks: In what situations is initiating structure desirable? In what situations is consideration desirable?

The model has two general propositions:

1. Leader behavior is acceptable and satisfying to subordinates to the extent that the subordinates see such behavior as either an immediate source of satisfaction or as instrumental to future satisfaction.
2. Leader behavior will be motivational to the extent that (a) it makes satisfaction of subordinate needs contingent on effective performance, and (b) it complements the environment of subordinates by providing the coaching, guidance,

---

16. See, for instance, Robert W. Rice, "Psychometric Properties of the Esteem For the Least Preferred Coworker (LPC Scale)," *Academy of Management Review,* January 1978, pp. 106–18; and Chester A. Schriesheim, Brendan D. Bannister, and William H. Money, "Psychometric Properties of the LPC Scale: An Extension of Rice's Review," *Academy of Management Review,* April 1979, pp. 287–90.

17. Robert J. House, "A Path-Goal Theory of Leader Effectiveness," *Administrative Science Quarterly,* September 1971, pp. 321–38.

18. Robert J. House and Terence R. Mitchell, "Path-Goal Theory of Leadership," *Journal of Contemporary Business,* Autumn 1974, p. 86.

support, and rewards necessary for effective performance and which may otherwise be lacking in subordinates or in their environment.[19]

In addition, two sets of contingency variables moderate the relationship between the leader's behavior and the subordinate's output. These are (1) personal characteristics of the subordinates, and (2) environmental pressures and task demands. The model's relationships are summarized in Figure 11–4. Given these two general propositions and two sets of moderating variables, the model would make hypotheses such as the following regarding the behavioral dimensions a leader should use:

> *Consideration* with subordinates who score low on the Locus of Control Scale (those who believe that their rewards are contingent on their own behavior) and *initiating structure* with subordinates who score high on the Locus of Control Scale (those who believe their rewards are the result of luck or another's behavior)

19. Ibid., p. 84.

FIGURE 11–4   Summary of Path-Goal Relationships

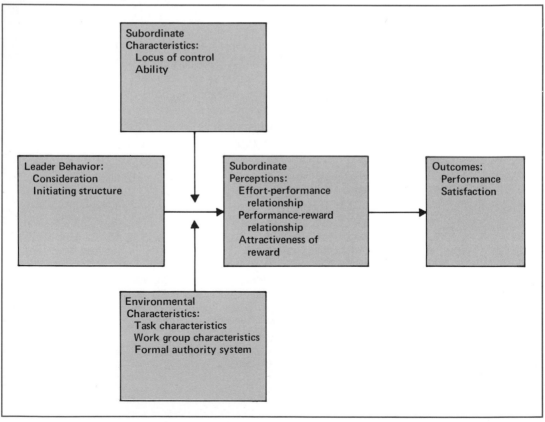

Initiating structure with highly authoritarian subordinates

Less *initiating structure* as the subordinate's perception of his or her abilities relative to task demands increases

Less *initiating structure* where the routine nature of the task, clear group norms, or objective controls of the formal authority system already make goals and paths apparent

Less *initiating structure* and more *consideration* with subordinates who find their work tasks dissatisfying, fatiguing, frustrating, or stress-inducing.

In summary, the path-goal model proposes that consideration is most helpful to subordinates in structured situations and less helpful in unstructured ones; and that initiating structure will lead to greater satisfaction when the tasks are ambiguous or stressful than when they are highly structured and well laid out. Where the tasks to be done are not clear, subordinates appreciate the leader clarifying the path to goal achievement. High consideration, on the other hand, results in high employee satisfaction when subordinates are performing structured or routine tasks. In clearly defined and structured tasks, efforts by the leader to explain tasks that are already clear will be seen by the subordinates as redundant or even insulting.

Does research confirm the path-goal model? Because the model is fairly new and has undergone modifications, it's difficult to draw any definitive conclusions. As one reviewer noted after surveying the research, "One is left with the feeling that the findings are stronger for the consideration hypotheses than the structuring hypotheses and stronger for satisfaction as a criterion than for performance."[20] Yet, given the criticisms of Fiedler's model and the support for an expectancy theory of motivation, it appears that the direction the path-goal model is taking holds promise.

Leader-Participation Model

The most recent addition to the contingency approach is the leadership-participation model proposed by Victor Vroom and Phillip Yetton.[21] It relates leadership behavior and participation to decision making. Recognizing that task structures have varying demands for routine or nonroutine activities, these researchers suggest that leader behavior must adjust to reflect the task structure. Vroom and Yetton's model is normative—it provides a sequential set of rules that should be followed in determining the form and amount of participation in decision making, as determined by different types of situations. As shown in Figure 11–5, the model is a decision tree incorporating eight contingencies and five alternative leadership styles.

20. Terence R. Mitchell, "Organizational Behavior," in *Annual Review of Psychology,* Vol. 30, ed. M. R. Rosenzweig and L. W. Porter (Palo Alto, Calif.: Annual Reviews, 1979), p. 265.

21. Victor H. Vroom and Phillip W. Yetton, *Leadership and Decision Making* (Pittsburgh: University of Pittsburgh Press, 1973).

FIGURE 11–5 Leader-Participation Model

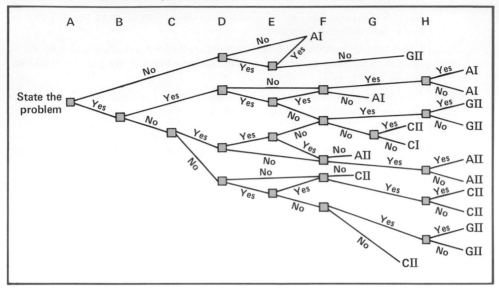

The model assumes that any of five behaviors may be feasible in a given situation:

AI. You solve the problem or make a decision yourself using information available to you at that time.

AII. You obtain the necessary information from subordinates, then decide on solution to the problem yourself. You may or may not tell subordinates what the problem is in getting the information from them. The role played by your subordinates in making the decision is clearly one of providing the necessary information to you, rather than generating or evaluating alternative solutions.

CI. You share the problem with relevant subordinates individually; getting their ideas and suggestions without bringing them together as a group. Then *you* make the decision which may or may not reflect your subordinates' influence.

CII. You share the problem with your subordinates as a group, collectively obtaining their ideas and suggestions. Then, you make the decision which may or may not reflect your subordinates' influence.

GII. You share the problem with your subordinates as a group. Together you generate and evaluate alternatives and attempt to reach an agreement (consensus) on a solution.

Although these five decision behaviors closely parallel the autocratic-democratic continuum depicted in Figure 11–2, the Vroom-Yelton model goes beyond that model by suggesting a specific way of analyzing problems by means of eight contingency questions. By answering "Yes" or "No" to these questions, the leader can arrive at which of the five decisions behaviors is preferred—that is, how much participation should be used.

The eight questions must be answered in order from A to H:

A. If the decision were accepted, would it make a difference which course of action were adopted?

B. Do I have sufficient information to make a high-quality decision?

C. Do subordinates have sufficient additional information to result in a high-quality decision?

D. Do I know exactly what information is needed, who possesses it, and how to collect it?

E. Is acceptance of the decision by subordinates critical to effective implementation?

F. If I were to make the decision by myself, is it certain that it would be accepted by my subordinates?

G. Can subordinates be trusted to base solutions on organizational considerations?

H. Is conflict among subordinates likely in the preferred solution?

Again, referring to Figure 11–5, based on the answers to questions A through H, the leader follows the decision tree until reaching its end. The designation at the end of the branch (either AI, AII, CI, CII, or GII) tells the leader what to do.

To date the research testing the leader-participation model has been encouraging,[22] but considerably more investigations are needed to test the model's normative propositions against effectiveness data. It does, however, confirm existing empirical evidence that leaders use participatory methods (1) when the quality of the decision is important; (2) when it is important that subordinates accept the decision and it is unlikely that they will do so unless they are allowed to take part in it; and (3) when subordinates can be trusted to pay attention to the goals of the group rather than simply to their own preferences.

This model has also confirmed that leadership research should be directed at the situation rather than the person. It probably makes more sense to talk about autocratic and participative *situations,* rather than autocratic and participative *leaders.* This, importantly, is a fundamental deviation from Fiedler's viewpoint. The Fiedler model emphasizes changing the situation to match the inherent characteristics of the leader. The leader's style is basically assumed to be inflexible. Vroom and Yetton would disagree. They demonstrate that leaders are not rigid, but adjust their style to different situations.

The cartoon in Figure 11–6 proposes adjusting the individual to the coat, rather than vice versa. We can think of the "coat" as analogous to the "situation." In terms of leadership, if an individual's leadership style range is very narrow, as Fiedler proposes, we are required to place individuals into the appropriate "size of coat" if they are to lead successfully. If Vroom and Yetton are right, then all the leader has to do is assess the "coat" that is available and

22. See, for example, Victor H. Vroom and Arthur G. Jago, "On the Validity of the Vroom-Yetton Model," *Journal of Applied Psychology,* April 1978, pp. 151–62; and Charles Margerison and Richard Glube, "Leadership Decision-Making: An Empirical Test of the Vroom and Yetton Model," *Journal of Management Studies,* February 1979, pp. 45–55.

FIGURE 11–6

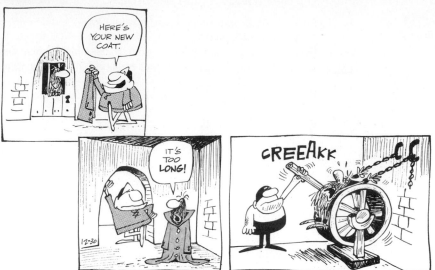

Source: Brant Parker and Johnny Hart, *Let There Be Reign* (Greenwich, Conn: Fawcett Books, 1972).

adjust his or her style accordingly. Whether we adjust the coat to fit the person (à la Fiedler) or fix the person to fit the coat (à la Vroom and Yetton) is an issue requiring further investigation.

Sometimes Leadership Is Irrelevant!

In keeping with the contingency spirit, we want to conclude this section by offering this notion: The belief that *some* leadership style *will always* be effective *regardless* of the situation may not be true. Leadership may not always be important. Data from numerous studies collectively demonstrate that, in many situations, whatever behaviors leaders exhibit are irrelevant. Certain individual, job, and organizational variables can act as "substitutes for leadership," negating the formal leader's ability to exert either positive or negative influence over subordinate attitudes and effectiveness.[23]

For instance, characteristics of subordinates such as their experience, training, "professional" orientation, or need for independence can neutralize the effect of leadership. These characteristics can replace the need for a leader's support or ability to create structure and reduce task ambiguity. Similarly, jobs that are inherently unambiguous and routine or that are intrinsically satisfying may place less demands on the leadership variable. Finally, organizational characteristics like explicit formalized goals, rigid rules and procedures, or cohesive work groups can act in the place of formal leadership.

23. This section is adapted from Steven Kerr and John M. Jermier, "Substitutes for Leadership: Their Meaning and Measurement," *Organizational Behavior and Human Performance*, December 1978, pp. 375–403.

The above comments should not be surprising. After all, in Chapter 3 and subsequent chapters, we have introduced independent variables that have been documented to impact on employee performance and satisfaction. Yet supporters of the leadership concept have tended to place an undue burden on this variable for explaining and predicting behavior. It is too simplistic to consider subordinates as guided to goal accomplishments based solely on the behavior of their leader. It is important, therefore, to recognize explicitly that leadership is merely another independent variable in our overall OB model. In some situations it may contribute a lot to explaining employee productivity, absence, turnover, and satisfaction; but in other situations, it may contribute little toward that end.

LOOKING FOR COMMON GROUND: WHAT DOES IT ALL MEAN?

The topic of leadership certainly doesn't lack for theories. But from an overview perspective, what does it all mean? Let's try to identify commonalities among the leadership theories and attempt to determine what, if any, practical value the theories hold for application to organizations.

Careful examination discloses that the concepts of "task" and "people"— often expressed in more elaborate terms that hold substantially the same meaning—permeate most of the theories.[24] The task dimension is called just that by Fiedler, but it goes by the name of "initiating structure" for the Ohio State group and the path-goal supporters, "production-orientation" by the Michigan researchers, and "concern for production" by Blake and Mouton. The people dimension gets similar treatment, going under such aliases as "consideration," and "employee-oriented" or "relationship-oriented" leadership. It seems clear that leadership behavior can be shrunk down to two dimensions—task and people—but researchers continue to differ as to whether the orientations are two ends of a single continuum (you could be high on one or the other but not both) or two independent dimensions (you could be high or low on both).

Although one well-known scholar argues that virtually every theory has also "wrestled with the question of how much a leader should share power with subordinates in decision-making,"[25] there is far less support for this contention. The autocratic-participative continuum and the leadership-participation model both directly address this issue, but the task-people dichotomy appears to be far more encompassing.

How should we interpret the findings presented in this chapter? Some traits have shown, over time, to be modest predictors of leadership effectiveness. But the fact that a manager possessed intelligence, dominance, self-confidence, or the like would by no means assure us that his or her subordinates

24. Barbara Karmel, "Leadership: A Challenge to Traditional Research Methods and Assumptions," *Academy of Management Review*, July 1978, pp. 477–79.

25. Schein, *Organizational Psychology*, p. 132.

would be productive and satisfied employees. The ability of these traits to predict leadership success is just not that strong.

The early task-people approaches (i.e., the Ohio State, Michigan, and managerial grid theories) also offer us little substance. The strongest statement one can make based on these theories is that leaders who rate high in people orientation should end up with satisfied employees. The research is too mixed to make predictions regarding employee productivity or the effect of a task orientation on productivity and satisfaction.

The wealth of research on the Fiedler model has failed to confirm the theory in its entirety, but parts of it are supported. When category I, IV, V, or VIII situations exist, the utilization of the LPC instrument to assess whether there is a leader-situation match and the use of that information to predict employee productivity and satisfaction outcomes seems warranted.

The path-goal model represents an up-to-date task-people approach. Its use of individual and task characteristics as moderating variables has met with reasonable success, especially in predicting satisfaction. Yet the theory itself is "relatively new to the literature of organizational behavior. Consequently, path-goal theory is offered more as a tool for directing research and stimulating insight than as a proven guide for managerial action."[26]

The autocratic-participative continuum and its modern-day equivalent, the Vroom-Yetton leadership-participation model, offer a diversity of leadership styles. Although studies to validate the Vroom-Yetton model are still scarce, the early results are encouraging. One investigation, for example, found that leaders who were high in agreement with the model had subordinates with higher productivity and higher satisfaction than those leaders who were in low agreement with the model.[27] A major reservation, in addition to the need for more confirming studies, is the complexity of the model itself. With five styles, eight contingency variables, and eighteen possible outcomes, it would be difficult to use as a guide for practicing managers. One might additionally question whether, under the stress of day-to-day activities, managers could be expected to follow the rational, conscious process the model requires. Of course, from our descriptive perspective, we might answer "It doesn't matter." What does matter is that where we find leaders who follow the model, we should expect also to find productive and satisfied employees.

IMPLICATIONS FOR PERFORMANCE AND SATISFACTION

Leadership plays a central part in understanding group behavior, for it is the leader who usually provides the direction toward goal attainment. Therefore, a more accurate predictive capability should be valuable in improving group performance.

26. House and Mitchell, "Path-Goal Theory," p. 94.

27. Margerison and Glube, "Leadership Decision-Making."

In this chapter we have described a transition in approaches to the study of leadership—from the simple trait orientation to increasingly complex and sophisticated models, such as those proposed by House and by Vroom and Yetton. With the increase in complexity has also come an increase in our ability to explain and predict behavior.

Predictive ability increased as a result of the recognition that inclusion of situational factors was critical. Recent efforts have moved beyond mere recognition toward specific attempts to isolate these situational variables. We can expect further progress to be made with leadership models, but the last decade has seen us take several large steps—large enough that we now can make moderately effective predictions as to who can best lead a group and explain under what conditions a given approach (task-oriented or people-oriented) is likely to lead to high performance and satisfaction.

FOR DISCUSSION

1. Trace the development of leadership research.

2. Discuss the strengths and weaknesses in the trait approach to leadership.

3. "Behavioral theories of leadership are static." Do you agree or disagree? Discuss.

4. What is the managerial grid? Contrast its approach to leadership with the Ohio State and Michigan groups.

5. What are the contingencies in Fiedler's contingency model?

6. Develop an example where you operationalize the Fiedler model.

7. What are the contingencies of the path-goal model? What are the conclusions obtained from this model?

8. Describe the leader-participation model. Using the model, what is the preferred leadership style for a prison guard? For a surgeon in the operating room? For a high school principal? For the manager of research and development at Eastman-Kodak?

9. When might leaders be irrelevant?

10. Which leadership theories, or parts of theories, appear to demonstrate reasonable predictive capability? Can you integrate them into a single synthesized theory?

FOR FURTHER READING

GHISELLI, E., *Explorations in Management Talent.* Pacific Palisades, Calif.: Goodyear, 1971. Reports on the development, validation, and usefulness of traits for identifying successful managers.

HUNT, J. G., and L. L. LARSON, *Crosscurrents in Leadership.* Carbondale, Ill.: Southern Illinois University Press, 1979. The most recent in an ongoing set of edited papers coming out of Southern Illinois' leadership conferences.

MCGREGOR, D., *The Human Side of Enterprise.* New York: McGraw-Hill, 1960. Classic treatise that argues that the traditional theories of management concerning human nature and the control of human behavior in the organizational setting are composed of unrealistic and limiting assumptions.

MINER, J. B., "The Uncertain Future of the Leadership Concept: An Overview," *Organization and Administrative Sciences,* Summer-Fall, 1975, pp. 197–208. The leadership concept has outlived its usefulness and should be abandoned in favor of a theory of control.

REDDIN, W. J., *Managerial Effectiveness.* New York: McGraw-Hill, 1970. Presents the author's 3-D Theory, with its four basic styles of leader behavior.

STOGDILL, R. M., *Handbook of Leadership: A Survey of Theory and Research.* Riverside, N.J.: Free Press, 1974. A comprehensive review of important experimental and questionnaire research on leadership for the past several decades.

POINT

FIEDLER AND CHEMERS

Leaders make a difference

Adapted and edited from Fred E. Fiedler and Martin M. Chemers, "Leadership and Management," in Contemporary Management: Issues and Viewpoints, *ed. Joseph W. McGuire (Englewood Cliffs, N.J.: Prentice-Hall, 1974), pp. 362–78. With permission.*

There can be very little question that an organization's success and failure—indeed, its very survival—depends in large part on the leadership it is able to attract. As a result, we heap rewards and honors on our leaders for the success of their organizations, and we make them bear the brunt of failure. If the team loses, the coach gets fired. On the other hand, we are willing to pay some of our leaders ten, twenty, or even more times the salary of the nonsupervisory employee. And we also spend billions of dollars yearly on recruitment, selection, and training of leaders, managers, and supervisors. Clearly, the problems of leadership are far from academic.

We shall here define the leader as the individual in the group who has the task of directing and coordinating task-relevant group activities. In groups that do not have a designated leader, he is the one who carries the primary responsibility for performing these functions in the group.

Modern leadership theory has had two major concerns. The first involves who becomes a leader or how one attains a position of leadership. This concern has resulted in hundreds of studies devoted to searching out leadership traits. The second major problem pertains to the question of leadership effectiveness—or how one becomes an effective leader. This second concern has spawned numerous studies of leader selection, leadership tests, research on effective and ineffective leader behavior, and leadership styles. It has influenced the philosophy and method of leadership training for supervisors and managers in business and industry. In discussing the theories and research on leadership, it is important that we clearly distinguish between leadership *position* and leadership *effectiveness*. Whether we like it or not, it is important to recognize that the attainment of a leadership position may be purely fortuitous. A person may be the leader because he is the most charming or able member of the group, because his family owns 51 per cent of the stock, or simply because he was the only person available at the time. Whether he will be comparatively more successful than others is a distinct and separate question.

How do you get to be a leader? The simplest answer is to get someone to follow you. This is accomplished by having material or psychological resources that the followers want—superior intelligence, a strong personality, money to hire employees, or control over organizational resources, such as a military commander might have. Although the trend in the United States is against nepotism, most leaders throughout the world attain leadership positions at least in part by being born into the right family. Warner and Abegglen reported in 1955 that 48 percent of American business executives came from families that owned substantial stock in the company. The proportion in many countries outside the United States is undoubtedly higher.

Also, consider the many supervisory positions in American government and industry that require specific types of training and education. How many managers of a highway department do not have a degree in civil engineering? Many production managers have to have college training, it is almost impossible to become a judge without being a lawyer, and it is difficult, if not impossible, to rise to high positions in the military services without college or military academy training.

Personality attributes clearly do play a part in determining who becomes a leader. However, we should be fully aware of the fact that the attainment of a leadership position may be as much a factor of a person's education, economics, politics, or genealogy as of his personal attributes.

Leadership also depends to a considerable degree upon being at the right place at the right time. It also helps to be visible. Studies support that the visibility and participation of the individual determines to a large extent his leadership status.

Who, then, becomes a leader? Two major generalizations are in order.

1. People tend to become leaders if they are somewhat superior to other members in their group in the particular abilities, skills, or control over resources that assist group members to satisfy their needs or the group to achieve its goals.

2. People tend to become leaders if their particular assignment or personality attributes make them more visible than others in the group.

Let us now turn to the second major question in leadership theory—namely, how to be an effective leader.

First of all, the data suggest very strongly that both the task-motivated as well as the relationship-motivated types of persons can be effective leaders *if they are placed in the right situation*. In other words, every leader can be effective in some situations and ineffective in others.

Second, we cannot really talk about a good or a poor leader since the data show that the effectiveness of the leader is determined in large part by the situation. Hence, we can only speak about a leader who is effective in one situation but ineffective in another.

COUNTER →←POINT

PFEFFER

Do leaders really matter?

Adapted and edited from Jeffrey Pfeffer, "The Ambiguity of Leadership." Academy of Management Review, *January 1977, pp. 104–11. With permission.*

Hall asked a basic question about leadership: "Is there any evidence of the magnitude of the effects of leadership?" Surprisingly, he could find little evidence. Given the resources that have been spent studying, selecting, and training leaders, one might expect that the question of whether or not leaders matter would have been addressed earlier.

There are at least three reasons why it might be argued that the observed effects of leaders on organizational outcomes would be small. First, those obtaining leadership positions are selected, and perhaps, only certain, limited styles of behavior may be chosen. Second, once in the leadership position, the discretion and behavior of the leader are constrained. And third, leaders can typically affect only a few of the variables that may impact organizational performance.

Persons are selected to leadership positions. As a consequence of this selection process, the range of behaviors or characteristics exhibited is reduced, making it more problematic to empirically discover the effect of leadership. There are many types of constraints on the selection process. The attraction literature suggests that there is a tendency for persons to like those they perceive as similar. In critical decisions such as the selection of persons for leadership positions, compatible styles of behavior probably will be chosen.

Selection of persons is also constrained by the internal system of influence in the organization. As Zald noted, succession is a critical decision, affected by political influence and by environmental contingencies faced by the organization.

Finally the selection of persons to leadership positions is affected by a self-selection process. Organizations and roles have images, providing information about their character. Persons are likely to select themselves into organizations and roles based upon their preferences for the dimensions of the organizational and role characteristics as perceived through these images. The self-selection of persons would tend to work along with organizational selection to limit the range of abilities and behaviors in a given organizational role.

Analyses of leadership have frequently presumed leadership style or leader behavior was an independent variable that could be selected or trained at will to conform to what research would find to be optimal. Even theorists who took a more contingent view of appropriate leadership behavior generally assumed that with proper training, appropriate behavior could be produced. Fiedler, noting how hard it was to change behavior, suggested changing the situational characteristics rather than the person, but this was an unusual suggestion in the context of prevailing literature which suggested that leadership style was something to be strategically selected according to the variables of the particular leadership theory.

But the leader is embedded in a social system, which constrains behavior. The leader has a role set, in which members have expectations for appropriate behavior and persons make efforts to modify the leader's behavior. Pressures to conform to the expectations of peers, subordinates, and superiors are all relevant in determining actual behavior.

Leaders, even in high-level positions, have unilateral control over fewer resources and fewer policies than might be expected. Investment decisions may require approval of others, while hiring and promotion decisions may be accomplished by committees. Leader behavior is constrained both by the demands of others in the role set and by organizationally prescribed limitations on the sphere of activity and influence.

Many factors that may affect organizational performance are outside a leader's control, even if he or she were to have complete discretion over major areas of organizational decision. For example, consider the executive in a construction firm. Costs are largely determined by operation of commodities and labor markets; and demand is largely affected by interest rates, availability of mortgage money, and economic conditions that are affected by governmental policies over which the executive has little control. School superintendents have little control over birth rates and community economic development, both of which profoundly affect school system budgets. While the leader may react to contingencies as they arise, or may be a better or worse forecaster, in accounting for variation in organizational outcomes, he or she may account for relatively little compared to external factors.

Second, the leader's success or failure may be partly due to circumstances unique to the organization but still outside his or her control. Leader positions in organizations vary in terms of the strength and position of the organization. The choice of a new executive does not fundamentally alter a market and financial position that has de-

veloped over years and affects the leader's ability to make strategic changes and the likelihood that the organization will do well or poorly. Organizations have relatively enduring strengths and weaknesses. The choice of a particular leader for a particular position has limited impact on these capabilities.

Two studies have assessed the effects of leadership changes in major positions in organizations. Lieberson and O'Connor examined 167 business firms in thirteen industries over a twenty-year period, allocating variance in sales, profits, and profit margins to one of four sources: year (general economic conditions), industry, company effects, and effects of changes in the top executive position. They concluded that compared to other factors, administration had a limited effect on organizational outcomes.

Using a similar analytical procedure, Salancik and Pfeffer examined the effects of mayors on city budgets for thirty major U.S. cities. Data on expenditures by budget category were collected for 1951–68. Variance in amount and proportion of expenditures was apportioned to the year, the city, or the mayor. The mayoral effect was relatively small, with the city accounting for most of the variance, although the mayor effect was larger for expenditure categories that were not as directly connected to important interest groups. Salancik and Pfeffer argued that the effects of the mayor were limited both by absence of power to control many of the expenditures and tax sources, and by construction of policies in response to demands from interest in the environment.

Leadership is associated with a set of myths reinforcing a social construction of meaning that legitimates leadership-role occupants, and attributes social causality to leadership roles, thereby providing a belief in the effectiveness of individual control. In analyzing leadership, this mythology and the process by which such mythology is created and supported should be separated from analysis of leadership as a social influence process, operating within constraints.

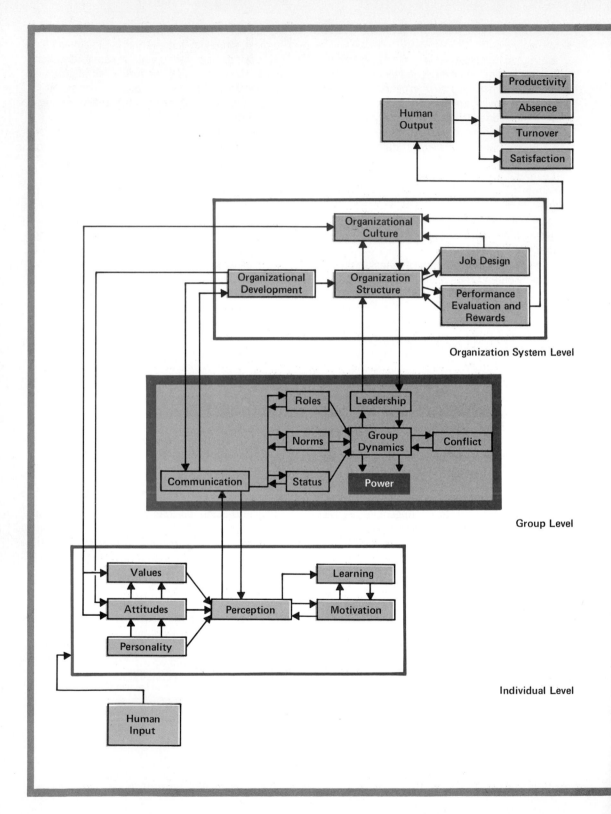

Human
Output

Productivity

Absence

Turnover

Satisfaction

Organizational
Culture

Job Design

Organizational
Development

Organization
Structure

Performance
Evaluation and
Rewards

Organization System Level

Roles

Leadership

Norms

Group
Dynamics

Conflict

Communication

Status

Power

Group Level

Values

Learning

Attitudes

Perception

Motivation

Personality

Individual Level

Human
Input

CHAPTER 12

Power

AFTER STUDYING THIS CHAPTER, YOU SHOULD BE ABLE TO—

Define and explain the following key terms and concepts:

Assertiveness
Blocking
Coalitions
Coercive power
Dependence
Elasticity of power
Exchange of benefits
Expert power
Ingratiation
Knowledge power
Opportunity power

Personal power
Persuasive power
Position power
Power
Rationality
Referent power
Reward power
Sanctions
Uncertainty
Upward appeal

Understand:

The nature of power
Four bases of power
Four sources of power
Eight power tactics and their contingencies
How power is achieved
The importance of dependency in power relationships

> You can get much farther with a kind word and a gun than you can with a kind word alone.
>
> —AL CAPONE

The subject of power has been described by Bertrand Russell as "the fundamental concept in social science . . . in the same sense in which Energy is the fundamental concept in physics."[1] In spite of the almost universal acceptance among both academics and management practitioners of the importance of power, it has only very recently received the attention it deserves. The most frequently cited publication on power is more than twenty years old,[2] but that should not be true for long. I can think of no OB concept where more progress was made during the latter part of the 1970s than in power. For instance, recent publications have clarified terminology,[3] given us new knowledge on tactics,[4] and increased our understanding as to what happens to powerholders as a result of using power.[5]

The 1980s should see a continuation of interest in the topic of power. The evidence indicates that the acquisition and distribution of power is a natural process in any group. Power determines what goals the group will pursue and how the group's resources will be distributed among its members. These, in turn, play an important part in determining how effective the group will be. An understanding of power, therefore, is a requisite for all students of OB.

A DEFINITION OF POWER

Power refers to a capacity that A has to influence the behavior of B, so that B does something he or she would not otherwise do. This definition implies (1) a

1. Bertrand Russell, *Power: A New Social Analysis* (London: Allen & Unwin, 1938), p. 12.

2. J. R. P. French, Jr., and Bertram Raven, "The Bases of Social Power," *Studies in Social Power,* ed. D. Cartwright (Ann Arbor: University of Michigan, Institute for Social Research, 1959), pp. 150–67.

3. Samuel B. Bachrach and Edward J. Lawler, *Power and Politics in Organizations* (San Francisco: Jossey-Bass, 1980).

4. David Kipnis, Stuart M. Schmidt, and Ian Wilkinson, "Intraorganizational Influence Tactics: Explorations in Getting One's Way," *Journal of Applied Psychology,* August 1980, pp. 440–52.

5. David Kipnis, *The Powerholders* (Chicago: University of Chicago Press, 1976).

potential that need not be actualized to be effective, (2) a *dependence* relationship, and (3) that B has some *discretion* over his or her own behavior. Let's look at each of these points more closely.

Power may exist but not be used. It is, therefore, a capacity or potential. Arthur Fonzerelli, on the television series "Happy Days," has power. Everyone is afraid of "The Fonz," yet he has never actually had to use his power to get others to comply with his wishes. They respond in fear that he *might* use his physical force but, as long as no one "calls his bluff," his capacity to influence others is as effective as if he actually used physical force. Our point again is that one can have power but not impose it.

Probably the most important aspect of power is that it is a function of dependence. The greater B's dependence on A, the greater is A's power in the relationship. Dependence, in turn, is based on alternatives that B perceives and the importance that B places on the alternative(s) that A controls. A person can have power over you only if he or she controls something you desire. If you want a college degree, have to pass a certain course to get that degree, and your current instructor is the only faculty member in the college that teaches that course, he or she has power over you. Your alternatives are highly limited and you place a high degree of importance on obtaining a passing grade. Similarly, if you're attending college on funds totally provided by your parents, you probably recognize the power that they hold over you. You are dependent on them for financial support. But once you're out of school, have a job, and are making a solid income, your parents' power is reduced significantly. Who among us, though, has not known or heard of the rich relative that is able to control a large number of family members merely through the implicit or explicit threat of "writing them out of the will"?

For A to get B to do something he or she otherwise would not do means that B must have the discretion to make choices. At the extreme, if B's job behavior is so programmed that he is allowed no room to make choices, he obviously is constrained in his ability to do something other than what he is doing. For instance, job descriptions, group norms, organizational rules and regulations, as well as community laws and standards constrain people's choices. As a nurse, you may be dependent on your supervisor for continued employment. But in spite of this dependence, you're unlikely to comply with her request to perform heart surgery on a patient or steal several thousand dollars from petty cash. Your job description and laws against stealing constrain your ability to make these choices.

CONTRASTING LEADERSHIP AND POWER

A careful comparison of our description of power with our description of leadership in the previous chapter should bring the recognition that the two concepts are closely intertwined. Leaders use power as a means of attaining group goals. Leaders achieve goals, and power is a means for facilitating their achievement.

What differences are there between the two terms? One difference relates to goal compatibility. Power does not require goal compatibility, merely dependence. Leadership, on the other hand, requires some congruence between the goals of the leader and the led. The other difference deals with the direction that research on the two concepts has taken. Leadership research, for the most part, emphasizes style. It seeks answers to questions like: How supportive should a leader be? How much decision making should be shared with subordinates? In contrast, the research on power has tended to encompass a broader area and focus on tactics for gaining compliance. It has gone beyond the individual as exerciser because power can be used by groups as well as individuals to control other individuals or groups.

BASES AND SOURCES OF POWER

Where does power come from? What is it that gives an individual or group influence over others? The early answer to these questions was a five-category classification scheme identified by French and Raven.[6] They proposed that there were five bases or sources of power which they termed coercive, reward, expert, legitimate, and referent power. Coercive power depends on fear; reward power derives from the ability to distribute anything of value (typically money, favorable performance appraisals, interesting work assignments, friendly colleagues, and preferred work shifts or sales territories); expert power refers to influence that derives from special skills or knowledge; legitimate power is based on the formal rights one receives as a result of holding an authoritative position or role in an organization; and referent power develops out of others' admiration for one and their desire to model their behavior and attitudes after that person. While French and Raven's classification scheme provided an extensive repertoire of possible bases of power, their categories created ambiguity because they confused bases of power with sources of power.[7] The result was much overlapping. We can improve our understanding of the power concept by separating bases and sources so as to develop clearer and more independent categories.

Bases of power refers to what the powerholder has that gives him or her power. Assuming you're the powerholder, your bases are what you control that enables you to manipulate the behavior of others. There are four power bases—coercive power, reward power, persuasive power, and knowledge power.[8] We'll amplify on each in a moment.

How are *sources* of power different from bases of power? The answer is that sources tell us where the powerholder gets his or her power bases. That is, sources refer to how you come to control the bases of power. There are four sources—the position you hold, your personal characteristics, your expertise,

6. French and Raven, "Bases of Social Power."

7. Bachrach and Lawler, *Power and Politics,* pp. 34–36.

8. Adapted from ibid. and Amitai Etzioni, *Comparative Analysis of Complex Organizations* (New York: Free Press, 1961).

and the opportunity you have to receive and obstruct information.[9] Each of these will also be discussed in a moment.

Let us now turn back to the four bases of power and define them.

Bases of Power

Coercive Power. The coercive base depends on fear. One reacts to this power out of fear of the negative ramifications that might result if one fails to comply. It rests on the application, or the threat of application, of physical sanctions such as infliction of pain, deformity, or death; the generation of frustration through restriction of movement; or the controlling through force of basic physiological or safety needs.

In the 1930s, when John Dillinger went into a bank, held a gun to the teller's head, and asked for the money, he was incredibly successful at getting compliance with his request. His power base? Coercive. A loaded gun gives its holder power because others are fearful that they will lose something which they hold dear—their life.

> Of all the bases of power available to man, the power to hurt others is possibly most often used, most often condemned, and most difficult to control . . . the state relies on its military and legal resources to intimidate nations, or even its own citizens. Businesses rely upon the control of economic resources. Schools and universities rely upon their right to deny students formal education, while the church threatens individuals with loss of grace. At the personal level, individuals exercise coercive power through a reliance upon physical strength, verbal facility, or the ability to grant or withhold emotional support from others. These bases provide the individual with the means to physically harm, bully, humiliate, or deny love to others.[10]

At the organizational level, A has coercive power over B if A can dismiss, suspend, or demote B, assuming that B values his or her job. Similarly, if A can assign B work activities that B finds unpleasant or treat B in a manner that B finds embarrassing, A possesses coercive power over B.

Reward Power. The opposite of coercive power is the power to reward. People comply with the wishes of another because it will result in positive benefits; therefore, one who can distribute rewards that others view as valuable will have power over them. Our definition of rewards is here limited to only material rewards. This would include salaries and wages, commissions, fringe benefits, and the like.

Persuasive Power. Persuasive power rests on the allocation and manipulation of symbolic rewards. If you can decide who is hired, manipulate the mass media, control the allocation of status symbols, or influence a group's norms, you have persuasive power. For instance, when a teacher uses the class climate to control a deviant student, or when a union steward arouses the members to use

9. Bachrach and Lawler, *Power and Politics,* pp. 34–36.

10. Kipnis, *Powerholders,* pp. 77–78.

their informal power to bring a deviant member into line, you are observing examples of persuasive power being used.

Knowledge Power. Knowledge, or access to information, is the final base of power. We can say that when an individual in a group or organization controls unique information, and when that information is needed to make a decision, that individual has knowledge-based power.

To summarize the above, the bases of power refer to what the power-holder controls that enables him or her to manipulate the behavior of others. The coercive base of power is the control of punishment; the reward base is the control of material rewards; the persuasive base is the control of symbolic rewards; and the knowledge base is the control of information.

Sources of Power

Position Power. In formal groups and organizations, probably the most frequent access to one or more of the power bases is one's structural position. A teacher's position includes significant control over symbols, a secretary frequently is privy to important information, and the head coach of an NFL team has substantial coercive resources at his disposal. All of these bases of power are achieved as a result of the formal position each holds within their structural hierarchy.

Personal Power. Personality traits were discussed in Chapter 4 and again in the previous chapter on leadership. They reappear within the topic of power when we acknowledge the fact that one's personal characteristics can be a source of power. If you are articulate, domineering, physically imposing, or possessing of that mystical quality called "charisma," you hold personal characteristics that may be used to get others to do what you want.

Expert Power. Expertise is a means by which the powerholder comes to control specialized information (rather than the control itself, which we have discussed as the knowledge base of power). Those who have expertise in terms of specialized information can use it to manipulate others. Expertise is one of the most powerful sources of influence, especially in a technologically oriented society. As jobs become more specialized, we become increasingly dependent on "experts" to achieve goals. So, while it is generally acknowledged that physicians have expertise and hence expert power—when your doctor talks, you listen—you should also recognize that computer specialists, tax accountants, solar engineers, industrial psychologists and other specialists are able to wield power as a result of their expertise.

Opportunity Power. Finally, being in the right place at the right time can give one the opportunity to exert power. One need not hold a formal position in a group or organization to have access to information that is important to others or be able to exert coercive influence. An example of how one can use an opportunity to create a power base is the story of Lyndon Johnson, when he was a student at Southwestern Texas State Teachers College. He had a job as special assistant to the college president's personal secretary.

As special assistant, Johnson's assigned job was simply to carry messages from the president to the department heads and occasionally to other faculty members. Johnson saw that the rather limited function of messenger had possibilities for expansion; for example, encouraging recipients of the messages to transmit their own communications through him. He occupied a desk in the president's outer office, where he took it upon himself to announce the arrival of visitors. These added services evolved from a helpful convenience into an aspect of the normal process of presidential business. The messenger had become an appointments secretary, and, in time, faculty members came to think of Johnson as a funnel to the president. Using a technique which was later to serve him in achieving mastery over the Congress, Johnson turned a rather insubstantial service into a process through which power was exercised.[11]

Johnson eventually broadened his informal duties to include handling the president's political correspondence, preparing his reports for state agencies, and even came regularly to accompany the college president on his trips to the state capital—the president eventually relying on his young apprentice for political counsel. Certainly this represents an example of someone using an opportunity to redefine his job and to give himself power.

Summary

The foundation to understanding power begins by identifying where power comes from (sources) and, given that one has the means to exert influence, what it is that one manipulates (bases). Figure 12–1 visually depicts the relationship between sources and bases. Sources are the means. Individuals can use their position in the structure, rely on personal characteristics, develop expertise, or take advantage of opportunities to control information. Control of one or more of these sources allows the powerholder to manipulate the behavior of others via coercion, reward, persuasion, or knowledge bases. To reiterate,

11. Doris Kearns, "Lyndon Johnson and the American Dream," *The Atlantic Monthly,* May 1976, p. 41.

FIGURE 12–1   Sources and Bases of Power

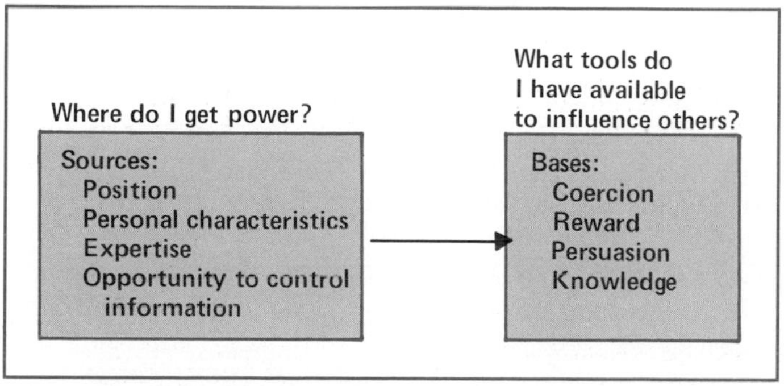

sources are *where* you get power. Bases are *what* you manipulate. Those who seek power must develop a source of power. Then, and only then, can they acquire a power base.

DEPENDENCY AND UNCERTAINTY

Earlier in this chapter it was said that probably the most important aspect of power is that it is a function of dependence. In this section, it will be shown how dependency, along with uncertainty, is central to understanding power. We'll make our point by using propositions.

The greater B's dependency on A, the greater power A has over B. When you possess anything that others require but that you alone control, you make them dependent upon you and, therefore, you gain power over them.[12] Dependency, then, is inversely proportional to the alternative sources of supply. If something is plentiful, possession of it will not increase your power. If everyone is intelligent, intelligence gives no special advantage. Similarly, among the super-rich, money is no longer power. But as the old saying goes, "in the land of the blind, the one-eyed man is king!" If you can create a monopoly by controlling information, prestige, or anything that others crave, they become dependent on you. Conversely, the more that you can expand your options, the less power you place in the hands of others. This explains, for example, why most organizations develop multiple suppliers rather than giving their business to only one. It also explains why so many of us aspire for financial independence. Financial independence reduces the power that others can have over us.

An example of the role dependency plays in a work group or an organization is the case of Mike Milken, the thirty-year-old head of the corporate bond department at a major New York City brokerage firm.[13] A native Californian, Milken grew disenchanted with New York and decided to return to southern California and a warmer climate. But Milken made so much money for his employer that they were not about to let him go. The solution: Rather than lose his trading skills to some competitor with West Coast connections, the company agreed to move its entire bond department. Milken and the staff of twenty people working for him were, in the spring of 1978, all moved to Los Angeles. The cost of setting up this office, moving employees and their families, and absorbing housing subsidies all being part of the price Mike Milken's employer was willing to pay to keep his skills.

A more recent example took place in professional basketball during the fall of 1981. Earvin "Magic" Johnson, the 22-year-old super-star on the Los Angeles Lakers team, chose one Wednesday evening to blast his coach's system. He told the press that he could not play under his coach, Paul Westhead,

12. R. E. Emerson, "Power-Dependence Relations," *American Sociological Review*, Vol. 27 (1962), pp. 31–41.

13. Sharon Johnson, "Mohammed and the Mountain," *New York Times*, January 29, 1978, p. F5.

and demanded to be traded. Within 24 hours, the Lakers' owner fired West-head.

Westhead's record was not in question. He had led the Lakers to the NBA championship during the 1979–80 season. At the time of his firing, the team was only a half-game behind their conference leader with a 7–4 win-loss record. The issue really was: Who was dispensable? In the summer of 1981, Johnson had signed a 25-year, $25 million contract with the Laker organization. West-head, on the other hand, was operating under a far less lucrative 4-year pact. Johnson was a major asset to the Laker team and his 25-year contract made it almost impossible for him to be traded. No other team was willing to assume such a contractual obligation. The Laker owner had little choice but to fire the coach. Regardless of the fact that a professional coach is the formal "boss" over his team's members, this example dramatizes that a player or any employee (who has no legitimate position power) can still be extremely influential if the "team's" options are severely restricted.

A concept referred to as the "elasticity of power" can help to illustrate the interrelationship between power and dependency. In economics, considerable attention is focused on the elasticity of demand, which is defined as the relative responsiveness of quantity demanded to change in price. This concept can be modified to explain the strength of power.

Elasticity of power is defined as the relative responsiveness of power to change in available alternatives. One's ability to influence others is viewed as being dependent on how these others perceive their alternatives.

As shown in Figure 12–2, assume we have two individuals. Mr. A's power

FIGURE 12–2   Elasticity of Power

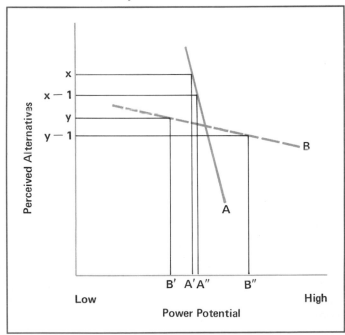

elasticity curve is relatively inelastic. This would describe, for example, an employee who believed that he had a large number of employment opportunities outside his current organization. Fear of being fired would have only a moderate impact on Mr. A, for he perceives that he has a number of other alternatives. Mr. A's boss finds that threatening A with termination has only a minimal impact on influencing A's behavior. A reduction in alternatives (from X to $X-1$) only increases the power of A's boss slightly (A' to A''). However, Mr. B's curve is relatively elastic. He sees few other job opportunities. His age, education, present salary, or lack of contacts may severely limit his ability to find a job somewhere else. As a result, Mr. B is dependent on his present organization and boss. If B loses his job (Y to $Y-1$), he may face prolonged unemployment, and it shows itself in the increased power of B's boss. As long as B perceives his options as limited and B's boss holds the power to terminate his employment, B's boss will hold considerable power over him. In such a situation, it is obviously important for B to get his boss to *believe* that his options are considerably greater than they really are. If this is not achieved, B places his fate almost entirely in the hands of his boss and makes him captive to almost any demands the boss devises.

Higher education provides an excellent example of how this elasticity concept operates. In universities where there are strong pressures for the faculty to publish, we can say that a department head's power over a faculty member is inversely related to that member's publication record. The more recognition the faculty member receives through publication, the more mobile he or she is. That is, since other universities want faculty who are highly published and visible, there is an increased demand for his or her services. Although the concept of tenure can act to alter this relationship by restricting the department head's alternatives, those faculty members with little or no publications have the least mobility and are subject to the greatest influence from their superiors.

To the extent that a low-ranking member has important knowledge not available to high-ranking members, the low-ranking member is likely to have power over the high-ranking members. This statement is the natural result when we combine our previous statement regarding dependency with what we have previously discussed about knowledge and expertise. It explicitly states that one does not have to hold a legitimate hierarchical role in a group or organization in order to have power. Individuals who are low-ranking in the hierarchy can develop a strong and potent power base by acquiring knowledge that high-ranking participants are dependent upon. This may be achieved by destroying the procedure manuals that describe how a job is done, refusing to train people in your job or even to show others exactly what you do, creating specialized language and terminology that inhibits others from understanding your job, or operating in secrecy so the activity will appear more complex and difficult than it really is.

A person difficult to replace has greater power than has an easily replaceable person. This statement also evolves out of the role dependency plays in power positions. The more unique your skills, the greater advantage you have in influencing others in ways that are personally satisfying. This applies to occupational categories as well as to unique individual talents:

In the late 1950s, when there were relatively few engineers to service an expanding American economy, engineers had great prestige and power. They could force employers to provide them with large salaries and benefits, by threatening to withhold their services. By the 1970s, however, many persons had become engineers and consequently the bargaining power of engineers with employers was practically nil.[14]

The same thing happened among elementary and secondary school teachers. In the 1940s and 1950s, there was a significant shortage. Today, literally hundreds of thousands of individuals with teaching credentials look in vain for teaching jobs. School administrators no longer fear that competent teaching replacements cannot be found. In contrast, if you had a degree in accounting in the early 1980s, you found yourself in a powerful position in negotiating with your employer or prospective employers. In the early 1980s, at least, accountants were more difficult to replace than elementary or secondary teachers.

The ability to reduce group uncertainty increases an individual's potential power. Just as dependency is an effective approach for developing power, the evidence suggests that individuals who can reduce the uncertainties that their group or organization faces possess a valuable resource that can create power.

Organizations seek to avoid uncertainty.[15] Those individuals who can absorb the organization's uncertainty will have influence in the organization. In a French factory, one researcher noticed that maintenance engineers exerted considerable power in spite of their generally low rank in the hierarchy.[16] Why? The researcher found that the only major remaining uncertainty confronting the organization was the breakdown of machinery—and only the maintenance engineers could control this uncertainty.

Another researcher studied departmental power in a group of industrial organizations and found that the marketing department was consistently rated as the most powerful.[17] He concluded that the most critical uncertainty facing these firms was selling their products. This might suggest that during a labor strike, the organization's negotiating representatives have increased power or that engineers, as a group, would be more powerful at IBM than at Procter & Gamble. These inferences appear to be generally valid. Labor negotiators *do* become more powerful within the personnel area and the organization as a whole during periods of labor strife. An organization such as IBM, which is heavily technologically oriented, is highly dependent on its engineers in order to maintain its product superiority. And, at IBM, engineers are clearly the most powerful group At Procter & Gamble, marketing is the name of the game, and marketers are the most powerful occupational group.

14. Kipnis, *Powerholders,* p. 159.

15. Richard M. Cyert and James G. March, *A Behavioral Theory of the Firm* (Englewood Cliffs, N.J.: Prentice-Hall, 1963).

16. Michel Crozier, *The Bureaucratic Phenomenon* (Chicago: University of Chicago Press, 1964).

17. Charles Perrow, "Departmental Power and Perspective in Industrial Firms," in *Power in Organizations,* ed. M. N. Zald (Nashville, Tenn.: Vanderbilt University Press, 1970).

POWER TACTICS

This section is a logical extension of our previous discussion. We've reviewed *where* power comes from and *what* it is that powerholders manipulate. Now, we go the final step—to power tactics. Tactics tell us *how* to manipulate the bases. The following discussion will show you how employees translate their power bases into specific actions.

One of the few elements of power that has gone beyond anecdotal evidence or armchair speculation is the topic of tactics. Recent research indicates that there are standardized ways by which powerholders attempt to get what they want.[18]

When 165 managers were asked to write essays describing an incident in which they influenced either their bosses, co-workers, or subordinates, a total of 370 power tactics grouped into 14 categories were identified. These answers were condensed, rewritten into a 58-item questionnaire, and given to over 750 employees. These respondents were not only asked how they went about influencing others at work but also the possible reasons for influencing the target person. The results, which are summarized below, give us considerable insight into power tactics—how employees influence others and the conditions under which one tactic is chosen over another.

The findings identified eight tactical dimensions:

1. *Assertiveness*—setting deadlines, demanding compliance with requests, repeated reminders, ordering the individual to do what was asked, pointing out that rules required compliance
2. *Ingratiation*—includes low-profile and nonobtrusive behaviors such as acting humble, making the other person feel important, being friendly prior to making a request
3. *Rationality*—presenting information to support a request, using logic, explaining the reasons for the request
4. *Sanctions*—preventing a salary increase, promising a salary increase, threatening to give an unsatisfactory performance appraisal or to withhold a promotion
5. *Exchange of benefits*—trading favors, reminding target of previous favors done for him
6. *Upward appeal*—making a formal appeal to higher levels, obtaining the informal support of higher-ups, sending the target to see the powerholder's superior
7. *Blocking*—engaging in a work slowdown, threatening to discontinue working with the target person, ceasing to be friendly to the target
8. *Coalitions*—getting the support of co-workers or subordinates to back up the request

As we might predict, the researchers found that employees do not rely on the eight tactics equally. Some are more popular than others—ingratiation and rationality are the most frequently applied—and usage depends on contingency variables such as the status of the target, the goal of the powerholder, the level in the organization of the powerholder, the size of the work unit, and the existence or absence of unions.

18. Kipnis, Schmidt, and Wilkinson, "Intraorganizational Influence Tactics."

If the target is the boss, powerholders tended to rely on rationality. With co-workers, the most popular tactics were ingratiation, exchange of benefits, and upward appeal. When trying to influence subordinates, the most frequently used tactics were assertiveness, ingratiation, sanctions, exchange of benefits, and upward appeal.

Respondents were given a set of goals or situations and asked to identify which tactics they used. If the goal was to assign work to a target, assertiveness was most preferred. When trying to convince a target to accept new ideas, rationality was most likely to be relied upon. If the goal was to improve the target's job performance, both assertiveness and rationality were used. Finally, when respondents sought personal assistance from the target, ingratiation tactics were most popular.

The respondent's own level in the organization was closely associated with use of power tactics. The higher the respondent's job status, the more likely they were to use rationality and assertiveness tactics when influencing both their superiors and subordinates. Respondents with high job status also used sanctions more frequently and sought aid from their superiors less frequently when influencing their subordinates. Apparently, as the respondents' own job status rose, they were more likely to use more direct tactics and be less dependent upon superiors.

The findings suggest that as the number of persons in a work unit increase, higher reliance is placed on strong and impersonal means of control. In influencing subordinates in large work units, the respondents more frequently used assertiveness, sanctions, and upward appeal.

Lastly, if the organization was unionized, respondents were more likely to use ingratiation tactics to influence their subordinates, to avoid the use of assertiveness when influencing co-workers, and to use rationality tactics less frequently and blocking tactics more frequently when influencing bosses.

The above findings are by no means easy to assimilate. The tactics that a powerholder uses varies with his or her goals and degree of control over the target. But in spite of the complexity of the conclusions, our ability to explain and predict when individuals are likely to use which power tactics is certainly enhanced as a result of this research.

POWER IN GROUPS: COALITIONS

Those "out of power" and seeking to be "in" will first try to increase their power individually. Why spread the spoils if one doesn't have to? But if this proves ineffective, the alternative is to form a coalition. There *is* strength in numbers.

The natural way to gain influence is to become a powerholder. Therefore, those who want power will attempt to build a personal power base. But in many instances, this may be difficult, risky, costly, or impossible. In such cases, efforts will be made to form a coalition of two or more "outs" who, by joining together, can each better themselves at the expense of those outside the coalition.

In the late 1960s, college students found that by joining together to form a "student power group," they could achieve ends that had been impossible individually. Historically, employees in organizations who were unsuccessful in bargaining on their own behalf with management resorted to labor unions to bargain for them. In recent years, even some managers have joined unions after finding it difficult to individually exert power to attain higher wages and greater job security.

Can we predict how large a coalition will be? Yes! Preference will be given to keeping it as small as possible. Large coalitions are more difficult to mobilize initially and to maintain over time than smaller ones. Larger ones are harder to coordinate and there are increased opportunities for conflicts between prospective members. Therefore, coalitions tend to be just large enough to exert the power necessary to achieve their goals and will resist inclusion of excess members.[19]

Finally, can we predict when coalitions are more likely to develop? We propose that the more routine the tasks of a group, the greater the likelihood that coalitions will form. The more that the work that people do is routine, the greater their substitutability for each other and, thus, the greater their dependence. To offset this dependence, they can be expected to resort to a coalition. We see, therefore, that unions appeal more to low-skill and nonprofessional workers than to skilled and professional types. Of course, where the supply of skilled and professional employees is high relative to their demand or where organizations have standardized traditionally unique jobs, we would expect even these incumbents to find unionization attractive.

IMPLICATIONS FOR PERFORMANCE AND SATISFACTION

The understanding of power requires comprehending the role that dependency and uncertainty play in power dynamics and familiarity with power sources and bases.

Those individuals who can make others dependent upon them—either actually or as perceived—will increase their power over these others. Because groups avoid uncertainty, individuals who appear to possess the ability to reduce uncertainty will also gain power. This explains why group members withhold information or keep their activities shrouded in secrecy. This approach can make one's activities appear more complex and important than they may well be. The *perception* that one's activities are critical to the group's effectiveness and reduce external threats to the group is more important than whether the activities *actually* perform these functions.

19. W. H. Riker, *The Theory of Political Coalitions* (New Haven, Conn.: Yale University Press, 1962).

Performance

Knowledge-based power is the most strongly and consistently related with effective performance. For example, in a study of five organizations, knowledge was the most effective base for getting others to perform as desired.[20] Competence appears to offer wide appeal and its use as a power base results in high performance by group members.

In contrast, position power does *not* appear to be related to performance differences. In spite of position being the most widely given reason for complying with a superior's wishes, it does not seem to lead to higher performance, though the findings are far from conclusive. Among blue-collar workers, one researcher found significantly positive relations between position power and four of six production measures. However, position power was not related with average earnings or performance against schedule.[21] Another study could find no relationship between the use of position power and high efficiency ratings.[22] One's position is effective for exacting compliance, but there is little evidence to suggest that it leads to higher levels of performance. This may be explained by the fact that position power tends to be fairly constant, especially within a given organization.

The use of reward and coercive power has a significant inverse relationship to performance. People hold a negative view of reward and coercion as reasons for complying with a superior's requests. This view is reflected in the finding that these bases are associated with lower performance.[23] Further, research finds the use of coercive power to be negatively related to group effectiveness.[24]

Satisfaction

We find that knowledge power is strongly and consistently related with satisfaction. The evidence overwhelmingly indicates that this base is most satisfying to subjects of the power.[25] Knowledge-based power obtains both public and private compliance, and avoids the problem of making subjects comply merely be-

20. Jerald G. Bachman, D. G. Bowers and P. M. Marcus, "Bases of Supervisory Power: A Comparative Study in Five Organizational Settings," in *Control in Organizations*, ed. Arnold S. Tannenbaum (New York: McGraw-Hill, 1968), p. 236.

21. K. Student, "Supervisory Influence and Work-Group Performance," *Journal of Applied Psychology*, Vol. 52 (1968), pp. 188–94.

22. John Ivancevich, "An Analysis of Control, Bases of Control, and Satisfaction in an Organizational Setting," *Academy of Management Journal*, December 1970, pp. 427–36.

23. Jerald G. Bachman, "Faculty Satisfaction and the Dean's Influence: An Organizational Study of Twelve Liberal Arts Colleges," *Journal of Applied Psychology*, February 1968, pp. 55–61.; and Jerald G. Bachman, C. G. Smith, and J. A. Slesinger, "Control, Performance and Satisfaction: An Analysis of Structure and Individual Effort," *Journal of Personality and Social Psychology*, August 1966, pp. 127–36.

24. Bachman, Bowers, and Marcus, "Bases of Supervisory Power."

25. See, for example, footnotes 23 and 24.

cause the powerholder has the "right" to request compliance. Additionally, our value system is built on the idea of merit and competence, and knowledge power appears to most closely align with these values. If individuals find knowledge power to be most compatible with American values, it should logically give the greatest satisfaction.

Finally, the use of coercive power is inversely related to individual satisfaction. Coercion not only creates resistance, it is generally disliked by individuals. Studies of college teachers and sales personnel found coercion the least-preferred power base.[26] A study of insurance company employees also drew the same conclusion.[27]

FOR DISCUSSION

1. What is power? How is it different from leadership?

2. Contrast French and Raven's power classification to the bases and sources presented in this chapter.

3. What is the difference between a source of power and a base of power?

4. Contrast power tactics with power bases and sources. What are some of the key contingency variables that determine which tactic a powerholder is likely to use?

5. "Knowledge power and expert power are the same thing." Do you agree or disagree? Discuss.

6. What is a coalition? When is it likely to develop? How large will it be?

7. Which power bases are best for stimulating high performance? Explain.

8. Which power bases produce the highest satisfaction among subjects? Explain.

9. Based on the information presented in this chapter, what would you do as a new college graduate entering a new job to maximize your power and accelerate your career progress?

FOR FURTHER READING

CHRISTIE, R., and F. GEIS, *Studies in Machiavellianism.* New York: Academic Press, 1970. Scholarly attempt to define and measure Machiavellianism. Found high Machs manipulate more, win more, are persuaded less, and persuade others more.

26. See footnote 23.
27. Ivancevich, "Analysis of Control."

KORDA, M., *Power!* New York: Random House, 1975. Offers an insightful, though nonscholarly, view of the workings of organizations and how knowledge of power can be used to promote one's self-interest.

KOTTER, J. P., "Power, Dependence, and Effective Management," *Harvard Business Review,* July–August 1977, pp. 125–36. Describes common characteristics of managers who have been successful at acquiring considerable power and using it to manage their dependence on others.

MACHIAVELLI, N., *The Prince,* ed. T. G. Gergin. New York: Appleton-Century-Crofts, 1964. The classic treatise analyzing what practices had brought success in the past and deducing from them what principles ought to be followed for success in the present.

PFEFFER, J., *Power in Organizations.* Marshfield, Mass.: Pitman, 1981. The most up-to-date and comprehensive source on the topic of power.

ZALD, M. N., ed., *Power in Organizations.* Nashville, Tenn.: Vanderbilt University Press, 1970. A collection of papers and commentaries that serve to examine the role power and politics play upon control, decision making, and effecting and inhibiting change.

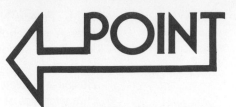

MCCLELLAND AND BURNHAM

A case for the power-oriented manager

What makes or motivates a good manager? The question is so enormous in scope that anyone trying to answer it has difficulty knowing where to begin. Some people might say that a good manager is one who is successful; and by now most business researchers and businessmen themselves know what motivates people who successfully run their own small businesses. The key to their success has turned out to be what psychologists call "the need for achievement"; the desire to do something better or more efficiently than it has been done before. Any number of books and articles summarize research studies explaining how the achievement motive is necessary for a person to attain success on his own.

But what has achievement motivation got to do with good management? There is no reason on theoretical grounds why a person who has a strong need to be more efficient should make a good manager. While it sounds as if everyone ought to have the need to achieve, in fact, as psychologists define and measure achievement motivation, it leads people to behave in very special ways that do not necessarily lead to good management.

For one thing, because they focus on personal improvement, on doing things better by them-selves, achievement-motivated people want to do things themselves. For another, they want concrete short-term feedback on their performance so that they can tell how well they are doing. Yet a manager, particularly one in a large complex organization, cannot perform all the tasks necessary for success by himself or herself. He must manage others so that they will do things for the organization. Also, feedback on his subordinate's performance may be a lot vaguer and more delayed than it would be if he were doing everything himself.

The manager's job seems to call more for someone who can influence people than for someone who does things better on his own. In motivational terms, then, we might expect the successful manager to have a greater "need for power" than need to achieve.

To measure the motivations of managers, good and bad, we studied a number of individual managers from different large U.S. corporations who were participating in management workshops designed to improve their managerial effectiveness.

The general conclusion of these studies is that the top manager of a company must possess a high need for power, that is, a concern for influencing people. However, this need must be disciplined and controlled so that it is directed toward the benefit of the institution as a whole and not toward the manager's personal aggrandizement. Moreover, the top manager's need for power ought to be greater than his need for being liked by people.

In examining the motive scores of over fifty

managers of both high and low morale units in all sections of the same large company, we found that most of the managers—over 70 percent—were high in power motivation compared with men in general. This finding confirms the fact that power motivation is important for management. (Remember that as we use the term "power motivation," it refers not to dictatorial behavior, but to a desire to have impact, to be strong and influential.) The better managers, as judged by the morale of those working for them, tended to score even higher in power motivation. But the most important determining factor of high morale turned out not to be how their power motivation compared to their need to achieve but whether it was higher than their need to be liked. This relationship existed for 80 percent of the better sales managers as compared with only 10 percent of the poorer managers. And the same held true for other managers in nearly all parts of the company.

In the research, product development, and operations divisions, 73 percent of the better managers had a stronger need for power than a need to be liked (or what we term "affiliation motive") as compared with only 22 percent of the poorer managers. Why should this be so? Sociologists have long argued that, for a bureaucracy to function effectively, those who manage it must be universalistic in applying rules. That is, if they make exceptions for the particular needs of individuals, the whole system will break down.

The manager with a high need for being liked is precisely the one who wants to stay on good terms with everybody, and, therefore, is the one most likely to make exceptions in terms of particular needs. If a male employee asks for time off to stay home with his sick wife to help look after her and the kids, the affiliative manager agrees almost without thinking, because he feels sorry for the man and agrees that his family needs him.

When President Ford remarked in pardoning ex-President Nixon that he had "suffered enough," he was responding as an affiliative manager would, because he was empathizing primarily with Nixon's needs and feelings. Sociological theory and our data both argue, however, that the person whose need for affiliation is high does not make a good manager. This kind of person creates poor morale because he or she does not understand that other people in the office will tend to regard exceptions to the rules as unfair to themselves, just as many U.S. citizens felt it was unfair to let Richard Nixon off and punish others less involved than he was in the Watergate scandal.

In summary, the good manager in a large company does not have a high need for achievement, as we define and measure that motive, although there must be plenty of that motive somewhere in his organization. The top managers shown here have a high need for power and an interest in influencing others, both greater than their interest in being liked by people. The manager's concern for power should be socialized—controlled so that the institution as a whole, not only the individual, benefits. Men and nations with this motive profile are empire builders; they tend to create high morale and to expand the organizations they head.

COUNTER ⋈ POINT

LEAVITT AND LIPMAN-BLUMEN

A case for the relational manager

Both the changing world and our own common sense indicate that the relational side of U.S. organizations needs shoring up. Although direct observers of the management scene have been sending similar messages for a long time, their case is even stronger in today's world.

We shall approach our subject from the perspective of recent research on *achieving styles.*

Our approach starts by dividing achieving styles into two major categories: *direct* and *relational. Direct* styles are get-it-done, task-oriented styles. Direct types of people do it themselves, organize and compete to win it—no matter what the "it" happens to be. *Relational styles,* in contrast, always involve intervening relationships with other people. Relational managers help, support, and back up other people—often getting their kicks from contributing to the success of others, or from a true sense of belonging.

Trying to convince tough-minded managers that they ought to become less direct and more relational may be like trying to convince them to give up their private offices. Most of us around organizations give a perfunctory nod to the notion that we ought to run a happy ship, but the bottom line is our unit's measurable, observable performance.

We do not (repeat, not) assert that relational behavior is necessarily the road to executive success in most U.S. organizations at this time. The direct models are still the ones that make it almost everywhere. Data from contemporary research indicate that people who now get to the top in management are strongly power-motivated. They do not typically show strong needs for affiliation—for close, cozy groups.

But the organizational world is not fixed; it is slowly changing. So it seems quite possible that researchers will "discover" some years from now that successful managers are more relational than they had believed and less competitive or power-oriented.

Some relevant questions we have been worrying about include these:

—Do competitive, power-driven people now succeed because of the inherent nature of organized work, or because that's the way we set up our organizations in the old days and changing now is very painful?

—Does the direct, competitive, power image of the executive at least partly reflect the rigid old organization's effort to attract people like itself from the shrinking population of young people who still share those standards?

Let us elaborate on the assertion that times are indeed changing in a direction calling for more *relational* managerial styles.

Consider the following findings and current trends:

1. *Despite the widespread macho mythology about competitiveness in the executive suite, re-*

search points out that competitiveness does not seem to be the key to success. Other, more "intrinsic" styles called "work" (preference for getting on with the work) and "mastery" (an interest in mastering skills and the like) seem to play a far bigger role.

2. *Young people are shifting their values and interests (not radically, but incrementally) away from careers as their central life focus and toward a concern about general "life-style."* Some of what that means is an interest in long weekends, sailboats, and a temperate climate. It also seems to mean a wish for a more pleasant and challenging work environment.

3. *The hunger for warm, affectionate relationships appears to be growing in the United States.* Many of the traditional institutions that provided people with a sense of membership and community have been declining. And faith in them has been declining more rapidly.

4. *American managers now tend to see Japanese organizations as competent and innovative, not as industrial copycats.* Most scholars who have tried to pinpoint the key difference between Japanese and American management styles emphasize the *relational* quality of Japanese organizations. Japanese managers seem to build stronger social bonds among their employees. They invest more in company-related social activities. They are far less individually competitive (at least overtly) within their organizations.

5. *Firms using strongly relational styles often are successful in the United States.* Recent studies of American companies, derived from earlier observations of Japanese organizations, suggest the advantages, including the cost effectiveness, of a relational milieu. The research indicates that even within the same industry, many companies with "relational" cultures seem to work at least as effectively as more internally competitive firms even when judged by the usual financial and economic criteria.

6. *Women are moving into management.* Organizations now have access to a large number of people in our society who traditionally have been trained to a very high level of relational orientation and skill.

7. *Divorce between the individual and the organization is becoming more difficult.* Selection and promotion procedures increasingly are coming under public scrutiny. Partly in response to the Freedom of Information Act, managers are confronting demands for opening their personnel evaluation files, for laying bare their previously well-guarded personnel decisions. As the difficulty of justifying their hiring and firing practices increases, managers begin to place greater emphasis on "getting along" with their staffs.

8. *More and more, the tasks of contemporary organizations (particularly in high technology industries) require teamwork.* Teamwork becomes a term with much more immediate organizational meaning than it ever had before. And effective teamwork requires both competent individuals and a collaborative spirit. Buying collections of individual stars does not necessarily produce great team performance unless those stars can be bonded together with some strong relational glue.

9. *Where growth has slowed, the direct/competitive model is less functional.* The traditional reward of quick promotion for the aggressive young executive begins to dry up as growth rates decelerate. Satisfactory alternative rewards are hard to find, particularly for those preselected to view the world competitively. Since opportunities for relational rewards are largely independent of organizational growth, more relational people might very well create many of their own rewards, even in a leveled-off organization.

While the above forces drive toward relational organizations, one can also argue that sometimes these, plus other strong forces, appear to be driving in the opposite direction. Increased government regulation requires more impersonal, nonrelational lock-stepped uniformity of rewards and control procedures. And innovations in informational technology point toward a console-to-console world without much need for human interaction.

But if such depersonalizing forces are growing, doesn't that only increase the relevance of the relational issue? For after all, human beings continue to be the basic units in organizations and they still need and seek human interaction.

Taken together, the changes we are viewing seem to dictate a prescription for incremental, modest, but real shifts toward more relational strategies.

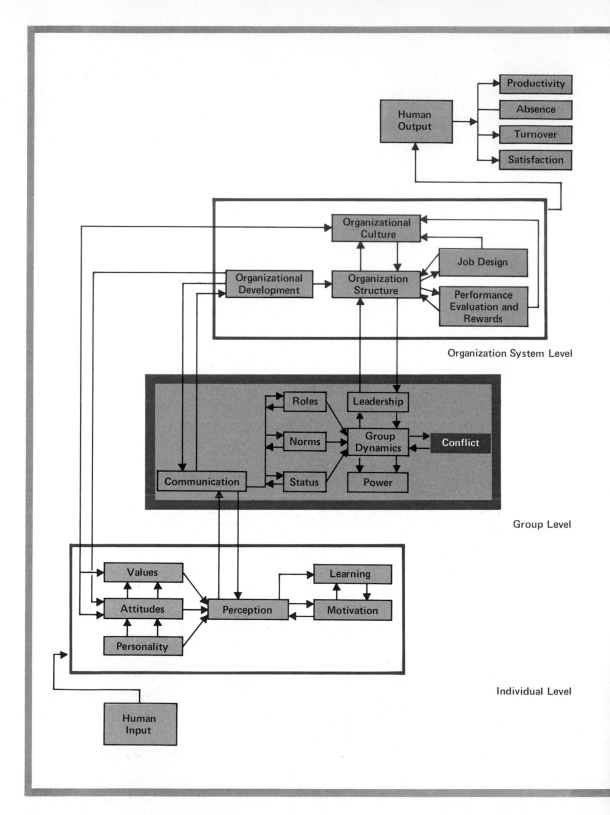

Human Output

- Productivity
- Absence
- Turnover
- Satisfaction

Organization System Level

- Organizational Culture
- Organizational Development
- Organization Structure
- Job Design
- Performance Evaluation and Rewards

Group Level

- Roles
- Norms
- Status
- Communication
- Leadership
- Group Dynamics
- Conflict
- Power

Individual Level

- Values
- Attitudes
- Personality
- Perception
- Learning
- Motivation

Human Input

CHAPTER 13
Conflict

AFTER STUDYING THIS CHAPTER, YOU SHOULD BE ABLE TO—

Define and explain the following key terms and concepts:

Accommodation
Avoidance
Behavioral view
Collaboration
Competition
Conflict
Dysfunctional conflict

Felt conflict
Functional conflict
Interactionist view
Perceived conflict
Sharing
Traditional view

Understand:

The difference between the traditional, behavioral, and
    interactionist views
The conflict process
The difference between functional and dysfunctional conflict
The sources of conflict
Five methods for reducing conflicts
The benefits and disadvantages of conflict

> Part of my job is to keep the five guys who hate me away from the five guys who are undecided.
>
> —CASEY STENGEL

It has been proposed that conflict is a theme that has occupied the thinking of man more than any other—with the exception of God and love.[1] It has been only recently, though, that conflict has become a major area of interest and research for students of organizational behavior. The evidence suggests that this interest has been well-placed—the type and intensity of conflict *does* affect group behavior.

In this chapter we shall define conflict, review three different ways of looking at it, present a process model of conflict, and consider the impact of conflict on group behavior.

A DEFINITION OF CONFLICT

There has been no shortage of definitions for conflict.[2] In spite of the divergent meanings the term has acquired, several common themes underlie most definitions. Conflict must be *perceived* by the parties to it. Whether conflict exists or not is a perception issue. If no one is aware of a conflict, it is generally agreed that no conflict exists. Of course, conflicts perceived may not be real while many situations that otherwise could be described as conflictive are not because the group members involved do not perceive the conflict. For a conflict to exist, therefore, it must be perceived. Additional commonalities among most conflict definitions are the concepts of *opposition, scarcity,* and *blockage,* and the assumption that there are two or more parties whose interests or goals appear to be incompatible. Resources—whether money, jobs, prestige, power, or whatever—are not unlimited, and their scarcity encourages blocking behavior. The parties are therefore in opposition. When one party blocks the goal achievement of another, a conflict state exists.

Differences between definitions tend to center around *intent* and whether

1. Robert D. Luce and Howard Raiffa, *Games and Decisions* (New York: John Wiley, 1957).

2. Clinton F. Fink, "Some Conceptual Difficulties in the Theory of Social Conflict," *Journal of Conflict Resolution,* December 1968, pp. 412–60.

conflict is a term limited only to *overt acts*. The intent issue is a debate over whether blockage behavior must be a determined action or whether it could occur as a result of fortuitous circumstances. As to whether conflict can only refer to overt acts, some definitions, for example, require signs of manifest fighting or open struggle as criteria for the existence of conflict.

Our definition of conflict acknowledges awareness (perception), opposition, scarcity, and blockage. Further, we assume it to be a determined action, which can exist at either the latent or overt level. We define conflict to be *a process in which an effort is purposely made by A to offset the efforts of B by some form of blocking that will result in frustrating B in attaining his goals or furthering his interests.*

While the above definition may, at first glance, seem rather esoteric, the terms and concepts that are used will become increasingly clear later in this chapter when we describe the stages that lead to conflict.

TRANSITIONS IN CONFLICT THOUGHT

It is entirely appropriate to say that there has been "conflict" over the role of conflict in groups and organizations. One school of thought has argued that conflict must be avoided—that it indicates a malfunctioning within the group. We call this the *traditional* view. Another school of thought, the *behavioral* view, argues that conflict is a natural and inevitable outcome in any group; and that it need not be evil, but rather has the potential to be a positive force in determining group performance. The third, and most recent perspective, proposes not only that conflict *can* be a positive force in a group, but explicitly argues that some conflict is *absolutely necessary* for a group to perform effectively. We label this third school the *interactionist* approach. Let us take a closer look at each of these views.[3]

The Traditional View

The early approach to conflict assumed that conflict was bad. Conflict was viewed negatively, and it was used synonymously with terms like violence, destruction, and irrationality in order to reinforce its negative connotation. Conflict, by definition, was viewed as harmful and was to be avoided.

The traditional view was consistent with the attitudes that prevailed about group behavior in the 1930s and 1940s. From findings provided by studies like those done at Hawthorne, it was argued that conflict was a dysfunctional outcome resulting from poor communication, a lack of openness and trust between people, and the failure of managers to be responsive to the needs and aspirations of their employees.

The view that all conflict is bad certainly offers a simple approach to look-

---

3. This section has been adapted from Stephen P. Robbins, *Managing Organizational Conflict: A Nontraditional Approach* (Englewood Cliffs, N.J.: Prentice-Hall, 1974), pp. 11–25.

ing at the behavior of people who create conflict. Since all conflict is to be avoided, we need merely direct our attention to the causes of conflict and correct these malfunctionings in order to improve group and organizational performance. Although research studies now provide strong evidence to dispute that this approach to conflict reduction results in high group performance, most of us still evaluate conflict situations utilizing this outmoded standard.

The Behavioral View

The behavioral position argued that conflict was a natural occurrence in all groups and organizations. Since conflict was inevitable, the behavioral school advocated acceptance of conflict. They rationalized its existence: It cannot be eliminated, and there are even times when conflict may benefit a group's performance. The behavioral view dominated conflict theory from the late 1940s through the mid-1970s.

The Interactionist View

The current view toward conflict is the interactionist perspective. While the behavioral approach *accepted* conflict, the interactionist approach *encourages* conflict on the grounds that a harmonious, peaceful, tranquil, and cooperative group is prone to becoming static, apathetic, and nonresponsive to needs for change and innovation. The major contribution of the interactionist approach, therefore, is encouraging group leaders to maintain an ongoing minimum level of conflict—enough to keep the group viable, self-critical, and creative.

Given the interactionist view, and it is the one we shall take in this chapter, it becomes evident that to say conflict is all good or all bad is inappropriate and naïve. Whether a conflict is good or bad depends on the type of conflict. Specifically, it's necessary to differentiate between functional and dysfunctional conflicts.

DIFFERENTIATING FUNCTIONAL
FROM DYSFUNCTIONAL CONFLICTS

The interactionist view does not propose that *all* conflicts are good. Rather, some conflicts support the goals of the group and improve its performance; these are functional, constructive forms of conflict. Additionally, there are conflicts that hinder group performance; these are dysfunctional or destructive forms.

Of course, it is one thing to argue that conflict can be valuable for the group, but how does one tell if a conflict is functional or dysfunctional?

The demarcation between functional and dysfunctional is neither clear nor precise. No one level of conflict can be adopted as acceptable or unacceptable under all conditions. The type and level of conflict that creates healthy and positive involvement toward one group's goals may, in another group or in the same group at another time, be highly dysfunctional.

The important criterion is group performance. Since groups exist to attain a goal or goals, it is the impact that the conflict has on the group, rather than on any singular individual, that defines functionality. The impact of conflict on the individual and on the group is rarely mutually exclusive, so the ways that individuals perceive a conflict may have an important influence on its effect on the group. However, this need not be the case and when it is not, our orientation will be to the group. For us to appraise the impact of conflict on group behavior—to consider its functional and dysfunctional effects—we shall consider whether the individual group members perceive the conflict as good or bad to be irrelevant. A group member may perceive an action as dysfunctional, in that the outcome is personally dissatisfying to him or her. However, for our analysis, it would be functional if it furthers the objectives of the group.

THE CONFLICT PARADOX

If some conflict has been proven to be beneficial to a group's performance, why do most of us continue to look at conflict as undesirable? The answer is that we live in a society that has been built upon the traditional view. Tolerance of conflict is counter to most cultures in developed nations. In North America, the home, school, and church are generally the most influential institutions during the early years when our attitudes are forming. These institutions, for the most part, have historically reinforced anticonflict values and emphasized the importance of getting along with others.

The home has historically reinforced the authority pattern through the parent figure. Parents knew what was right and children complied. Conflict between children or between parents and children has generally been actively discouraged. The traditional school systems in developed countries reflected the structure of the home. Teachers had *the* answers and were not to be challenged. Disagreements at all levels were viewed negatively. Examinations reinforced this view: Students attempted to get their answers to agree with those the teacher had determined were right. The last major influencing institution, the church, also has supported anticonflict values. The religious perspective emphasizes peace, harmony, and tranquility. Church doctrines, for the most part, advocate acceptance rather than argument. This is best exemplified by the teachings of the Roman Catholic Church. According to its beliefs, when the Pope speaks officially (ex cathedra) on religious matters, he is infallible. Such dogma has discouraged questioning the teachings of the Church.

Should we be surprised, then, that the traditional view of conflict continues to receive wide support in spite of the evidence to the contrary?

Let us now proceed to move beyond definitions and philosophy, to describe and analyze the evolutionary process leading to conflict outcomes.

CONFLICT PROCESS

The conflict process can be thought of as comprising four stages: potential opposition, cognition and personalization, behavior, and outcomes. The process is diagrammed in Figure 13–1.

Stage I: Potential Opposition

The first step in the conflict process is the presence of conditions that create opportunities for conflict to arise. They *need not* lead directly to conflict, but one of these conditions is necessary if conflict is to arise. For simplicity's sake, these conditions (which also may be looked at as causes or sources of conflict) have been condensed into three general categories: communication, structure, and personal variables.

Communication. The communicative source represents those opposing forces that arise from semantic difficulties, misunderstandings, and "noise" in the communication channels. Much of this discussion can be related back to our comments on communication and communication networks in Chapter 10.

One of the major myths that most of us carry around with us is that poor communication is the reason for conflicts—"if we could just communicate with each other, we could eliminate our differences." Such a conclusion is not unreasonable, given the amount of time each of us spends communicating. But, of course, poor communication is certainly not the source of *all* conflicts, though there is considerable evidence to suggest that problems in the communication process act to retard collaboration and stimulate misunderstanding.

FIGURE 13–1 The Conflict Process

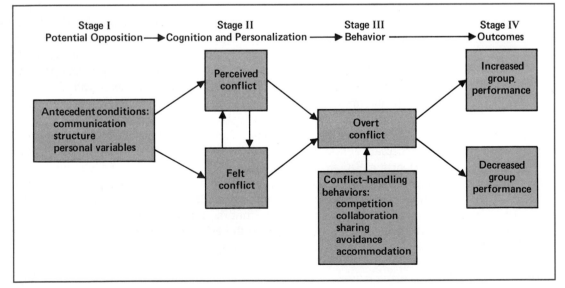

A review of the research suggests that semantic difficulties, insufficient exchange of information, and noise in the communication channel each are barriers to communication and potential antecedent conditions to conflict.[4] Specifically, evidence demonstrates semantic difficulties arise as a result of differences in training, selective perception, and inadequate information about others. Research has further demonstrated a surprising finding: The potential for conflict increases when either too little or too much communication takes place. Apparently, an increase in communication is functional up to a point, whereupon it is possible to overcommunicate with a resultant increase in the potential for conflict. Too much information as well as too little can lay the foundation for conflict. Further, the channel chosen for communicating can have an influence on stimulating opposition. The filtering process that occurs as information is passed between members, and the divergence of communications from formal or previously established channels, offer potential opportunities for conflict to arise.

Structure. The term structure is used, in this context, to include variables such as size; degree of routinization, specialization, and standardization in the tasks assigned to group members; heterogeneity of members; leadership styles; reward systems; and the degree of dependence between groups.

Research indicates that size and specialization act as a force to stimulate conflict. The larger the group and the more specialized its activities, the greater the likelihood of conflict. Tenure and conflict have been found to be inversely related. The potential for conflict tends to be greatest where group members are younger and where turnover is high.

There is some indication that a close style of leadership—tight and continuous observation with general control of the others' behaviors—increases conflict potential, but the evidence is not particularly strong. Too much reliance on participation may also stimulate conflict. Research tends to confirm that participation and conflict are highly correlated, apparently because participation encourages the promotion of differences. Reward systems, too, are found to create conflict when one member's gain is at another's expense. Finally, if a group is dependent on another group (in contrast to the two being mutually independent) or if interdependence allows one group to gain at another's expense, opposing forces are stimulated.[5]

Personal Variables. Personal factors include the individual value systems that each person has and the personality characteristics that account for individual idiosyncracies and differences.

The evidence indicates that certain personality types—for example, individuals who are highly authoritarian, dogmatic, and who demonstrate low esteem—lead to potential conflict. Most important, and probably the most overlooked variable in the study of social conflict, is differing value systems. In

4. Ibid., pp. 39–40.
5. Ibid., pp. 49–50.

Chapter 3, we argued that values are the initial foundation upon which individual behavior is built. It seems reasonable that differences in value structure are an important explanation for why conflicts occur. Value differences, for example, are the best explanation of such diverse issues as prejudice, disagreements over one's contribution to the group and the rewards one deserves, or assessments of whether this particular book is any good. The fact that John dislikes blacks and Dana believes John's position indicates his ignorance; that an employee thinks he is worth $30,000 a year but his boss believes him to be worth $24,000; and that Ann thinks this book is interesting to read while Jennifer views it as a "crock of . . . ," are all value judgments. And differences in value systems are important sources for creating the potential for conflict.

Stage II: Cognition and Personalization

If the conditions cited in Stage I generate frustration, then the potential for opposition becomes actualized in the second stage. The antecedent conditions can only lead to conflict when one or more of the parties are affected by, and cognitive of, the conflict.

As we noted in our definition of conflict, perception is required. Therefore, one or more of the parties must be aware of the existence of the antecedent conditions. However, because a conflict is perceived does not mean that it is personalized. In other words, "A may be aware that B and A are in serious disagreement . . . but it may not make A tense or anxious, and it may have no effect whatsoever on A's affection towards B."[6] It is at the felt level, when individuals become emotionally involved, that parties experience anxiety, tenseness, frustration, or hostility.

Stage III: Behavior

We are in the third stage of the conflict process when a member engages in action that frustrates the attainment of another's goals or prevents the furthering of the other's interests. This action must be intended; that is, there must be a knowing effort to frustrate another. At this juncture, the conflict is out in the open.

Overt conflict covers a full range of behaviors—from subtle, indirect, and highly controlled forms of interference to direct, aggressive, violent, and uncontrolled struggle. At the low range, this overt behavior is illustrated by the student who raises his or her hand in class and questions a point the instructor has made. At the high range, strikes, riots, and wars come to mind.

Stage III is also where most conflict-handling behaviors are initiated. Once the conflict is overt, the parties will develop a method for dealing with the conflict. This does not exclude conflict-handling behaviors from being initiated in Stage II, but in most cases, these techniques for reducing the frustration are

6. Louis R. Pondy, "Organizational Conflict: Concepts and Models," *Administrative Science Quarterly*, September 1967, p. 302.

used when the conflict has become observable rather than as preventive measures. One author has identified five such orientations: competition, collaboration, avoidance, accommodation, and sharing.[7]

Competition. When one party seeks to achieve her goals or further her interests, regardless of the impact on the parties to the conflict, she competes and dominates. These win-lose struggles, in formal groups or in an organization, frequently utilize the formal authority of a mutual superior as the dominant force, and the conflicting parties each will use their own power bases in order to resolve a victory in their favor.

Collaboration. When the parties to conflict each desire to satisfy fully the concern of all parties, we have cooperation and the search for a mutually beneficial outcome. In collaboration, the behavior of the parties is aimed at solving the problem, at clarifying the differences rather than accommodating various points of view. The participants consider the full range of alternatives; the similarities and differences in viewpoint become more clearly focused; and the causes or differences become outwardly evident. Because the solution sought is advantageous to all parties, collaboration is often thought of as a win-win approach to resolving conflicts. It is, for example, a frequent tool of marriage counselors. Behavioral scientists, who value openness, trust, authenticity, and spontaneity in relationships, are also strong advocates of a collaborative approach to resolving conflicts.

Avoidance. A party may recognize that a conflict exists but react by withdrawing, or suppressing the conflict. Indifference or the desire to evade overt demonstration of disagreement can result in withdrawal: The parties acknowledge physical separation and each stakes out a territory that is distinct from the other's. If withdrawal is not possible or desirous, the parties may suppress, that is, withhold their differences. When group members are required to interact because of the independence of their tasks, suppression is a more probable outcome than withdrawal.

Accommodation. When the parties seek to appease their opponent, they may be willing to place their opponent's interests above their own. In order that the relationship can be maintained, one party is willing to be self-sacrificing. We refer to this behavior as accommodation. When husbands and wives have differences, it is not uncommon for one to accommodate the other by placing their spouse's interest above their own.

Sharing. When each party to the conflict must give up something, sharing occurs, resulting in a compromised outcome. In sharing, there is no clear winner or loser. Rather, there is a rationing of the object of the conflict or, where the object

7. Kenneth W. Thomas, "Conflict and Conflict Management," in *Handbook of Industrial and Organizational Psychology,* ed. M. Dunnette (Chicago: Rand McNally, 1976).

is not divisible, one rewards the other by yielding something of substitute value. The distinguishing characteristic of sharing, therefore, is that it requires each party to give up something. Negotiations between unions and management represent a situation where sharing is required in order to reach a settlement and agree upon a labor contract.

Stage IV: Outcomes

The interplay between the overt conflict behavior and conflict-handling behaviors result in consequences. As the model demonstrates, they may be functional in that the conflict has resulted in an improvement in the group's performance. Conversely, group performance may be hindered and we would describe the outcome as dysfunctional.

Functional Outcomes. How might conflict have acted as a force to increase group performance? It is hard to visualize a situation where open or violent aggression could be functional. But there are a number of instances where it is possible to envision how low or moderate levels of conflict could improve the effectiveness of a group. Because it is often difficult to think of instances where conflict can be constructive, let us consider some examples, then look at the research evidence.

Conflict is constructive when it improves the quality of decisions, stimulates creativity and innovation, encourages interest and curiosity among group members, provides the medium through which problems can be aired and tensions released, and fosters an environment of self-evaluation and change. The evidence suggests that conflict can improve the quality of decision making by allowing all points, particularly the ones that are unusual or held by a minority, to be weighed in important decisions. Conflict is an antidote for groupthink. It does not allow the group passively to "rubber stamp" decisions that may be based on weak assumptions, inadequate consideration to relevant alternatives, or other debilities. Conflict challenges the status quo and therefore furthers the creation of new ideas, promotes reassessment of group goals and activities, and increases the probability that the group will respond to change.

Research studies in diverse settings confirm the functionality of conflict. Consider the following findings.

The comparison of six major decisions during the administrations of four different U.S. presidents found that conflict reduced the chance that groupthink would overpower policy decisions. The comparisons demonstrated that conformity among presidential advisers was related to poor decisions, while an atmosphere of constructive conflict and critical thinking surrounded the well-developed decisions.[8]

The bankruptcy of the Penn Central Railroad has been generally attributed to mismanagement and a failure of the company's board of directors to question actions taken by management. The board was composed of outside

---

8. Irving L. Janis, *Victims of Groupthink* (Boston: Houghton Mifflin, 1972).

directors who met monthly to oversee the railroad's operations. Few questioned the decisions made by the operating management, though there was evidence that several board members were uncomfortable with many decisions made by the management. Apathy and a desire to *avoid* conflict allowed poor decisions to stand unquestioned.[9] This, however, should not be surprising since a review of the relationship between bureaucracy and innovation has found that conflict encourages innovative solutions.[10] The corollary of this finding also appears true: Lack of conflict results in a passive environment with reinforcement of the status quo.

Not only do better and more innovative decisions result from situations where there is some conflict, there is evidence indicating that conflict can be positively related to productivity. It was demonstrated that, among established groups, performance tended to improve more when there was conflict among members than when there was fairly close agreement. The investigators observed that when groups analyzed decisions that had been made by the individual members of that group, the average improvement among the high-conflict groups was 73 percent greater than that of those groups characterized by low-conflict conditions.[11] Others have found similar results: Groups composed of members with different interests tend to produce higher quality solutions to a variety of problems than do homogeneous groups.[12]

Similarly, studies of professionals—systems analysts and research and development scientists—support the constructive value of conflict. An investigation of twenty-two teams of systems analysts found that the more incompatible groups were likely to be more productive.[13] Research and development scientists have been found to be most productive where there is a certain amount of intellectual conflict.[14]

Conflict can even be constructive on sports teams and in unions. Studies of sports teams indicate that moderate levels of group conflict contribute to team effectiveness and provide an additional stimulus for high achievement.[15] This

9. P. Binzen and J. R. Daughen, *Wreck of the Penn Central* (Boston: Little, Brown, 1971).

10. V. A. Thompson, "Bureaucracy and Innovation," *Administrative Science Quarterly,* Vol. 10 (1965), pp. 1–20.

11. J. Hall and M. S. Williams, "A Comparison of Decision-Making Performances in Established and Ad-Hoc Groups," *Journal of Personality and Social Psychology,* February 1966, p. 217.

12. Richard L. Hoffman, "Homogeneity of Member Personality and Its Effect on Group Problem-Solving," *Journal of Abnormal and Social Psychology,* January 1959, pp. 27–32; Richard L. Hoffman and Norman R. F. Maier, "Quality and Acceptance of Problem Solutions by Members of Homogeneous and Heterogeneous Groups," *Journal of Abnormal and Social Psychology,* March 1961, pp. 401–7.

13. R. E. Hill, "Interpersonal Compatibility and Work Group Performance Among Systems Analysts: An Empirical Study," *Proceedings of the Seventeenth Annual Midwest Academy of Management Conference,* Kent, Ohio, April 1974, pp. 97–110.

14. Donald C. Pelz and Frank Andrews, *Scientists in Organizations* (New York: John Wiley, 1966).

15. Hans Lenk, "Konflikt und Leistung in Spitzensportmann-schafter: Isozometrische Strukturen von WettKämpfachtern in Ruden," *Soziale Welt,* Vol. 15 (1964), pp. 307–43.

was seen in the performance of the New York Yankees baseball teams during 1977 and 1978. The teams were consistently confronted with internal conflicts, yet they both won the World Series. An examination of local unions found that conflict between members of the local was positively related to the union's power and to member loyalty and participation in union affairs.[16] These findings might suggest that conflict within a group indicates strength rather than, in the traditional view, weakness.

Dysfunctional Outcomes. The destructive consequences of conflict upon a group or organization's performance are generally well known. A reasonable summary might state: Uncontrolled opposition breeds discontent, which acts to dissolve common ties, and eventually leads to destruction of the group. And, of course, there is a substantial body of literature to document how conflict—the dysfunctional varieties—can reduce group effectiveness.[17] Among the more undesirable consequences are a retarding of communication, reductions in group cohesiveness, and subordination of group goals to the primacy of infighting between members. At the extreme, conflict can bring group functioning to a halt and potentially threaten the group's survival.

This discussion has again returned us to the issue of what is functional and what is dysfunctional. Research on conflict has yet to identify those situations where conflict is more likely to be constructive than destructive. However, the difference between functional and dysfunctional conflict is important enough for us to go beyond the substantive evidence and propose at least two hypotheses. The first is that extreme levels of conflict—exemplified by overt struggle or violence—are rarely, if ever, functional. Functional conflict is probably most often characterized by low to moderate levels of subtle and controlled opposition. Second, the type of group activity should be another factor determining functionality. We hypothesize that the more creative or unprogrammed the decision-making tasks of the group, the greater the probability that internal conflict is constructive. Groups that are required to tackle problems requiring new and novel approaches—as in research, advertising, and other professional activities—will benefit more from conflict than groups performing highly programmed activities—for instance, those of work teams on an automobile assembly line.

IMPLICATIONS FOR PERFORMANCE AND SATISFACTION

Many people assume that conflict is related to lower group and organizational performance. This chapter has demonstrated that this assumption is frequently

16. Arnold Tannenbaum, "Control Structure and Union Functions," *American Journal of Sociology,* May 1956, pp. 127–40.

17. For an excellent source of studies that focus on the dysfunctional consequences of conflict, see the *Journal of Conflict Resolution.*

FIGURE 13–2 Conflict and Unit Performance

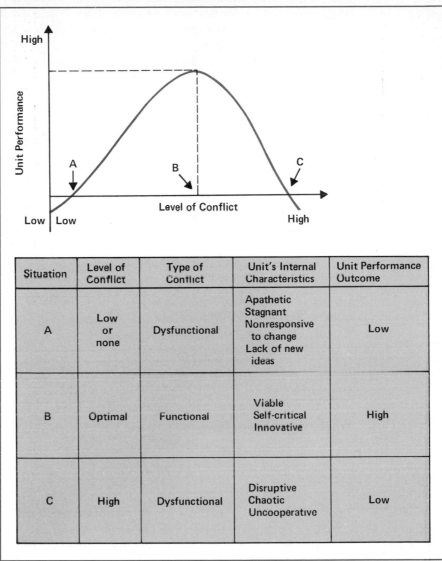

Situation	Level of Conflict	Type of Conflict	Unit's Internal Characteristics	Unit Performance Outcome
A	Low or none	Dysfunctional	Apathetic Stagnant Nonresponsive to change Lack of new ideas	Low
B	Optimal	Functional	Viable Self-critical Innovative	High
C	High	Dysfunctional	Disruptive Chaotic Uncooperative	Low

fallacious. Conflict can be either constructive or destructive to the functioning of a group or unit. As shown in Figure 13–2, levels of conflict can be either too high or too low. Either extreme hinders performance. An optimal level is where there is enough conflict to prevent stagnation, stimulate creativity, allow tensions to be released, and initiate the seeds for change; yet not so much as to be disruptive or deter coordination of activities.

Inadequate or excessive levels of conflict can hinder the effectiveness of a group or an organization, resulting in reduced satisfaction of group members, increased absence and turnover rates, and eventually lower productivity. On the other hand, when conflict is at an optimal level, complacency and apathy should be minimized; motivation should be enhanced through the creation of a challenging and questioning environment with a vitality that makes work interesting; and there should be the needed turnover to rid the organization of misfits and poor performers.

FOR DISCUSSION

1. Name, discuss, and contrast three views on conflict.

2. Is conflict good or bad? Discuss.

3. What are the components in the conflict process model? From your own experiences, give an example of how a conflict proceeded through the four stages.

4. Discuss five conflict resolution techniques. What are the strengths and weaknesses of each.

5. "The larger the group, the greater the likelihood of conflict." Do you agree or disagree? Discuss.

6. "As an organization becomes more structured, it tends to eliminate creativity." Do you agree or disagree? Discuss.

7. "Participation is an excellent method for identifying differences and resolving conflicts." Do you agree or disagree? Discuss.

8. What is the difference between functional and dysfunctional conflict? What determines functionality?

FOR FURTHER READING

DEUTSCH, M., *The Resolution of Conflict: Constructive and Destructive Processes*. New Haven, Conn.: Yale University Press, 1973. Explores the factors that determine whether the outcome of conflict will be fruitful or destructive.

FILLEY, A. C., *Interpersonal Conflict Resolution*. Glenview, Ill.: Scott, Foresman, 1975. Analyzes the conflict process and describes the Integrative Decision Making method of conflict resolution through problem solving.

HARRISON, F., "A Conceptual Model of Organizational Conflict," *Business and Society*, Winter 1980, pp. 30–40. Presents a comprehensive and integrated model of organizational conflict.

KATZ, D., and R. L. KAHN, *The Social Psychology of Organizations*, 2nd ed., pp. 611–51. New York: John Wiley, 1978. Sophisticated analysis of the conflict process, its effects, and the management of conflict.

KILMANN, R. H., and K. W. THOMAS, "Four Perspectives on Conflict Management: An Attributional Framework for Organizing Descriptive and Normative Theory," *Academy of Management Review,* January 1978, pp. 59–68. Identifies four perspectives on conflict derived from the process versus structure distinction and the internal versus external attributions distinction.

MURRAY, V. V., "Some Unanswered Questions on Organizational Conflict," *Organization and Administrative Sciences,* Winter 1974–75, pp. 35–53. Reviews organizational conflict literature, discussing gaps and fallacies.

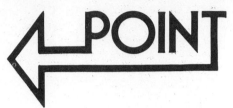

POINT

FILLEY

The case for problem solving

The thesis presented here is somewhat one-sided, though I hope not naïvely so. It suggests that problem-solving and collaborative methods can, and generally should, be used in situations where parties are mutually dependent, where support for and implementation of agreement is required, and where the use of creative resources by the parties involved is important. It does not deny that power-oriented methods of conflict resolution are popular, or that people use different methods for different kinds of conflicts, or that there are some positive consequences to be gained from conflict, or that there are some situations where problem solving may prove too costly to use. Ultimately, a contingency model of conflict resolution methods will be developed. Until then, the positive consequences of problem solving as a resolution strategy seem to be sufficiently documented to emphasize its use.

The first premise may help one to understand the relative frequency with which power-oriented rather than problem-solving methods are used for conflict resolution. The premise states that *knowledge is unlimited, but our perceptions are very limited.* In the present context, this suggests that there is a way to resolve a conflict to the mutual satisfaction and benefit of the parties, but that perceptions of the situation encourage power-oriented behavior.

Power-oriented methods divide a fixed pie of 100 percent, or what is otherwise called a "zero-sum" situation—one party's gain is the other party's loss. Most conflicts occur because the people involved perceive the situation in this way. For example, conflicts frequently occur about two solutions with no discussion or identification of the goals involved. This "my way (solution) versus your way (solution)" leads naturally to power-oriented behavior.

Perceptions of fixed-sum situations also induce bargaining and compromise. The actual bargaining behavior by the parties and their effectiveness will depend upon such conditions as personality of the bargainers, status differences, and knowledge of bargaining strategies and tactics.

In contrast with power-oriented methods, problem-solving methods assume that it is possible to find a solution to the conflict that will benefit both parties. They do not assume any zero-sum situation since the gain of one party is not equal to the loss of the other; instead, both parties may gain with the outcome.

Their use of problem solving is encouraged when the parties take a "we versus the problem" focus and seek to maximize the payoff to both parties. There is no great mystery to this process. It involves identifying the goals or values that each party wants to achieve with the present preferred alternatives, and then an exhaustive search for solutions that meet such combined goals.

Problem-solving methods involve the application of facts and logic to solving problems that are created by conflictive situations. They evoke intellectual intensity rather than emotional intensity or power. Where a conflict is present and the perceptions, attitudes, feelings, situation, and process produce power-oriented relations between the parties, *conflict management* may alter these conditions, allowing the use of problem-solving methods.

To be illustrative rather than exhaustive, the following are possible changes and conditions that might allow problem-solving methods of conflict-resolution to replace power-oriented methods. *Perceptual*—identifying the problem in terms of goals rather than two solutions; identifying the existence of mutually beneficial solutions; changing the focus of attention to the problem rather than the other party; identifying the costs of not agreeing; identifying the costs of self-sacrifice or domination. *Attitudinal*—enhancing desirability of mutually acceptable solutions by demonstrating the negative effects of losing on self-esteem and pointing out the unwillingness of the loser to support the agreement; enhancing trust between parties by increasing mutuality of influence and by sharing relevant information. *Affective*—establishing positive feelings by each party about themselves and others through clinical or fact-gathering methods; minimizing feelings of anger, threat, or defensiveness by depersonalizing the problem and by using neutral language. *Situational*—reducing time pressure; dividing neutral spatial arrangements; increasing proximity and interaction of the parties; equalizing or ignoring power differences.

In addition, changes may be made in the process. Communication between parties can be clarified to ensure common meaning; issues can be stated specifically and not generalized; problems may be jointly defined by the parties; feedback can be made descriptive; process stages of problem identification, solution generation, and evaluation may be separated; problem statements may be redefined in terms of needs rather than solutions; and process rules may proscribe forcing, acquiescing, or avoiding behaviors.

The items stated above should suggest that it is possible to manage the resolution of conflictive solutions so that problem-solving rather than power-oriented methods are used. Limited perceptions by the parties of both the process and the content considerations involved may be altered to more fully utilize their creative capacities. Such alteration may benefit from the use of a third party who can help manage conflict more effectively.

It seems reasonable to suggest that where parties in an organization are mutually dependent upon each other, cooperation is functional and desirable. Where conflicts occur, it seems that problem solving is a preferred strategy over force or compromise, since it will evoke greater cooperation between the parties in the end.

There is nothing startling in this view. It suggests why, even though individuals have fixed patterns of resolution behavior, problem-solving is the most frequently used resolution strategy between superiors and subordinates. It suggests why managers reporting incidents of effective and ineffective conflict resolution mention problem-solving as a major type of effective resolution and forcing as a major type of ineffective resolution. Or, it explains why people engaged in group decisions who disagree openly and then resolve their differences by problem-solving make better decisions than the average or the best member of the group.

Problem-solving methods are also preferred where commitment and implementation of an agreement by the parties is desired. Capitulation or compromise of personal goals engendered through forcing strategies is not likely to generate high levels of support for an agreement. Problem-solving methods, which provide for achievement of each party's goals, will generate higher levels of support. Thus, as suggested earlier, where cooperation between parties is necessary because of their mutual dependency, where the use of creative resources by the parties is important, and where support for and implementation of the agreement is necessary, problem-solving methods of conflict resolution appear to have advantages over power-oriented methods.

COUNTER ✕ POINT

ROBBINS

Problem solving: a special case

Let me begin by briefly noting those points on which Professor Filley and I are in agreement. These include his recognition of the popularity of power-oriented methods and the positive consequences that can be gained from conflict, his awareness that there are situations where the cost of problem solving exceeds its benefits and, finally, his belief that we are moving toward a contingency model for managing conflict.

However, acknowledging that we have areas of agreement does not mean that I believe Professor Filley has correctly assessed the realities in conflict management. In this article, I propose that he (1) has failed to consider why it is that power-oriented methods are so popular; (2) implies that problem solving has reasonably wide application potential, a position that is difficult to support; (3) has failed to place problem solving into its proper perspective—that is, as merely one tool in a manager's conflict resolution tool chest; and (4) ignores the substantial progress we have made toward the contingency framework that both of us agree is a desirable goal.

Does it not occur to Professor Filley that the reason individuals rely so heavily on power-oriented methods is that they work? Organizations operate with limited resources. Promotion opportunities are not free goods. Neither are pay raises.

Not everyone can be expected to be appraised as an outstanding performer. Similarly, not everyone's "bright" ideas can be implemented. Since most activities that create conflicts in organizations are due to resource scarcity, the desire to assume them to be something other than "zero-sum-based" must be seen as idealistic. Individuals become quickly aware of the zero-sum aspect of organizational life and, hence, rely heavily on power-oriented resolution techniques for effectively resolving conflicts.

Problem solving can be an effective method for dealing with conflicts as long as certain conditions are met. It assumes that the conflicting parties have the potential to achieve a better solution through collaboration. If conflicts are based on communicative sources—ambiguity, distortion, the inadequate passage of information, or channel overflow—problem solving is a natural and effective remedy. But the organization structure and differences in individual and group value systems are also major sources of conflict. When problem solving is used with value conflicts, for example, it leads not to reduced levels of conflict but, rather, to heightened levels. Problem solving acts to identify and widen differences, resulting in the conflict parties entrenching deeper into the conflicting positions.

The major difference between Professor Filley and myself appears to lie in our estimates of the percent of conflict situations that meet the requirements for successful problem solving. While I have no empirical data to support this point, observation leads me to conclude that probably less

TABLE 1 Resolution Techniques

Technique	Brief Definition	Strengths	Weaknesses
Problem solving (also known as confrontation or collaboration)	Seeks resolution through face-to-face confrontation of the conflicting parties. Parties seek mutual problem definition, assessment, and solution.	Effective with conflicts stemming from semantic misunderstandings. Brings doubts and misperceptions to surface. Good where insights of diverse people are sought; where concerns are too important to be compromised; to gain commitment from others through involvement.	Can be time-consuming. Inappropriate for most noncommunicative conflicts, especially those based on different value systems.
Superordinate goals	Introduces common goals that two or more conflicting parties each desire that cannot be reached without cooperation of those involved. Goals must be highly valued, unattainable without the help of all parties involved in the conflict, and commonly sought.	When used cumulatively and reinforced, develops "peacemaking" potential, emphasizing dependency and cooperation.	Difficult to devise.
Expansion of resources	Makes more of the scarce resource available.	Each conflicting party can be victorious.	Resources rarely exist in such quantities as to be easily expanded.
Avoidance	Includes withdrawal and suppression.	Easy to do. Natural reaction to conflict. May allow parties to cool down.	No effective resolution. Conflict not eliminated. Temporary.
Smoothing	Plays down differences while emphasizing common interests.	All conflict situations have points of commonality within them. Cooperative efforts are reinforced. Preserves harmony and avoids disruptions.	Differences are not confronted and remain under the surface. Temporary.
Compromise	Requires each party to give up something of value. Includes external or third-party interventions, negotiation, and voting.	No clear loser. Consistent with democratic values. Gives an expedient solution when under time pressures.	No clear winner. Power oriented—influenced heavily by relative strength of parties. Temporary.
Authoritative command	Imposes solution from a superior holding formal positional authority.	Very effective in organizations since members recognize and accept authority of superiors. Good in emergencies and where unpopular courses of action need implementation (i.e., cost cutting, discipline).	Cause of conflict is not treated. Does not necessarily bring agreement. Temporary.
Altering the human variable	Changes the attitudes and behavior of one or more of the conflicting parties. Includes use of education, sensitivity and awareness training, and human relations training.	Results can be substantial and permanent. Has potential to alleviate the source of conflict.	Most difficult to achieve. Slow and costly.
Altering structural variables	Changes structural variables. Includes transferring and exchanging group members, creating coordinating positions, developing an appeals system, and expanding the group or organization's boundaries.	Can be permanent. Usually within the authority of a manager.	Often expensive. Forces organization to be designed for specific individuals and thus requires continual adjustment as people join or leave the organization.

than 10 percent of all situations where conflict levels are too high can be effectively resolved through problem solving. Problem solving should, therefore, be viewed for what it is—a single tool in the manager's tool chest. With communicative conflicts, problem solving is generally the preferred method. On the other hand, there are more effective methods for dealing with the resolution of structural and value-laden conflicts.

We have made considerable progress in isolating a number of conflict resolution techniques and identifying the situations in which each tends to be most effective (see Table 1).

The technique chosen should be contingent on the source of the conflict and the cost-benefit of its usage. I agree with Professor Filley that in those instances where problem solving can be effective, it should be used. Unfortunately, to look at the conditions in which problem solving is most effective as anything other than special cases does not seem to be consistent with organizational realities.

CASE IIIA ⟶ Welcome to the School Board

Vacaville is a small community in southern Texas. Its 22,000 residents are primarily farmers or operators of small businesses. The Vacaville School Board is made up of the mayor; two members of the city council; the superintendent of Vacaville schools; and eight members, at large, elected for four-year terms by Vacaville voters.

The school board is a relatively stable body. Paul Gomez has been the mayor of Vacaville for eleven years. A rancher, Gomez spends about ten hours a week on his mayoral duties, for which he is paid $5,000 a year. The two city council members have each been on the board for more than eight years. Jack deNuervo, the school superintendent, has held his same job for nearly twenty-six years, currently earns $29,000 annually, but has reached sixty-five years of age and has advised the board that he will be retiring. The remaining eight at-large members have staggered terms. Every year two come up for reelection.

In the November 1980 election, long-time at-large board member Mary Cardoza was defeated by a wealthy businessman, J. T. Thomas. The election campaign had been bitter. Thomas spent over $30,000 to defeat Cardoza. In contrast, Cardoza reported spending less than $2,000 on her campaign. Name calling had risen to unheard-of levels. Thomas's campaign was built almost exclusively on attacking what he referred to as "Cardoza's free-spending and liberal views on education," rather than selling himself. However, he did consistently tell the voters through his television, radio, and newspaper ads that, if elected, he was committed to "cutting truancy and getting tough with those students causing discipline problems."

It was obvious to everyone who attended the first meeting of 1981, which coincidentally was also the first one where Thomas sat as a board member, that the days of short and tranquil meetings were over. That January 12 meeting began at 7:00 P.M. and disbanded (a more appropriate term than adjourned) four-and-a-half hours later. For the record, no one who was there could remember any previous board meeting running longer than two hours.

The fireworks began almost immediately. Gomez and deNuervo had expected Thomas to be trouble. They anticipated that he would propose some new and strict policies for governing the schools and they certainly expected him to be active in the selection of deNuervo's successor. What they hadn't expected was the coalition Thomas had formed with the other at-large members. When Thomas spoke, it was obvious he was not speaking as a lonely voice. His comments were consistently echoed by the other at-large members.

The first item on the January 12 agenda had been a routine capital expenditure request. DeNuervo was requesting $4,200 to purchase three new IBM typewriters that would replace three old manual models. DeNuervo held little discussion on the request, assuming routine approval. He nearly fell out of his chair when the request was defeated 8 to 4.

The second item on the agenda was approval of a job offer to fill a vacancy in the fine arts department at the high school. Board members had had an opportunity to review the candidate's file earlier. But deNuervo was more cautious now. Rather than call for a quick vote, he wanted to hear from each member. It soon became obvious that while the candidate was fully qualified, one small thing was bothering Thomas. It seems that in the late 1960s, when the candidate had been a college freshman, he had been arrested for participating in an antiwar demonstration. After nearly two hours of debate surrounding the candidate's character, deNuervo realized that the battle was lost. All at-large members were dominated by Thomas. Whichever way he voted, so would the others. The final vote was predictable. The candidate was rejected 8 to 4.

At 11:15 P.M., deNuervo realized he was going to have to end the meeting but he was determined to handle one last item—the appointments to the superintendent's screening and selection committee. This committee would be made up of three board members and their task would be to find deNuervo's replacement. Each of the board members was given a piece of paper and told to write three names on it. Those three board members with the highest votes would comprise the committee. Not surprisingly, the three highest vote-getters were Thomas and two other at-large members.

When deNuervo got home that night and related what had happened at the meeting to his wife, she replied, "I'm not surprised. I've heard gossip that Thomas has promised all the at-large members that if they support him on the board, he will fully finance their reelection campaigns. He apparently has also told them that if they go against him—ever—he would actively support their opponents."

Questions

1. Describe the power interactions in this case.
2. There is conflict between the at-large members and the others. What is the source of this conflict? How could the conflict be resolved?
3. Use Fiedler's leadership model to explain Thomas's apparent success as a leader. Can Thomas be classified as a high or low LPC leader? Why?
4. If you were deNuervo, what could you do to counteract or defuse Thomas's power?

CASE IIIB ⟶ A Man Has Got to Know His Place

Scott Korman was not your ordinary doctoral student. At age thirty-five, he was ten years older than most other students in the Ph.D. program. Unlike his contemporaries, he held no teaching assistantship. In fact, he made no secret that he did not need financial assistance as did his peers. Scott's Pierre Cardin shirts, Gucci loafers, and $40,000 Mercedes didn't do much toward helping him blend into the role of the struggling student.

Scott's background is well-known around the university. He had his B.A. and M.A. degrees in English literature from Stanford University by the time he was twenty-three. Scott then took a job at a junior college in Virginia and taught English literature and creative writing. In his spare time, he wrote. His first novel was published when Scott was twenty-seven. It was favorably received by critics and the book-buying public. The book sold nearly 60,000 copies in hardback and over 2 million in paperback. At twenty-nine, Scott published his second novel. Selected by several major book clubs, this novel sold over 300,000 in hardback, and 3 million in paperback. It was also sold to Hollywood for $500,000, though it never was made into a film. His third novel, published last year, was on the best-seller list for twenty-two weeks. The paperback rights alone were purchased for $1.6 million.

Success to Scott was more than selling lots of books and making millions of dollars. Scott wanted the academic life. He dreamed of being a professor of creative writing at a quality eastern university and sharing his ideas with young people. But such a goal requires a doctoral degree—the Ph.D. So Scott has decided to go back to school to earn his doctorate.

The first semester back was difficult for Scott. It was not easy for him to sublimate a lot of his opinions on writing. Unfortunately, many of his ideas did not agree with those held by his professors. But he was learning to play the student role. The more pressing problem was something Scott couldn't control. That was the way the faculty reacted to him. Not surprisingly, they were not used to having a best-selling author around, especially as a lowly graduate student. One young assistant professor, who himself could not have been much over twenty-six years old, told Scott directly, "You don't belong here. You don't have any talent. Your books may sell a lot and you may be the darling of Madison Avenue, but I'm going to do everything I can to see that you never get your degree."

At one level, Scott felt like laughing. Why would these people—established academics with all the appropriate credentials—care that he had written three successful novels? He wasn't a novelist here; he was a student! At another level, Scott realized that whether he got a Ph.D. or not rested with the professors in his department and they apparently didn't enjoy playing second fiddle, in reputation, to a graduate student.

Questions

1. Analyze Scott's dilemma in terms of the various types of role conflict and in relation to status incongruence.
2. Analyze Scott's situation in terms of interpersonal conflict and power.
3. Utilizing the material on power, explain why some professors are not excited by Scott's presence in the program.
4. What could Scott do to increase the likelihood of obtaining his Ph.D.?

CASE IIIC → Tip Says No Way

Marc Lattoni supervises an eight-member cost accounting department in a large metals fabricating plant in Albuquerque, New Mexico. He was promoted about six months ago to his supervisory position after only a year as an accountant. It was no secret that Marc got the promotion predominantly due to his education—he has an M.B.A., whereas no one else in the department has a college degree. The transition to supervisor went smoothly, and there was little in the way of problems until this morning.

Business had been prospering at the plant for some time, and the need for an additional cost accountant in the department to handle the increased workload was becoming increasingly apparent. In fact, it had been on Marc's mind for over a month. Department members were complaining about the heavy workload. Overtime had become commonplace and the large amount of overtime was adversely affecting the department's efficiency statistics. Marc believed that he would have little or no trouble supporting his request for a new full-time position with his boss.

Marc believed the search for the new employee would be relatively hassle free. This was because he had already spotted an individual who he thought would fill the new slot nicely. The individual he had in mind was currently working in the production control department of the plant.

Unofficially, Marc had talked with the production control supervisor and the plant's personnel director, and the three had agreed that Ralph Simpson, a young black clerk in production, would be an excellent candidate to move into cost accounting. Ralph had been with the company for eight months, had shown above-average potential, and was only six units shy of his bachelor's degree (with a major in accounting) which he was earning at night at the state university.

Marc had met with Ralph earlier in the week and discussed the possibility that cost accounting might have a vacancy. Ralph told Marc that he would be very interested in pursuing the position. After further discussing the subject over lunch, all unofficially, Marc said that, although he could make no promises, he was prepared to recommend Ralph for the job. However, Marc emphasized that it would be a week to ten days before a final decision was made and the announcement made official.

This morning, Marc came into his office as usual around five minutes to eight. As he began reviewing some audit reports, there was a heavy knock on his door. Before Marc could get the words "Come in" out of his mouth, the door flew open and in stormed Tip O'Malley, one of the accountants in the cost department.

Tip O'Malley is fifty-eight years old and has been at the plant since its opening twenty-six years ago. He was born and raised in a small town in the deep South. From his angered red face, it was obvious to Marc that Tip was not paying a social call.

"What's this I hear that some black guy is joining our department. The grapevine is saying that black down in production control is coming up here. Well, let me tell you something. I've never worked with a black and I never will. I have *no* intention of working in the same department as any black!"

Questions

1. Analyze the actions on this case in terms of formal and informal communication.
2. Analyze the power relationship between Marc and Tip.
3. What is the source of the conflict?
4. What conflict resolution techniques would be relevant in handling this situation?
5. Which techniques do you recommend for Marc? Why?

CASE IIID → Getting Off to a Good Start

Sue Reynolds is twenty-two years old and will be receiving her B.S. degree in Human Resource Management from the University of Hartford at the end of this semester. She has spent the past two summers working for Connecticut Mutual, filling in on a number of different jobs while employees took their vacations. She has received and accepted an offer to join CM on a permanent basis upon graduation, as a supervisor in the policy renewal department.

Connecticut Mutual is a large insurance company. In the headquarters office alone, where Sue will work, they employ 5,000 employees. The company believes strongly in the personal development of its employees. This translates into a philosophy, emanating from the top executive offices, of trust and respect for all CM employees.

The job Sue will be assuming requires her to direct the activities of twenty-two clerks. Their jobs require little training and are highly routine. A clerk's responsibility is to ensure that renewal notices are sent on current policies, to tabulate any changes in premium from a standardized table, and to advise the sales division if a policy is to be canceled as a result of nonresponse to renewal notices.

Sue's group is composed of all females, ranging from nineteen to sixty-two years of age, with a median age of twenty-three. For the most part, they are high school graduates with little prior working experience. The salary range for policy renewal clerks is $920 to $1,070 per month. Sue will be replacing a long-time CM employee, Mabel Fincher. Mabel is retiring after thirty-seven years with CM, the last fourteen spent as a policy renewal supervisor. Since Sue had spent a few weeks in Mabel's group last summer, she was familiar with Mabel's style and also knew most of the group members. She anticipated no problems from any of her soon-to-be employees, except possibly for Lillian Lantz. Lillian was well into her fifties, had been a policy renewal clerk for over a dozen years, and—as the "grand old lady"—carried a lot of weight with group members. Sue concluded that without Lantz' support her job could prove very difficult.

Sue is determined to get her career off on the right foot. As a result, she has been doing a lot of thinking about the qualities of an effective leader.

Questions

1. What are the critical factors that will influence Sue's success as a leader? Would these factors be the same if success were defined as group satisfaction rather than group productivity?
2. Do you think that Sue can *choose* a leadership style? If so, describe the style you think would be most effective for her. If not, why?
3. What suggestions might you make to Sue to help her win over or control Lillian Lantz?

EXERCISE IIIA →

Status Ranking Task

Instructions: Rank the following occupations according to the prestige which is attached to them in the United States. Place a "1" in front of the occupation which you feel to be most prestigious, etc., all the way to "15," least prestigious.

____Author of novels
____Newspaper columnist
____Policeman
____Banker
____U.S. Supreme Court Justice
____Lawyer
____Undertaker
____State governor
____Sociologist
____Scientist
____Public school teacher
____Dentist
____Psychologist
____College professor
____Physician

Now form a group of from six to twelve participants. The objective of this group will be to create a consensus group ranking. The ranking of each occupation must be agreed upon by each member before it becomes a part of the group's decision. Members should try to make each ranking one with which *all* members agree at least partially. Two ground rules: no averaging, and no "majority rule" votes. The group should take no more than thirty minutes to complete its task. When a group decision has been reached, turn to page 534 for the correct answer (based on national studies) and further directions.

Source: J. W. Pfeiffer and J. E. Jones, *A Handbook of Structured Experiences for Human Relations Training*, Vol. 2 (Revised). San Diego, CA: University Associates Press, 1974. Used with permission.

EXERCISE IIIB →

Leadership Questionnaire

The following items describe aspects of leadership behavior. Respond to each item according to the way you would be most likely to act if you were the leader of a work group. Circle whether you would be likely to behave in the described way always (A), frequently (F), occasionally (O), seldom (S), or never (N).

If I were the leader of a work group . . .

A F O S N___ 1. I would most likely act as the spokesman of the group.

A F O S N___ 2. I would encourage overtime work.

A F O S N___ 3. I would allow members complete freedom in their work.

A F O S N___ 4. I would encourage the use of uniform procedures.

A F O S N___ 5. I would permit the members to use their own judgment in solving problems.

A F O S N___ 6. I would stress being ahead of competing groups.

A F O S N___ 7. I would speak as a representative of the group.

A F O S N___ 8. I would needle members for greater effort.

A F O S N___ 9. I would try out my ideas in the group.

A F O S N___10. I would let the members do their work the way they think best.

A F O S N___11. I would be working hard for a promotion.

A F O S N___12. I would be able to tolerate postponement and uncertainty.

A F O S N___13. I would speak for the group when visitors were present.

A F O S N___14. I would keep the work moving at a rapid pace.

A F O S N___15. I would turn the members loose on a job and let them go to it.

A F O S N___16. I would settle conflicts when they occur in the group.

A F O S N___17. I would get swamped by details.

A F O S N___18. I would represent the group at outside meetings.

A F O S N___19. I would be reluctant to allow the members any freedom of action.

A F O S N___20. I would decide what shall be done and how it shall be done.

A F O S N___21. I would push for increased production.

A F O S N___22. I would let some members have authority which I could keep.

A F O S N___23. Things would usually turn out as I predict.

A F O S N___24. I would allow the group a high degree of initiative.

A F O S N___25. I would assign group members to particular tasks.

A F O S N___26. I would be willing to make changes.

A F O S N___27. I would ask the members to work harder.

A F O S N___28. I would trust the group members to exercise good judgment.

A F O S N___29. I would schedule the work to be done.

A F O S N___30. I would refuse to explain my actions.
A F O S N___31. I would persuade others that my ideas are to their advantage.
A F O S N___32. I would permit the group to set its own pace.
A F O S N___33. I would urge the group to beat its previous record.
A F O S N___34. I would act without consulting the group.
A F O S N___35. I would ask that group members follow standard rules and
regulations.
T___   P___

Turn to page 534 for scoring directions and key.

Source: J. W. Pfeiffer and J. E. Jones, *A Handbook of Structured Experiences for Human Relations Training,* Vol. I, (Revised). San Diego, CA: University Associates Press, 1969. Used with permission.

EXERCISE IIIC ⟶

Power-Orientation Test

Instructions. For each statement, circle the number that most closely resembles your attitude.

Statement	Disagree			Agree	
	A lot	A little	Neutral	A little	A lot
1. The best way to handle people is to tell them what they want to hear.	1	2	3	4	5
2. When you ask someone to do something for you, it is best to give the real reason for wanting it rather than giving reasons that might carry more weight.	1	2	3	4	5
3. Anyone who completely trusts anyone else is asking for trouble.	1	2	3	4	5
4. It is hard to get ahead without cutting corners here and there.	1	2	3	4	5
5. It is safest to assume that all people have a vicious streak, and it will come out when they are given a chance.	1	2	3	4	5
6. One should take action only when it is morally right.	1	2	3	4	5

7. Most people are basically good and kind.	1	2	3	4	5
8. There is no excuse for lying to someone else.	1	2	3	4	5
9. Most men forget more easily the death of their father than the loss of their property.	1	2	3	4	5
10. Generally speaking, men won't work hard unless they're forced to do so.	1	2	3	4	5

Turn to page 535 for scoring directions and key.

Source: Richard Christie and Florence L. Geis, *Studies in Machiavellianism.* © Academic Press 1970. Reprinted by permission.

PART IV

The Organization System

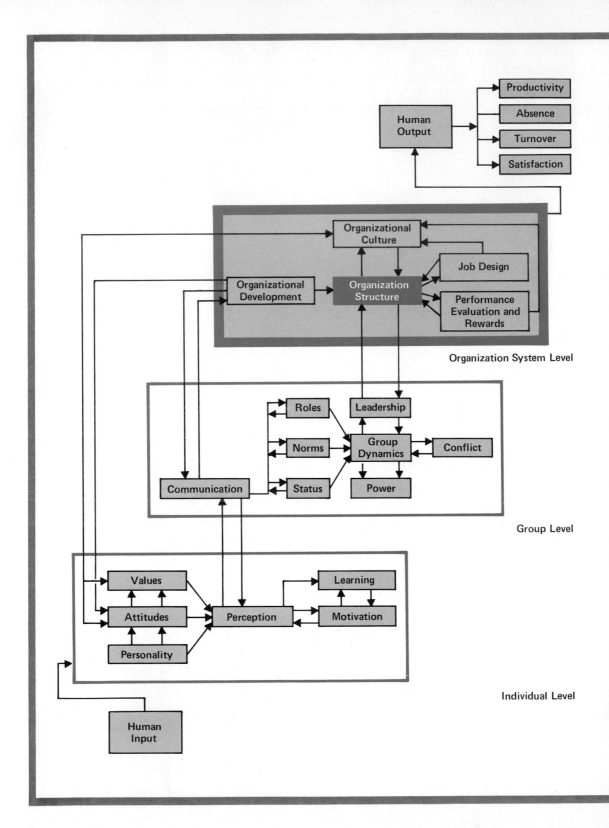

CHAPTER 14
Organization Structure

AFTER STUDYING THIS CHAPTER, YOU SHOULD BE ABLE TO—

Define and explain the following key terms and concepts:

Adhocratic structure	Mechanistic structure
Authority	Organic structure
Bureaucratic structure	Power-control
Centralization	Product structure
Complexity	Simple structure
Decentralization	Size
Environment	Spatial differentiation
Formalization	Span of control
Functional structure	Staff authority
Horizontal differentiation	Structure
Line authority	Technology
Matrix	Vertical differentiation

Understand:

The three components that make up organization structure
The factors that determine structure.
The difference between mechanistic and organic structures
A classification scheme for identifying different structures

> One man's red tape is another man's system.
>
> —DWIGHT WALDO

Jerry Nichols's job is pretty good. He's got an attractively furnished office on the top floor of a Houston skyscraper, a nice view, his own secretary, the prestige that goes with being a security analyst with a major brokerage firm, and a salary bonus package that earns him better than $60,000 a year—not bad for a twenty-eight-year-old guy who has been out of school for less than five years.

In contrast to a blue-collar assembly-line worker, Jerry Nichols has a lot of freedom on his job. But in absolute terms, Jerry and the more than 100 million other North Americans who go to work every Monday have a number of restrictions imposed on them by their organizations that limit and regulate their attitudes and behavior. Most employees have a job description that says what they are supposed to do. The organization has rules telling Jerry and the millions of employees like Jerry what they can and cannot do. There is an authority hierarchy that defines who everyone's boss is and the formal channels through which communications are to pass. These are examples of structural characteristics that most organizations have. In this chapter, we want to demonstrate how an organization's *structure* effects the attitudes and behavior of its members.

WHAT IS STRUCTURE?

An organization's structure is made up of three components. The first has to do with the amount of vertical, horizontal, and spatial differentiation. This is called *complexity*. Next, is the degree to which rules and procedures are utilized. This is referred to as *formalization*. The third is *centralization*, which considers where decision-making authority lies. Let's briefly elaborate on each of these components.

Complexity

Complexity can be broken down into three parts. *Horizontal differentiation* considers the degree of horizontal separation between units. *Vertical differentiation* refers to the depth of the organizational hierarchy. *Spatial differentiation* encompasses the degree to which the location of an organization's facilities and personnel are geographically dispersed. The more that an organization is differentiated along these dimensions, the more complex it is.

Horizontal Differentiation. Horizontal differentiation refers to the degree of differentiation between units based on the orientation of members, the nature of the tasks they perform, and their education and training. We can state that the larger the number of different occupations within an organization that require specialized knowledge and skills, the more horizontally complex that organization is. Why? Because diverse orientations make it more difficult for organizational members to communicate and more difficult for management to coordinate their activities. For instance, when organizations create specialized groups or expand departmental designations, they differentiate groups from each other, making interactions between those groups more complex. If the organization is staffed by people who have similar backgrounds, skills, and training, they are likely to see the world in more similar terms. Conversely, diversity increases the likelihood that they will have different goal emphases, time orientations, and even a different work vocabulary. Job specialization reinforces differences—the chemical engineer's job is clearly different from that of the personnel recruitment interviewer. Their training is different. The language they use on their respective jobs is different. They are typically assigned to different departments which further reinforces their divergent orientations.

Vertical Differentiation. Vertical differentiation refers to the depth of the structure. Differentiation increases, and hence complexity, as the number of hierarchial levels in the organization increases. The more levels that exist between top management and operatives, the greater the potential for communication distortion, the more difficult it is to coordinate the decisions of managerial personnel, and the more difficult it is for top management to oversee closely the actions of operatives.

Vertical and horizontal differentiation should not be construed as independent of each other. Vertical differentiation may be best understood as a response to an increase in horizontal differentiation. As work is divided into smaller parts, it becomes increasingly necessary to coordinate tasks. Since high horizontal differentiation means members will have diverse training and background, it may be difficult for the individual units to see how their tasks fit into the greater whole. The bricklayers on a large construction site may see themselves as merely laying bricks, not putting up a building. Someone must supervise their tasks to see that they are done according to the architect's plan and consistent with the time schedule. The result is a need for increased coordination which shows itself in the development of vertical differentiation.

Spatial Differentiation. An organization can perform the same activities with the same horizontal and vertical arrangement in multiple locations. Yet, this existence of multiple locations increases complexity. Therefore, the third element in complexity is spatial differentiation, which refers to the degree to which the location of an organization's offices, plants, and personnel are geographically dispersed.

A manufacturing company horizontally differentiates when it separates the marketing function from production. Yet, if essentially identical marketing activities are carried on in six geographically dispersed sales offices—Seattle, Los Angeles, Atlanta, New York, Toronto, and Brussels—while all production is done in a large factory in Cleveland, this organization is more complex than if both the marketing and production activities were performed at the same facility in Cleveland. The spatial concept applies similarly with vertical differentiation. If an organization's senior executives reside in one city, middle managers in a half-dozen cities, and lower-level managers in a hundred different company offices around the world, complexity has increased. Why? Because communication, coordination, and control is easier where spatial differentiation is low.

A final point: Spatial differentiation considers distance as well as numbers. If the state of Delaware had two regional welfare offices located in Dover and Wilmington, these offices would be approximately 45 miles apart. If the state of Alaska had two comparably sized offices in Anchorage and Fairbanks, these offices would be separated by 350 miles. Although the number of offices is the same in both cases, the Delaware welfare organization would be less complex due to the smaller distance involved.

Formalization

Formalization refers to the degree to which jobs within the organization are standardized. If a job is highly formalized, then the job incumbent has a minimum amount of discretion over what is to be done, when it is to be done, and how he or she should do it. Employees can be expected always to handle the same input in exactly the same way, resulting in a consistent and uniform output. There are explicit job descriptions, lots of organizational rules, and clearly defined procedures covering work processes in organizations where there is high formalization. Where formalization is low, job behaviors are relatively nonprogrammed and employees have a great deal of freedom to exercise discretion in their work. Since an individual's discretion on the job is inversely related to the amount of behavior that is preprogrammed by the organization, the greater the standardization, the less input the employee has into how his or her work is to be done. Standardization not only eliminates the possibility of employees engaging in alternative behaviors, but even removes the need for employees to consider alternatives.

The degree of formalization can vary widely between organizations and within organizations. Certain jobs, for instance, are well known to have little formalization. College book travelers—the representatives of publishers who call on professors to inform them of their company's new publications—have a great deal of freedom in their jobs. They have no standard sales "spiel," and the extent of rules and procedures governing their behavior may be little more than the requirement that they submit a weekly sales report and some suggestions on what pluses to emphasize for the various new titles. At the other extreme, there are clerical and editorial positions in the same publishing houses where employ-ees are required to "clock in" at their work station by 8:00 A.M. or be docked a half-hour of pay and, once at that work station, to follow a set of precise proce-dures dictated by management.

It is generally true that the narrowest of unskilled jobs—those that are sim-plest and most repetitive in nature—are most amenable to high degrees of for-malization. The greater the professionalization of a job, the less likely it is to be highly formalized. Yet there are obvious exceptions. Public accountants and consultants, for instance, typically are required to keep detailed hour-by-hour records of their activities so their companies can appropriately bill clients for their services. In general, however, the relationship holds. The jobs of lawyers, engineers, social workers, librarians, and like professionals tend to rate low on formalization.

Formalization not only differs with whether the jobs are unskilled or pro-fessional, but also by level in the organization and by functional department. Employees higher in the organization are increasingly involved in activities that are less repetitive and require more unique solutions. The discretion that man-agers have increases as they move up the hierarchy so that formalization is low-est at the highest levels of the organization.

The kind of work that people are engaged in also influences the degree of formalization. Jobs in production are typically more formalized than those in sales or research. Why? Because production tends to be concerned with stable and repetitive activities. Such jobs lend themselves to standardization. In con-trast, the sales department must be flexible in order to respond to changing needs of customers, while research must be flexible if it is to be innovative.

Centralization

Centralization refers to the degree to which decision making is concentrated at a single point in the organization. The concept includes only formal authority—that is, the rights inherent in one's position. Typically, it is said that if top man-agement makes the organization's key decisions with little or no input from low-er-level personnel, then the organization is centralized. In contrast, the more that lower-level personnel provide input or are actually given the discretion to make decisions, the more decentralized the organization. As we shall point out, an or-ganization characterized by centralization is an inherently different structural ani-mal than one where decision making has been pushed down to those managers who are closest to the action.

A small but important point needs to be made before we move on. While they are sometimes confused with one another, the concept of centralization is distinctly different from that of spatial differentiation. Centralization is concerned with the dispersion of authority to make decisions within the organization, not geographic dispersion. While it is generally true that organizations with high spa-tial differentation also tend to be decentralized (because it's hard for headquar-ters management in New York to oversee and understand the unique problems in its office in Vancouver, for instance), this need not be the case. Information technology can allow top management to stay on top of problems in geographically dispersed locations and make the key decisions that effect personnel in those locations. Conversely, an organization operating entirely in a single building can be decentralized if top management delegates authority to its lower-level managers.

WHY DO STRUCTURES DIFFER?

We have identified three components which, when "mixed and matched," create different structural forms. For instance, an organization that is highly complex, formalized, and decentralized certainly has a different structure from an organization of similar size and function that is low in complexity, has few rules and procedures governing personnel, and where decision making is centralized in the top executive suites.

Before we review the various forms that structures can take, we need to understand those forces that influence the form that is chosen. Management is the obvious decision-making body for choosing structure. But there are forces that limit management's choices. In the following pages, we shall present the major forces that researchers have identified as causes or determinants of an organization's structure.

Size

A quick glance at the organizations we deal with regularly in our lives would lead most of us to conclude that size would have some bearing on an organization's structure. The 900,000 employees of the Bell System, for example, do not neatly fit into one building, nor into several departments supervised by a couple of managers. It's pretty hard to envision 900,000 people being organized in any manner other than that which would be labeled as high in complexity. On the other hand, a local telephone answering service that employs ten people and generates less than $300,000 a year in service fees is not likely to need decentralized decision making or formalized procedures and regulations.

A little more thought suggests that the same conclusion—size influences structure—can be arrived at through a more sophisticated reasoning process. As an organization hires more operative employees, it will attempt to take advantage of the economic benefits from specialization. The result will be increased horizontal differentiation. Grouping like functions together will facilitate intragroup efficiencies, but will cause intergroup relations to suffer as each performs its different activities. Management, therefore, will need to increase vertical differentiation to coordinate the horizontally differentiated units. This expansion in size is also likely to result in spatial differentiation. All of this increase in complexity will reduce top management's ability to directly supervise the activities within the organization. The control achieved through direct surveillance, therefore, will be replaced by the implementation of formal rules and regulations. This increase in formalization may also be accompanied by still greater vertical differentiation as management creates new units to coordinate the expanding and diverse activities of organizational members. Finally, with top management further removed from the operating level, it becomes difficult for senior executives to make rapid and informative decisions. The solution is to substitute decentralized decision making for centralization. Following this reasoning, we see changes in size leading to major structural changes.

But does it actually happen this way? Does structure change directly as a result in a change in the total number of employees? A review of the evidence indicates that size has a significant influence on some but certainly not all elements of structure.

Size appears to impact on complexity at a decreasing rate.[1] That is, increases in organization size are accompanied by initially rapid and subsequently more gradual increases in differentiation. The biggest effect, however, is on vertical differentiation.[2] As organizations increase their number of employees, more levels are added, but at a decreasing rate.

The evidence is quite strong linking size and formalization.[3] There is a logical connection between the two. Management seeks to control the behavior of its employees. This can be achieved by direct surveillance or by the use of formalized regulations. While not perfect substitutes for each other, as one increases, the need for the other should decrease. Because surveillance costs should increase very rapidly as an organization expands in size, it seems reasonable to expect that it would be less expensive for management to substitute formalization for direct surveillance as size increases.

There is also a strong inverse relationship between size and centralization.[4] In small organizations, it's possible for management to exercise control by keeping decisions centralized. As size increases, management is physically unable to maintain control in this manner and, therefore, is forced to decentralize.

Technology

The term *technology* refers to how an organization transfers its inputs to outputs. Every organization has one or more technologies for converting financial, human, and physical resources into products or services. The Ford Motor Company, for instance, predominantly uses an assembly-line process to make its products. On the other hand, colleges may use a number of instruction technol-

1. Peter M. Blau, "A Formal Theory of Differentiation in Organizations," *American Sociological Review,* April 1970, pp. 201–18.

2. Dennis S. Mileti, David F. Gillespie, and J. Eugene Haas, "Size and Structure in Complex Organizations," *Social Forces,* September 1977, pp. 208–17.

3. William A. Rushing, "Organizational Size, Rules, and Surveillance," in *Organizations: Structure and Behavior,* ed. Joseph A. Litterer, 3rd ed. (New York: John Wiley, 1980), pp. 396–405; and Y. Samuel and B. F. Mannheim, "A Multi-dimensional Approach toward a Typology of Bureaucracy," *Administrative Science Quarterly,* June 1970, pp. 216–28.

4. See, for example, Peter M. Blau and Richard A. Schoenherr, *The Structure of Organizations* (New York: Basic Books, 1971); and John Child and Roger Mansfield, "Technology, Size, and Organization Structure," *Sociology,* September 1972, pp. 369–93.

ogies—the ever-popular formal lecture method, the case analysis method, the experiential exercise method, the programmed learning method, and so forth.

There is no agreement on a universal technology classification.[5] If there is a common denominator among those classifications that attempt to describe the processes or methods that organizations use to transform inputs into outputs it is the *degree of routineness*. By this we mean that technologies tend toward either routine or nonroutine activities. The former are characterized by automated and standardized operations. This describes such diverse processes as mass production assembly lines or repetitive clerical tasks. Nonroutine activities are customized. They include such varied operations as furniture restoring, custom shoemaking, or NASA's efforts at developing the space shuttle. As shown in Figure 14–1, we can think of all technologies as falling somewhere along a routine-nonroutine continuum.

Some researchers argue that there is a *technological imperative,* that is, that technology *causes* structure.[6] A more moderate position is that technology *constrains* managers. If managers have a considerable degree of choice over their organization's technology, then there is little basis for the imperative argument. Technology would only control structure to the degree that managers chose a technology that demanded certain structural dimensions. For instance, it has been argued that organizations choose the domain in which they will operate and, hence, the activities that they will engage in.[7] If an organization decides to offer consulting advice tailored to the needs of its clients, it is not likely to use the routine-oriented mass production technology. Similarly, the fact that Volkswagen of America chose to build a manufacturing facility in Pennsylvania that could produce at least 400 cars a day which could, in turn, retail in the $7,000-to-$9,000 price range pretty well eliminated any technology other than one relying heavily on routinized mass production activities. Had VW of America decided to produce only 4 cars a day at that plant and charge $100,000 or more a piece for each car (which more accurately describes the production facility at Rolls Royce), then routine mass production might not be at all appropriate. The point is that "choice of domain, and a set of activities and tasks, tend to constrain the organization's technology, but the domain is still chosen."[8] The counterpoint, of course, is that even though domain is chosen, technology is still a major influence on structure. For instance, research laboratories are typically low in formalization, while claims departments in insurance companies are typically high on this structural dimension. A good part of this structural difference

5. The most frequently referenced technology categories have been offered by Joan Woodward, *Industrial Organization: Theory and Practice* (London: Oxford University Press, 1965); Charles Perrow, "A Framework for the Comparative Analysis of Organizations," *American Sociological Review,* April 1967, pp. 194–208; and James D. Thompson, *Organizations in Action* (New York: McGraw-Hill, 1967).

6. Woodward, *Industrial Organization;* and Perrow, *Framework.*

7. Jeffrey Pfeffer, *Organizational Design* (Arlington Heights, Ill.: AHM Publishing Corp., 1978), p. 99.

8. Ibid.

FIGURE 14–1 Technology Classification with Representative Examples

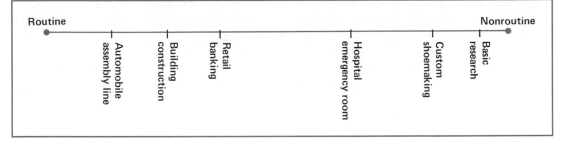

can be traced to the fact that research labs use nonroutine technologies and claims departments activities are standardized and routine.

What relationships have been found between technology and structure? Although the relationship is not overwhelmingly strong, we do find that routine technology is positively associated with low complexity. The greater the routineness, the fewer the number of occupational groups.[9] Similarly, as the work becomes more sophisticated, customized, and nonroutine, more problems occur that require management's attention. Closer supervision results and, with it, more vertical levels are necessary in the structure. So nonroutine technology is likely to lead to high complexity.

The technology-formalization relationship is stronger. Studies consistently show routineness to be associated with the presence of rule manuals, job descriptions, and other formalized documentation.[10]

Finally, the technology-centralization relationship is less straightforward. It seems logical that routine technologies would be associated with a centralized structure, whereas nonroutine technologies, which rely more heavily on the knowledge of specialists, would be characterized by delegated decision authority. This position has met with some support.[11] However, a more generalizable conclusion is that the technology-centralization relationship is moderated by the degree of formalization.[12] Formal regulations and centralized decision making are both control mechanisms and management can substitute them for each other. Routine technologies should be associated with centralized control if there is a minimum of rules and regulations. However, if formalization is high, routine technology can be accompanied by decentralization. So, we would predict that routine technology would lead to centralization, but only if formalization is low.

9. Jerald Hage and Michael Aiken, "Routine Technology, Social Structure, and Organizational Goals," *Administrative Science Quarterly,* September 1969, pp. 366–77.

10. Donald Gerwin, "Relationships between Structure and Technology at the Organizational and Job Levels," *Journal of Management Studies,* February 1979, pp. 70–79.

11. Andrew Van De Ven, André Delbecq, and Richard Koenig, Jr., "Determinants of Coordination Modes within Organizations," *American Sociological Review,* April 1976, pp. 322–38.

12. Jerald Hage and Michael Aiken, "Relationship of Centralization to Other Structural Properties," *Administrative Science Quarterly,* June 1967, pp. 72–92.

Environment

An organization's environment represents anything outside the organization itself. The problem of defining an organization's environment, however, is often quite difficult. "Nature has neatly packaged people into skins, animals into hides, and allowed trees to enclose themselves with bark. It is easy to see where the unit is and where the environment is. Not so for social organizations."[13] We'll define the environment as composed of those institutions or forces that affect the performance of the organization, but over which the organization has little control. These typically include suppliers, customers, government regulatory agencies, and the like. But keep in mind that it is not always clear who or what is included in any specific organization's relevant environment.

The environment-structure relationship has received a large amount of attention. The reason for this attention is quite simple: Organizations must adapt to their environments if they are to succeed because organizations are dependent on their environments if they are to survive. They must identify and follow their environments, sense changes in those environments, and make appropriate adjustments as necessary. But changing environments produce uncertainty if management can't predict in what ways their environments are moving. And management doesn't like uncertainty. As a result, management will try to eliminate or at least minimize the impact of environmental uncertainty. Alterations in the organization's structural components are a major tool that management has for controlling environmental uncertainty. The environmental imperative would propose, therefore, that the degree of environmental uncertainty is *the* determinant of structure. If uncertainty is high, the organization will be designed along flexible lines in order to adapt to rapid changes. If uncertainty is low, management will opt for a structure that will be most efficient and offer the highest degree of managerial control—characterized by high complexity, high formalization, and centralization.

Does the evidence support the above predictions? The answer is "Yes." Environmental uncertainty and organizational complexity are inversely related. This is particularly true for departments within organizations.[14] Those departments within the organization that are most dependent on the environment—like marketing or research and development—are typically the lowest in complexity.

Similarly, formalization and environmental uncertainty are inversely related.[15] That is, certain and stable environments lead to high formalization. Why? Because stable environments create a minimal need for rapid response and economies exist for organizations that standardize their activities.

13. Jeffrey Pfeffer and Gerald R. Salancik, *The External Control of Organizations: A Response Dependence Perspective* (New York: Harper & Row, 1978), p. 29.

14. Paul Lawrence and Jay W. Lorsch, *Organization and Environment: Managing Differentiation and Integration* (Boston: Harvard Business School, Division of Research, 1967).

15. See, for example, Robert B. Duncan, "Characteristics of Organizational Environments and Perceived Environmental Uncertainty," *Administrative Science Quarterly*, September 1972, pp. 313–27.

Centralization is also affected by the environment. If the environment is large and multifaceted, it becomes difficult for management to monitor. As a result, the structure tends to become decentralized.[16] This explains why the marketing function in organizations is typically decentralized. If a firm has a large number of customers and the needs of these customers are prone to rapid changes, management must be able to respond rapidly if it is to keep its customers satisfied. This can best be achieved by pushing key decisions down to the local marketing managers who are closest to the customer. Decentralization allows for more rapid response.

Power-Control

An increasingly popular and insightful approach to the question of what causes structure is to look to a political explanation. Size, technology, and environment—even when combined—can at best explain only 50 to 60 percent of the variability in structure.[17] There is a growing body of evidence that suggests that power and politics can explain why an organization's structure is the way it is better than any of the previous three factors. More specifically, the power-control explanation states that an organization's structure is the result of a power struggle by internal constituencies who are seeking to further their interests.[18] Like all decisions in an organization, the structural decision is not fully rational. Managers do not necessarily choose those alternatives that will maximize the organization's interest. They choose criteria and weight them so that the "best choice" will meet the minimal demands of the organization, and also satisfy or enhance the interests of the decision maker. Size, technology, and environmental uncertainty act as constraints by establishing parameters and defining how much discretion is available. Almost always, within the parameters, there is a great deal of room for the decision maker to maneuver. The power-control position, therefore, argues that those in power will choose a structure that will maintain or enhance their control. Consistent with this perspective, we should expect structures to change very slowly, if at all. Significant changes would occur only as a result of a political struggle in which new power relations evolve. But this rarely occurs. Transitions in the executive suite are usually peaceful. They are evolutionary rather than revolutionary. However, major shake-ups in top management occasionally do occur. Not surprisingly, they are typically followed by major structural changes.

Predictions based on the power-control viewpoint differ from those based on the three previous approaches in that those approaches were basically contingency models: Structures change to reflect changes in size, technology, or en-

16. Henry Mintzberg, *The Structuring of Organizations* (Englewood Cliffs, N.J.: Prentice-Hall, 1979), pp. 273–76.

17. John Child, "Organization Structure, Environment and Performance: The Role of Strategic Choice," *Sociology*, January 1972, pp. 1–22; and Derek S. Pugh, "The Management of Organization Structures: Does Context Determine Form?" *Organizational Dynamics*, Spring 1973, pp. 19–34.

18. Pfeffer, *Organizational Design*.

vironmental uncertainty. The power-control approach, however, is essentially noncontingent. It assumes little change within the organization's power coalition. Hence, it would propose that structures are relatively stable over time. More importantly, power-control advocates would predict that after taking into consideration size, technology, and environmental factors, those in power would choose a structure that would best serve their personal interests. What type of structure would that be? Obviously one that would be low in complexity, high in formalization, and centralized. These structural dimensions will most likely maximize control in the hands of senior management. A structure with these properties becomes the single "one best way" to organize. Of course, *best* in this context refers to "maintenance of control" rather than enhancement of organizational performance.

Is the power-control position an accurate description? The evidence suggests that it explains a great deal of why organizations are structured the way they are.[19] This will become clearer in the next section when we review the various forms that structures can take and then note how accurately the power-control predictions describe the structural design of most organizations in North America.

HOW STRUCTURES DIFFER: A CLASSIFICATION SCHEME

It is possible, by mixing and matching the three structural dimensions, to form a variety of structural forms. The more popular of these forms are the simple, bureaucratic, functional, product, and adhocratic structures. Each of these will be briefly described in this section. First, however, we shall present two general models of structural design: the mechanistic and organic structures.[20] Like the routine-nonroutine dichtomy used in our discussion of technology, these structures can be seen as two extremes along a continuum (see Figure 14–2).

A mechanistic structure is characterized by high complexity, high formalization, and centralization. It performs routine tasks, relies heavily on programmed behavior, and is relatively slow in responding to the unfamiliar. An

19. Ibid.

20. Tom Burns and G. M. Stalker, *The Management of Innovation* (London: Tavistock, 1960).

FIGURE 14–2 Mechanistic–Organic Continuum

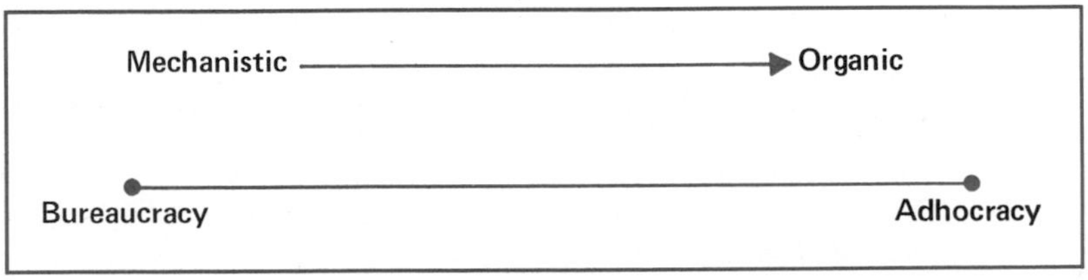

Mechanistic ————————————→ Organic

Bureaucracy   Adhocracy

FIGURE 14–3 Structure of Fashion Flair Stores

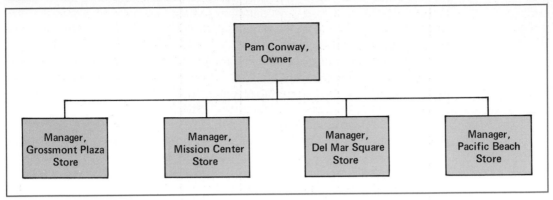

organic structure is just the opposite. It is flexible and adaptive, characterized by low complexity, low formalization, and decentralization. No organization is purely mechanistic or purely organic, but rather moves toward one or the other. As shown in Figure 14–2, bureaucracy is as close as one can get to operationalizing the mechanistic design, while adhocracy closely aligns with the organic model. We'll discuss these structural forms, along with several others, in the following section.

The Simple Structure

What might the following organizations have in common: a small retail store, an electronics firm run by a hard-driving entrepreneur, a new Planned Parenthood office, and a city in the midst of a race riot? They probably all utilize the simple structure.

The simple structure is characterized most by what it is not rather than what it is. The simple structure is not elaborated.[21] It is low in complexity, has little formalization, and has authority centralized in a single person. Figure 14–3 shows an example of the simple structure: the Fashion Flair retail stores. Notice that this organization is flat or low on vertical differentiation. Decision making is basically informal—all important decisions are centralized in the hands of the senior executive who, because of the organization's low complexity, is able readily to obtain key information and can act rapidly when required. This senior executive is the owner-manager at Fashion Flair.

When are you likely to find a simple structure? At least five conditions can be noted.

When the organization is small or is in its formative stage of development. Small size usually means less repetitive work, so standardization is less attractive. Informal communication is convenient. As long as the structure remains small,

---

21. Henry Mintzberg, "Structure in 5's: A Synthesis of the Research on Organization Design," *Management Science,* March 1980, p. 331.

the "one-man show" can effectively oversee all activities, be knowledgeable about key problems, and carry out all important decisions. Similarly, the new organization tends to adapt the simple structure because it has not had the time to elaborate its structure.

When the environment is rapidly changing but is easily comprehensible. A rapidly changing environment requires an organic form in order that the organization can react to its unpredictable contingencies. A single person can assimilate and monitor an easily comprehensible environment.

When the organization faces high hostility or a crisis. Regardless of size, when an organization suddenly confronts a hostile environment, survival instincts emerge. Top management will want control. Standard operating procedures are usually shelved and decisions are centralized. The net effect is a temporary flattening of the organization.

When the senior manager is also the owner. Consistent with the power-control position, you would expect owner-managers to want to maintain control of their organization. These individuals also have the power to maintain a structure that allows them the greatest control. The simple structure concentrates decision making in a single place and owner-managers find this attractive.

When the senior executive either wants to hoard power or his subordinates thrust the power upon him. When the top executive hoards power and purposely avoids high formalization in order that he can maximize the impact of his discretion, he may design a simple structure for his organization. Additionally, even if the senior executive doesn't crave power, if subordinates don't want to be involved with decision making, they force it back upon the executive. The result is the same as if the power was sought by the executive: Decision making becomes centralized in one person at the top and the organization takes on simple structure characteristics.

The Bureaucratic Structure

The best-known and one of the most popular forms of structure is *bureaucracy.* While to many the term bureaucracy conjures up a host of attributes implying inefficiency—red tape, paper shuffling, rigid application of rules, redundance of effort—bureaucracy is in fact, a very efficient way of organizing certain tasks.

When we talk of bureaucracy, we refer to a structure that has the following characteristics:

Division of labor—Each person's job is broken down into simple, routine, and well-defined tasks.

Well-defined authority hierarchy—There is a multilevel formal structure, with a hierarchy of positions or offices. Each lower office is under the supervision and control of a higher one.

High formalization—To ensure uniformity and to regulate the behavior of jobholders, there is heavy dependence on formal rules and procedures.

Impersonal nature—Sanctions are applied uniformly and impersonally to avoid involvement with individual personalities and personal preferences of members.

Employment decisions based on merit—Selection and promotion decisions are based on technical qualifications, competence, and performance of the candidate.

Career tracks for employees—Members are expected to pursue a career in the organization. In return for this career commitment, employees are given permanent employment; that is, they are retained even if they "burn out" or their skills become obsolete.

Distinct separation of members' organizational and personal lives—To prevent the demands and interests of personal affairs from interfering with the rational impersonal conduct of the organization's activities, the two are kept completely separate.[22]

While the above individual characteristics represent the ideal or perfect bureaucracy, cumulatively they are a fairly accurate description of most large organizations. Whether you are describing the structure of Mobil Oil, the American Broadcasting Company, Bristol-Myers, the New York City school system, or the U.S. Army, these organizations and thousands of others substantially meet all the characteristics we attribute to bureaucracy. In structural terms, they are highly complex and highly formalized. Whether they are centralized or decentralized typically depends on the type of people they employ. If employees are professionals or hold specialized skills, the bureaucracy will be decentralized. Otherwise, authority is typically kept centralized.

When are you likely to find a bureaucratic structure? When organizations are large in size, use routine technology, and have a stable and easily comprehensible environment. These characteristics are relatively widespread as evidenced by the popularity of bureaucracy as a structural form. The vast majority of large organizations are bureaucratic structures and, for all but a few, bureaucracy represents the most efficient way for them to organize. It has achieved its widespread popularity because it works best with the type of technologies and environments that most large organizations have. Additionally, it is also consistent with maintaining control in the hands of the organization's power elite.

The Functional Structure

The distinguishing feature of the functional structure is that similar and related occupational specialties are grouped together. Activities such as marketing, accounting, manufacturing, and personnel are grouped under a functional head who reports to a central headquarters. Figure 14–4 shows a typical functional structure for a manufacturing firm.

The functional structure is extremely popular, undoubtedly due to its compatability with the bureaucratic structure. That is, the functional structure maximizes the economies from specialization. By putting like specialties together you get economies of scale, you minimize duplication of personnel and equipment,

22. Max Weber, *The Theory of Social and Economic Organizations,* ed. Talcott Parsons, trans. A. M. Henderson and Talcott Parsons (New York: Free Press, 1947).

FIGURE 14-4 Functional Structure in a Manufacturing Organization

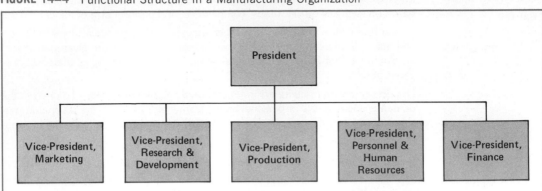

and employees are likely to feel comfortable and satisfied because they are part of a homogeneous group where their peers all talk "the same language."

The functional structure is most likely to be evident in organizations that deal in a single product or service. Conversely, it is unlikely to be used in multiproduct or multimarket organizations. Why? Because as an organization diversifies by adding products or markets, the functional specialists must spread their talent. In such cases, the advantages of specialization begin to be more than offset by the problems of diversification. In terms of our structural dimensions, we can say that the increase in horizontal differentiation facilitates within-unit efficiencies but increases the difficulty of coordinating interunit relations.

The Product Structure

In addition to organizing by function, you can structure an organization around product lines. Figure 14–5 shows the product structure at General Motors. Employees belong to a specific product division—like Chevrolet, Pontiac, Cadillac, or Saginaw Steering Gear. Within each product structure is typically something resembling a functional structure.

The major advantage to the product form is accountability. The product manager is responsible for all facets surrounding the product. Instead of the marketing manager having fifteen different product lines to oversee, each product structure will have its own marketing manager with sole responsibility for marketing his or her division's product. In this way, product control is centralized with the product manager. The drawbacks, of course, are the need to coordinate activities between product structures and the duplication of functions within the various structures. Whereas in the functional structure a department of five people might be able to handle the entire organization's purchasing activities, if that organization is structured around ten product divisions, each will probably require a purchasing agent, thus doubling the number of personnel engaged in purchasing. You are likely to find product structures, therefore, when management has a diverse set of product lines and believes that the extra costs of duplicating activities is more than offset by the benefits that accrue when all activities related to a certain product are centralized and coordinated by a single product manager.

The Adhocratic Structure

What bureaucracy is to the mechanistic form, adhocracy is to the organic. The term *adhocracy* refers to any structure that is essentially a flexible, adaptive, responsive system organized around unique problems to be solved by groups of relative strangers with diverse professional skills. In terms of our structural dimensions, adhocracies would be characterized as having moderate to low complexity, low formalization, and decentralized decision making.

An adhocracy may be a temporary project group, a task force, or a committee. For instance, if Procter & Gamble wanted to develop and design a new product—say a toothpaste—they would likely rely on an adhocratic structure. Personnel with expertise in finance, marketing, manufacturing, cost accounting, product design, research, and other relevant areas would be tapped from their functional departments and temporarily assigned the task of creating the product, designing its package, determining its market, computing its manufacturing costs, and assessing its profit margin. Once the problems had been fully worked out of the product and it was ready to be produced in quantity, the adhocratic structure would be disbanded and the toothpaste would be integrated into the permanent functional structure.

The term adhocracy would also be appropriately applied to what has been called the *matrix structure*. Essentially, the matrix combines the functional and product structures. Ideally, it seeks to gain the strengths of each, while avoiding their weaknesses. That is, the strength of the functional structure lies in putting like specialists together, which minimizes the number necessary; and it allows the pooling and sharing of specialized resources across products. Its major disadvantage is the difficulty of coordinating the tasks of diverse functional specialists so their activities are completed on time and within budget. The product structure, on the other hand, has exactly the opposite benefits and disadvantages. It facilitates the coordination among specialties to achieve on-time completion and meet budget targets. Further, it provides clear responsibility for all activities related to a product, but with duplication of activities and costs.

Figure 14–6 shows the matrix form as used in a College of Administrative Sciences. The academic departments of accounting, economics, and so forth are functional units. Additionally, specific programs (i.e., products) are overlaid on the functions. In this way, members in a matrix structure have a dual assignment: to their functional department and to their product group. For instance, a professor of accounting may report to the director of undergraduate programs as well as to the chairman of the accounting department.

When would management use an adhocratic structure like the matrix? When flexibility is important for the organization's success. The matrix provides a focus on one person for all matters concerning the product, offers high human resource flexibility, and has the mechanisms to generally allow rapid response to product needs and client desires.

FIGURE 14–5 General Motors Corporation

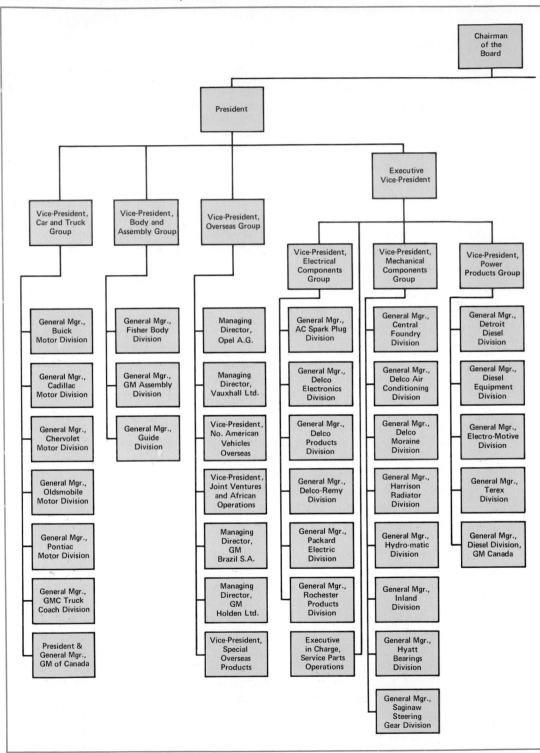

Source: Abridged organization through courtesy of General Motors, September 1980

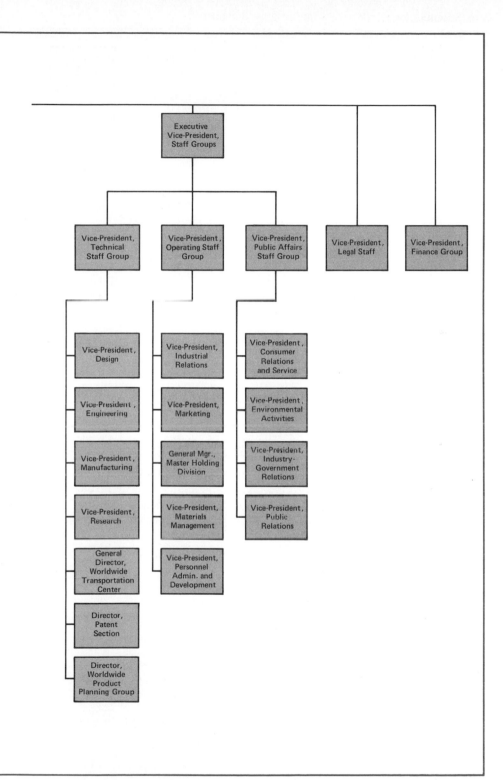

FIGURE 14–6   Matrix Structure for a College of Administrative Sciences

Academic Departments \ Programs	Undergraduate	Master's	Ph.D.	Research	Executive Programs	Community-Service Programs
Accounting						
Administrative and Environmental Studies						
Economics						
Finance						
Marketing						
Organizational Behavior						
Political Sciences						
Quantitative Methods						

KEY STRUCTURAL VARIABLES AND THEIR RELEVANCE TO OB

Now we move to the crux of our concern: relating structure to performance and satisfaction. This is no trivial task. The research on the structure-performance relationship, for instance, has been described as "among the most vexing and ambiguous in the field of management and organizational behavior."[23] Seven structural variables have received the bulk of the attention. As a result, the following analysis reviews the evidence as it relates only to these variables.[24] This is not a major shortcoming, however, since these seven include the essence of what we have called "organization structure."

23. Dan R. Dalton, William D. Tudor, Michael J. Spendolini, Gordon J. Fielding, and Lyman W. Porter, "Organization Structure and Performance: A Critical Review," *Academy of Management Review*, January 1980, p. 60.

24. This section has drawn on the findings and insights provided in Lyman W. Porter and Edward E. Lawler III, "Properties of Organization Structure in Relation to Job Attitudes and Job Behavior," *Psychological Bulletin*, July 1965, pp. 23–51; Lawrence R. James and Allan P. Jones, "Organization Structure: A Review of Structural Dimensions and Their Conceptual Relationships with Individual Attitudes and Behavior," *Organizational Behavior and Human Performance*, June 1976, pp. 74–113; Chris J. Berger and Larry L. Cummings, "Organizational Structure, Attitudes, and Behaviors," in *Research in Organizational Behavior*, Vol. 1, ed. Barry M. Staw (Greenwich, Conn.: JAI Press, 1979), pp. 169–208; and Dalton et al., "Organization Structure," pp. 49–64.

Size

If we look at the organization as a whole, there is evidence to tentatively suggest that job satisfaction tends to decrease with size. This is intuitively logical since larger size results in fewer opportunities for individuals to participate in decision making, less proximity and identification with organizational goals, and less clarity between individual effort and an identifiable outcome. Increased organizational size also appears to lead to higher absenteeism, though not necessarily greater turnover. The larger size offers less opportunity for an employee to identify with his or her organization but evidence suggests that larger organizations tend to pay better than smaller ones. The result is that individuals do not leave the larger organization but they do have a propensity to absent themselves more frequently from work. Interestingly, these findings may be moderated by the degree of decentralization. If increased size is accompanied by increased delegation of authority, the negative impact of size tends to be reduced.

The attention paid to the impact of size on performance and attitudes has not been focused solely at the total organization level. Concern has also been given to subunit size, that is, to the size of intraorganizational work units. There appears to be a definite positive relationship between subunit size and both absenteeism and turnover. This is in contrast to total organization size which, as we noted above, tends to be related only to absenteeism. Regarding job satisfaction, there seems to be no systematic and consistent relationship attributable to subunit size.

Organizational Level

Is satisfaction or performance affected by an employee's position in the vertical hierarchy? For instance, are senior executives more satisfied with their jobs than operatives or low-level supervisors?

In terms of structural variables, the most frequently investigated characteristic has been level in the organizational hierarchy. Although the evidence is far from conclusive, the bulk of the evidence finds that as we go up the hierarchy, we generally find more satisfied employees. Although one can debate causality, it seems unlikely that satisfied employees are getting more promotions than grumpy employees. It is far more logical to conclude that as one moves up in the organization, pay, formal authority, status, accouterments, and other rewards increase and, with them, job satisfaction.

Line versus Staff

The distinction is typically made in organizations between individuals with line authority and those with staff authority. Line personnel possess command authority, while staff personnel support and advise the line. Does this difference affect the attitudes and behavior of those involved?

The early evidence indicated that staff personnel derived less satisfaction from their jobs. This might have been due to the fact that staff jobs were more specialized and offered less opportunity for decision making. More recent studies suggest that there are no consistent, important differences in the satisfaction levels of persons in line and staff positions. It's possible that the traditional distinction between line and staff has in recent years become blurred in many organizations. It is not unusual nowadays for staff personnel to exert tremendous power over line managers as a result of their technical expertise. Therefore, while staff personnel may not enjoy positional authority, their satisfaction is not adversely affected because they have other power sources.

Span of Control

The term "span of control" refers to the number of subordinates who report directly to a manager. Does this variable influence employee performance or satisfaction?

A review of the research indicates that it is probably safe to say that there is no evidence to support a relationship between span of control and performance. While it is intuitively attractive to argue that large spans might lead to higher employee performance because these spans provide more distant supervision, more opportunity for personal initiative, and better communication, the research fails to support this notion. At this point it is impossible to state that any particular span of control is best for producing high performance or high satisfaction among subordinates. The most we can say is that there is some, but slight, evidence that a manager's job satisfaction increases as the number of subordinates he or she supervises increases.

Horizontal Differentiation

There have not been many studies that have looked at the horizontal differentiation—performance relationship. The preponderance of evidence suggests a positive relationship—that is, the greater the specialization, the higher the performance—but because the measures of performance tend to be questionable and several studies find no association, a realistic conclusion would be that the relationship between horizontal differentiation and performance has not been clearly demonstrated.

Evidence for the impact of horizontal differentiation on satisfaction is only a little more encouraging. Horizontal differentiation has generally been regarded as leading to lower satisfaction in that a large segment of the work force is turned off and alienated by having to do narrowly defined and repetitive tasks. However, as we shall show in the next chapter on job design, this conclusion must be moderated by individual differences. Some people prefer structured and narrowly defined work tasks, while others value autonomy and freedom. Again, a clear relationship between horizontal differentiation and satisfaction has not been demonstrated.

Vertical Differentiation

Are there significant differences in terms of employee performance and satisfaction in tall organizations (with many vertical levels) versus flat organizations? There are mixed findings on the performance dimension. Both positive and negative relationships are reported in reviews of the research, making it difficult to generalize. On the satisfaction dimension, it appears that vertical differentiation does matter. High-level managers in tall organizations and lower-level managers in flat organizations experience more satisfaction than their opposites.

Centralization

The last independent variable we shall look at is centralization. Although we must qualify our generalizations, there do seem to be some meaningful relationships between centralization and our dependent variables.

The evidence supports the conclusion that centralization is negatively related with performance. Although these studies were done with managerial and professional personnel—therefore limiting our ability to generalize to blue collar and nonprofessional employees—the evidence is nevertheless consistent.

There is limited evidence that—for a large segment of the work force—decentralization generates less job alienation, less dissatisfaction with work, greater satisfaction with supervision, and greater communication frequency among co-workers at the same level in the organization. Yet, even though centralization and satisfaction appear to be inversely related, this conclusion is likely to be moderated by individual differences and the type of tasks that employees perform. For instance, we would predict that this inverse relationship is likely to be stronger among professionals than among blue-collar workers.

IMPLICATIONS FOR PERFORMANCE AND SATISFACTION

This chapter has defined organization structure, explained its causes, presented a number of different ways in which structures may be designed, and then reviewed the evidence linking organization structure to performance and satisfaction. Our position is that an organization's internal structure contributes to explaining and predicting behavior. That is, in addition to individual differences and group factors, the structural relationships in which people work have an important bearing on employee attitudes and behavior.

In spite of our claim that structure is important, much of the research from which we have drawn our conclusions has fatal flaws. For instance, measures of performance and satisfaction are frequently open to question, as are definitions and instruments used to measure such variables as size and centralization. Additionally, some studies include only professionals, while others include only blue-collar workers. It is not surprising, therefore, that we find conflicting results and qualified conclusions.

The previous section summarized the best-known detailed reviews of the implications of structure on performance and satisfaction. In this section, let's extend the evidence and draw some general conclusions that—though certainly not definitively supported in the literature—nevertheless appear defensible.

Figure 14–7 visually depicts what we have discussed in this chapter. Size, technology, environment, and power-control determine the type of structure an organization will have. Complexity, formalization, and centralization represent the structural components that can be manipulated to form various structural designs. The better-known of these designs include the simple structure, bureaucracy, the functional form, the product form, and adhocracy. Let us now offer some general thoughts.

For a large proportion of the population, high structure—that is, high complexity, high formalization, and centralization—leads to reduced job satisfaction. High vertical differentiation tends to alienate lower-level employees because vertical communication becomes more difficult and one can feel like "low man on the totem pole." On the other hand, upper management undoubtedly finds that the rewards that go with their position enhance job satisfaction.

Specialization would also tend to be inversely related to satisfaction, especially where jobs have been divided into extremely minute tasks. This conclusion would have to be moderated to reflect individual differences among employees. While most prefer autonomy, not *all* do.

For individuals who value autonomy and self-actualization, large size, when accompanied by high centralization, results in lower satisfaction. As we

FIGURE 14–7 Organization Structure Model

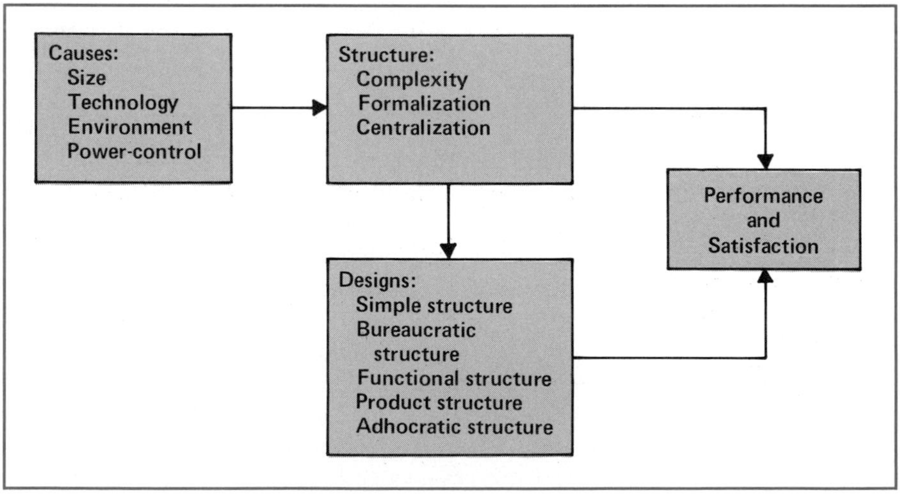

have noted, there are fewer opportunities to participate in decision making, less proximity and identification with organizational goals, and less feeling that individual effort is linked to an identifiable outcome. In other words, the larger the organization, the more difficult it is for the individual to see the impact of his or her contribution to the final goods or service produced.

Product structures and adhocracies increase cohesiveness among unit members, and more closely aligns their authority with the responsibility for completion of a particular assignment. For certain types of activities, these structures are undoubtedly superior from management's standpoint. For instance, if tasks are nonroutine and there exists a great deal of environmental uncertainty, the organization can be more responsive when structured along organic rather than mechanistic lines. But these more responsive structures provide both advantages and disadvantages to employees. They rarely have restrictive job descriptions or excessive rules and regulations, nor do they require workers to obey commands that are issued by distant executives. But they usually have overlapping layers of responsibility and play havoc with individuals who need the security of doing standardized tasks. To maximize employee performance and satisfaction, individual differences should be taken into account.[25] Individuals with a high degree of bureaucratic orientation tend to place a heavy reliance on higher authority, prefer formalized and specific rules, and prefer formal relationships with others on the job. These people are better suited to mechanistic structures. Those individuals with a low degree of bureaucratic orientation would be better suited to organic structures.[26]

25. Paul M. Nemiroff and David L. Ford, Jr., "Task Effectiveness and Human Fulfillment in Organizations: A Review and Development of a Conceptual Contingency Model," *Academy of Management Review,* October 1976, pp. 69–82.

26. Ibid., p. 74.

FOR DISCUSSION

1. What is meant by the term organization structure?

2. Describe the factors that determine how complex an organization is.

3. Which one of the following *most* determines structure: size, technology, environment, power-control? Explain.

4. Define and give examples of what is meant by the terms technology and environment.

5. Define a bureaucracy. Identify its key components. How prevalent is this structural form?

6. Which one of the following structures is least centralized: simple, bureaucratic, product? Why?

7. Under what conditions would management likely choose (a) a mechanistic structure? (b) an organic structure?

8. "Employees prefer to work in flat, decentralized organizations." Do you agree or disagree? Discuss.

9. What is the relationship between each of the following and employee performance and satisfaction: (a) size? (b) organizational level? (c) line versus staff? (d) span of control? (e) horizontal differentiation? (f) vertical differentiation? (g) centralization?

10. Do you think most employees prefer high formalization? Support your position.

FOR FURTHER READING

KATZ, D., and R. L. KAHN, *The Social Psychology of Organizations,* 2nd ed. New York: John Wiley, 1978. Highly sophisticated analysis of organizational design and processes from a systems perspective.

MINTZBERG, H., *The Structuring of Organizations,* chaps. 17–21. Englewood Cliffs, N.J.: Prentice-Hall, 1979. Describes the primary structural designs available to management.

ROBBINS, S. P., *Organization Theory: The Structure and Design of Organizations.* Englewood Cliffs: Prentice-Hall, 1983. Comprehensive discussion of topics introduced in this chapter.

SCOTT, W. G., "Organization Theory: A Reassessment," *Academy of Management Journal,* June 1974, pp. 242–54. Proposes that the values underlying current organization theory are no longer valid. Suggests a radical model based on current realities.

THOMPSON, J. D., *Organizations in Action*. New York: McGraw-Hill, 1967. Classic treatise in which the author argues that the fundamental problem facing organizations is uncertainty.

WHETTON, D. A., "Sources, Responses, and Effects of Organizational Decline," in *The Organization Life Cycle: Issues in the Creation, Transformations, and Decline of Organizations,* ed. J. Kimberly and R. H. Miles, pp. 342–74. San Francisco: Jossey-Bass, 1980. Organization theory has a growth bias. Decline is the forgotten stepchild—the other side of the growth-decline curve.

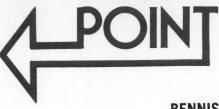

BENNIS

The coming death of bureaucracy

Adapted and edited from Warren G. Bennis, "The Coming Death of Bureaucracy," Think, November–December 1966, pp. 30–35. Reprinted by permission from Think Magazine, published by IBM, copyright 1966 by International Business Machines Corporation.

A short while ago, I predicted that we would, in the next twenty-five to fifty years, participate in the end of bureaucracy as we know it and in the rise of new social systems better suited to the twentieth-century demands of industrialization. This forecast was based on the evolutionary principle that every age develops an organizational form appropriate to its genius, and that the prevailing form, known by sociologists as bureaucracy and by most businessmen as "damn bureaucracy," was out of joint with contemporary realities. I realize now that my distant prophecy is already a distinct reality so the prediction is already foreshadowed by practice.

I should like to make clear that by bureaucracy I mean a chain of command structured on the lines of a pyramid—the typical structure that coordinates the business of almost every human organization we know of: industrial, governmental, of universities and research and development laboratories, military, religious, voluntary.

The bureaucratic "machine model" was developed as a reaction against the personal subjugation, nepotism and cruelty, and the capricious and subjective judgments which passed for managerial practices during the early days of the In-

dustrial Revolution. Bureaucracy emerged out of the organizations' need for order and precision and the workers' demands for impartial treatment. It was an organization ideally suited to the values and demands of the Victorian era. And just as bureaucracy emerged as a creative response to a radically new age, so today new organizational-shapes are surfacing before our eyes.

There are at least four relevant threats to bureaucracy:

1. *Rapid and unexpected change*—Bureaucracy's strength is its capacity to efficiently manage the routine and predictable in human affairs. Bureaucracy, with its nicely defined chain of command, its rules and its rigidities, is ill adapted to the rapid change out the environment now demands.

2. *Growth in size*—While, in theory, there may be no natural limit to the height of a bureaucratic pyramid, in practice the element of complexity is almost invariably introduced with great size.

3. *Increasing diversity*—Today's activities require persons of very diverse, highly specialized competence.

Hurried growth, rapid change, and increase in specialization pit these three factors against the components of the pyramid structure, and we should expect the pyramid of bureaucracy to begin crumbling.

4. *Change in managerial behavior*—There is, I believe, a subtle but perceptible change in the philosophy underlying management behavior. Real change seems under way because of:

a. A new concept of *man,* based on increased knowledge of his complex and shifting needs, which replaces an oversimplified, innocent, push-button idea of man.

b. A new concept of *power,* based on collaboration and reason, which replaces a model of power based on coercion and threat.

c. A new concept of *organizational values,* based on humanistic-democratic ideals, which replaces the depersonalized mechanistic value system of bureaucracy.

The real push for these changes stems from the need not only to humanize the organization, but to use it as a crucible of personal growth and development of self-realization.

The social structure of organizations of the future will have some unique characteristics. The key word will be "temporary." There will be adaptive, rapidly changing *temporary* systems. These will be task forces organized around problems-to-be-solved by groups of realtive strangers with diverse professional skills. The groups will be arranged on an organic rather than a mechanical model; they will evolve in response to a problem rather than to programmed role expectations. The executive thus becomes a coordinator or "linking pin" between various task forces. He must be a man who can speak the polyglot jargon of research, with skills to relay information and to mediate between groups. People will be evaluated not vertically according to rank and status, but flexibly and functionally according to skill and professional training. Organizational charts will consist of project groups rather than stratified functional groups. (This trend is already visible in the aerospace and construction industries, as well as many professional and consulting firms.)

Adaptive, problem-solving, temporary systems of diverse specialists, linked together by coordinating and task-evaluating executive specialists in an organic flux—this is the organization form that will gradually replace bureaucracy as we know it. As no catchy phrase comes to mind, I call this an organic-adaptive structure. Organizational arrangements of this sort may not only reduce intergroups conflicts; they may also induce honest-to-goodness creative collaboration.

The organic-adaptive structure should increase motivation and thereby effectiveness, because it enhances satisfactions intrinsic to the task. There is a harmony between the educated individual's need for tasks that are meaningful, satisfactory, and creative in a flexible organizational structure.

In these new organizations of the future, participants will be called upon to use their minds more than at any other time in history. Fantasy, imagination, and creativity will be legitimate in ways that today seem strange. Social structures will no longer be instruments of psychic repression but will increasingly promote play and freedom on behalf of curiosity and thought.

COUNTER POINT

MIEWALD

The greatly exaggerated death of bureaucracy

Adapted and edited from Robert D. Miewald, "The Greatly Exaggerated Death of Bureaucracy." © 1970 by the Regents of the University of California. Reprinted from California Management Review, *Vol. 13, No. 2, pp. 65–69 by permission of the Regents.*

The inevitable revolution in the conditions of life within the organization is heralded by experts in administrative theory. Warren Bennis, in particular, seems to have caught the fancy of many by describing this coming breakthrough in terms of some exciting predictions about the death of bureaucracy and the evolution of a "postbureaucratic" managerial system. Certainly there can be no doubt that the organization is changing, but will the change in direction leave the specter of bureaucracy far behind? Quite the contrary, it can be argued that the forces of bureaucratization were never in finer fettle, and, indeed, that the very same theorists who are singing the dirge have had much to do with the rejuvenation of bureaucracy.

The perspective of all modern scholars on the subject of bureaucracy is probably conditioned by the extent of their exposure to the pioneering work of Max Weber. Genius though he was, Weber was not prescient; he could not have foreseen all the many forms that the essence of bureaucracy could take. His formulation of the concept of bureaucracy has provided an invaluable tool for the analysis of organizational problems in a society that is making the adjustment to industrialization. However, rather than making the superficial assumption that "postindustrial" means "postbureaucratic," it might be wiser for today's students to inquire whether bureaucracy can adjust to the new age which, so the sociologists and economists insist, we have recently entered. Bennis, for example, believes that the transition in administrative thought from mechanical to organic models will be fatal to bureaucracy. But is bureaucracy restricted to the mechanical? In many cases it would appear that external bureaucratic constraints have simply been replaced by more subtle influences on the individual. The end result in either case is the same: a high degree of predictability about human behavior within the large, complex organization.

For Weber, any historical bureaucracy was merely a concrete manifestation of the inexorable process of "demystification," which was conquering the world. This process is independent of specific forms; the true essence of bureaucratization feeds upon that which will make affairs of men more amenable to rational calculation. Given the administrative technology of the nineteenth century and his familiarity with the authoritarian tendencies of the Germans, it is little wonder that Weber described the bureaucratic instrument as he did. He would hardly have been surprised, however, to learn that more sophisticated means of controlling behavior had been invented. Weber's main scholarly concern, then, was with the progressive rationalization of the world and its impact on human relationships.

Bureaucracy, in the Weberian scheme of things, is only "the most rational offspring" of the social phenomenon called discipline. This neutral, impersonal force permitted large numbers of people to be coordinated in efforts aimed at the methodical accomplishment of formal goals. If the worker can be indoctrinated to accept the discipline of the organization, then his behavior can be calculated, along with nonhuman production factors, in a formula for optimum productivity. As Weber noted, it was the recognition of the need for such calculation in terms of the human resources that accounted for the success of the American brand of management. A rational discipline, in short, is the underlying strength of the bureaucratic structure.

And now we may ask, how does the so-called postbureaucratic situation differ from the administrative style that one might reasonably expect in a completely demystified milieu? Of course, as most laymen can testify, it does not differ at all in any significant sense, and one might want to argue that in the most critical areas, the postbureaucratic system is nothing more than the Weberian model with all the more sophisticated modifications. Despite all the agonized contortions that management specialists have put themselves through in the twentieth century, the remarkable fact remains that there has been no substantial change in their basic premises. The guiding belief is still that those regularities exist which, on one level or another, may be learned and acted upon. Whether the knowledge is embodied in the "bounded rationality" of a formal bureaucratic structure or in the professional's internalized determinants of behavior, administration is nothing more than the pursuit of a limited concept of rational discipline.

In reviewing the literature of a half-century of management science, one comes to the conclusion that bureaucracy is not dead, but rather that the most controversial element of the Weberian model is gradually being replaced by a less artificial and more effective variation. This troublesome element is the nature of authority in an organization based on knowledge. Management science, at whatever stage in its growth, has not been concerned with eliminating bureaucracy, but instead with improving it by finding a way around the dilemma of knowledge and authority in an organization with a unilinear definition of rationality. The language used by several generations of theorists retains the same flavor.

It must be emphasized that Weber himself would not have been relieved by the claims of those who say the struggle against bureaucracy is over. In a brilliant analysis of Weber's political sociology, Wolfgang Mommsen argues that Weber attached the highest priority to the free development of the individual personality. He was, of course, too much a product of his culture to endorse the glorification of the irrational, but he did regard the conclusions that arose from his many sociological studies with despair; the universal rationalization of life was depriving the personality of its grand role as the final arbiter of values. In more familiar Weberian terminology, the process of demystification was robbing the charismatic impulse of its vitality, of its creative force in society. During his lifetime, Weber's personal preference for a dynamic society in which the individual retains the largest possible number of options was being made obsolete by the irresistible drive toward greater predictability of behavior.

It is not too much to say, then, that Weber would conclude that bureaucracy is still alive and well. And this is the essential point that students of administration must come to realize if they are going to attack effectively the multiple crises of our era. To find specific elements of Weber's model of bureaucracy poorly adjusted to our times is a reasonable concession to the fact that conditions do change. But this is not the same as eliminating bureaucracy, for, in the most profound sense, bureaucracy will be with us as long as men insist that there is only one perception of reality by which rationality can be measured.

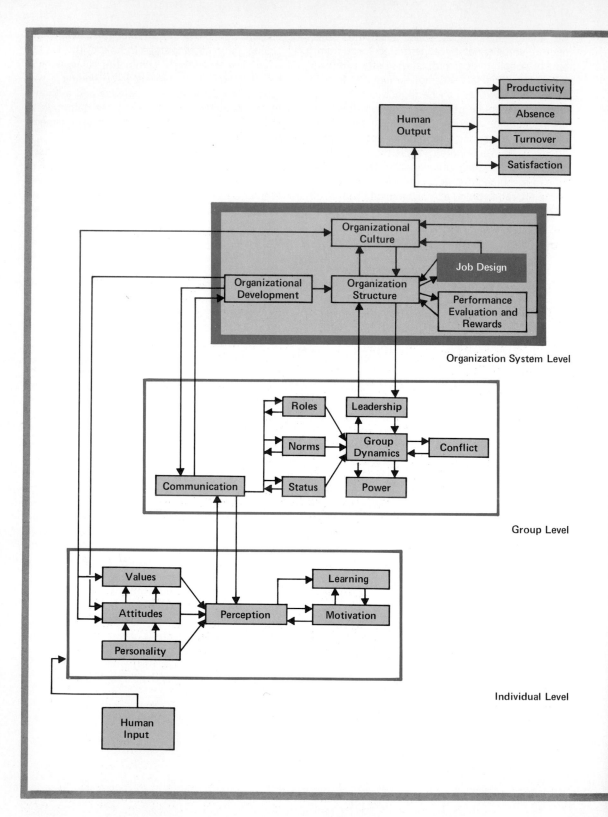

CHAPTER 15

Job Design

AFTER STUDYING THIS CHAPTER, YOU SHOULD BE ABLE TO—

Define and explain the following key terms and concepts:

Autonomous work teams
Autonomy
Feedback
Flex-time
Growth need strength
Integrated work teams
Job characteristics model
Job design
Job enlargment
Job enrichment
Job redesign

Job rotation
Motivating potential score
Quality circles
Scientific management
Shorter workweek
Skill variety
Sociotechnical systems
Task identity
Task significance
Work modules

Understand:

What is job design
The evolution of job design
The characteristics that make jobs different
Current design options available to management

> On too many jobs, nine-to-five seems like five-to-life.
>
> —S.P.R.

Jobs are different. On that point there can be little debate. It's also true that individuals perceive certain jobs as more desirable than others. However, what *you* consider to be a routine and boring job, someone *else* is very likely to view as quite satisfying. So while jobs can be objectively differentiated, we cannot say that everyone would find the job of theatre critic for the *Chicago Sun Times* interesting and challenging. Nor can we say that filing credit card applications alphabetically for eight hours a day, five days a week, at the American Express office in New York would be universally considered a dull job. As we learned in Part 2 of this book, individuals have different needs and preferences. This should show up in their preference for jobs. And, of course, it does. In fact, most organizations go to a great deal of trouble to select individuals who will fit smoothly into the organization and the job vacancy to be filled. The evidence indicates that certain individuals are attracted to and selected by certain types of organizations.[1] Those entrepreneurial individuals who like to see things happen fast, like to take risks, and are more loners than team players are typically turned off by large mechanistic organizations—and such organizations can be expected to be turned off by this type of individual. This is consistent with the literature on personnel selection. Organizations use tests, interviews, and other selection devices to find the right match between the organization's characteristics and an applicant's personal and background attributes. But additionally, research demonstrates that job characteristics mediate the relationship between organization structure and employee reactions.[2] That is, structural properties affect the characteristics of employees' jobs. So, for instance, organization structures that are highly formalized and centralized tend to be negatively associated with employee descriptions of the amount of autonomy, variety, and feedback in their jobs.[3]

The way jobs are designed, therefore, influences employee performance

1. See, for example, Greg R. Oldham and J. Richard Hackman, "Relationships between Organizational Structure and Employee Reactions: Comparing Alternative Frameworks," *Administrative Science Quarterly*, March 1981, pp. 66–83.

2. Ibid.

3. Jon L. Pierce and Randall B. Dunham, "An Empirical Demonstration of the Convergence of Common Macro-and-Micro-Organization Measures," *Academy of Management Journal*, September 1978, pp. 410–18.

FIGURE 15–1

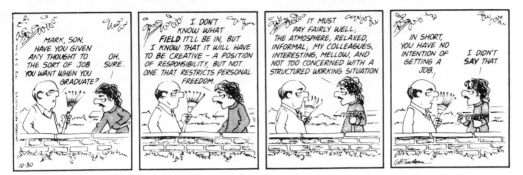

Source: Copyright 1973, G. B. Trudeau. Distributed by Universal Press Syndicate.

and satisfaction. But how? Given that jobs are different, what are these differences? And how do these differences affect employee performance and satisfaction? These are questions this chapter seeks to answer.

WHAT IS JOB DESIGN?

The term *job design* refers to the way that tasks are combined to form complete jobs. Some jobs are routine because the tasks are standardized and repetitive; others are nonroutine. Some require a large number of varied and diverse skills; others are narrow in scope. Some jobs constrain employees by requiring them to follow very precise procedures; others allow employees substantial freedom in how they do their work. Our point is that jobs differ as to the way their tasks are combined.

A term closely aligned with job design is *job redesign*. When jobs are changed, then job redesign takes place. More specifically, job redesign refers to any activities that involve the alteration of specific jobs (or interdependent systems of jobs) that seeks to increase both the quality of an employee's work experience and on-the-job productivity.[4] In the following pages, we shall discuss job design and then propose various redesign options available to management. Particular attention will be focused on how given redesign options affect employee productivity, absence, turnover, and satisfaction.

HISTORICAL DEVELOPMENT OF JOB DESIGN

It's very hard to pick up any recent business periodical and *not* find an article about some company or government agency introducing a four-day workweek,

4. J. Richard Hackman, "Work Design" in *Improving Life at Work,* ed. J. Richard Hackman and J. Lloyd Suttle (Santa Monica, Calif.: Goodyear, 1977), p. 98.

flexible work hours, Japanese-style participation groups, autonomous work teams, or some similar job redesign. This may lead you to think of job design as a relatively new topic. This is far from the case.

The content and design of jobs has interested engineers and economists for centuries. In its early years, job design was really nothing more than a synonym for job specialization. In 1776, for instance, Adam Smith articulated in his *Wealth of Nations* the economic efficiencies that could be achieved by dividing jobs into smaller and smaller pieces so each worker could perform a minute and specialized task. Undoubtedly one of the most important early efforts at job design was undertaken at the turn of this century by Frederick Taylor in what has become known as the Scientific Management movement.

Scientific Management

In the early 1900s, Frederick Taylor proposed scientific management principles designed to maximize production efficiency. He sought to replace the seat-of-the-pants approach for determining each element of a worker's job with a scientific approach. The centerpiece of scientific management was the elimination of time and motion waste. How was this done? By carefully studying jobs to determine the most efficient way it could be completed. Jobs were partitioned into small and simple segments and the workers were given specific instructions on how each segment was to be done.

The results of Taylor's efforts—in economic terms—were nothing short of spectacular. He was consistently able to achieve productivity improvements in the range of 200 percent or more. Many workers, however, did not like the jobs designed according to the dictates of scientific management. They found the repetitive work depersonalized, boring, and unchallenging. Because their jobs often represented small "cogs" in a big "wheel," employees increasingly complained that their work was meaningless. To offset the boredom of their highly repetitive jobs, workers would do things that were not always in the best interest of the organization. They came to work late, they took three- or four-day weekends, and they quit to find more interesting work.

Probably one of the most publicized reactions to overspecialized jobs was the action by automobile assembly-line workers in the early 1970s at the Lordstown, Ohio, Chevrolet plant. Workers were found to be welding empty soda pop bottles inside doors, purposely gouging the paint on cars as they went by, and engaging in other dysfunctional behaviors. The Lordstown workers, it was said, were frustrated and looking for ways to overcome the dull, repetitive, and unchallenging tasks they were assigned. Welding a bottle inside a door or putting a deep scratch into a car's paint without getting caught provided a diversionary outlet.

The Lordstown events occurred in the early 1970s, but the recognition that a good thing—work simplification—could be carried too far began to get attention in the late 1940s and early 1950s. As a result of insights from psychologists, sociologists, and other social scientists, attention began to shift to the human needs of people. The jobs themselves had been engineered to be efficiently performed by robotlike workers. But people are not robots. They have needs and feelings. No matter how well-engineered a job is, if the design fails to consider the human element, the economies of specialization could be more than offset by the diseconomies of employee dissatisfaction. And on many jobs, this is exactly what was happening. So attention became increasingly focused on job design approaches that would make work less routine and more meaningful.

Job Enlargement

One of the first approaches was to expand jobs horizontally, or what we call *job enlargement.* Increasing the number and variety of tasks that an individual performed resulted in jobs with more diversity. Instead of only sorting the incoming mail by department, for instance, a mail sorter's job could be enlarged to include physically delivering the mail to the various departments or running outgoing letters through the postage meter.

Efforts at job enlargement met with less than enthusiastic results. As one employee who experienced such a redesign on his job remarked to your author, "Before I had one lousy job. Now, through enlargement, I have three!"

So, while job enlargement attacked the lack of diversity in overspecialized jobs, it did little to instill challenge or meaningfulness to a worker's activities. Job enrichment was introduced to deal with the shortcomings of enlargement.

Job Enrichment

Job enrichment refers to the vertical expansion of jobs. It increases the degree to which the worker controls the planning, execution, and evaluation of his or her job. An enriched job organizes tasks so as to allow workers to do a complete activity, increases the employee's freedom and independence, increases responsibility, and provides feedback so individuals will be able to assess and correct their own performance.

Reports of organizations implementing job enrichment programs have been well publicized and the importance of the concept requires that it be given an expanded discussion. Such a discussion will be undertaken later in this chapter. From an historical perspective, it is sufficient to note that job enrichment essentially developed in the 1960s as a response to employee dissatisfaction and productivity problems that excessive specialization created. The interest it initiated continues through to today.

Sociotechnical Systems

Another job design innovation of the 1960s was the concept of sociotechnical systems. Like job enlargement and enrichment, this approach represented a response to the overly narrow scientific management view of job design.

Sociotechnical systems is more a philosophy toward job design than a specific technique. Its central theme is that job design must address both the technical and the social aspects of the organization if work systems are to produce greater employee productivity and higher personal fulfillment for organization members. Every job has technological aspects. But technical tasks are performed in an environment influenced by a culture, a set of values, and generally acceptable organization practices. Redesign efforts that look only at the technical aspects of a job are likely to overlook critical factors that influence employee performance and satisfaction.

Advocates of sociotechnical systems provided no explicit guidance in exactly how the work, the social surroundings, and the organization interact. Their suggestions, however, did rely heavily on group-oriented approaches to work. The idea of work teams, which we shall discuss later in this chapter, evolved out of the sociotechnical systems philosophy. The notion that there are a number of interrelated factors that eventually influence the success or failure of a job design effort—which we shall discuss in the next section—undoubtedly is also rooted in sociotechnical systems.

Summary

Scientific management, job enlargement and enrichment ideas, and the sociotechnical systems philosophy have each left their imprint on current job design efforts. But where are we today? If there is presently one overwhelming influence on the design of jobs, it is clearly the job characteristics model which developed during the 1970s. This model offers us some very tangible "handles" from which to guide and implement job redesign efforts. Importantly, it also allows us to look at a particular job and to predict how the structure of that job will influence the performance and satisfaction of its incumbent.

THE JOB CHARACTERISTICS MODEL

The most complete framework we have available for analyzing a job's design is the job characteristics model.[5] It identifies five job characteristics, their interrelationships, and their predicted impact on employee productivity, motivation, and satisfaction.

Core Dimensions

According to the model, any job can be described in terms of five core job dimensions which are defined as follows:

1. *Skill variety*—the degree to which a job requires a variety of different activities so the worker can use a number of different skills and talents.
2. *Task identity*—the degree to which the job requires completion of a whole and identifiable piece of work.

5. J. Richard Hackman and Greg R. Oldham, "Development of the Job Diagnostic Survey," *Journal of Applied Psychology*, April 1975, pp. 159–70.

3. *Task significance*—the degree to which the job has a substantial impact on the lives or work of other people.
4. *Autonomy*—the degree to which the job provides substantial freedom, independence, and discretion to the individual in scheduling the work and in determining the procedures to be used in carrying it out.
5. *Feedback*—the degree to which carrying out the work activities required by the job results in the individual obtaining direct and clear information about the effectiveness of his or her performance.

Interrelationships

Figure 15–2 presents the model. Notice how the first three dimensions—skill variety, task identity, and task significance—combine to create meaningful work. That is, if these three characteristics exist in a job, we can predict the incumbent will view the job as being important, valuable, and worthwhile. Notice, too, that jobs that possess autonomy give the job incumbent a feeling of personal responsibility for the results; and that if a job provides feedback, the employee

FIGURE 15–2 The Job Characteristics Model

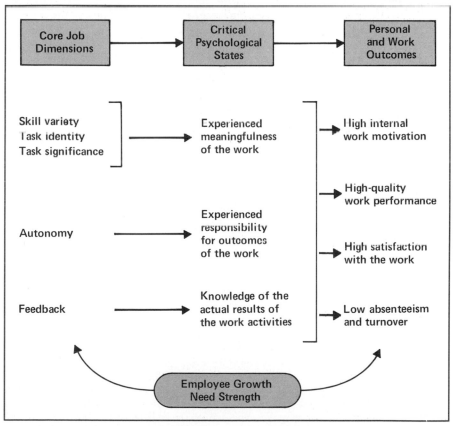

Source: J. Richard Hackman, "Work Design," in *Improving Life at Work*, ed. J. R. Hackman and J. L. Suttle (Santa Monica, Calif.: Scott, Foresman and Company, 1977), p. 129.

will know how effectively he or she is performing. From a motivational stand-point, the model says that internal rewards are obtained by an individual when he *learns* (knowledge of results) that he *personally* (experienced responsibility) has performed well on a task that he *cares about* (experienced meaningful-ness).[6] The more that these three psychological states are present, the greater will be the employee's motivation, performance, and satisfaction; and the lower his absenteeism and likelihood of leaving the company. As the model shows, the links between the job dimensions and the outcomes are moderated or ad-justed for by the strength of the individual's growth need, that is, by the employ-ee's desire for self-esteem and self-actualization. This means that individuals with a high growth need are more likely to experience the psychological states when their jobs are enriched than are their counterparts with a low growth need. Moreover, they will respond more positively to the psychological states, when they are present, than will low growth need individuals.

Predictions from the Model

The core job dimensions can be combined into a single predictive index, called the motivating potential score (MPS). Its computation is shown in Figure 15–3.

Jobs that are high on motivating potential must be high on at least one of the three factors that lead to experiencing meaningfulness, and they must be high on both autonomy and feedback. If jobs score high on motivating poten-tial, the model predicts that motivation, performance, and satisfaction will be positively affected, while the likelihood of absence and turnover is lessened.

The job characteristics model is still undergoing testing. For instance, there is increasing evidence that task identity fails to add to the model's predictive ability; that skill variety may be redundant with autonomy; and that merely add-ing all the variables rather than adding some and multiplying by others may achieve equally predictive scores.[7] Yet the overall evidence is certainly encour-aging. Future "fine-tuning" of its components and relationships will enhance its predictive accuracy, but we can still make the following statements with relative confidence:

1. People who work on jobs with high core job dimensions are more motivated, satisfied, and productive than those who do not.
2. People with strong growth needs respond more positively to jobs that are high in motivating potential than do those with weak growth needs.
3. Job dimensions operate through the psychological states in influencing person-al and work outcome variables, rather than influencing them directly.[8]

6. Hackman, "Work Design," p. 129.

7. See Randall B. Dunham, "Measurement and Dimensionality of Job Characteristics," *Journal of Applied Psychology,* August 1976, pp. 404–09; Jon L. Pierce and Randall B. Dunham, "Task Design: A Literature Review," *Academy of Management Review,* January 1976, pp. 83–97; and Denise M. Rousseau, "Technological Differences in Job Characteristics, Employee Satisfaction, and Motivation: A Synthesis of Job Design Research and Sociotechnical Systems Theory," *Organizational Behavior and Human Performance,* October 1977, pp. 18–42.

8. Hackman, "Work Design," pp. 132–33.

FIGURE 15–3 Computing a Motivating Potential Score

$$\text{Motivating Potential Score} = \left[\frac{\text{Skill variety} + \text{Task identity} + \text{Task significance}}{3} \right] \times \text{Autonomy} \times \text{Feedback}$$

A little more speculative are predictions that are based on integration of the job characteristics model and types of organization structure.[9] Researchers defined organization structures as mechanistic or organic, job design as simple or complex, and employee growth need strength as low or high. They then sought to determine how the mix of these variables influenced worker response. It was found that employee satisfaction, motivation, and performance were highest when there was congruence across the variables—that is, when organic structure, complex jobs, and high growth needs were combined or when mechanistic structure, simple jobs, and low growth needs were combined. The lowest levels of satisfaction, motivation, and performance occurred where high growth need individuals were in simple jobs and mechanistic structures. While further research is needed to confirm these findings, it is a beginning to the linking of job characteristics, individual differences, and organizational structures.

Summary

Any job can be analyzed using the job characteristics model. The data from this analysis can then be aggregated to compute the job's MPS score. This score, when coupled with knowledge of the job incumbent's growth need strength and the overall organization's structure, can allow us to make predictions about the employee's satisfaction, motivation, and performance.

Of course, from a normative standpoint, the model can also guide us in the design of jobs. It suggests that if an employee's growth need strength is low, standardized and simplified jobs should not be a barrier to high performance and satisfaction. But if growth need strength is high, management should consider forming natural work units to increase task identity and task significance; combining tasks to increase skill variety and task significance; involving the employee more with clients or customers to increase skill variety, autonomy, and feedback; giving the employee more say and responsibility in planning and evaluating his or her work to increase autonomy; and opening communication channels, especially channels flowing directly from the job itself, to increase feedback.[10]

9. Jon L. Pierce, Randall B. Dunham, and Richard S. Blackburn, "Social Systems Structure, Job Design, and Growth Need Strength: A Test of a Congruency Model," *Academy of Management Journal,* June 1979, pp. 223–40.

10. Hackman, "Work Design," pp. 136–40.

CURRENT REDESIGN OPTIONS

A number of redesign options have been suggested for improving the quality of work life. Some have been widely adopted, while others have never acquired much of a following. In this section we shall review various redesign options available to management.

Job Rotation

Job rotation allows workers increased skill variety by permitting them to shift jobs periodically. When an activity no longer is challenging, the employee would be rotated to another job, at the same level, that has similar skill requirements. The shifts can include as few as two people—the rotation being merely an exchange of jobs. However, the organization can provide much more elaborate rotation designs where a dozen or more employees are involved. The latter case would describe, for instance, the practices in the headquarters of some of the largest U.S. banks. New college graduates are hired with the idea that in three or four years they will be able to assume managerial positions in the bank. Their training consists of spending four to six months in all the key areas of the bank— operations, lending, trusts, and so forth. At about the time they have gained a reasonable understanding of an activity, they are rotated to a new area.

The strength of job rotation is that it reduces boredom through diversifying the employee's activities. Of course, it can also have indirect benefits for the organization since employees with a wider range of skills give management more flexibility in scheduling work, adapting to changes, and filling vacancies. The drawbacks to job rotation center around costs, disruptions, and its rather limited impact on enhancing job meaningfulness. Shifting people around has costs. Even though the same skill levels are assumed, productivity is typically adversely effected in the short term. The loss of efficiencies derived through experience can be substantial. Job rotations also create disruptions. Members of the work group have to adjust to the new employee. The supervisor may also have to spend more time answering questions and monitoring the work of the recently rotated employee. Finally, rotation is a weak solution to jobs that score low on motivating potential. Since job rotation doesn't really change the job, merely the job-employee mix, employees are unlikely to have experienced greater meaningfulness from their work by having done four boring jobs during a given year instead of one.

Work Modules

If you can conceive of extremely rapid job rotation, to the point where one would assume new activities every few hours, you can comprehend the technique of work modules. The work modules concept has been suggested as a solution to meet the problem of fractionated, boring, and programmed work, at an acceptable price, with undiminished quality and quantity of product.[11]

11. Robert L. Kahn, "The Work Module," *Psychology Today*, February 1973, pp. 35–39.

Professor Robert Kahn of the University of Michigan has defined a work module as a time task unit, equal to approximately two hours of work at a given task. A normal forty-hour-a-week job would then be defined in terms of four modules a day, five days a week, for between forty-eight and fifty weeks a year.

Through the use of modules, it would be possible to increase work diversity and give employees a greater opportunity to determine the nature of their jobs. Employees could request a set of modules that would together constitute a day's work. Additionally, those tasks that are characteristically seen as undesirable could be spread about, for example, by having everyone take a module or two each day. The result would be that people would change activities through changing work modules.

One benefit of work modules includes letting employees pick their work tasks, thus taking into account individual job preferences. Further, it provides a way for the more boring and undesirable tasks to get completed without totally demoralizing those people who must do them. Finally, since employees would be allowed some say in the choice of modules, the job would be constructed to meet the needs of the individual, rather than forcing people to fit a particularly defined job.

However, work modules would present the same cost and disruption obstacles as job rotation. Considerable time and money are involved in planning and executing the changeover. Bookkeeping and payroll computation costs increase. Conflicts can also develop over the question of equity and allocation of modules.

Are there any organizations that have tried work modules? If there are, they have received no publicity. The closest approximation that your author is familiar with is the practice in some firms of allowing workers in a specific group of jobs to trade activities each day after lunch. But these are isolated practices representing fewer than 100 employees in corporations that employ tens of thousands.

Job Enrichment

We introduced job enrichment earlier as the vertical expansion of jobs. In this section we shall discuss the concept at greater length. As you will see, job enrichment is important because it fulfills almost all of the requirements for high motivation potential as defined by the job characteristics model.

A job is enriched by allowing the worker to assume some of the tasks executed by his or her supervisor. Enriched jobs are vertically expanded so that employees take on additional responsibility to plan, execute, and inspect their work. Successful job enrichment should, in addition to increasing responsibility, also increase the freedom and independence of employees, organize tasks so as to allow workers to do a complete activity, and provide feedback so individuals will be able to correct their own performance.

A successful job enrichment program should ideally increase employee satisfaction. But since organizations do not exist to create employee satisfaction as an end, there must also be direct benefits to the organization. There is evidence that job enrichment produces lower absenteeism and reduced turnover costs; but on the critical issue of productivity, the evidence is inconclusive. In some situations, job enrichment has increased productivity; in others, productivity has been decreased. However, when it decreases, there does appear to be consistently conscientious use of resources and a higher quality of product or service. In other words, in terms of efficiency, for the same input a higher quality of output is obtained.

There is no shortage of examples where job enrichment has been implemented. Enriched jobs have been introduced at organizations as diverse as Texas Instruments,[12] Bankers Trust,[13] the Buick Division of General Motors,[14] and Travelers Insurance.[15] Just what enrichment efforts might look like can be seen in the following descriptions of its implementation within the Buick Product Engineering group and in key punching operations at Travelers Insurance.

Buick Product Engineering. The Buick Product Engineering group decided in the early 1970s to analyze the job of Assembler for enriching. An Assembler is a skilled hourly mechanic, responsible for performing experimental changes in fleet cars as ordered by the Design Engineers and for keeping the fleet cars in top operating condition. The Product Engineering group included forty-five Assemblers.

The Assembler's content of daily tasks was restructured and redefined, but the job description itself was not changed. Job modifications included such things as allowing the Assembler to:

Correct any deficiencies discovered and to record the action on a work sheet (this job modification was selected as the most practical for initial introduction)

Choose his own work assignment

Contact the Design Engineers directly

Inspect his own work

Establish his own completion dates and job hour content.

Presentations concerning the proposed job restructuring were made to departmental management, the Design Engineers, and the union. An informal approach was used to introduce the program to the Assemblers. Each foreman handled implementation according to his assessment of the best way to approach his employees. He determined the feelings in his own group and in most cases introduced additional job modifications on a man-to-man basis. Accep-

---

12. E. D. Week, "Job Enrichment 'Cleans Up' at Texas Instruments," in *New Perspectives in Job Enrichment* ed. J. R. Maher (New York: Van Nostrand Reinhold, 1971).

13. W. Philip Kraft and Kathleen L. Williams, "Job Redesign Improves Productivity," *Personnel Journal,* July 1975, pp. 393–97.

14. F. J. Schotters, "Job Enrichment at Buick Products Engineering," *GM Personnel Development Bulletin,* No. 22, June 4, 1973.

15. J. Richard Hackman, G. R. Oldham, R. Janson, and K. Purdy, "A New Strategy for Job Enrichment," *California Management Review,* Summer 1975, pp. 57–71.

tance of the project was fostered by the Assemblers themselves, who often "sold" the program to each other through informal discussions.

One of the ways that each supervisor tracked project progress was by recording the reactions from his Assemblers. In some cases implementation of the job modifications was too fast and negative feedback occurred—"How come I have to write these tickets? Did they take all the pencils away from the engineers?"

During the early stages of the program, some Design Engineers also expressed objections to the redefined duties. However, as communication between Assemblers and Design Engineers improved and as additional phases of job restructuring were introduced, most difficulties were worked out through face-to-face discussion.

This interpersonal approach prevented the program from becoming a "management directive" and resulted in management credibility and in employee acceptance of the project.

Since implementation of the job enrichment program, the following changes have been observed by Product Engineering supervision:

> Productivity has increased nearly 13 percent (as measured by increased work tickets per Assembler per month).

> Petty grievances have been virtually eliminated.

> Fleet cars are kept in better mechanical condition because Assemblers have shown initiative in discovering and repairing such discrepancies as rattles, steering gear whine, defective exhaust systems, and engine starting problems.

> Departmental morale has improved considerably, along with increased pride and interest in the work.

> Communication and personal relationships between and among Assemblers, foremen, and Design Engineers have increased and improved. (Assemblers now call or visit engineers to discuss projects personally.)

Travelers Insurance. This large insurance company was displeased with the performance of its keypunch operators. Output seemed inadequate, the error rate excessive, and absenteeism too high. A review of the job found it to rate low on the core job dimensions identified in the job characteristics model. The following changes were introduced:

1. The random assignment of work was replaced by assigning to each operator continuing responsibility for certain accounts.
2. Some planning and control functions were combined with the central task of keypunching.
3. Each operator was given several channels of direct contact with clients. When problems arose, the operator, not the supervisor, took them up with the client.
4. Operators were given the authority to set their own schedules, plan their daily work, and correct obvious coding errors on their own.
5. Incorrect cards were returned by the computer department to the operators who punched them, and the operators corrected their own errors. Weekly computer printouts of errors and productivity were sent directly to the operator rather than the supervisor.

The above enrichment efforts led to some impressive results. Fewer key-punch operators were needed, the quantity of output increased, error rates and absenteeism were reduced, and job attitudes improved. The changes reportedly saved Travelers over $90,000 a year.

Integrated Work Teams

If job enlargement is practiced at the group rather than individual level, you have integrated work teams. For jobs that require teamwork and cooperation, this approach can increase diversity for team members.

What would an integrated work team look like? Basically, instead of performing a single task, a large number of tasks would be assigned to a group. The group then would decide the specific assignments of members and be responsible for rotating jobs among the members as the tasks required. The team would still have a supervisor who would oversee the group's activities. You see the frequent use of integrated work teams in such activities as building maintenance and construction. In the cleaning of a sizeable office building, it is not unusual for the foreman to identify the tasks to be completed and then to let the maintenance workers, as a group, choose how the tasks will be allocated. Similarly, a road construction crew frequently decides, as a group, how its various tasks are to be completed.

Autonomous Work Teams

Autonomous work teams represent job enrichment at the group level. The work that the team does is deepened through vertical integration. The team is given a goal to achieve and then is free to determine work assignments, rest breaks, inspection procedures, and the like. Fully autonomous work teams even select their own members and have the members evaluate each other's performance. As a result, supervisory positions take on decreased importance and may even be eliminated. The autonomous work team concept has been applied at a General Foods pet food plant in Topeka, Kansas, and at a plant of Shaklee Corporation in Norman, Oklahoma, that manufactures health powders and pills.

General Foods. The Topeka pet food plant was built in 1971 especially to accommodate the autonomous work team concept.[16] Teams have from seven to fourteen members and hold collective responsibility for large segments of the production process. The team's responsibilities include the functions of the traditional departments in a plant—maintenance, quality control, industrial engineering, and personnel. For instance, teams do their own screening of applicants to locate replacements who are qualified and who will fit into the teams. Workers make job assignments, schedule coffee breaks, and even decide team members' pay raises.

16. Richard E. Walton, "From Hawthorne to Topeka and Kalmar," in *Man and Work in Society,* ed. E. L. Cass and F. G. Zimmer (New York: Van Nostrand Reinhold, 1975), pp. 118–19.

A unique feature at the Topeka plant is the absence of job classification grades. All operators have a single classification and earn pay increases based on their ability to master an increasing number of jobs. Because no limits are placed on how many team members can qualify for the higher pay brackets, employees are encouraged to teach each other their jobs.

When the experiment began, team leaders were appointed to facilitate team development and decision making. However, after several years, the teams became so effective at managing themselves that the team leader positions were being eliminated.

What impact did this work environment have on the employees' and the plant's performance? Several years following its introduction, employees were generally praising the variety, dignity, and influence that they enjoyed. They liked the team spirit, open communication, and opportunities to expand their mastery of job skills. While the experiment was not without criticizers, most employees believed that the work system as a whole was better than any other they knew about. From the management side, the plant operated with 35 percent fewer employees than similar plants organized along traditional lines. Additionally, the experiment resulted in higher output, minimum waste, avoidance of shutdowns, lower absenteeism, and lower turnover.

Shaklee Corporation. Shaklee adopted a similar job design format in 1979 at its Oklahoma plant that produces nutritional products, vitamins, and other pills.[17] About 190 of the plant's production employees were organized into teams with 3 to 15 members. As in the Topeka operation, the team members set their own production schedules, decide what hours to work, select new team members from a pool approved by the personnel department, and even initiate discharges if necessary. The results have been impressive. The company reports that units produced per hour of labor are up nearly 200 percent over other plants, two-thirds of which increase they attribute to the autonomous work team concept (the rest is explained by better equipment). Management states that the Oklahoma plant can produce the same volume as their more traditional facilities but at 40 percent of the labor costs.

Quality Circles

The most recent addition to job redesign alternatives has been the quality circle. Originally begun in the United States and exported to Japan in the 1950s, the quality circle has recently been imported back to the United States.[18] As it developed in Japan, the quality circle concept is frequently mentioned as one of the techniques that Japanese firms utilize which has allowed them to make better-quality products at lower costs than their American counterparts. In fact, this

17. "The New Industrial Relations," *Business Week,* May 11, 1981, p. 96.
18. Ibid., p. 86.

concept has grown so popular in Japan, one expert estimates that approximately one out of every nine Japanese workers is involved in a quality circle.[19]

What is a quality circle? It is a voluntary group of workers—primarily a normal work crew—who have a shared area of responsibility.[20] They meet together weekly, on company time and on company premises, to discuss their quality problems, investigate causes, recommend solutions, and take corrective actions. They take over the responsibility for solving quality problems, and they generate and evaluate their own feedback. Of course, it is not presumed that employees inherently have this ability. Therefore, part of the quality circle concept includes teaching participating employees group communication skills, various quality strategies, and measurement and problem-analysis techniques.

Quality circles are expanding rapidly in the United States in large and small companies alike. Honeywell, Inc., for instance, has 350 quality circles involving about 4,000 employees.[21] Hughes Aircraft credits quality circles for saving $45,000 a year from reduction of defects and another $48,000 from redesign suggestions made by a quality circle group.[22]

The quality circle integrates job redesign with the idea of extensive employee participation. In terms of the job characteristics model, the concept increases skill variety, task identity, autonomy, and feedback.

Shorter Workweek

There has been increasing interest in recent years in the use of shorter workweeks. A number of innovative programs have been proposed; workweeks of three 12-hour days, four 9-hour days, and four 10-hour days have been the most widely implemented. For our discussion, we shall concern ourselves with the four-day, forty-hour program, or what is often just called 4-40.

The 4-40 program was conceived to allow workers more leisure time and more shopping time, and to permit them to travel to and from work at non-rush-hour times. It was suggested that such a program would increase employee enthusiasm, morale, and commitment to the organization; increase productivity and reduce costs; reduce machine downtime in manufacturing; reduce overtime, turnover, and absenteeism; and make it easier for the organization to recruit employees. These positive outcomes have been postulated in spite of the fact that the four-day week does not impact upon any of the core dimensions in the job characteristics model.

It has been proposed that the four-day workweek may positively affect productivity in situations in which the work process requires significant start-up

19. "A Quality Concept Catches on Worldwide," *Industry Week,* April 16, 1979, p. 125.

20. Ed Yager, "Quality Circle: A Tool for the '80's," *Training and Development Journal,* August 1980, p. 62.

21. "The New Industrial Relations," p. 92.

22. "A Quality Concept Catches on Worldwide," p. 125.

and shutdown periods.[23] When start-up and shutdown times are a major factor, productivity standards take these periods into consideration in determining the time required to generate a given output. Consequently, in such cases, the four-day workweek will increase productivity even though performance of the workers is not affected, because the improved work scheduling reduces non-productive time. Performance results under the 4-40 program, however, appears to be somewhat mixed.

An investigation of 470 clerical and supervisory employees in an accounting function found that 62 percent of the workers saw their jobs as more tiring under the 4-40 program, and managers complained about the difficulties of co-ordinating workloads. However, there was a 10 percent reduction in overtime, and 78 percent of the employees did not want to revert to the traditional five-day workweek once the program had been operating for six months. Although analysis of productivity figures indicated that they were unaffected either positively or negatively, supervisors were generally unenthusiastic about the program. Fifty-one percent of them saw it as detrimental to their work areas; only 18 percent saw it as beneficial.[24]

What is the effect of a shorter workweek when it has been established for at least a year? One study, taken over thirteen months, using experimental and controlled subjects, found that workers utilizing the four-day workweek were more satisfied with their personal worth, social affiliation, job security, and pay; experienced less anxiety and stress; and performed better with regard to productivity than the control group members working the five-day week.[25] A study in a medium-sized pharmaceutical company employing over 200 people found workers generally positive toward the shorter workweek, but these attitudes did change over time.[26] After one year, the effects of the four-day week on the worker's home lives were perceived as significantly less positive than when they were first reported.

While one must be careful in generalizing from such mixed findings, the evidence does indicate that the shorter workweek is effective in improving morale, reducing dissatisfaction, and reducing absenteeism and turnover figures in the early months after implementation. However, after approximately one year, some of these advantages may disappear. Employees begin to complain more frequently about increased fatigue and the difficulty of coordinating their jobs with their personal lives—the latter a problem more particularly for working mothers.

23. Eugene J. Calvasina and W. Randy Boxx, "Efficiency of Workers on the Four-Day Workweek," *Academy of Management Journal,* September 1975, pp. 604–10.

24. James C. Goodale and A. K. Aaagaard, "Factors Relating to Varying Reactions to the 4-Day Work Week," *Journal of Applied Psychology,* February 1975, pp. 33–38.

25. John M. Ivancevich, "Effects of the Shorter Workweek on Selected Satisfaction and Performance Measures," *Journal of Applied Psychology,* December 1974, pp. 717–21.

26. Walter R. Nord and Robert Costigain, "Worker Adjustment to the Four-Day Week: A Longitudinal Study," *Journal of Applied Psychology,* August 1973, pp. 60–66.

Flex-time

During the past decade, the introduction of flexible work hours—or flex-time—has been widely practiced. In contrast to the shorter work week, flex-time actually increases an employee's autonomy.

Flex-time allows employees some discretion over when they arrive at work and leave. Employees have to work a specific number of hours a week, but are free to vary the hours of work within certain limits. Each day consists of a common core, usually six hours, with a flexibility band surrounding the core. For example, the core may be 10:00 A.M. to 4:00 P.M., with the office actually opening at 7:30 A.M. and closing at 6:00 P.M. All employees are required to be at their jobs during the common core period, but they are allowed to accumulate their other two hours before and/or after the core time. Some flex-time programs allow extra hours to be accumulated and turned into a free day off each month.

Flex-time has been implemented in a number of diverse organizations. A recent survey, for instance, indicated that approximately 13 percent of all U.S. companies were using some varient of flex-time.[27]

Employee reactions to flex-time programs have not been universally supportive; however, far more of the evidence is positive than negative. Let's review some of that evidence.

One analysis of 445 organizations that had initiated a flex-time program found 48 percent reporting productivity gains. These gains averaged 12 percent and were primarily attributed to improved morale and lower absenteeism.[28] A comprehensive evaluation of 79 separate flex-time applications, mostly in business firms, found it to be a low-cost design option that was favorably received by the operative workers, first-line supervisors, and managers.[29] A similar evaluation of 74 public sector applications of flex-time also demonstrated positive results.[30] Favorable behavioral and attitudinal effects dominated the studies.

The response to flex-time of 150 clerical workers in a large British insurance company is probably fairly generalizable. Workers perceived that they had greater freedom, had a better integration of work and leisure, found it easier to start and leave early, and enjoyed the opportunity to build up credit toward taking time off. On the negative side, workers were required to punch in and out on time clocks, a procedure that had not been required prior to the flex-time program, and they disliked having to make up time if they missed a train or had

27. Stanley D. Nollen, "Does Flex-time Improve Productivity?" *Harvard Business Review,* September-October 1979, pp. 12, 16–18, 22.

28. Ibid.

29. Robert T. Golembiewski and Carl W. Proehl, Jr., "A Survey of the Empirical Literature on Flexible Workhours: Character and Consequences of a Major Innovation," *Academy of Management Review,* October 1978, pp. 837–53.

30. Robert T. Golembiewski and Carl W. Proehl, Jr., "Public Sector Applications of Flexible Workhours: A Review of Available Experience," *Public Administration Review,* January-February 1980, pp. 72–85.

to take time off to visit the doctor or dentist. However, negative factors were generally minimal.[31]

JOB REDESIGN OPTIONS AND JOB CHARACTERISTICS

Figure 15–4 summarizes the redesign options we have discussed in terms of their ability to meet the criteria identified in the job characteristics model. A quick glance tells us that there is a great deal of difference between the various techniques.

The shorter workweek, as previously noted, does not positively effect any of the five job characteristics. Flex-time, at best, only enhances autonomy.

The other techniques all increase skill variety. Whether they increase task significance is difficult to assess without knowing more about the work content in question.

Figure 15–4 indicates that job enrichment, autonomous work teams, and quality circles are significantly superior to the other options *in terms of the job characteristics model.* Of course, there are other reasons why management may decide to redesign jobs in addition to increasing their motivation potential; and there is nothing in Figure 15–4 to indicate cost-benefit considerations. The various options we have proposed differ significantly in their implementation costs. Obviously, autonomous work teams must generate considerably more benefits than job rotation if they are to justify the greater time, effort, and cost to implement them. Nevertheless, for employees who possess a high growth need, their performance and satisfaction should be higher when working in enriched jobs, on autonomous work teams, or participating in quality circles.

31. Martin G. Evans, "The Impact of Flex-Time in a Large British Insurance Company," Working Paper 73-12, University of Toronto, Faculty of Management Studies, 1973.

FIGURE 15–4 Job Characteristics Provided by Various Job Redesign Options

Redesign Option	Skill Variety	Task Identity	Task Significance	Autonomy	Feedback
Job enlargement	X		?		
Job rotation	X		?		
Work modules	X		?	X	
Job enrichment	X	X	?	X	X
Integrated work teams	X		?		
Autonomous work teams	X	X	?	X	X
Quality circles	X	X	?	X	X
Shorter workweek					
Flex time				X	

IMPLICATIONS FOR PERFORMANCE AND SATISFACTION

The way that jobs are designed will influence the performance and satisfaction of the individuals performing those jobs. But the effect has been shown to be moderated by individual differences, particularly growth need strength. This has led us to the conclusion that employee performance and satisfaction will be higher where workers are matched with the appropriate structures and job characteristics.

For employees with a high growth need, the most favorable outcomes should be achieved when they work in organic structures doing complex jobs. Redesign options such as job enrichment, autonomous work teams, and quality circles are compatible with high employee growth need.

For employees low on growth need, performance and satisfaction are likely to be highest when matched with a mechanistic structure and simple jobs. This type of individual is likely to perform quite effectively in the repetitive tasks typically associated with assembly-line work and standardized clerical activities.

FOR DISCUSSION

1. Contrast job design in 1903 and in 1983.

2. Which current redesign options do you think have been most influenced by the sociotechnical systems movement? Explain.

3. What is the job characteristics model?

4. Why must a job, to score high on motivating potential, have both high autonomy and feedback?

5. "Employees should have jobs that give them autonomy and diversity." Do you agree or disagree? Discuss.

6. Contrast job enlargement with job enrichment.

7. What are the advantages and disadvantages to the shorter work-week?

8. What are the advantages and disadvantages of flex-time?

9. Do you think that in twenty years most jobs will score high on motivating potential? Explain.

10. "Want to find out if a person likes his job? Ask him if he would stay with it if he inherited $5 million tomorrow!" What percent of today's labor force do you think would continue working at their present job if they were suddenly independently wealthy? Do you see any common characteristics either in the persons or jobs of those who would choose to continue their present work?

COHEN, A. R., and H. GADON, *Alternative Work Schedules.* Reading, Mass.: Addison-Wesley, 1978. Introduces and reviews the evidence on flex-time, the shorter workweek, and other alternative work schedule ideas.

DAVIS, L. E., "Job Design: Overview and Future Direction," *Journal of Contemporary Business,* Spring 1977, pp. 85–102. Presents the evolution of job design and offers some predictions concerning its future directions.

FEIN, M., "Job Enrichment: A Re-Evaluation," *Sloan Management Review,* Fall 1973, pp. 69–88. Argues that most job enrichment applications are either commonsense job redesign or occurred among a select group of employees; there are few, if any, genuine cases where the technique has been applied successfully to a large, heterogeneous work force.

LAWLER, E. E. III, and L. L. CUMMINGS, "Task Design," in *Point and Counterpoint in Organizational Behavior,* ed. B. Karmel, chap. 5. Hinsdale, Ill.: Dryden Press, 1980. Two scholars debate the role of individual differences in predicting the outcomes of job design.

NORTON, D. D., D. MASSENGIL, and H. L. SCHNEIDER, "Is Job Enrichment a Success or Failure?" *Human Resource Management,* Winter 1979, pp. 28–37. Reviews job enrichment and presents a contingency view of when it is related to success.

SCHRANK, R. "How to Relieve Worker Boredom," *Psychology Today,* July 1978, pp. 79–80. Jobs should be designed to allow employees to "schmooze"—to talk, fool around, and do other things unrelated to their assigned work.

A job design scenario: route one

Adapted from J. Richard Hackman, "The Design of Work in the 1980s," Organizational Dynamics, Summer 1978 (New York: AMACOM, a division of American Management Associations, 1978), pp. 3–17. With permission.

How will work be designed by the end of the 1980s? If you assume many individuals are presently underutilized and underchallenged at work, you get what I call the "Route One" scenerio. If people are underutilized by the work they do, it should lead to increases in the level of challenge that is built into jobs and in the degree of control jobholders have in managing their own work. Jobs would be changed to make them fit better for the people who do them. Let me expand on the Route One scenerio or the "fitting jobs to people" viewpoint.

It seems to me indisputable that numerous jobs have become increasingly simplified and routinized in the last several decades, even as members of the U.S. work force have become better educated and more ambitious in their expectations about what life will hold for them. The result is a poor fit between large numbers of people and their work. These people, whom one author calls "the reserve army of the underemployed," have more to offer their employers than those employers seek, and they have personal needs and aspirations that cannot be satisfied by the work they do.

It also is indisputable that many people do not seek challenge and meaning in their work but instead aspire to a secure job and a level of income that permits them to pursue personal interests and satisfactions off the job. Do the underutilized and underchallenged workers comprise three quarters of the work force or only one quarter?

We cannot say for sure. What we can say—and this statement may be much more important—is that for some unknown millions of people, work is neither a challenge nor a personally fulfilling part of life. And the organizations that employ them are obtaining only a portion of the contribution that these people could be making.

The core idea of Route One is to build increased challenge and autonomy into the work for the people who perform it. By creating job conditions that motivate employees *internally,* gains might be realized both in the productive effectiveness of the organization and in the personal satisfaction and well-being of the work force.

Specifically, the aspiration would be to design work so that employees experience the work as inherently meaningful, feel personal responsibility for the outcomes of the work, and receive, on a regular basis, trustworthy knowledge about the results of their work activities. My research suggests that when all three of these conditions are met, most people are internally motivated to do a good job—that is, they get a positive internal "kick" when they do well, and feel bad when they do poorly. Such feelings provide an incentive for trying to perform well and, when performance is excellent, leads to feelings of satisfaction with the work and with one's self.

We still have much to learn about how to design jobs, but if we can find most of the answers during the next few years, the shape of work in the next decade could turn out to be quite different from what it is today. Assuming that we follow Route One, and do so competently and successfully, here are some speculations about the design and management of work in the mid-1980s.

1. Responsibility for work will be pegged clearly at the organizational level at which the work is done. No longer will employees experience themselves as people who merely execute activities that "belong" to someone else (such as a line manager). Instead, they will feel, legitimately, that they are both responsible and accountable for the outcomes of their own work. Moreover, the resources and the information needed to carry out the work (including feedback about how well the work is being done) will be provided directly to employees, without being filtered first through line and staff managers.

2. Explicit consideration will be given to questions of employee motivation and satisfaction when new technologies and work practices are invented and engineered, on a par with the consideration now given to the employee's intellectual and motor capabilities.

3. Organizations will be leaner, with fewer hierarchical levels and fewer managerial and staff personnel whose jobs are primarily documentation, supervision, and inspection of work done by others.

4. Last, if the previous predictions are correct, eventually a good deal of pressure will be brought to bear on the broader political and economic system to find ways to make effective use of the human resources that are no longer needed to populate work organizations.

COUNTERPOINT

HACKMAN

A job design scenario: route two

Adapted and edited from J. Richard Hackman, "The Design of Work in the 1980s," Organizational Dynamics, Summer 1978, pp. 3–17.

If you assume that people are more adaptable than we traditionally give them credit for, you get what I call "Route Two." If people gradually adapt and adjust to almost any work situation, even one that initially seems to underutilize their talents greatly, it should lead to greater control of work procedures and closer monitoring of work outcomes by management to increase the productive efficiency of the work force. This Route Two scenario proposes fitting people to the jobs.

If we take Route Two, the idea is to design and engineer work for maximum economic and technological efficiency and then do whatever must be done to help people adapt and adjust in personally acceptable ways to their work experiences. No great flight of imagination is required to guess what work will be like if we follow Route Two; the sprouts of this approach are visible now. Work is designed and managed in a way that clearly subordinates the needs and goals of people to the demands and requirements of fixed jobs. External controls are employed to ensure that individuals do in fact behave appropriately on the job. These include close and directive supervision, financial incentives for correct performance, tasks that are engineered to minimize the possibility of human mistakes, and information and control systems that allow management to monitor the performance of the work system as closely and continuously as possible. And,

throughout, productivity and efficiency tend to dominate quality and service as the primary criteria for assessing organizational performance.

If we continue down Route Two, what might we predict about the design and management of work by the end of the 1980s? Here are my guesses:

1. Technological and engineering considerations will dominate decision making about the design of jobs. Technology is becoming increasingly central to many work activities, and that trend will accelerate. Also, major advances will be achieved in techniques for engineering work systems to make them ever more efficient. Together, these developments will greatly boost the productivity of individual workers and, in many cases, result in tasks that are nearly "people proof" (that is, work that is arranged virtually to eliminate the possibility of error because of faulty judgment, lapses of attention, or misdirected motivation). Large numbers of relatively mindless tasks, including many kinds of inspection operations, will be automated out of existence. The change from person to machine will both increase efficiency and eliminate many problems that arise from human frailties.

Accompanying these technological advances will be a further increase in the capability of industrial psychologists to analyze and specify in advance the knowledge and skills that will enable a person to perform almost any task that can be designed satisfactorily. Sophisticated employee assessment and placement procedures will be used to select people and assign them to tasks, and only rarely will an individual be put into a job for which he or she is not fully qualified.

The result of all these developments will be a quantum improvement in the efficiency of most work systems, especially those that process physical materials or paper. And while employees will receive more pay for less work, they will also experience substantially less discretion and challenge in their work activities.

2. Work performance and organizational productivity will be closely monitored and controlled by managers using highly sophisticated information systems. Integrated circuit microprocessors will provide the hardware needed to gather and summarize performance data for work processes that presently defy cost-efficient measurement. Software will be developed to provide managers with data about work performance and costs that are far more reliable, more valid, and more current than is possible with existing information systems. Managers increasingly will come to depend on these data for decision making and will use them to control production processes vigorously and continuously.

Because managerial control of work will increase substantially, responsibility for work outcomes will lie squarely in the laps of managers, and the gap between those who do the work and those who control it will grow. There will be accelerated movement toward a two-class society of people who work in organizations, with the challenge and intrinsic interest of managerial and professional jobs increasing even as the work of rank-and-file employees becomes more controlled and less involving.

3. Desired on-the-job behavior will be elicited and maintained by extensive and sophisticated use of extrinsic rewards. Since (if my first prediction is correct) work will be engineered for clarity and simplicity, there will be little question about what each employee should (and should not) do on the job. Moreover (if my second prediction is correct), management will have data readily at hand to monitor the results of each employee's work on a more or less continuous basis. All that will be required then, are devices to ensure that the person actually does what he or she is *supposed* to do.

Because many jobs will be routinized, standardized, and closely controlled by management, it is doubtful that employee motivation to perform appropriately can be created and maintained from intrinsic rewards (people working hard and effectively because they enjoy the tasks or because they obtain internal reinforcement from doing them well). So management will have to use extrinsic rewards (such as pay or supervisory praise) to motivate employees, providing such rewards for behavior that is in accord with the wishes of management.

4. Most organizations will sponsor programs to aid employees in adapting to life at work under Route Two conditions, including systematic "attitude development" programs to foster high job satisfaction and organizational commitment. Sophisticated procedures for helping employees and their families deal with alcohol, drug abuse, and domestic problems also will be offered by many organizations. These latter programs will become much more prevalent (and necessary) than they are at present, I believe, because of some unintended spin-offs of the movement toward the productive efficiencies of Route Two.

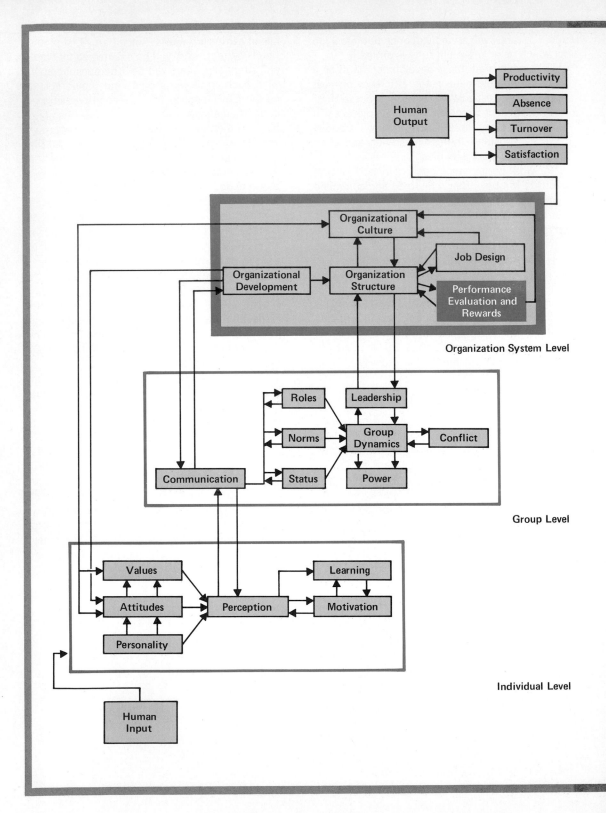

CHAPTER 16
Performance Evaluation and Rewards

AFTER STUDYING THIS CHAPTER, YOU SHOULD BE ABLE TO—

Define and explain the following key terms and concepts:

Absolute standards
Leniency error
Low differentiation
Merit

Objectives
Relative standards
Similarity error

Understand:

The importance of performance evaluation
The purposes of performance evaluation
What should be evaluated
How it should be evaluated
The criteria by which rewards are distributed
The types of rewards
The importance attributed to the performance-reward relationship
How rewards condition behavior

Would you study differently for a course if your goal was *to learn as much as you could about the subject* rather than *to make a high grade on the tests in the course?* When I ask that question of students, I frequently get an affirmative answer. When I inquire further, I am typically told that making a high grade is only partially determined by knowledge of the material. You also need to know what the instructor thinks is important. I have been told by many a student that, "If you want to do well in a course, you do best to study what the instructor tests for." In some cases, that approach will also result in learning as much as you can about the subject. But in many courses, studying to make a high grade means studying much differently than if you were studying for general knowledge.

Let me propose another question. Assume you are taking two similar classes, both with enrollments of about twenty. In one class, the grade is determined totally by your scores on the midterm and final. In the other class, the midterm and final each count only 25 percent, with the remaining 50 percent being allocated for class participation. Would your in-class behavior be different in the two classes? I would predict that most students would talk more—ask questions, answer questions, offer examples, elaborate on points made by the instructor—in the class where participation was so highly weighted.

The above paragraphs are meant to illustrate how the system's evaluation and reward practices influence behavior. Studying and in-class behavior are modified to take into consideration the criteria that the instructor evaluates and the linking of those evaluations to desirable rewards (i.e., high grades). It's not unusual, in fact, for the more experienced student to behave five different ways in five different classes in order to obtain five high grades. The reason studying and in-class behaviors vary is certainly in large measure directly attributable to the different performance evaluation and reward systems that instructors use.

What applies in the school context also applies to employees at work. In this chapter, we shall show how performance evaluation and reward systems influence the attitudes and behaviors of people in organizations.

PERFORMANCE EVALUATION

Why do organizations evaluate the performance of their employees? *How* do they do these evaluations? *What* measurement problems can occur to subvert the intentions of objective evaluations? These are the key questions addressed in this section.

Purposes of Performance Evaluation

Performance evaluation serves a number of purposes in organizations. Management uses evaluations for *general personnel decisions.* Evaluations provide input into such important decisions as promotions, transfers, and terminations. Evaluations *identify training and development needs.* They pinpoint employee skills and competencies that are currently inadequate but for which programs can be developed to remedy. Performance evaluations can be used as *a criterion against which selection and development programs are validated.* Newly hired employees who perform poorly can be identified through performance evaluation. Similarly, the effectiveness of training and development programs can be determined by assessing how well those employees who have participated do on their performance evaluation. Evaluations also fulfill the purpose of *providing feedback to employees* on how the organization views their performance. Finally, performance evaluations are used as the *basis for reward allocations.* Decisions as to who gets merit pay increases and other rewards are determined by performance evaluations.

Each of these functions of performance evaluation is important. Yet their importance to us depends on the perspective we're taking. Several clearly are most relevant to personnel management decisions. But our interest is in organizational behavior. As a result, we shall be emphasizing performance evaluation in its role as a determinant of reward allocations.

Performance Evaluation and Motivation

In Chapter 6, considerable attention was given to the expectancy model of motivation. We argued that this model currently offers the best explanation of what conditions the amount of effort an individual will exert on his or her job. A vital component of this model is performance, specifically the effort-performance and performance-reward linkages. Do people see effort leading to performance, and performance to the rewards that they value? Clearly, they have to know what is expected of them. They need to know how their performance will be measured. Further, they must feel confident that if they exert an effort within their capabilities that it will result in a satisfactory performance as defined by the criteria by which they are being measured. Finally, they must feel confident that if they perform as they are being asked, they will achieve the rewards they value.

In brief, if the objectives that employees are seeking are unclear, if the criteria for measuring those objectives are vague, and if the employees lack confidence that their efforts will lead to a satisfactory appraisal of their performance, or believe that there will be an unsatisfactory payoff by the organization when their performance objectives are achieved, we can expect individuals to work considerably below their potential.

Performance Standards

Every job in an organization should have set standards that clarify what is expected of the job's incumbent. These performance standards should be clear and objective enough to be understood and measured; they should not be articulated in ambiguous phrases such as "a full day's work" or "a good job." Vague standards tell us nothing. The expectations a manager has in terms of work performance by her subordinates must be clarified enough in her mind so that she will be able to communicate these expectations to her subordinates and, at some later date, appraise their performance against these previously established standards.

Unfortunately, too many jobs have vague performance standards. Ideally, standards should be tangible, measurable, and verifiable. This means that, wherever possible, we should avoid qualitative objectives and substitute quantifiable statements. For example, a quantitative objective might be "to cut, each day, 3,500 yards of cable to standard five-foot lengths, with a maximum scrap of 50 yards," or "to prepare, process, and transfer to the treasurer's office all accounts payable vouchers within three working days from the receipt of the invoice." Performance standards like these can be measured, verified, and they are tangible.

Methods of Performance Evaluation

Three different approaches exist for doing evaluations. Employees can be appraised against (1) absolute standards, (2) relative standards, or (3) objectives.

Absolute Standards. The use of absolute standards means employees are *not* compared with each other. Evaluators may write essays describing the employee's strengths and weaknesses. In more elaborate evaluations, the rater may check off "Yes" or "No" responses to a previously prepared list of traits or behaviors that the employee demonstrates.

The common thread through all evaluation methods that use the absolute standard is that the employee is judged against a rigid standard rather than against the performance of other employees. When a college instructor gives grades that are based on 90 and above equalling an "A," 80 and above a "B," and so forth—and makes no adjustment for how the class does as a whole—an absolute standard approach is being used. This approach avoids problems like trying to rank-order five people in a small department whose performance levels are nearly identical. On the other hand, the use of absolute standards tends to result in high evaluations. That is, evaluators lean toward packing their subjects into the high part of the scale. This, in fact, happens in many organizations.

Take the case of the U.S. Army captain who could not understand why he had been passed over for promotion. He had seen his file and knew that his average rating by his superior was 86. Given his knowledge that the rating system defined "outstanding performance" as 90 or above, "good" as 80 or above, "average" as 70 or above, and "inadequate performance" as anything below 70, he was at a loss to understand why he had not been promoted, given his near-outstanding performance evaluation. The officer's confusion was somewhat resolved when he found out the "average" rating of captains in the United States Army was 92!

Relative Standards. The second category of evaluation methods compares employees against each other. These methods use relative rather than absolute measuring devices. For instance, employees may be order-ranked into classification groups such as "top one-fifth" or "second one-fifth." Another approach is merely to rank a given set of employees from highest to lowest. If you are evaluating thirty employees using individual ranking, then only one can be "best" and someone must be relegated to last.

Relative standards overcome one objection of absolute standards in that there can be no bias toward inflating everyone's evaluation. If a department has only five employees, relative standards require that they be compared against each other and ranked. This, of course, can be a major drawback. When the number of individuals being evaluated is small or when there is little actual variability among those being evaluated, relative standards may generate unrealistic appraisals. If, for instance, there are eleven individuals in a department working as different levels of effectiveness, by definition, five of them must be "below average." Ironically, if two of the below-average workers leave, then one of the previously "above average" performers must fall into the below-average category. Because comparisons are relative, an employee who is mediocre may score high only because he is the "best of the worst." In contrast, an excellent employee who is matched against "stiff" competition may be evaluated poorly when in absolute terms her performance is quite outstanding.

Objectives. The third approach to evaluation makes use of objectives. Employees are evaluated by how well they accomplish a specific set of objectives that have been determined to be critical in the successful completion of their jobs.

This approach works well where the organization—from the top down—is strongly committed to setting objectives and rewarding people based on their success in achieving their objectives. The use of objectives gives performance evaluation a results-oriented emphasis and provides motivation because employees know exactly what is expected of them.

Problems in the Search for Objectivity

No single evaluation method is perfect. While organizations may seek to make performance evaluation an objective process in which the evaluator is free from personal biases, prejudices, and idiosyncracies, there are a number of measurement problems that can arise to subvert these best of intentions. To the degree that the following factors are prevalent, an employee's evaluation will not accurately reflect his or her actual performance level.

Leniency Error. Every evaluator has his or her own value system which acts as a standard against which appraisals are made. Relative to the true or actual performance an individual exhibits, some evaluators mark high and others low. The former is referred to as positive leniency error, and the latter as negative leniency error. When evaluators are positively lenient in their appraisal, an individual's performance becomes overstated; that is, rated higher than it actually should. Similarly, a negative leniency error understates performance, giving the individual a lower appraisal.

If all individuals in an organization were appraised by the same person, there would be no problem. Although there would be an error factor, it would be applied equally to everyone. The difficulty arises when we have different raters with different leniency errors making judgments. For example, assume a situation where both Jones and Smith are performing the same job for different supervisors, but they have absolutely identical job performance. If Jones's supervisor tends to err toward positive leniency, while Smith's supervisor errs toward negative leniency, we might be confronted with two dramatically different evaluations.

Halo Error. The halo effect or error, as we noted in Chapter 5, is the tendency for an evaluator to let the assessment of an individual on one trait influence his or her evaluation of that person on other traits. For example, if an employee tends to be conscientious and dependable, we might become biased toward that individual to the extent that we will rate him or her high on many desirable attributes.

People who design teaching appraisal forms for college students to fill out in evaluating the effectiveness of their instructor each semester must confront the halo effect. Students tend to rate a faculty member as outstanding on all criteria when they are particularly appreciative of a few things he or she does in the classroom. Similarly, a few bad habits—like showing up late for lectures, being slow in returning papers, or assigning an extremely demanding reading requirement—might result in students evaluating the instructor as "lousy" across the board.

Similarity Error. When the evaluator rates other people giving special consideration to those qualities that he perceives in himself, he is making a similarity error. For example, the evaluator who perceives himself as aggressive may evaluate others by looking for aggressiveness. Those who demonstrate this characteristic tend to benefit, while others are penalized.

Again, this error would tend to wash out if the same evaluator appraised all the people in the organization. However, interrater reliability obviously suffers when various evaluators are utilizing their own similarity criteria.

Low Differentiation. It is possible that, regardless of whom the appraiser evaluates and what traits are used, the pattern of evaluation remains the same. It is possible that the evaluator's ability to appraise objectively and accurately has been impeded by social differentiation, that is, the evaluator's style of rating behavior.

It has been suggested that evaluators may be classified as (1) high differentiators, who use all or most of the scale, or (2) low differentiators, who use a limited range of the scale.[1]

Low differentiators tend to ignore or suppress differences, perceiving the universe as more uniform than it really is. High differentiators, on the other hand, tend to utilize all available information to the utmost extent and thus are better able to define perceptually anomalies and contradictions than low differentiators.[2]

This finding tells us that evaluations made by low differentiators need to be carefully inspected, and that the people working for a low differentiator have a high probability of being appraised as significantly more homogeneous than they really are.

Forcing Information to Match Nonperformance Criteria. While rarely advocated, it is not a totally infrequent practice to find the formal evaluation taking place *following* the decision as to how the individual has been performing! This may sound illogical, but it merely recognizes that subjective, yet formal, decisions are often arrived at prior to the gathering of objective information to support that decision. For example, if the evaluator believes that the evaluation should not be based on performance, but rather seniority, he may be unknowingly adjusting each "performance" evaluation so as to bring it into line with the employee's seniority rank. In this and other similar cases, the evaluator is increasing or decreasing performance appraisals to align with the nonperformance criteria actually being utilized.

Inflationary Pressures. One of the interesting social phenomena taking place in recent years has been the gradual inflation in the appraisal of individuals. As "equality" values have grown in importance in our society, there has been a tendency to make less rigorous evaluation and to reduce negative repercussions from the evaluation by generally inflating or upgrading appraisals. Although little research has been done on this subject in industry, clearly an excellent example has been the inflation of grades in colleges and universities throughout the United States. A study of 197 colleges and universities found that between 1960 and 1974, grade-point averages had risen about one-half of a letter grade.[3] In the spring of 1975, at Yale University, almost 43 percent of all marks given were

1. Abraham Pizam, "Social Differentiation—A New Psychological Barrier to Performance Appraisal," *Public Personnel Management,* July–August 1975, pp. 244–47.

2. Ibid., pp. 245–46.

3. Malcolm Scully, "Inflated Grades Worrying More and More Colleges," *Chronicle of Higher Education,* May 19, 1975, p. 1.

"A" grades. At Dartmouth, 60 percent of the class of 1975 earned degrees with some kind of academic honor.[4] On a broader level, a report of the Carnegie Council on Policy Studies in Higher Education shows that in 1969, 7 percent of undergraduate grades were "A's" and 47 percent were "B's." In 1976, the "A's" had increased to 19 percent and the "B's" to 55 percent.[5]

While it can be argued that students are more intelligent now or try harder, evidence does not support this contention. In fact, based on results of standardized tests, today's students are significantly weaker than those of ten or twenty years ago. The most widely adopted conclusions suggest that (1) faculty are less rigorous in their grading as a result of the drop in demand for higher education, and (2) as student bodies become more diverse in terms of socioeconomic and intellectual abilities, there is a trend to shift grades upward rather than judge all students on the traditional criteria.

Inappropriate Substitutes for Performance. It is the unusual job where the definition of performance is absolutely clear and direct measures are available for appraising the incumbent. In many jobs it is difficult to get consensus on what is "a good job," and it is even more difficult to get agreement on what criteria will determine performance. For a saleswoman, the criterion may be the dollar sales in her territory, but even this criterion is affected by factors such as economic conditions and actions of competitors—factors outside the saleswoman's control.

As a result, the evaluation is frequently made by using substitutes for performance; criteria that hopefully closely approximate performance and act in its place. Many of these substitutes are well chosen and give a good approximation of actual performance. However, the substitutes chosen are not always appropriate. It is not unusual, for example, to find organizations using criteria such as enthusiasm, neatness, positive attitudes, conscientiousness, promptness, and congeniality as substitutes for performance. In some jobs, one or more of the criteria listed in the previous sentence *are* part of performance. Obviously, enthusiasm does enhance the effectiveness of a teacher. You're more likely to listen to and be motivated by a teacher who is enthusiastic than one who is not. And increased attentiveness and motivation typically lead to increased learning. But enthusiasm may in no way be relevant to effective performance for many accountants, watch repairpersons, or copyeditors. So what may be an appropriate substitute for performance in one job may be totally inappropriate in another.

Sharing Performance Evaluation Results

We have thus far argued that organizations seek objectivity when they evaluate the performance of their employees, but there are factors that distort evaluations and make high objectivity difficult. We have also noted that individuals should

4. "Yale Students to Have Their 'F's' Recorded Again," *New York Times,* January 18, 1976, p. 1.

5. "The 'B' Comes to Animal House," *Fortune,* June 18, 1979, p. 44.

know what is expected of them, the specific criteria by which they will be appraised, and how they will be measured against these criteria. Regardless of how the appraisal data is gathered, there usually comes a time when the results of the evaluation are shared with the employee. This sharing may be an ongoing process (i.e., daily output reports with comparative data on actual units produced and the goal for the day), but it is usually reserved for the annual or semiannual employee performance review. (Unfortunately, sometimes it is *never* shared with the employee.) This review often takes place *only* because the personnel department requires it as part of the individual's salary appraisal.

One of the most challenging tasks facing a manager is learning how to present an accurate appraisal to his or her subordinate and then having the subordinate accept the appraisal in a constructive manner. Appraising another person's performance is one of the most emotionally charged of all management activities. The impression the subordinate receives about his assessment has a strong impact on his self-esteem and, very importantly, on his subsequent performance. Of course, conveying good news is considerably less difficult for both the manager and the subordinate than revealing that performance has been below expectations. In this context, the discussion of the evaluation can have negative as well as positive motivational consequences. Statistically speaking, half of all employees are below median, yet evidence tells us that the average employee's estimate of her own performance level generally falls around the 75th percentile.[6] A survey of over 800,000 high school seniors also found that people seem to see themselves as better than average. Seventy percent rated themselves above average on leadership; and when asked to rate themselves on "ability to get along with others," none rated themselves below average, 60 percent rated themselves in the top 10 percent, and 25 percent saw themselves among the top one percent! Similarly, a survey of 500 clerical and technical employees found that 58 percent rated their own performance as falling in the top 10 percent of their peers doing comparable jobs and a total of 81 percent placed themselves in the top 20 percent![7]

The above evidence indicates that truthful evaluations will frequently place the manager in a situation where the subordinate's perception of her own performance overstates the manager's appraisal. Thus, to the extent that evaluation influences the behavior of organizational members, an organization's performance evaluation process can demotivate those employees who perceive the evaluation as unjust.

REWARDS

Our knowledge of motivation tells us that people do what they do to satisfy needs. Before they do anything, they look for the payoff or reward. Because many of these rewards—salary increases, promotions, and preferred job assign-

6. Ronald J. Burke, "Why Performance Appraisal Systems Fail," *Personnel Administration,* June 1972, pp. 32–40.

7. "How Do I Love Me? Let Me Count the Ways," *Psychology Today,* May 1980, p. 16.

ments, to name a few—are organizationally controlled, we should consider rewards as an important force influencing the behavior of employees.

Effect of Rewards on Behavior

We react to rewards. As we learned in Chapter 7, those behaviors that are rewarded are reinforced and encouraged. A change in rewards is also likely to change behavior. These realities are certainly exemplified by the U.S. tax system.

In February 1981, the newly elected President Reagan pledged that the taxing power of the federal government "must not be used to regulate the economy or bring about change." This might be nice in theory, but the fact remains that changes in the tax system will bring about changes in the behavior of taxpayers. The tax system was designed to encourage certain types of behaviors and discourage others. Over time, the designers' intentions have gone a long way in shaping the way we live. Look at the evidence.

The tax system encourages you, among other things, to secure your future, help the "organized" needy, pursue distant job opportunities, own a home, have children, conserve energy, invest in certain risky ventures, and have your tax forms completed by a professional. You receive deductions for pension plan payments; donations to charities, universities, political candidates, and others that the government has identified as needy; moving expenses related to taking a job in a different location; interest expense, which is the major proportion of an individual's house payment; a fixed deduction for each child you support; costs related to better insulating your home; write-offs from investments in such risky ventures as cattle, oil, and films; and the cost of having a tax professional do your returns for you. Of course, by encouraging some behaviors, the government officials who participate in writing our tax code also discourage other behaviors. This is evident, for example, when they do not allow deductions for the cost of renting an apartment, sending a child to college, or directly buying groceries for a needy family in your neighborhood. The tax system has identified certain behaviors that it wants to reward through making them tax deductible, while discouraging others. President Reagan's efforts to cut taxes, for instance, will certainly change the spending and saving habits of millions of Americans. Our point is that the U.S. tax system—by the way it specifies rewards—conditions the behavior of taxpayers. An organization's reward system has the same effect on employees.

Perceptions of Rewards

It is impossible to overemphasize the fact that perceived rewards condition behavior. Regardless of what the organization *says* it rewards, people will respond to what behaviors they *perceive* are rewarded.

The manager who continually assures workers that suggestions for doing their job are encouraged, yet ridicules any and all suggestions, impresses upon his subordinates by his behavior that he does not reward suggestions. Similarly, managers may articulate sincere displeasure with those workers who "apple polish," but if workers perceive that this behavior is rewarded, they will have their "polishing rags" always close at hand.

Examples abound of people adjusting their behavior to the criteria they perceive as actually being rewarded. In a public employment agency, the interviewer's job is to match jobs and workers. One researcher found that in such an agency, interviewers were evaluated and rewarded by a simple measure—the number of interviews they conducted. Not surprisingly, interviewers were far more interested in the number of interviews they conducted each day than with the placement of clients in jobs.[8] Similarly, a consultant was investigating police effectiveness in a small city and could not explain why officers rarely stopped their patrol cars. All day long they cruised back and forth at top speed along the highway that ran through the city. They began at one end, turned around, and went back at full speed. This back and forth behavior went on, day after day. The consultant was puzzled: What did this behavior have to do with police performance? His puzzlement was resolved when he found that the city council thought high mileage on patrol cars was a good measure of police effectiveness.[9]

Determinants of Rewards

Most organizations believe that their reward system is designed to reward merit. The problem is that we find differing definitions of merit. Some define merit as being "deserving," while to others merit is being "excellent."[10] "One person's merit is another person's favoritism."[11] A consideration of "deserving" may take into account such factors as intelligence, effort, or seniority. The problem is that what is deserving may differ from what is excellent—a problem that is exacerbated by the difficulty of defining excellence. If excellence refers to performance, we concede how unsatisfactory have been our efforts to measure performance. Creation of quantifiable and meaningful performance measures of almost all white-collar and service jobs, and many blue-collar jobs, have eluded us. Thus, while few will disagree with the viewpoint that the merit concept for distributing rewards is desirable, what constitutes merit is highly debatable.

In the next several pages we shall briefly assess the role of performance as a prerequisite for rewards, and then discuss other popular criteria by which rewards are distributed. In Chapter 6, we argued that motivation will be highest

8. Peter M. Blau, *The Dynamics of Bureaucracy,* rev. ed. (Chicago: University of Chicago Press, 1963).

9. "The Cop-Out Cops," *The National Observer,* August 3, 1974.

10. Enid F. Beaumont, "A Pivotal Point for the Merit Concept," *Public Administration Review,* September–October 1974, pp. 426–30.

11. David Stanley, "The Merit Principle Today," *Public Administration Review,* September–October 1974, p. 425.

when performance and rewards are closely linked. But, in reality, performance is only *one* of many criteria upon which organizational rewards are distributed.

Performance. Performance is results measurement. It merely asks the question: Did you get the job done? To reward people in the organization, therefore, requires some agreed-upon criterion for defining their performance. Whether this criterion is valid or not in representing performance is not relevant to our definition; as long as rewards are allocated based on factors that are directly linked to doing the job successfully, we are using performance as the determinant. For many jobs, productivity is used as a single criterion. But as jobs become less standardized and routine, productivity becomes more difficult to measure and, hence, the defining of performance becomes increasingly complex.

Another difficult issue with performance is differentiating between quantity and quality. For example, an individual may generate a high output, but his performance standards may be quite low. Hence, where controls are not instituted to protect against such abuses, we often find quantity replacing quality.

Effort. It is not uncommon for a report card in grammar school to include effort as one of the categories used in grading students. Organizations rarely make their rewarding of effort that explicit, yet it is certainly a major determinant in the reward distribution.

The rewarding of effort represents the classical example of rewarding means rather than ends. In organizations where performance is generally of low caliber, rewarding of effort may be the only criterion by which to differentiate rewards. For example, a major eastern university was attempting to increase its research efforts and had designated the objective of obtaining grants or funded research as a critical benchmark toward this end. Upon selection of this objective, all faculty members were informed that rewards for the coming year were going to be based on performance in obtaining grants. Unfortunately, after the first year of the program, even though approximately 20 percent of the faculty had made grant applications, none were approved. When the time came for performance evaluation and the distribution of rewards, the dean chose to give the majority of the funds available for pay raises to those faculty members who had applied for grants. Here is a case where performance, defined in terms of obtaining funded research grants, was zero, so the dean chose to allocate rewards based on effort.

The above example is much less rare than one might think. On the assumption that those who try should be encouraged, in many cases effort can count *more than* actual performance. The employee who is clearly perceived by her superiors to be working less than at her optimum can often expect to be rewarded less than some other employee who, while producing less, is giving out a greater effort. Even where it is clearly stated that performance is what will be rewarded, people who make evaluations and distribute rewards are only human. Therefore, they are not immune to sympathizing with those who try hard, but with minimal success, and allowing this to influence their evaluation and reward decisions.

Seniority. Seniority, job rights, and tenure dominate most civil service systems in the United States, and while they do not play as important a role in business corporations, the length of time on the job is still a major factor in determining the allocation of rewards. Seniority's greatest virtue is that, relative to other criteria, it is easy to determine. We may disagree as to whether the quality of Smith's work is higher or lower than that of Jones, but we would probably not have much debate over who has been with the organization longer. So seniority represents an easily quantifiable criterion that can be substituted for performance.

Skills Held. Another practice that is not uncommon in organizations is to allocate rewards based on the skills of the employee. Regardless of whether the skills are used, those individuals who possess the highest skills or talents will be rewarded commensurately. Where such practices are used, it is not unusual to see individuals become "credential crazy." The requirement that an individual needs a college degree in order to attain a certain level within the organization is utilizing skills as a determinant of rewards. Similarly, the requirement that an individual has to pass certain skill tasks by demonstrating an acceptable score in order to maintain a particular position in the organization is again using skills as a reward criterion. If it is necessary for a secretary to demonstrate that he or she can take shorthand at 120 words per minute to be eligible for consideration as secretary to a department head, and if department heads do all their dictation into a dictating machine rather than giving it directly to the secretary, we see an example of a skill being utilized as a reward criterion when, in effect, it is irrelevant.

When individuals enter an organization, their skill level is usually a major determinant of the compensation they will receive. In such cases, the marketplace or competition has acted to make skills a major element in the reward package. These externally imposed standards can evolve from the community or from occupational categories themselves. In other words, the relationship of demand and supply for particular skills in the community can significantly influence the rewards the organization must expend to acquire those skills. Also, the demand-supply relationship for an entire occupational category throughout the country can affect rewards.

Job Difficulty. The complexity of the job can be a criterion by which rewards are distributed. For example, those jobs that are highly repetitive and can be learned quickly may be viewed as less deserving in rewards than those that are more complex and sophisticated. Jobs that are difficult to perform, or are undesirable due to stress or unpleasant working conditions, may have to carry with them rewards that are higher in order to attract workers to these activities.

Discretionary Time. The greater the discretion called for on a job, all other things being equal, the greater the impact of mistakes and the greater the need for good judgment. In a job that has been completely programmed—that is, where each step has been procedurized and there is no room for decision making by the incumbent—there is little discretionary time. Such jobs require less judgment, and lower rewards can be offered to attract people to take these positions. As discretion time increases, greater judgmental abilities are needed, and rewards must commensurately be expanded.

Reward Determinants in Practice

Motivation theory argues for linking rewards to performance. If we accept that pay is a primary reward in organizations, there is little evidence that organizations actually use performance as the single most important determinant of pay. A more realistic conclusion would be that pay is allocated at least as much for effort as for accomplishment.[12] A survey of nearly 9,000 workers, consisting of management, salaried, and hourly employees, suggests some interesting predictors of pay.[13] For management positions, education proved to be the best predictor of compensation. The job level held and the age of the incumbent were also relatively good predictors of actual pay. "It appears that the better educated, higher level, older managers, who have been with the company somewhat longer, are better paid."[14] Among salaried employees, age was the most closely related variable to pay, closely followed by education and job level. Length of time on the job was the major predictor for hourly workers. Those hourly workers who had been with the company the longest were the highest paid. The researchers concluded:

> One inference that seems resasonable from all these data is that the amount of an employee's pay is likely to be determined by many factors, a large portion of which seem to be from those such as age, education, tenure, and job level. It is possible, however, that such factors have little or no relation to actual effectiveness or job performance.
>
> This finding casts considerable doubt that employee performance is related to pay.[15]

A survey of 493 large manufacturing and service companies provides further evidence to suggest that rewards are not based on performance criteria.[16] As Figure 16–1 shows, pay increases in these companies tended to be more influenced by external factors such as the national cost-of-living index and community pay policies than by individual worker productivity.

---

12. See, for example, Lyman W. Porter and Edward E. Lawler III, *Managerial Attitudes and Performance* (Homewood, Ill.: Richard D. Irwin, 1968), p. 158; and Jay R. Schuster, Barbara Clark, and Miles Rogers, "Testing Portions of the Porter and Lawler Model Regarding the Motivational Role of Pay," *Journal of Applied Psychology*, June 1971, pp. 187–95.

13. W. W. Ronan and G. J. Organt, "Determinants of Pay and Pay Satisfaction," *Personnel Psychology*, Winter 1973, pp. 503–20.

14. Ibid., p. 511.

15. Ibid., p. 513.

16. David A. Weeks, *Compensating Employees: Lessons of the 1970's*, Report No. 707 (New York: The Conference Board, 1976), pp. 12–14.

FACTORS DETERMINING PAY INCREASES	EMPLOYEE CATEGORY				
	Officers and Executives	Exempt Salaried	Nonexempt Salaried	Nonunion Hourly	Union Hourly
Worker productivity	4	7	5	3	9
Company's financial results	1	2	3	5	7
Company's financial prospects	2	3	4	4	5
Internal equity among groups	6	5	6	6	8
Increases of industry leaders	5	6	8	7	4
Area surveys	3	1	1	1	6
Ability to hire	7	8	7	10	10
National bargaining settlements	9	10	10	8	2
Union demands	10	9	9	9	1
Cost-of-living index	8	4	2	2	3

Note: Importance rating determined by frequency of mentions in first, second, or third place in a ranking from 1 to 10. Sample composed of manufacturing (44%), banking and insurance (38%), utility (15%), and retail (3%) firms.

Source: Adapted from David A. Weeks, *Compensating Employees: Lessons of the 1970's.* Report No. 707 (New York: The Conference Board, 1976), pp. 12-14.

Types of Rewards

Rewards are a vital component in determining the level of effort that an individual is willing to exert on his or her job. When employees see little or no relation between their performance and rewards—for example, they observe pay raises being granted for nonperformance reasons—rewards no longer act as motivators to high performance. Even though many organizations, by choice or tradition or contract, allocate rewards on nonperformance criteria, we should recognize that rewards hold their greatest impact on worker motivation and productivity when they are designed to pay off for performance.

The types of rewards that an organization can allocate are more complex than is generally thought. Obviously, there is direct compensation. But there are also indirect compensation and nonfinancial rewards. Each of these types of rewards can be distributed on an individual, group, or organization-wide basis. Figure 16–2 presents a structure for looking at rewards.

Intrinsic rewards are those that individuals receive for themselves. They are largely a result of the worker's satisfaction with his or her job. As noted in

FIGURE 16–2 Types of Rewards

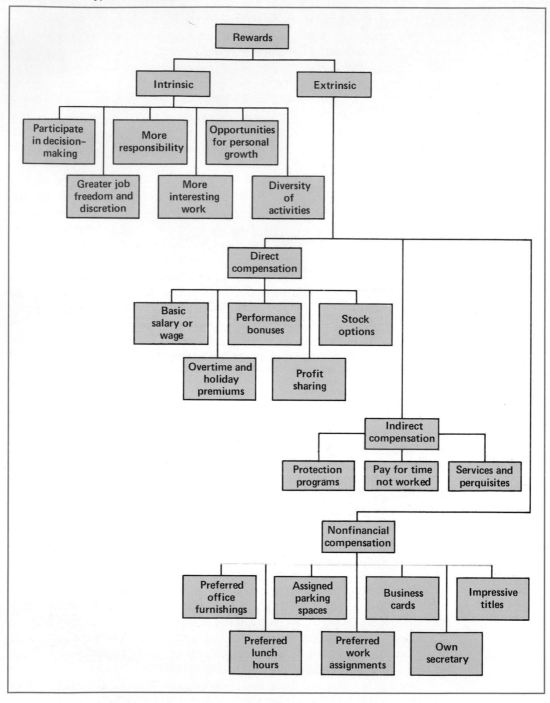

Chapter 15, techniques like job enrichment or any efforts to redesign or restructure work to increase its personal worth to the employee may make his or her work more intrinsically rewarding.

As previously noted, extrinsic rewards include direct compensation, indirect compensation, and nonfinancial rewards. Of course, an employee expects some form of direct compensation: a basic wage or salary, overtime and holiday premium pay, bonuses based on performance, profit sharing, and/or possibly opportunities to purchase stock options. Employees will expect their direct compensation generally to align with their assessment of their contribution to the organization and, additionally, will expect it to be relatively comparable with the direct compensation given to other employees with similar abilities and performance.

The organization will provide employees with indirect compensation: insurance, pay for holidays and vacations, services, and perquisites. Inasmuch as these are generally made uniformly available to all employees at a given job level, regardless of performance, they are really not motivating rewards. However, where indirect compensation is controllable by management and is used to reward performance, then it clearly needs to be considered as a motivating reward. To illustrate: If a company-paid membership in a country club is not available to all middle- and upper-level executives, but only to those who have shown particular performance ratings, then it is a motivating reward. Similarly, if company-owned automobiles and aircraft are made available to certain employees based on their performance rather than their "entitlement," we should view these indirect compensations as motivating rewards for those who might deem these forms of compensation as attractive.

As with direct compensation, indirect compensation may be viewed in an individual, group, or organizational context. However, if rewards are to be linked closely with performance, we should expect individual rewards to be emphasized. On the other hand, if a certain group of managers within the organization have made a significant contribution to the effective performance of the organization, a blanket reward such as a membership in a social club might be appropriate. Again, is is important to note that since rewards achieve the greatest return when they are specifically designed to meet the needs of each individual, and since group and organizational rewards tend to deal in homogeneity—that is, they tend to treat all people alike—these types of rewards must, by definition, be somewhat less effective than individual rewards. The only exceptions to that statement are those instances where there is a high need for cohesiveness and group congeniality. In such instances, individuals may find group rewards more personally satisfying than individual rewards.

The classification of nonfinancial rewards tends to be a smorgasbord of desirable "things" that are potentially at the disposal of the organization. The creation of nonfinancial rewards is limited only by managers' ingenuity and ability to assess "payoffs" that individuals with the organization find desirable and that are within the managers' jurisdiction.

The old saying "One man's food is another man's poison" certainly applies to rewards. What one employee views as highly desirable, another finds superfluous. Therefore, *any* reward may not get the desired result; however, where selection has been done assiduously, the benefits to the organization by way of higher worker performance should be impressive.

Some workers are very status conscious. A paneled office, a carpeted floor, a large walnut desk, or a private bathroom may be just the office furnishing that stimulates an employee toward top performance. Status-oriented employees may also value an impressive job title, their own business cards, their own secretary, or a well-located parking space with their name clearly painted underneath the "Reserved" sign.

Some employees value having their lunch at, say, 1 P.M. to 2 P.M. If lunch is normally from 11 A.M. to 12 noon, the benefit of being able to take their lunch at another, more desirable time can be viewed as a reward. Having a chance to work with congenial colleagues or achieving a desired work assignment or an assignment where the worker can operate without close supervision are all rewards that are within the discretion of management and, when carefully aligned to individual needs, can provide stimulus for improved performance.

IMPLICATIONS FOR PERFORMANCE AND SATISFACTION

The understanding of an organization's evaluation procedure and reward system are important in attempting to explain and predict the behavior of individuals within the organization. People do not work gratis. They expect payoffs: salary, fringe benefits, promotion opportunities, recognition, social contact, and so forth. If employees perceive that their efforts will be accurately appraised and if they further perceive that the rewards they value are closely linked to their appraisals, the organization will have optimized the motivational properties from its evaluation and reward procedures and policies. More specifically, based on the contents of this chapter and our discussion of motivation in Chapter 6, we can conclude that rewards are likely to lead to high employee performance and satisfaction when they are (1) perceived as equitable by the employee, (2) tied to performance, and (3) tailored to the needs of the individual. These conditions should foster a minimum of dissatisfaction among employees, reduced withdrawal patterns, and increased organizational commitment. If these conditions do not exist, the probability of withdrawal behavior increases, and the prevalence of marginal or barely adequate performance increases. If workers perceive that their efforts are not recognized or rewarded, and if they view their alternatives as limited, they may continue working, but perform at a level considerably below their capability.

FOR DISCUSSION

1. How can an organization's performance evaluation system affect employee behavior?

2. How can an organization's reward system affect employee behavior?

3. Why do organizations evaluate employees?

4. What qualities should effective performance standards contain?

5. What is (a) leniency error? (b) halo error? (c) similarity error?

6. Contrast absolute standards with relative standards. What are the advantages and disadvantages of each?

7. If the average employee believes he is performing at the 75th percentile, what does this imply for employee performance reviews?

8. Identify and discuss popular criteria by which organizations distribute rewards.

9. Do organizations reward performance? Do they reward merit? Explain.

10. Some organizations have a personnel policy that pay information be kept secret. Not only is pay information not given out by management but employees are also discouraged from talking about their pay with co-workers. How do you think this practice affects employee behavior?

FOR FURTHER READING

COLBY, J., and R. WALLACE, "Performance Appraisal: Help or Hindrance to Employee Productivity?" *Personnel Administration*, October 1975, pp. 37–39. Performance appraisal should be consistent with the employee's self-image and be done on a year-round basis.

DAVIS, C., and A. FRANCIS, "The Many Dimensions of Performance Measurement: There Is More to Performance Than Profits or Growth," *Organizational Dynamics*, Winter 1975, pp. 51–65. In any organization, performance measurement involves conflicting objectives, agonizing choices, and continuing tradeoffs between criteria and contributors.

HAMMER, T. H., "Relationships between Local Union Characteristics and Worker Behavior and Attitudes," *Academy of Management Journal*, December 1978, pp. 560–77. The union can be a moderating variable effecting the reward-performance and reward-satisfaction relationship.

KEARNEY, W. J., "Pay for Performance? Not Always," *MSU Business Topics*, Spring 1979, pp. 5–16. The best workers cannot always be compensated appropriately. Identifies the barriers to paying for performance.

LAWLER, E. E., III, *Pay and Organizational Effectiveness*. New York: McGraw-Hill, 1971. An important book which considers the facts and fantasies underlying the impact of pay on performance.

THOMPSON, P. H., and G. W. DALTON, "Performance Appraisal: Managers Beware," *Harvard Business Review*, January–February 1970, pp. 149–57. The performance evaluation and feedback systems that management perceives as fair and optimal too often lead to widespread discouragement, cynicism, and alienation.

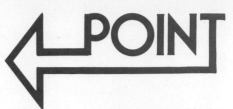

POINT

OLSEN and BENNETT

Performance appraisal as a management technique

Adapted and edited from Leif O. Olsen and Addison C. Bennett, "Performance Appraisal: Management Technique or Social Process? Part I, Management Technique," Management Review, *December 1975.* © 1975 by AMACOM, a division of American Management Associations. All rights reserved.

The objectives of performance appraisal are praiseworthy and utilitarian. Judged by its goals, performance appraisal is a concept that appears compatible with our values as well as with our beliefs concerning the perfectability of man. It has its roots in the solid American tradition of achievement of success through hard work and self-improvement. In addition, it helps reinforce the omnipotence of management and define the present and future status of employees in the organization. Often, at the moment of its introduction into an organization, it has seemed to possess all the irresistible characteristics associated with an idea whose time has come. But has it really been an idea whose time has come or have we been infatuated with its technique?

The focus of performance appraisal as usually applied is on changing the behavior of the individual for the benefit of the organization. Let us trace its recent development so we can better anticipate its future development. Let us consider performance appraisal as having two dimensions: one, the manner in which judgment is applied to the *evaluation* of an employee's performance; the other, the means used to achieve *changes* in the

employee's performance. Progress on either of these dimensions is, in our opinion, associated with the stage of development of other management processes in the organization.

At the first stage, performance appraisal is dominated by a perception of the organization as a "machine designed for the attainment of productivity." While the organization is considered complex, intricate, and even dynamic, it is still perceived as a machine.

This perception affects the processes used in the management of the organization. For example, employees are considered components of the machine, consequently no employee is irreplaceable. If a component does not function properly, it is replaced with another. Furthermore, since the organization is a machine, there is no reason why productivity cannot be measured with scientific objectivity and accuracy. As a result, performance appraisal tends to emphasize measurement and minimize motivation.

The emphasis given to measurement can be illustrated by such "merit rating" techniques as graphic rating scales, check lists, and forced-choice rating devices. The factors chosen for rating are likely to be related to the processes by which work is thought to be performed but often have little relevance to the results the employee is supposed to accomplish. We see the inclusion of such factors as "accuracy," "dependability," and "attendance." In some cases, the factors tend to go beyond the legitimate context of the relationship between the organization and employee. Such extensions result in confusion with

444

respect to the main issue of what exactly is being appraised.

The focus in the first stage is almost exclusively on the needs of the organization. Improvements of employee performance are sought for the purpose of accomplishing organizational objectives: Employee needs are considered subordinate to the needs of the organization, and the present and future existence of the organization is paramount. Performance appraisal is generally characterized by one-way communication, with employees given the opportunity to explain performance inadequacies. All too frequently this also permits condemnation of these inadequacies by the superior—with all its accompanying trauma.

The task the employee performs, and any objectives he is to accomplish, are established by management. There is minimal participation by the individual in determining his work goals. The employee, more often than not, is told what to do, how, and when. And when his performance is reviewed, it is the past that is reviewed—a past that cannot be altered.

In the second stage, performance appraisal reflects the influence of the increasing degree of participation occurring in our society and our more advanced knowledge of human behavior and motivation. In this stage the employee is perceived as a human being whose needs must be considered. However, the organization still remains the paramount entity.

The guiding thought at this stage is that employees must fit into the organization; they are expected to contribute to the organization first, with individual growth and development being viewed as a byproduct of value to both the organization and the individual.

While in the second stage, performance appraisal has a number of characteristics similar to those of the first stage, it also possesses characteristics that reflect acceptance of recent advances in our knowledge of human behavior. The second stage, for example, is characterized by a greater recognition that satisfaction of the employee's needs for fulfillment and self-actualization through work is essential to the well-being of the organization. We also see a shift in emphasis from an evaluation of such factors as the personality of the employee and *how* he does his job to a performance appraisal based on *what* is actually accomplished by the employee. The appraisal process now places importance on whether the employee is accomplishing the results desired, and efforts are made to allow employees to participate in formulating these work objectives. The supervisor, however, still has the final word regarding work objectives and how they are to be achieved.

Further, fewer managers appraise performance by means of a critical review of the past and more use the development of commitments for the future as a way of enhancing motivation and providing a framework for productive behavior. An essential part of this framework is the need for effective employee-manager communication. This increased emphasis on communication is another important characteristic of the second stage. The value of what the employee has to say and the importance of providing the opportunity for him to say it are both recognized.

Perhaps the most important characteristic of this stage is recognition of employees as members of society with full rights equal to those of all members. Despite this, they still have limited rights *within* the organization in which they work. Frequently, for example, they do not have the right to know the salary range for their positions or to have access to other types of data relevant to them as members of the organization. Also, they do not have the right to determine how they shall be compensated but are required to accept whatever mix of direct compensation and benefits the organization has developed, regardless of how it suits their individual needs or desires. Most important of all, as far as motivation and development are concerned, they do not have the right of full participation in the determination of what is to be achieved from their work and how. At this stage, performance appraisal emphasizes such approaches as performance standards and goal setting.

COUNTER ⊲⊳ POINT

OLSEN and BENNETT

Performance appraisal as a social process

At the third stage of development, the employee is perceived and treated as a human being whose needs are paramount to him and of equal importance to those of the organization. The employee works for the organization, not by the necessity, but by choice. He is seen as an individual rather than a unit of the labor market. There is a greater concern for the employee's development as an individual in his own right rather than as a component of the organization. The primary objective of development is to enhance the employee's growth, for his benefit, with the expectation that his growth will also benefit the organization and society. In other words, what's good for John Doe is good for General Motors.

The manager's new role becomes one of providing supportive services to his employees to help them accomplish their part of the organization's objectives. To do this properly, the manager must have an understanding of human behavior and a knowledge of the skills required to do the work that must be done. The manager's role is to coordinate his employee's work with that of other groups and to provide the technical, material, and financial support that may be needed.

This redefinition of the roles of employee and manager results in their effective participation in the work of the organization. Since the employee has the responsibility for attaining specific results, he also has an obligation to participate in determining how and when these results are to be realized. This enhances the dignity of the employee and promotes his perception of himself as a contributor to the organization. This result is difficult to achieve in an authoritarian organization.

Another important effect of this changing employee-manager relationship is the increasing practice by the employee and the manager of *negotiating* the results to be obtained from the employee's work. Thereafter, evaluations of performance concentrate on the accomplishment of the objectives determined through these negotiations.

If what we are looking for is a means of achieving constructive changes in *future job behavior,* then acceptance of the process of negotiations within an organization is highly desirable.

Just what is negotiated between the employee and the manager? Very briefly, results! The use of negotiation assumes that the employee possesses the knowledge and skills to perform his job and that the manager, therefore, does not—nor should he have to—review with the employee the processes by which the employee will accomplish the results.

So, the employee commits himself to accomplish certain results. What does the manager commit himself to? The manager commits himself to providing the necessary materials, manpower, money, and whatever else is needed by the employee to accomplish the results.

What is unique about the negotiation approach, however, is not the commitments that are negotiated, but rather the process by which they come about. It is the process and its three primary principles of *equality of participation, freedom of discussion,* and *commitment to the future* that are the foundation for the commitment to change and to achieve.

It is reasonably safe to assume that the more two participants involved in a negotiation feel that they are on equal footing, the greater will be the amount of discussion that will take place.

Freedom of discussion is essential if we wish to bring about changes in the participants' attitudes that will result in a mutually arrived at agreement concerning future action. The participants are, in effect, planning for the future, and if they are to carry out these plans, they must be committed to them. It is discussion of near equals that will provide the basis needed for a joint commitment to achievement of long-term agreements.

In negotiating performance improvement, our concern with the past is limited to the guidance it can offer in helping us define the future. In brief, we should look on past performance as history that is used to help us to learn and to plot the future but not as a subject for negotiation. Negotiation counters the earlier-mentioned deficiencies in most performance appraisal processes by looking forward to what should be accomplished instead of back at the inadequacies of the past and by promoting greater freedom of discussion between the participants involved. Negotiation thereby moves toward the type of orientation that some organizations profess to want for their key people and managers, that of "putting them into business for themselves." Freedom and ability to negotiate in a meaningful and productive manner is an essential characteristic of entrepreneurial situations. In addition, negotiation becomes increasingly effective and realistic as the demands of people increase and they have sufficient job choice so they truly remain with an organization on a "consent" basis.

In addition, provision can be made for arbitration in those instances where negotiation between a manager and an employee breaks down. Just who should fill the role of "arbitrator" would be governed by such factors as the position of the individuals involved in negotiations and the position and personal attributes required on the part of the arbitrator.

Perhaps the single most important characteristic of this approach to performance appraisal is recognition of the fact that the employee not only has full rights as an individual in society, but that these rights do not change nor cease when he functions as a member of an organization. If we accept the extension of these rights from society into the organization, we then need to reexamine much of our present thinking about relationships between the employee and management. An acceptance of the "extension" concept also calls for an evaluation of reward structures and of methods of administering reward systems.

This third stage, while largely hypothetical as a total concept, integrates specific approaches that are neither novel nor unfamiliar. Its unique contribution is its attempt to recast the roles of the individual and the organization into patterns more consistent with the total environment in which both operate. This significant departure from past patterns of organizational behavior is in keeping with our main premise, namely, that performance appraisal must be viewed as a social process and, as such, must be in harmony with the social processes existing in the culture within which the organization functions.

In terms of this newly developed concept, are we really talking about performance appraisal? The answer is no. What we are talking about is a process that will achieve the objectives of performance appraisal yet avoid the detrimental side-effects that have been brought about by considering it as a technique rather than as a social process. *Performance appraisal as a managerial technique is dead.*

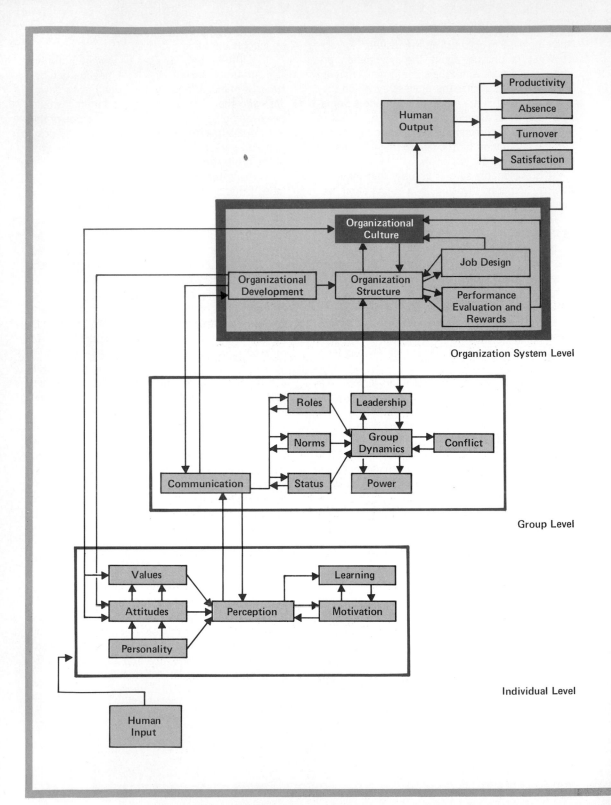

CHAPTER 17
Organizational Culture

AFTER STUDYING THIS CHAPTER, YOU SHOULD BE ABLE TO—

Define and explain the following key terms and concepts:

Collective socialization
Disjunctive socialization
Divestiture socialization
Encounter stage
Fixed socialization
Formal socialization
Individual socialization
Informal socialization

Investiture socialization
Metamorphosis stage
Organizational culture
Prearrival stage
Serial socialization
Socialization
Variable socialization

Understand:

The common characteristics making up organizational culture
The factors determining an organization's culture
The socialization process
The various socialization alternatives available to management

> In any organization, there are the ropes to skip and the ropes to know.
> —R. R. RITTI AND G. R. FUNKHOUSER

Just as individuals have personalities, so too do organizations. In Chapter 4, we found that individuals had relatively enduring and stable traits that helped us to predict their attitudes and behaviors. In this chapter, we propose that organizations, like people, can be characterized in terms such as aggressive, friendly, warm, innovative, relaxed, or conservative. These traits, in turn, can then be used to predict attitudes and behaviors of the people within these organizations.

The theme of this chapter is that there is a systems variable in organizations that, while hard to define or describe precisely, nevertheless exists and which employees generally describe in common terms. We call this variable *organizational culture*. Just as tribal cultures have totems and taboos that dictate how each member will act toward fellow members and outsiders, organizations have cultures that influence employees' actions toward clients, competitors, bosses, subordinates, and peers.[1] Just *what* organizational culture is and *how* organizations create their cultures will be discussed in the following pages.

WHAT IS CULTURE?

An organization's culture conveys important assumptions and norms governing values, activities, and goals. It tells employees how things are done and what's important. In the last decade we have made significant inroads toward developing some common understanding of organizational culture.

A Definition

There may be more disagreement about the appropriate label than the concept itself. That is, should the concept be called organizational culture, or personality, climate, or ambiance? The idea is the same, but researchers have used different labels to describe it. The most popular term used to describe an organization's personality is probably "organizational climate." However, this term lacks the richness of the concept discussed in this chapter. We prefer the broader term of

1. "Corporate Culture," *Business Week*, October 27, 1980, p. 148.

organizational culture not only to dramatize that organizations have different degrees of "warmth," but also to convey that organizations have traditions, values, customs, practices, and socialization processes that endure over long periods of time and that *do* influence the attitudes and behaviors of their members.

What do we specifically mean by organizational culture? We propose that it is a relatively uniform perception held of the organization; that it has common characteristics; that it is descriptive; that it can distinguish one organization from another; and that it integrates individual, group, and organization system variables.

First, organizational culture represents a common perception shared by the organization's members. Individuals with different backgrounds or at different levels in the organization tend to describe the organization's culture in similar terms.[2] They perceive a unique set of characteristics that are substantially organization-specific.

Second, there are five characteristics that researchers have identified as consistently tapping the essence of an organization's culture:[3]

1. *Individual autonomy*—includes individual responsibility, independence, and opportunities for exercising individual initiative
2. *Structure*—degree of formalization, centralization, and direct supervision
3. *Reward orientation*—factors of reward, promotion-achievement orientation, and emphasis upon profits and sales
4. *Consideration*—warmth and support provided by superiors
5. *Conflict*—degree of conflict present in interpersonal relationships between peers, as well as the willingness to be honest and open about interpersonal differences

Third, organizational culture is a descriptive term. It is concerned with how employees perceive the five characteristics, not whether they like them or not. This is important because it differentiates culture from job satisfaction.[4] Research on organizational culture has sought to measure how employees see their organization: Is it highly structured? Does it reward innovation? Does it stifle conflicts? Job satisfaction, on the other hand, seeks to measure affective responses to the work environment. That is, the former describes, while the latter evaluates.

Fourth, the evidence indicates that organizational cultures are distinct; that is, we can distinguish one organization from another in terms of culture. These cultural characteristics are relatively enduring over time and relatively static in their propensity to change.[5]

2. John A. Drexler, Jr., "Organizational Climate: Its Homogeniety within Organizations," *Journal of Applied Psychology,* February 1977, pp. 38–42.

3. John P. Campbell, Marvin D. Dunnette, Edward E. Lawler III, and Karl E. Weick, *Managerial Behavior, Performance, and Effectiveness* (New York: McGraw-Hill, 1970), p. 393.

4. Benjamin Schneider and Robert A. Snyder, "Some Relationships between Job Satisfaction and Organizational Climate," *Journal of Applied Psychology,* June 1975, pp. 318–28.

5. Garlie A. Forehand and B. Von Haller Gilmer, "Environmental Variations in Studies of Organizational Behavior," *Psychological Bulletin,* December 1964, p. 362.

Lastly, the concept of culture embraces individual, group, and organizational system level concepts. Autonomy taps an individual level variable. Consideration and conflict are group level characteristics. Structure and reward-orientation are organizational system dimensions.

In summary, we propose that every organization has its own unique culture. This culture includes long-standing, and often unwritten, rules and regulations; a special language that facilitates communication among members; shared standards of relevance as to the critical aspects of the work that is to be done; matter-of-fact prejudices; standards for social etiquette and demeanor; established customs for how members should relate to peers, subordinates, superiors, and outsiders; and other traditions that clarify to members what is appropriate and "smart" behavior within the organization and what is not.[6] As we shall show later in this chapter, employees who have been properly socialized to their organization's culture have learned how things are done, what matters, and which work-related behaviors and attitudes are acceptable and desirable and which ones are not.

Two Examples

Let's look at a couple of brief examples to illustrate just how an organization's culture influences employees and even the spouses of employees.

General Motors. General Motors has long been considered a conservative and risk-aversive organization. John DeLorean, a former senior executive at GM, described in the book, *On a Clear Day You Can See General Motors,* how he was pressured to act in ways consistent with GM's culture:

> . . . The Corporate rule was dark suits, light shirts and muted ties. I followed the rule to the letter, only I wore stylish Italian-cut suits, wide-collared off-white shirts and wide ties.
>
> "Goddammit, John," he'd [DeLorean's boss] yell. "Can't you dress like a businessman? And get your hair cut, too."
>
> My hair was ear length with sideburns. I felt both my clothes and hairstyle were contemporary but not radical, so I told him:
>
> "General Motor's business—selling annual styling changes—makes this a fashion business. And what the hell do you know about fashion? Most of these guys around here wear narrow-lapelled suits and baggy pants with cuffs that are four inches above their shoes."
>
> The fact that I had been divorced, was a health nut and dated generally younger actresses and models didn't set well with the corporate executives or their wives. And neither did my general disappearance from the corporate social scene. Dollie Cole, the second wife of then President Ed Cole, who himself was divorced, called me up after my second divorce when I was dating my wife Christina and told me, "They are all shook up on The Fourteenth Floor [where the top executives offices are located]. God! Don't get married again. You'd better cool it. All you've got to do is lay low and wait them out. Those guys will all be gone in five years. Don't kick away your career now."

---

6. John Van Maanen and Edgar H. Schein, "Toward a Theory of Organizational Socialization," in *Research in Organizational Behavior,* Vol. I, ed. Barry M. Staw (Greenwich, Conn.: JAI Press, 1979), p. 210.

Nevertheless, my clothing and lifestyle were increasingly rattling the cages of my superiors, as was the amount of publicity my personal and business lives were generating. I was being resented because my style of living violated an unwritten but widely revered precept that said no personality could outshine General Motors.[7]

Even though DeLorean had, at the age of forty-eight, risen to a position where he directed GM's Chevrolet, Buick, Oldsmobile, Pontiac, Cadillac, and GMC Truck and Coach Divisions—and was earning up to $650,000 a year—he quit in 1973. His complaint was that GM could not "accept or accommodate an executive who had made his mark in the corporation by being different and individualistic."[8] He went on to start the DeLorean Motor Co. which manufactures an innovative sports car in Northern Ireland.

U.S. Navy. The armed services are well known for their traditions. Did you know there's a book that describes these traditions and social customs for wives of Navy officers? There is, and it includes "useful bits of information every Navy wife needs but few really know,"[9] on topics such as hospitality, entertaining, and proper dress. The following excerpts suggest an organization that is rigid and formal:

> Anyone in civilian clothes may be as undignified and boorish as he likes, and the only reflections will be on him personally. But if an officer makes a public spectacle of himself, it reflects on the whole Service. So anything done in public which appears undignified, which gives a bad impression of the Navy, or which might be construed as conduct unbecoming a gentleman is frowned upon. To be untidy in dress or otherwise slovenly in appearance; to be rude or quarrelsome; to be overbearing or supercilious; to make a public display of affection; to be loud or boisterous, to be drunk or disorderly—these are all things that a Naval officer avoids.[10]

> . . . It is customary at small gatherings for the younger wives to rise when the wife of the senior officer enters the room and to remain standing as long as she does. If once seated, she gets up again, you need not rise also unless you wish to offer her some service, but it looks very rude for a group of young women to remain seated while an older one stands. If the senior officer's wife is anywhere near your age, or if she is sensitive of her years, you may offend rather than compliment her by rising. But unless you feel that it would be tactless to rise, you should do so.[11]

> . . . you should do all you can to fulfill the wishes of the wife of your husband's Commanding Officer *within the bounds of reason.* She is not priviledged to give you orders, and if she does, you are not obligated to carry them out; but as far as possible you should comply with her requests. If it is impossible for you to do so, or if you think she is imposing on you, you may courteously decline to do as she asks. But it is not only considered good manners to be as cooperative as possible, but it helps the morale of the ship if the wives all get along together. And no matter what your personal opinion of your Commanding Officer's wife may be,

7. J. Patrick Wright, *On a Clear Day You Can See General Motors* (Grosse Point, Mich.: Wright Enterprises, 1979), p. 9.

8. Ibid., p. 2.

9. Florence Ridgely Johnson, *Welcome Aboard: An Informal Guide for the Naval Officer's Wife,* 6th ed. (Annapolis, Md.: U.S. Naval Institute, 1964), p. vi.

10. Ibid., pp. 77–78.

11. Ibid., pp. 136–37.

don't criticize her or her husband while your husband is serving under him. It is death to morale.[12]

The above quotes were taken from a book published twenty years ago. While the Navy has changed since then, the rigid and formal culture depicted in these quotes is still largely unchanged. Traditions and customs are altered slowly. Of course, and this is extremely important, the fact that an organization's culture is relatively enduring means that it gives employees a sense of how to behave and what they ought to be doing. This, in turn, makes behavior in organizations more predictable.

SOCIALIZATION: HOW ORGANIZATIONS CREATE THEIR CULTURES

An organization's culture is not the result of any one input. The founding fathers of an organization typically have a major impact. Henry Ford at Ford Motor Company, Thomas Watson at IBM, J. Edgar Hoover at the FBI, Thomas Jefferson at the University of Virginia, and Edwin Land at Polaroid are examples of individuals and organizations who are closely linked. Watson's views, for instance, on research and development, product innovation, employee dress, and compensation policies are still evident at IBM although Watson died in 1956.

The present top management can also be expected to have a major impact on the organization's culture.[13] Through what they say and how they behave, senior executives establish norms that filter down through the organization as to whether risk taking is desirable; how much freedom managers should give their subordinates; what is appropriate dress; what actions will pay off in terms of pay raises, promotions, and other rewards; and the like.

In addition to the influence of the founding fathers and current senior executives, organizational culture is clearly affected by the organization's selection process. Organizations obviously do not hire everyone who applies. Who is hired and who is not is far from a random decision. Selection decisions include judgments as to whether the candidate will fit into the organization. And this attempt to ensure a proper match, whether purposely or inadvertently, contributes toward the creation of a uniform culture within the organization.[14] Examples of this phenomenon are widely evident. Corporations tend to recruit and select management personnel from within their own industry, thus enhancing

12. Ibid., pp. 92–93.

13. Renato Tagiuri and George H. Litwin, *Organizational Climate* (Boston: Harvard University Graduate School of Business Administration, 1968); and Jerome L. Franklin, "Down the Organization: Influence Processes across Levels of Hierarchy," *Administrative Science Quarterly*, June 1975, pp. 153–64.

14. Graeme Salaman, "The Sociology of Assessment: The Regular Commissions Board Assessment Procedure," in *People and Organizations: Media Booklet II* (Milton Keynes, England: Open University Press, 1974).

common perceptions.[15] The top Wall Street law firms still predominantly hire graduates from the prestigious eastern law schools, ensuring homogeniety of both partners and associates.[16] College fraternities and sororities assess potential members' socioeconomic status, personality, and physical appearance to find those "compatible" with the organization's image of itself. Personal contacts or "friends of friends" are a major source of job information for white-collar workers, which increases the likelihood that the organization will hire like-minded individuals.[17] It should not be surprising to learn that a study of the U.S. Federal Trade Commission found that the FTC attached more significance to regional background, old school ties, and political endorsements when recruiting attorneys than to their ability as reflected in grades or in the quality of law schools they attended.[18] These examples all confirm our contention that organizations use their personnel selection process to hire those who will fit in and accept the organization's values, norms, and customs, while at the same time screening out those who might challenge the system.

The indoctrinating of employees into the organization's culture is probably most evident, and undoubtedly most critical, when a new employee enters the organization. It is then that he or she is least familiar with the culture and is potentially most likely to disturb the values, norms, and customs that are currently in place. The organization, therefore, will want to process the new employee in order to get him or her to adapt to the organization's culture. We call this adaptation process *socialization*. Because organizations are constantly molding all employees so they reflect the organization's current culture, socialization is going on all the time. In the following pages, we shall demonstrate that the concept of socialization provides some important insights into *how* organizations create their cultures. We'll emphasize the most critical socialization stage: at time of entry into the organization. This is when the organization seeks to mold the outsider into an employee "in good standing." But keep in mind that the organization will be socializing every employee, although maybe not as explicitly, throughout his or her entire career in the organization.

What Is Socialization?

As we have already noted, socialization is a process of adaptation. It is the process by which employees come to understand the values, norms, and customs essential for assuming an organizational role and for becoming an accepted member of the organization. Those employees who fail to learn the essential or pivotal role behaviors risk being labeled "nonconformists" or "rebels" which often leads to expulsion. So socialization really performs two purposes. First, it

15. Jeffrey Pfeffer and H. Leblebici, "Executive Recruitment and the Development of Interfirm Organizations," *Administrative Science Quarterly,* December 1973, pp. 457–61.

16. Erwin O. Smigel, *The Wall Street Lawyer* (New York: Free Press, 1964).

17. Mark Granovetter, *Getting A Job: A Study of Contacts and Careers* (Cambridge, Mass.: Harvard University Press, 1974).

18. William Evan, *Organization Theory* (New York: John Wiley, 1976), p. 162.

reduces ambiguity for employees. They feel more secure because they know what is expected of them. Second, socialization provides benefits to the organization. It creates more uniform behavior in members, thus increasing understanding in communication, reducing conflicts, and requiring less direct employee supervision and fewer management controls.

⌈ The Socialization Process

Socialization can be conceptualized as a process made up of three stages: prearrival, encounter, and metamorphosis.[19] The first stage encompasses all the learning that occurs before a new member joins the organization. In the second stage, the new employee sees what the organization is really like and confronts the likelihood that expectations and reality may diverge. In the third stage, the relatively long-lasting changes take place. The new employee masters the skills required for his job, successfully performs his new roles, and makes the adjustments to his work group's values and norms.[20] This three-stage process impacts on the new employee's work productivity, commitment to the organization's objectives, and his or her decision to stay with the organization. Figure 17–1 depicts this process.

Prearrival. The *prearrival stage* explicitly recognizes that each individual arrives with a set of values, attitudes, and expectations. These cover both the work to be done and the organization. For instance, in many jobs, particularly professional work, new members will have undergone a considerable degree of prior socialization in training and in school. One major purpose of a business school, for example, is to socialize business students to what business is like, what to expect in a business career, and instill the kind of attitudes that professors believe will lead to successful assimilation in a firm. But prearrival socialization goes beyond the specific job. The selection process is used in most organizations to inform prospective employees about the organization as a whole. In addition, as noted previously, the selection process also acts to ensure the inclusion of the "right type"—those who will fit in. "Indeed, the ability of the individual to present the appropriate face during the selection process determines his ability to move into the organization in the first place. Thus, success depends on the degree to which the aspiring member has correctly anticipated the expectations and desires of those in the organization in charge of selection."[21]

Encounter. Upon entry into the organization, the new member enters the *encounter stage.* Here the individual confronts the possible dichotomy between

19. John Van Maanen and Edgar H. Schein, "Career Development," in *Improving Life at Work,* ed. J. Richard Hackman and J. Lloyd Suttle (Santa Monica, Calif.: Goodyear, 1977), pp. 58–62.

20. Daniel Charles Feldman, "The Multiple Socialization of Organization Members," *Academy of Management Review,* April 1981, p. 310.

21. Van Maanen and Schein, "Career Development," p. 59.

FIGURE 17–1 A Socialization Model

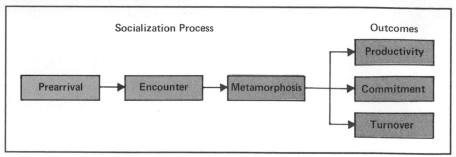

her expectations—about her job, her co-workers, her boss, and the organization in general—and reality. If expectations prove to have been more or less accurate, the encounter stage merely provides for a reaffirmation of the perceptions gained earlier. However, this is often not the case. Where expectations and reality differ, the new employee must undergo socialization that will detach her from her previous assumptions and replace these with another set that the organization deems desirable. At the extreme, a new member may become totally disillusioned with the actualities of her job, and resign. Proper selection should significantly reduce the probability of the latter occurrence.

Metamorphosis. Finally, the new member must work out any problems discovered during the encounter stage. This may mean going through changes—hence, we call this the *metamorphosis stage.* The ideas presented in the next section are designed to bring about the desired metamorphosis.

But what is a desirable metamorphosis? We can say that metamorphosis is complete, and the entry socialization process, when the new member has become comfortable with the organization and her job. She has internalized the norms of the organization and her work groups, and she understands and accepts these norms. The new member feels accepted by her peers as a trusted and valued individual. She is self-confident that she has the competence to complete her job successfully. She understands the system—not only her own tasks, but the rules, procedures, and informally accepted practices as well. Finally, she knows how she will be evaluated, that is, what criteria will be used to measure and appraise her work. She knows what is expected of her and what constitutes a job "well done." As Figure 17–1 shows, successful metamorphosis should have a positive impact on the new employee's productivity and her commitment to the organization, and reduce her propensity to leave the organization.

Socialization Methods

The management in organizations make decisions, either implicitly or explicitly, as to the way employees are to be socialized. The following represent various alternatives.[22] Notice, as you review these alternatives, how they contribute toward making an organizational culture consistent with the desires of the organization's management.

Formal or Informal? New employees may be put directly into their jobs, with no effort made to differentiate them for those who have been doing the job for a considerable length of time. Such cases represent examples of informal socialization—it takes place on the job and the new member gets little or no special attention. In contrast, socialization can be formal. The more formal the program, the more the new employee is segregated from the ongoing work setting and differentiated in some way to make explicit her newcomer's role.

The more formal a socialization program, the more likely it is that management has participated in its design and execution and, hence, the more likely that the recruit will experience the learning that management desires. In contrast, the more informal the program, the more success will depend on the new employee selecting the correct socialization agents. For example, if she chooses a co-worker who is highly knowledgeable about the job, accepts the system's values, and who is capable of transferring his knowledge, then socialization should be more successful than if the agent is marginally knowledgeable, a poor teacher, or holds deviant values. In most circumstances, laissez-faire socialization will increase the influence of the immediate work group on the new member.[23]

Whether a formal or an informal program is preferable will depend on management's goals. The more formal the program, the greater the likelihood that the recruit will acquire a known set of standards. That is, the new member is more likely to think and act like a GM executive, a management professor, or a U.S. Navy pilot. But an informal program is better for maintaining individual differences. Novel approaches to organizational problems and healthy questioning of the status quo are more likely to be generated by the person who has received informal socialization. And the informal program, because it takes place on the job, does not require transference of knowledge. The more that new members are removed from the day-to-day realities of the organization as part of the formal socialization process, the less they will be able to carry over, generalize, and apply the skills and norms learned in the socialization setting to the new job itself. Thus, there is likely to be more loss of learning from a formal program than from an informal program.

Of course, the idea of formal or informal programs represents two extremes along a continuum. Managers can make their programs more formal or more informal as they see necessary. In fact, a common practice in organizations is to use both. Employees begin with a relatively formal socialization to learn the key values, norms, and customs in the organization. Then they begin

22. This material is adapted with permission from John Van Maanen, "People Processing: Strategies of Organizational Socialization," *Organizational Dynamics,* Summer 1978, pp. 19–36. © 1978 by AMACOM, a division of American Management Associations.

23. Ibid., p. 24.

the informal socialization process on the job, where they learn the norms of their work group. The army recruit, for example, goes through six weeks of basic training—which is formal; followed up by the informal socialization that goes with becoming part of a working unit.

Individual or Collective? Another choice to be made by management is whether to socialize new members individually or to group them together and process them through an identical set of experiences.

The individual approach is likely to develop far less homogeneous views than collective socialization. As with the informal structure, individual socializing is more likely to preserve individual differences and perspectives. But socializing each person individually is expensive and time-consuming. It also fails to allow the new entrants to share their anxieties with others who are in similar circumstances.

Processing new members in collective groups allows the recruits to form alliances with others who can empathize with their adjustment problems. The recruits have people with whom they can interact and share what they are learning. The group shares problems and usually develop similar solutions. Therefore, collective socialization tends to form a common perspective on the organization among group members. College fraternity and sorority pledge classes are socialized collectively, and they tend to form consensus perspectives. Interestingly, because group socialization develops this consensual character, it allows the recruits, as a group, to deviate more from the standards held out by the organization than does the individual approach to socialization. It is easier for people to maintain a deviant position when they have others to support them. The group, therefore, is more likely than the individual to resist or redefine the organization's demands.

In practice, most large organizations find individual socialization impractical. They tend to rely on group socialization techniques. While small organizations, who have fewer new entrants to socialize, frequently use the individual approach, large organizations have moved to a collective approach because of its ease, efficiency, and predictability.

Fixed or Variable Time Period? A third major consideration for management is whether the transition from outsider to insider should be done on a fixed or variable time period. A fixed schedule reduces uncertainty for the new member since transition is standardized. She knows, for instance, that she is in a nine-month apprenticeship program. Each step of transition is clear. Successful completion of certain standardized steps means that she will be accepted to full-fledged membership. Variable schedules, in contrast, give no advanced notice of their transition timetable. Variability characterizes the socialization schedule for most professionals and managerial personnel.

Fixed schedules provide rigid conceptions of what is considered "normal" progress. Because the variable schedule does not, it requires new members to search for clues as to what is normal progress. They look for past patterns that might suggest when certain passages can and should be expected to take place or when tenure will be granted. Progress is then compared against these implied norms. Rumors and innuendos about who is going where and when characterize a variable schedule.

> Variable socialization processes give an administrator a powerful tool for influencing individual behavior. But the administration also risks creating an organizational situation marked by confusion and uncertainty among those concerned with their movement in the system. Fixed processes provide temporal reference points that allow people both to observe passages ceremonially and to hold together relationships forged during the socialization experiences. Variable processes, by contrast, tend to divide and drive apart people who might show much loyalty and cohesion if the process were fixed.[24]

Serial or Disjunctive? When an experienced organizational member, familiar with the new member's job, guides or directs a new recruit, we call this serial socialization. In this process, the experienced member acts as a tutor and model for the new employee. When the recruit does not have predecessors available to guide her or to model her behavior upon, we have disjunctive socialization.

Like our previous choices, both serial and disjunctive strategies have distinct advantages and disadvantages. Serial socialization maintains traditions and customs. Consistent use of this strategy will ensure a minimum amount of change within the organization over time. It also allows new members a look into the future by seeing in their more experienced colleague an image of themselves later in their career. However, each of these advantages has accompanying disadvantages. Stability and conformity may be achieved at the cost of stagnation and pressures to adhere to the status quo, even when conditions suggest the need for change. Similarly, a look into the future will have a positive effect on new employees only if they like what is seen. If the more experienced member is seen as frustrated, locked in, or caught up in some other negative context, the new employee may leave the organization rather than face what seems to be an agonizing future. This latter point indicates the importance of the experienced tutor in the serial process. If she is knowledgeable and enthusiastic, the recruit is likely to gain considerably from their working relationship. But if the tutor's morale is low, if she is a poor coach, or feels threatened by the recruit, serial socialization may, at worst, result in the loss of the new member. At best, it might result in socializing the employee with values that are counter to the interests of the organization.

The benefits and drawbacks to disjunctive socialization should be obvious from the above. It is likely to produce more inventive and creative employees because the recruit is not burdened by traditions. But this benefit must be weighed against the potential for creating deviants; that is, individuals who fail, due to an inadequate role model, to understand how their job is to be done and how it fits into the grand scheme of the organization.

Investiture or Divestiture? Our final consideration concerns whether our goal is to confirm or dismantle the incoming identity of the new member. Investiture

---

24. Ibid., p. 29.

rites ratify the usefulness of the characteristics that the person brings to the new job. This describes most high-level appointments in the organization. These individuals were selected on the basis of what they can bring to the job. The organization does not want to change these recruits, so entry is made as smooth and trouble-free as possible. If this is the goal, socialization efforts concentrate on reinforcing that "we like you just the way you are." This is frequently done by widely disseminating information on the new member's accomplishments. The recruit may be given a large degree of freedom to select her office furnishings, subordinates, and to make other decisions that will reflect on her performance. Elaborate initiation rites to confirm the new person's characteristics and "track record" are not unusual: news conferences, formal introduction of the candidate to influencial groups in the community, or visits to key people in the organization for ceremonial introductions and handshakes.

Far more often is the desire to strip away certain entering characteristics of a recruit. The selection process identified the candidate as a potential high performer; now it is necessary to make those minor modifications to improve the fit between the candidate and the organization. This fine-tuning may take the shape of requiring the recruit to sever old friendships; accepting a different way of looking at her job, peers, or the organization's purpose; doing a number of demeaning jobs to prove her commitment; or even undergoing harassment and hazing by more experienced personnel to verify that she fully accepts her role in the organization. One writer describes how a manager in an engineering company deliberately put each of his new engineers through an "upending experience" for the purpose of reducing their arrogance and making the point that they didn't have all the answers.

> He asked each new man to examine and diagnose a particular complex circuit, which happened to violate a number of textbook principles but actually worked very well. The new man would usually announce with confidence, even after an invitation to double-check, that the circuit could not possibly work. At this point the manager would demonstrate the circuit, tell the new man that they had been selling it for several years without customer complaint, and demand that the new man figure out why it did work. None of the men so far tested were able to do it, but all of them were thoroughly chastened and came to the manager anxious to learn where their knowledge was inadequate and needed supplementing. According to this manager, it was much easier from this point on to establish a good give and take relationship with his new man.[25]

This example is not atypical. First-year college students are frequently given extremely heavy workloads to shock them into the world of higher education. Similar divestiture practices occur for those entering military basic training, professional football, police cadet school, fraternal groups, religious cults, and self-realization groups, to name the more obvious. Such tactics build on the premise that if the organization is to instill a new set of values or norms, it first must shake up and possibly destroy those that are already in place.

If the goal of management is to produce similar employees, a divestiture

---

25. Edgar H. Schien, "Organizational Socialization and the Profession of Management," *Industrial Management Review,* Winter 1968, p. 5.

approach is likely to be used. It will achieve similar results with each recruit, and the process itself will promote a strong fellowship among those who have followed the same path to membership.

Conclusions

Our comments on socialization lead us to a number of conclusions:

1. An organization's socialization process is a significant determinant of the type of culture that an organization will have.
2. Socialization does not occur at one point, but is achieved more slowly over time.
3. Management can control, to a significant degree, the dominant values and norms within its organization by the type of socialization programs it establishes.
4. Successful organizational socialization frequently involves changes such as relinquishing certain attitudes, values, and behaviors; acquisition of new self-images, new involvements, new attitudes, and new values; and the learning of the required behavior patterns for effective performance.
5. Socialization does not produce conformity to a single standard, but rather decreases the extremes in behavior and attitudes.[26]

IMPLICATIONS FOR PERFORMANCE AND SATISFACTION

Figure 17–2 depicts organizational culture as an intervening variable. Employees form an overall subjective perception of the organization based on factors such as degree of autonomy, structure, reward orientation, warmth and support provided by supervisors, and willingness of management to tolerate conflict. This overall perception becomes, in effect, the organization's culture or personality. These favorable or unfavorable perceptions then affect employee performance and satisfaction.

Does culture have an equal impact on both employee performance and satisfaction: The evidence says "No." There is a relatively strong relationship

26. Several of these conclusions were suggested by Daniel Charles Feldman, "The Multiple Socialization of Organization Members: A Longitudinal Study," *Proceedings of the 41st Annual Academy of Management* (San Diego, 1981), p. 384.

FIGURE 17–2 How Organizational Culture Impacts Performance and Satisfaction

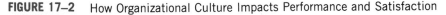

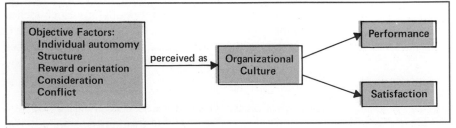

between culture and satisfaction, but this is moderated by individual differences.[27] In general, we propose that satisfaction will be highest when there is congruence between individual needs and the culture. For instance, an organization whose culture would be described as low in structure, having loose supervision, and which rewards people for high achievement is likely to have more satisfied employees if those employees have a high achievement need and prefer autonomy. Our conclusion, therefore, is that job satisfaction often varies according to the employee's perception of the organization's culture.

The relationship between culture and performance is less clear, although a number of studies find the two related.[28] But the relationship is moderated by the organization's technology.[29] Performance will be higher when the culture suits the technology. If the culture is informal, creative, and supports risk taking and conflict, performance will be higher if the technology is nonroutine. The more formally structured organizations that are risk-aversive, that seek to eliminate conflict, and that are prone to more task-oriented leadership will achieve higher performance when routine technology is utilized.

We should not overlook the influence socialization has on employee performance. An employee's performance depends to a considerable degree on knowing what he should or should not do. Understanding the right way to do a job indicates proper socialization. Further, the appraisal of an individual's performance includes how well the person fits into the organization. Can he get along with his co-workers? Does he have acceptable work habits? Does he demonstrate the right attitude? These qualities differ between jobs and organizations. For instance, on some jobs, employees will be evaluated higher if they are aggressive and outwardly indicate that they are ambitious. On another job, or on the same job in another organization, such an approach may be evaluated negatively. As a result, proper socialization becomes a significant factor in influencing both actual job performance and how it's perceived by others.

FOR DISCUSSION

1. How is organizational culture an integrative concept?

2. Contrast individual personality and organizational culture. How are they similar? How are they different?

3. What's the difference between job satisfaction and organizational culture?

4. Was John DeLorean's attitude and behavior good for General Motors? Explain.

27. Don Hellriegel and John W. Slocum, Jr., "Organizational Climate: Measures, Research, and Contingencies," *Academy of Management Journal,* June 1974, pp. 225–80.

28. Ibid.

29. Jay W. Lorsch and John J. Morse, *Organizations and Their Members* (New York: Harper & Row, 1974).

5. Is socialization brainwashing? Explain.

6. What benefits can socialization provide for the organization? For the new employee?

7. Explain the stages in the socialization process.

8. If management sought a culture characterized as innovative and autonomous, what might its socialization program look like?

9. If management sought a culture characterized as formalized and conflict-free, what might its socialization program look like?

10. Can you identify a set of characteristics that describe your college's culture? Compare them with several of your peers. How closely do they agree?

FOR FURTHER READING

BUCHANAN, B. II, "Building Organizational Commitment: The Socialization of Managers in Work Organizations," *Administrative Science Quarterly,* December 1974, pp. 533–46. Reviews which organizational experiences have the greatest impact on commitment. Major determinants of commitment for first-year employees were co-worker's attitudes toward the organization, initial job challenge, and pressures by the organization to adopt values or practices found personally repugnant.

FELDMAN, D. C., "A Practical Program for Employee Socialization," *Organizational Dynamics,* Autumn 1976, pp. 64–80. Offers a step-by-step description of the policies and practices required to make a socialization program successful.

JAMES, L. R., and A. P. JONES, "Organizational Climate: A Review of Theory and Research," *Psychological Bulletin,* December 1974, pp. 1096–112. Review of the literature to determine the extent to which organizational climate duplicates other organizational and individual domains.

LA FOLLETTE, W. R., "How Is the Climate in Your Organization?" *Personnel Journal,* July 1975, pp. 376–79. Knowledge of an organization's personality can help managers better understand the behavior and attitudes of their employees.

LOUIS, M. R., "Surprise and Sense Making: What Newcomers Experience in Entering Unfamiliar Organizational Settings," *Administrative Science Quarterly,* June 1980, pp. 226–51. Reviews what we know about the organizational entry experience.

SCHNEIDER, B., "Organizational Climates: An Essay," *Personnel Psychology,* Winter 1975, pp. 447–79. Presents evidence about the importance of the climate concept as an aid in understanding employee behavior in work organizations.

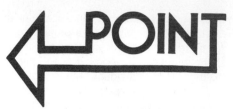

POWELL and BUTTERFIELD

The case for the subsystem climates in organizations

Adapted and edited from Gary N. Powell and D. Anthony Butterfield, "The Case for Subsystem Climates in Organizations," Academy of Management Review, *January 1978, pp. 151–57.*

Organizational climate (OC) has been a favorite topic of researchers on organizations for the past decade. Several researchers have recently suggested that organizations have many climates rather than one. This thesis represents a new development in the conceptualization of OC.

The purpose of this article is to provide further evidence for the existence of subsystem climates in organizations by reexamining the findings of past studies on climate and by reconsidering the proper unit of analysis for climate.

Organizational climate has been regarded as a property of the organization in most research studies. But about half of the two dozen studies surveyed in the present investigation performed analysis strictly at the individual level. Two-thirds of the studies drew climate perceptions from only one organization or without regard for organization. Some studies which did sample more than one organization still adhered to the individual as the unit of analysis.

The fact that many studies which were described as investigations of the organizational-level variable of climate actually examined the individual-level perceptions of climate indicates the state of confusion over the proper unit of analysis in climate research. Numerous attempts have been made to resolve the confusion. One researcher suggested that OC, operationalized as

individuals' perceptions of climate, may be just another name for job satisfaction. This proposition has since been rejected on theoretical and empirical grounds. In another attempt, a distinction was made between climate regarded as a property of organizations, or *organizational climate,* and as a property of individuals, or *psychological climate.* It was recommended that future research examine the relationship between organizational climate and psychological climate.

Payne and his associates made the most elaborate attempt to end the confusion. They identified three criteria which could be used to distinguish between various concepts pertaining to climate and satisfaction:

1. The unit of analysis—individual or organization

2. The element of analysis—job or group/organization

3. The nature of the measurement—descriptive or affective

When the element of analysis is specified as the organization and the nature of the measurement as descriptive, the two concepts which emerge are *organizational climate* for the organizational unit of analysis and *perceived organizational characteristics* for the individual unit of analysis.

Recent proposals settle the controversy in a sense. Rather than saying that climate is a property of either the organization or the individual, they say that it can be both. In a given study, its definition depends on the goals of the researcher.

In summary, climate has been viewed commonly as a property of organizations and frequently operationalized as a property of individuals. Recent theoretical discussions have held that climate can be a property of either the organization or an individual. The prospect that climate may be a property of subsystems of organizations such as work groups, functions, or positions has received relatively small recognition.

An organization is considered to have subsystem climates whenever at least one group (subsystem) of employees has different perceptions of the organization's climate than those of employees outside the subsystem. The perceived climate is a property more of the separate subsystems than of the organization as a whole. Thus the unique climate perceptions held by each subsystem may be defined as its subsystem climate. If managers in an organization perceive its climate differently than nonmanagers, their aggregate perceptions comprise the "managerial subsystem climate" (or simply managerial climate). Viewed in retrospect, the assumptions and findings of a number of climate studies point toward the existence of such subsystem climates.

Studies demonstrating differences in perceived climate within organizations support the existence of subsystem climates. Differences have been found between the climate perceptions of employees grouped by:

1. Level in organizational hierarchy
2. Line or staff position
3. Department/subunit
4. Biographical influences
5. Personality characteristics interacting with structural perceptions
6. Personality characteristics—activity/passivity, task orientation
7. Length of service—first/second generation

Once it is conceded that climate can exist at the individual level, three additional possiblities remain:

1. Climate exists independently at both the organizational and subsystem levels.
2. Climate exists at the subsystem and not the organizational level; organizational climate is simply the result of aggregating subsystem climates.

3. Climate exists at the organizational and not the subsystem level.

Alternative 3 has been assumed without examination in most climate studies. Recent advocates of the existence of subsystem climates in organizations have not distinguished between Alternatives 1 or 2. This article argues in favor of Alternative 1, that climate exists at the subsystem level and that OC exists independently from subsystem climates.

In addition to the climate studies cited, the existence of climate at the subsystem level is supported by consideration of the processes which affect perceptual responses. Perceptions are significantly affected by that part of the environment most immediately experienced by the employee, such as department, work group, hierarchical level, or reference group.

Because they do not have access to all its parts, it is difficult for employees to have global perceptions of the entire organization. But some employees may have perceptions based on a more global view than others. Employees who have been members of the organization longer, who are at higher levels in the organization, or whose jobs are boundary-spanning in nature and call for frequent interaction with members of other departments are more likely to recognize the OC. The more departments in which employees have worked, the more they may have an idea of the general climate of the organization beyond the individual departments. Conversely, the longer employees have been members of particular departments, the less they may have a view of the organization as a whole.

A conceptualization of organizations as having subsystem climates recognizes the possibilities of climate as both an individual and an organizational property. The climate perceived by a given individual qualifies as a subsystem climate, since each individual comprises a "finest grain" subsystem of the organization. When the organization is viewed as a subsystem of itself, its climate also qualifies as a subsystem climate, which might be called the "macro" subsystem climate. Thus we conclude that:

1. Climate is a property of subsystems in organizations. Subsystems may consist of organiza-

tional members taken individually, in groups formed on any basis, or as a whole.

2. As a conceptual construct, climate exists independently for separate subsystems. In fact, relationships may, but do not necessarily, exist between climates for separate subsystems. For example, the climate for new employees may not be completely divorced from the managerial climate as experienced by new employees who are also managers.

DREXLER

Climate is organization-specific

Adapted and edited from John A. Drexler, Jr., "Organizational Climate: Its Homogeneity Within Organizations," Journal of Applied Psychology, February 1977, pp. 38–42; © 1977 by the American Psychological Association. Reprinted/adapted by permission of the publisher and author.

Organizational climate, an element of organizational environments, is a construct that distinguishes among organizations and one that should have organization-specific variance. As such, it should be relatively homogeneous within organizations. Recently, confusion has been voiced over some current operationalizations and conceptualizations of this construct (i.e., multiple measurement—organizational attribute approach, perceptual measurement—organizational attribute approach, and perceptual measurement—individual attribute approach). For instance, if measures of organizational climate were limited to perceptual ones, the construct might more usefully be labeled "psychological climate."

Of interest is whether descriptive, but perceptually generated, measures of organizational conditions and procedures characterize organizations or whether they characterize variance at individual, group, or other levels of focus.

A related concern focuses on the appropriate level of explanation for the term *organization*. Specifically, what are the boundaries under which "climate" could be subsumed? Is climate, for example, defined at the level of an entire industrial plant or business enterprise, or might it be limited to some subsystems within either type of organization, such as a department or division? Theoretical and empirical work view policies and behaviors of highest-level managers as setting the climate for conditions and procedures within an organization. These conditions and procedures influence or constrain the behavior of managers at the next lower level. While behavior at this next level is constrained, these managers too may influence conditions and procedures for succeeding lower levels of management, adding to the constraints imposed from above. If this concept is correct, there should be differences in experienced climate across departments within the same organization, but if climate is an organizational attribute, subunit differences should be weaker than interorganizational differences.

The present study investigated (a) differences in climate among different organizations, (b) differences in climate across different organizations using groups that serve the same functions, (c) differences in climate among departments within the same organization, and (d) differences in the relative strengths of organization effects and department effects.

Data from persons in all types of work within 21 diverse industrial or business organizations were used. The climate data were average scores for work groups that ranged in size from 3 to 10. A total of 6,996 individuals comprised the 1,256 groups in the analyses.

The results supported the position that descriptive measures of organizational climate characterize organizations. Such measures have organization-specific variance and constitute organizational attributes. However, accepting the suggestion that perceptually generated measures of climate be called "psychological climate" would be misleading if it connotes a construct that is largely intraindividual. If, as demonstrated here, a large share of the variance in climate is organization specific, the term "organizational climate" remains more appropriate.

This is not to dismiss previous criticisms. The absence of clarity in the organizational-climate literature is valid. However, the solution is not necessarily to use other terms; organizational climate may still be used with certain measures, but only under rigorous requirements specifying the manner in which the construct is operationalized and conceptualized. For example, while the data used here were descriptive of specific organization-wide conditions and procedures, other studies have used affective responses to organizational environments. Whether these latter kinds of data would yield the same relationships found in the present study remains to be tested.

Additionally, climate may relate to properties of environments other than organizational ones, and climate measures may be aggregated at different levels of analysis. Depending on one's frame of reference, one could conceive of leadership climate, group climate, or departmental climate. These climates should include survey items with leadership, group, or departmental referents versus organizational ones. Further, the investigator may wish to exploit or explore the differences among individuals, groups, or functional units. In each case, the test should be whether the referent or the aggregation level yields discriminable climates.

In summary, the results reported in this study should encourage those researchers who consider organizational climate to be an organizational attribute: A large share of the variance in measures of climate that describe organization-wide conditions and procedures is organization specific. While there are differences in organizational climate across departments in the same organization, the departmental effects are much weaker than the organizational effects.

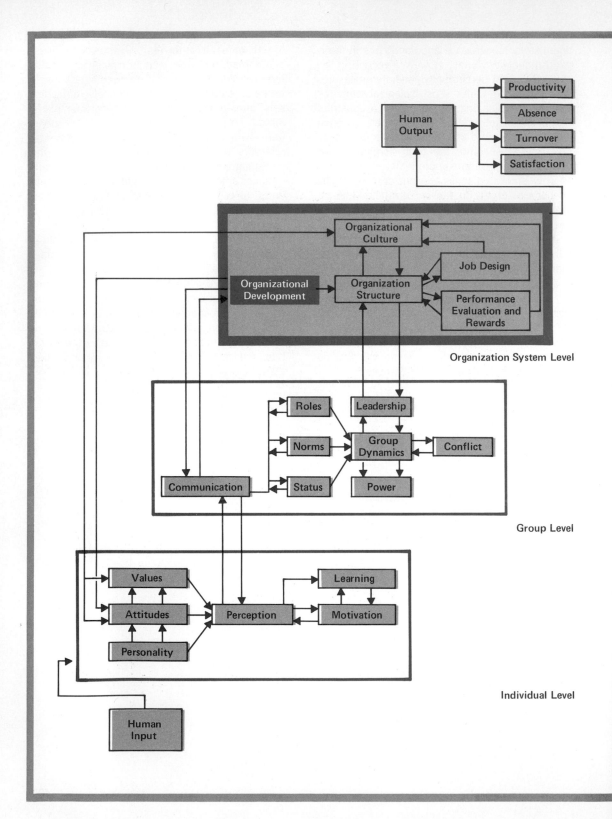

CHAPTER 18
Organizational Development

AFTER STUDYING THIS CHAPTER, YOU SHOULD BE ABLE TO—

Define and explain the following key terms and concepts:

Humanistic-democratic
    values
Intergroup development
MAPS
OB Mod
Organizational development
Problem solving
Process consultation

Sensitivity training
Survey feedback
Team building
Theory X
Theory Y
Transactional analysis

Understand

The nature of organizational development
The objectives of OD
The processes by which OD operates
The relationship of OD techniques and conflict resolution
    techniques
The difference between structural and human process techniques
Various techniques available for introducing behavioral change

> Most people hate any change that doesn't jingle in their pockets.
> —ANONYMOUS

In the 1960s, the term "organizational development" (OD) became increasingly popular to describe the facilitating of system-wide change in an organization. Today, the term is used for a variety of change-oriented activities. To some, it is merely a sexy name given to the sensitivity training or small-group discussion methods that gained popularity in the late 1950s. At the other extreme, it has been defined in such a general way as to encompass almost the entire management process. For example, OD has been described as "a complex network of events that enhances the ability of organizational members to manage the culture of their organization, to be creative in solving problems, and to assist their organization in adapting to the external environment."[1] A closer look finds that OD is a systems-oriented approach to change, with heavy emphasis on humanistic-democratic values, and the belief that facilitating the integration of individual and organizational objectives will increase the organization's effectiveness.

In this chapter we shall review the importance of change to an organization, consider the key objectives of OD, and then proceed to describe the smorgasbord of techniques that have been proposed for bringing about change.

CHANGE AND OD

We know that organizations exist in an environment of change. Technology, government regulation, competition, consumer tastes, and spending patterns are some of the more obvious factors that change over time and that organizations must adapt to if they are to survive. The issue is not whether organizations face change—they do! The issue is only one of degree. Those organizations that operate in a relatively certain environment need to be less concerned than those that operate in turbulent and dynamic environments. But how is organization-wide change brought about? Organizational development represents a process of preparing for and managing change. It acknowledges that change cannot take place in a vacuum—that changes in structure, technology, and people will

---

1. Wendell French, *The Personnel Management Process,* 3rd ed. (Boston: Houghton Mifflin, 1974), p. 56.

interact. If OD is successful, the attitudes and values of individuals, as well as the structure of the organization, will be more adaptive. When we review the popular OD techniques, we find that they draw heavily upon subjects touched on in our previous discussion of learning, motivation, group dynamics, conflict, organization structure, and job design.

In very general terms, planned change can be described as consisting of three stages: unfreezing, changing, and refreezing.[2]

1. *Unfreezing* creates the awareness of the need to change. The status quo is disturbed by reducing the strength of current values, attitudes, and/or behaviors.
2. *Changing* is the action-oriented stage. Specific changes are brought about through the development of new values, attitudes, and/or behaviors.
3. *Refreezing* stabilizes the change that has been brought about. The new state becomes the status quo and must be sustained.

Efforts to bring about change will frequently meet resistance. We have noted in previous chapters that people dislike uncertainty, yet change increases uncertainty. Individuals are required to trade in the known for the unknown. Employees want to know how a different work assignment, a transfer, or new co-workers will affect them. Individuals and groups fear that a change may adversely impact on their self-interest. As a result, employees will frequently create significant barriers to block change, even if this change may later prove to be beneficial to them.

Several classic studies have offered insight into how this resistance to change may be managed. A study designed to change food habits among housewives found that 32 percent of housewives exposed to a group-decision method changed to a new variety of meats, in contrast to only 3 percent of the women who received information through the lecture method.[3] The researcher concluded that involvement and group pressure reduced the housewives' resistance to change. Similarly, a experiment in a textile factory established three approaches for bringing about a change in work methods.[4] In the first group, the change was made autocratically by management and announced to the employees. The second involved employee participation through elected representatives. These representatives, with management, worked out the details of the change, then tried the new methods and trained others in the new procedures. In the third approach, there was full participation. All employees shared in the designing of new methods with management. The results of this experiment strongly favored the value of participation. In the first group, output actually dropped from the previous 60 units per hour to 48 units. However, the participation-by-representation group generated 68 units per hour and the total-participation group averaged 73 units per hour. Interestingly, when the members of

2. Kurt Lewin, *Field Theory in Social Science* (New York: Harper & Row, 1951).

3. Kurt Lewin, "Group Decision and Social Change," in *Readings in Social Psychology,* ed. G. E. Swanson, T. M. Newcome, and E. L. Hartley, 2nd ed. (New York: Holt, 1952), pp. 459–73.

4. Lester Coch and John R. P. French, Jr., "Overcoming Resistance to Change," *Human Relations,* November 1948, pp. 512–32.

autocratic and representative groups were later allowed total participation, their productivity increased to the level of the total participation group. As with the study to change food habits, this factory experiment attests to the value of participation in reducing resistance to change.

Though both of the above studies are more than thirty years old, their findings have not been overlooked by students of OD. As we shall see, OD techniques have a generous bias toward participatory methods. There is a strong belief held by those people actively engaged in OD that changes are more likely to be accepted by individuals who have been given a voice in determining the content and process of the change.

OD OBJECTIVES

Organizational development efforts are generally directed toward two ends: (1) improvement in an organization's effectiveness and (2) improvement in the satisfaction of its members. A major value issue underlying these objectives is that they can best be attained by humanizing organizations and encouraging the personal growth of people. When this is translated into operational language, we find the OD literature heavily laden with terms like collaboration, confrontation, authenticity, trust, support, and openness. For example, one author has defined the objectives of a typical OD program as follows:

1. To increase the level of trust and support among organizational members
2. To increase the incidence of confrontation of organizational problems, both within groups and among groups, in contrast to "sweeping problems under the rug"
3. To create an environment in which authority of assigned role is augmented by authority based on knowledge and skill
4. To increase the openness of communications laterally, vertically, and diagonally
5. To increase the level of personal enthusiasm and satisfaction in the organization
6. To find synergistic solutions to problems with great frequency
7. To increase the level of self- and group responsibility in planning and implementation[5]

The above description of OD objectives is heavily biased toward humanistic-democratic values. The change agent may be directive in OD; however, the literature emphasizes collaboration. Concepts like power, authority, control, conflict, and coercion are held in relatively low esteem among OD supporters. As a result, the OD techniques we shall review tend to emphasize power equalization (reducing hierarchical authority and control), the work group (rather than the individual), and the collaborative process.

5. Wendell French, "Organization Development: Objectives, Assumptions and Strategies," *California Management Review,* Winter 1969, p. 24.

One way to conceptualize the general orientation of OD researchers is to use the Theory X and Theory Y models proposed by Douglas McGregor.[6] He suggested two distinct views of human nature, one basically negative, labeled Theory X, and the other basically positive, labeled Theory Y. After viewing the way managers dealt with employees, McGregor concluded that a manager's view of human nature is based on a certain grouping of assumptions, and that managers tend to mold their behavior toward subordinates according to these assumptions.

Under Theory X, the four assumptions held by managers are:

1. Employees inherently dislike work and, whenever possible, will attempt to avoid it.
2. Since employees dislike work, they must be coerced, controlled, or threatened with punishment to achieve desired goals.
3. Employees will shirk responsibilities and seek formal direction whenever possible.
4. Most workers place security above all other factors associated with work, and will display little ambition.

In contrast to these negative views toward human nature, McGregor listed four other assumptions that he called Theory Y:

1. Employees can view work as being as natural as rest or play.
2. People will exercise self-direction and self-control if they are committed to the objectives.
3. The average person can learn to accept, even seek, responsibility.
4. Creativity—that is, the ability to develop innovative decisions—is widely dispersed throughout the population, and is not necessarily the sole province of those in management positions.

Theory X assumptions tend to be made by managers in organizations characterized by conformity, antagonism, and mistrust. In contrast, Theory Y is based on trust, openness, concern for others, and more respect for individuality. The Theory Y model can be said to best describe the philosophical bias and goals of OD researchers and practitioners.

But, of course, OD also is concerned with improving organizational performance. If it is true that the major hurdles to high organizational performance are dysfunctional conflicts, poor communication, structural rigidity, failure of members to know themselves and how they impact on others, and inadequate understanding of the attitudes and values of others, then OD should offer techniques for improving an organization's effectiveness. The OD techniques that we shall discuss are purported to increase member satisfaction and the meaningfulness of work. We shall review the evidence pertaining to these techniques, consider their ability to bring about change, and assess their effects on attitudes and behavior.

---

6. Douglas McGregor, *The Human Side of Enterprise* (New York: McGraw-Hill, 1960).

BASIC APPROACHES TO OD

The number of OD approaches is limited only by one's definition of OD. It may simply be a synonym for sensitivity training, in which case the topic is easily and quickly reviewed. Or it may encompass just about every possible idea that has been proposed to bring about change in individuals, groups, technology, or structure. In such a case, almost every topic we have covered in this book could be argued to be part of OD.

What we have tried to do is cull the more popular, interesting, and/or well-researched techniques for presentation here. For simplicity and clarity the techniques have been categorized as either structural or human process.[7]

Structural Techniques

The OD techniques that fall within the structural category affect work content and relationships among workers. The structural redesign techniques that we discussed in Chapter 15—job rotation, work modules, job enrichment, integrated and autonomous work teams, quality circles, the shorter workweek, and flextime—all represent structural OD techniques. That is, they represent planned structural interventions with the objectives of increasing individual satisfaction and organizational effectiveness. The result is that they could be properly discussed under the heading of "Redesign Options" or "Structural OD Techniques." We have chosen the former.

There is one important structural change technique that was not discussed in Chapter 15. That is MAPS—an acronym for Multivariate Analysis, Participation, and Structure.[8] Basically, MAPS begins with the development of a questionnaire by the change consultant in collaboration with effected organization members. This questionnaire gathers data on which colleagues best interact with, and member preferences concerning, the various task activities that the organization must complete. Both colleague and task variables are equally represented in the questionnaire because MAPS assumes both task and interpersonal compatibility are necessary for task effectiveness.

After the questionnaire is constructed and answered, the consultant determines the most relevant structural design alternatives using multivariate analysis. The design alternatives are then distributed to the members who will be effected. They then make the final decision as to which design, if any, they want to implement. The result is a structural design that is participatively determined and which meets both task and interpersonal constraints.

---

7. This categorization was adapted from Frank Friedlander and L. Dave Brown, "Organizational Development," in *Annual Review of Psychology* (Palo Alto, Calif.: Annual Reviews, 1974), pp. 313–41.

8. Ralph H. Kilmann and Bill McKelvey, "Organization Design: A Participative Multivariate Approach," *Administrative Science Quarterly*, March 1975, pp. 24–36.

Human Process Techniques

The vast majority of OD research has been directed at changing the attitude and behavior of individuals and groups through the processes of communication, decision making, and problem solving. Popular techniques include sensitivity training, survey feedback, process consultation, team building, and intergroup development. For the most part, each emphasizes participation and collaboration. Although not as popular, OB Modification and Transactional Analysis represent recent approaches that deserve discussion.

Sensitivity Training. It can go by a variety of names—laboratory training, sensitivity training, encounter groups, or T-groups (training groups)—but all refer to a method of changing behavior through unstructured group interaction. Members are brought together in a free and open environment in which participants discuss themselves and their interactive processes, loosely directed by a professional behavioral scientist. The group is process oriented, which means that individuals learn through observing and participating rather than being told. The professional creates the opportunity for participants to express their ideas, beliefs, and attitudes. He or she does not accept—in fact, overtly rejects—any leadership role.

The objectives of the T-groups are to provide the subjects with increased awareness of their own behavior and how others perceive them, greater sensitivity to the behavior of others, and increased understanding of group processes. Specific results sought include increased ability to empathize with others, improved listening skills, greater openness, increased tolerance of individual differences, and improved conflict resolution skills.

If individuals lack awareness of how others perceive them, then the successful T-group can effect more realistic self-perceptions, greater group cohesiveness, and a reduction in dysfunctional interpersonal conflicts. Further, it will ideally result in a better integration between the individual and the organization.

Research investigations into sensitivity training indicate that it can effectively change individual behavior. However, the impact of these changes on performance is inconclusive,[9] and the technique is not devoid of psychological risks. There have been cases reported of personality damage to those who were not adequately screened prior to participation. One study found that 19 percent, almost one out of five, of group participants suffered from negative psychological effects some six to eight months after the group met, and nearly one out of ten had suffered serious psychological harm.[10]

"The evidence, though still limited, is reasonably convincing that T-group training and the laboratory method do induce behavioral changes in the 'back-

---

9. John P. Campbell and Marvin D. Dunnette, "Effectiveness of T-Group Experience in Managerial Training and Development," *Psychological Bulletin,* August 1968, pp. 73–104.

10. Morton A. Lieberman, Irvin D. Yalom, and Matthew B. Miles, "Encounter: The Leader Makes a Difference," *Psychology Today,* March 1973, pp. 69–76.

home' setting."[11] But behavioral change means little unless we know what kind of change will be achieved. It has been argued by some, for instance, that there is no "typical" pattern of change; rather, there is a unique response for each individual.[12]

> If this is true, the present lack of knowledge about how individual differences variables interact with training program variables makes it nearly impossible for anyone to spell out ahead of time the outcomes to be expected from any given development program. That is, if training outcomes are truly unique and predictable, no basis exists for judging the potential worth of T-group training from an institutional or organizational point of view. Instead, its success or failure must be judged by each individual trainee in terms of his own personal goals.[13]

To summarize the results from sensitivity training, we find that the process changes behavior. Just specifically what that change means, however, in terms of on-the-job behavior, is still the subject of considerable debate.

Survey Feedback. One tool for assessing attitudes held by organizational members, identifying discrepancies among member perceptions, and solving these differences is the survey feedback approach.

Everyone in an organization can participate in survey feedback, but of key importance is the organizational family—the manager of any given unit and those employees who directly report to him or her. A questionnaire is usually completed by all members in the organization or unit. Organization members may be asked to suggest questions or may be interviewed to determine what issues are relevant. The questionnaire typically asks members for their perceptions and attitudes on a broad range of topics—such as decision-making practices; communication effectiveness; coordination between units; and satisfaction with the organization, job, peers, and their immediate supervisor.

The data from this questionnaire is tabulated with data pertaining to an individual's specific "family" and to the entire organization, and distributed to employees. This data then becomes the springboard for identifying problems and clarifying issues that may be creating difficulties for people. In some cases, the manager may be counseled by an external change agent about the meaning of the responses to the questionnaire and may even be given suggested guidelines for leading the organizational family in group discussion of the results. Particular attention is given to the importance of encouraging discussion and ensuring that discussions focus on issues and ideas, and not on attacking individuals.

Finally, group discussion in the survey feedback approach should result in members identifying possible implications of the questionnaire's findings. Are people listening? Are new ideas being generated? Can decision making, interpersonal relations, or job assignments be improved? Answers to questions like

---

11. John P. Campbell, Marvin D. Dunnette, Edward E. Lawler III, and Karl E. Weick, Jr., *Managerial Behavior, Performance, and Effectiveness* (New York: McGraw-Hill, 1970), p. 323.

12. D. R. Bunker, "Individual Applications of Laboratory Training," *Journal of Applied Behavioral Science,* April-June 1965, pp. 131–47.

13. Campbell et al., *Managerial Behavior,* p. 323.

these hopefully will result in the group agreeing upon commitments to various actions that will remedy the problems that are identified.

The survey feedback technique has gained a rapidly growing following. For instance, in 1977, more than 100,000 employees—ranging from production workers to senior management—participated.[14] General Electric surveyed 20,000 of its employees and found more than 50 percent were unhappy with promotion opportunities. As a result, unit managers at GE instituted regular monthly meetings and actively worked to improve communication. A year later, the number who were unhappy with promotion opportunities dropped to 20 percent even though not one person was promoted or changed jobs. The improvement, according to management, was due to an increased understanding of the situation.[15] A similar survey feedback program at the Parker Pen Company identified a number of problems and resulted in significant improvements in vacation and insurance benefits for employees, the introduction of a career opportunities program, as well as the development of a written policy manual to enhance communication and the consistency with which employees were treated.[16] Parker attributed improved upward and downward communication to the program, which resulted in higher morale and the expectation of increased productivity.

What does the general evidence demonstrate about survey feedback? We find that survey feedback meetings can lead to attitudinal changes by participants. Satisfaction, positive attitudes toward work and one's supervisor, and involvement in the organization have been shown to increase as a result of group discussion surrounding the survey results.[17] However, the manager of the organizational family can undermine the process. If the results are perceived as threatening, it has been suggested that managerial peer groups be formed to review and discuss findings before meeting with their subordinates in family groups.[18]

While the survey feedback approach changes attitudes, long-term changes in behavior have not resulted from mere group discussion of the results. There is, in fact, "little evidence that survey feedback alone leads to changes in individual behavior or organizational performance."[19] Discussion and involvement will

14. "A Productive Way to Vent Employee Gripes," *Business Week,* October 16, 1978, p. 168.

15. Ibid.

16. Douglas M. Soat, "An OD Strategy at Parker Pen," *Personnel,* March-April 1979, pp. 39–43.

17. See, for example, David G. Bowers, "O.D. Techniques and Their Results in 23 Organizations; the Michigan ICL Study," *Journal of Applied Behavioral Science,* January-February 1973, pp. 21–43; and L. D. Brown, "Research Action: Organizational Feedback, Understanding, and Change," *Journal of Applied Behavioral Science,* November-December 1972, pp. 697–774.

18. C. P. Alderfer and R. Ferriss, "Understanding the Impact of Survey Feedback," in *The Social Technology of Organizational Development,* ed. W. W. Burke and H. A. Hornstein (Fairfax, Va.: NTL Learning Resource Corp., 1972), pp. 234–43.

19. Friedlander and Brown, "Organizational Development," p. 327.

not bring about the desired changes if the discussion fails to initiate follow-up actions.[20]

Process Consultation. No organization operates perfectly. Managers often sense that their unit's performance can be improved, but they are unable to identify what can be improved and how it can be improved. The purpose of process consultation is for an outside consultant to assist a client, usually a manager, "to perceive, understand, and act upon process events" with which he or she must deal.[21] These might include, for example, work flow, informal relationships among unit members, and formal communication channels.

Process consultation (P.C.) is similar to sensitivity training in its assumption that organizational effectiveness can be improved by dealing with interpersonal problems, and in its emphasis on involvement. But P.C. is more task directed than sensitivity training.

Consultants in P.C. are there to "give the client 'insight' into what is going on around him, within him, and between him and other people."[22] They do not solve the organization's problems. Rather, the consultant is a guide or coach who advises on the process to help the client solve his or her own problems.

The consultant works with the client in *jointly* diagnosing what processes need improvement. The emphasis is on "jointly," because the client develops a skill at analyzing processes within his or her unit that can be continually called on long after the consultant is gone. Additionally, by having the client actively participate in both the diagnosis and the development of alternatives, there will be greater understanding of the process and the remedy, and less resistance to the action plan chosen.

Importantly, the process consultant need not be an expert in solving the particular problem that is identified. The consultant's expertise lies in diagnosis and developing a helping relationship. If the specific problem uncovered requires technical knowledge outside both the client and consultant's expertise, the consultant helps the client to locate such an expert and then instructs the client in how to get the most out of this expert resource.

Team Building. Organizations are made up of people working together to achieve some common end. Since people are frequently required to work in groups, considerable attention has been focused in OD on team building.

Team building can be applied within groups or at the intergroup level where activities are interdependent. For our discussion, we shall emphasize the intragroup level and leave intergroup development to the next section. As a re-

20. M. G. Miles et al., "The Consequences of Survey Feedback: Theory and Evaluation," in *The Planning of Change*, ed. W. G. Bennis, K. D. Benne, R. Chin, 2nd ed. (New York: Holt, Rinehart, & Winston, 1969), pp. 456–68.

21. Edgar H. Schein, *Process Consultation: Its Role in Organizational Development* (Reading, Mass.: Addison-Wesley, 1969), p. 9.

22. Ibid.

sult, our interest concerns applications to organizational families (command groups), as well as committees, project teams, and task groups.

Not all group activity has interdependence of functions. To illustrate, consider a football team and a track team:

> Although members on both teams are concerned with the team's total output they function differently. The football team's output depends synergistically on how well each player does his particular job in concert with his teammates. The quarterback's performance depends on the performance of his linemen and receivers, and ends on how well the quarterback throws the ball, and so on. On the other hand, a track team's performance is determined largely by the mere addition of the performances of the individual members.[23]

Team building is applicable to the case of interdependence, such as in football. The objective is to improve coordinative efforts of team members which will result in increasing the group's performance.

The activities included in team building can typically include goal setting, development of interpersonal relations among team members, role analysis to clarify each member's role and responsibilities, and team process analysis. Of course, team building may emphasize or exclude certain activities depending on the purpose of the development effort and the specific problems with which the team is confronted. Basically, however, team building attempts to use high interaction among group members to increase trust and openness.

It may be beneficial to begin by having members attempt to define the goals and priorities of the group. This will bring to the surface different perceptions of what the group's purpose may be. Following this, members can evaluate the group's performance—how effective are they in structuring priorities and achieving their goals? This should identify potential problem areas. This self-critique discussion of means and ends can be done with members of the total group present or, where large size impinges on a free interchange of views, may initially take place in smaller groups followed up by the sharing of their findings with the total group.

Team building can also address itself to clarifying each member's role in the group. Each role can be identified and clarified. Previous ambiguities can be brought to the surface. For some individuals it may offer one of the few opportunities they have had to think through thoroughly what their job is all about and what specific tasks they are expected to carry out if the group is to optimize its effectiveness.

Still another team building activity can be similar to that performed by the process consultant; that is, to analyze key processes that go on within the team to identify the way work is performed and how these processes might be improved to make the team more effective.

How successful is team building in improving group effectiveness? The evidence is mixed. A large portion of the studies that have sought to measure team building effectiveness relies heavily on anecdotal data. Reports indicate that it is

---

23. Newton Margulies and John Wallace, *Organizational Change: Techniques and Applications* (Glenview, Ill.: Scott, Foresman, 1973), pp. 99–100.

effective in increasing member involvement and participation in group activities and in improving the effectiveness of meetings.[24] Participant attitudes are affected by team building, but it is unclear "what effects group development has on actual task performance."[25]

Intergroup Development. A major area of concern in OD is the dysfunctional conflict that exists between groups. As a result, this has been a subject to which change efforts have been directed.

Intergroup development seeks to change the attitudes, stereotypes, and perceptions that groups have of each other. For example, in one company the engineers saw the accounting department as composed of shy and conservative types, and the personnel department as having a bunch of "smiley-types who sit around and plan company picnics." Such stereotypes can have an obvious negative impact on the coordinative efforts between the departments.

Though there are a number of approaches for improving intergroup relations,[26] a popular method emphasizes problem solving.[27] In this method, each group meets independently to develop lists of its perception of themselves, the other group, and how they believe the other group perceives them. The groups then share their lists, after which similarities and differences are discussed. Differences are clearly articulated, and the groups look for the causes of the disparities.

Are the groups' goals at odds? Were perceptions distorted? On what basis were stereotypes formulated? Have some differences been caused by misunderstandings of intentions? Have words and concepts been defined differently by each group? Answers to questions like these clarify the exact nature of the conflict. Once the causes of the difficulty have been identified, the groups can move to the integration phase—working to develop solutions that will improve relations between the groups.

Subgroups, with members from each of the conflicting groups, can now be created for further diagnosis and to begin to formulate possible alternative actions that will improve relations.

There is again little hard evidence upon which to evaluate the effectiveness of intergroup development methods like the problem-solving approach we have described. Reports of attitudes being positively influenced by the process exist, but little can be concluded as to the effect on individual behaviors or organization performance.[28]

24. Friedlander and Brown, "Organizational Development," p. 328.

25. Ibid., p. 329.

26. See, for example, E. H. Neilsen, "Understanding and Managing Intergroup Conflict," in *Managing Group and Intergroup Relations,* ed. J. W. Lorsch and P. R. Lawrence (Homewood, Ill.: Irwin-Dorsey, 1972), pp. 329–43.

27. R. R. Blake, J. S. Mouton and R. L. Sloma, "The Union-Management Intergroup Laboratory: Strategy for Resolving Intergroup Conflict," *Journal of Applied Behavioral Science,* No. 1, 1965, pp. 25–57.

28. Friedlander and Brown, "Organizational Development," p. 330.

OB Modification. A recent additon to the OD "tool chest" is Organizational Behavior Modification (OB Mod).[29] This technique attempts to integrate the reinforcement concepts of B. F. Skinner, which we discussed in Chapter 7, with the field of organizational behavior. Since most relevant organizational behavior is learned, OB Mod proposes that change agents can manipulate environmental contingencies to shape, change, and direct organizational behavior toward desired ends. Successful OB Mod will strengthen the likelihood that individuals will repeat desirable behaviors and weaken the likelihood they will engage in undesirable behaviors.

It has been argued that there has been an "almost total absence of the application of behavioral modification to organizational development," but that the "antecedent environment can be structured in such a way to increase the probabilities of more productive behaviors at every level of the organization and more positively reinforcing consequences can be made to follow goal congruent behaviors of the total organization."[30]

While there may be few specific usages of OB Mod in OD, reports on the general effectiveness of OB Mod for changing organizational behavior are encouraging. For instance, one study of production supervisors in a manufacturing firm found that the production rates in the departments where the supervisors had been trained in the OB Mod approach were significantly higher than those in departments where supervisors had not been given the training.[31] Additionally, the trained supervisors were successful in decreasing the number of complaints, reducing the group scrap rate, decreasing the number of overlooked defective pieces, and reducing the assembly reject rate.[32]

A survey of ten organizations using OB Mod—including Michigan Bell, General Electric, City of Detroit, B. F. Goodrich Chemical Company, and ACDC Electronics—found some impressive results.[33] For example, one unit of Michigan Bell reported that attendance performance had improved by 50 percent and productivity and efficiency were above standard; General Electric achieved a reduction in direct labor cost and an increase in worker productivity when OB Mod was used by 1,000 GE supervisors; Detroit saved over $1.5 million with garbage collection activity and achieved a significant reduction in citizen complaints; production increased over 300 percent at a B. F. Goodrich Chemical plant in Ohio; and ACDC obtained over a half-million dollars in cost

29. Fred Luthans and Robert Kreitner, *Organizational Behavior Modification* (Glenview, Ill.: Scott, Foresman, 1975).

30. Fred Luthans, "An Organizational Behavior Modification Approach to O.D.," paper presented at the Thirty-fourth Annual Meeting of the Academy of Management, Seattle, Washington, August 1974.

31. Robert Ottemann and Fred Luthans, "An Experimental Analysis of the Effectiveness of an Organizational Behavior Modification Program in Industry," Proceedings of the Thirty-fifth Annual Meeting of the Academy of Management, New Orleans, Lousiaina, August 1975, pp. 140–42.

32. Ibid.

33. W. Clay Hamner and Ellen P. Hamner, "Behavior Modification on the Bottom Line," *Organizational Dynamics,* Spring 1976, pp. 3–21.

reductions, reduced turnaround time on repairs from thirty to ten days, and increased attendance from 93.5 percent to 98.2 percent.

Transactional Analysis. Our final OD technique is also relatively new, but in contrast to OB Mod has been widely introduced in a broad spectrum of organizations. It is called Transactional Analysis (T.A.).

Transactional Analysis is both an approach for defining and for analyzing communication interactions between people and a theory of personality. The fundamental theory underlying T.A. holds that an individual's personality is made up of three ego states—the *parent,* the *child,* and the *adult.* These labels have nothing to do with age, but rather with aspects of the ego. The parent state is made up of one's attitudes and behavior incorporated from external sources. It is an ego state of authority and superiority. A person acting in his or her parent state is usually dominant, scolding, and otherwise authoritative.

The child contains all the impulses that are natural to an infant. Acting in this state, one can be obedient or manipulative; charming at one moment and repulsive the next. Whereas the parent acts as he or she was taught, the child is emotional and acts according to how he or she feels at the moment.

The adult state is objective and rational. It deals with reality and objectively gathers information. Since it reasons and is reasonable, its actions are almost computerlike—processing data, estimating probabilities, and making decisions. It is not prejudiced by the values of the parent or the natural urges of the child.

In T.A. theory, the parent and child ego states feel and react differently, while only the adult state thinks or processes transactional data logically before acting. Therefore, in most situations, the ideal interaction is an adult stimulus, followed by an adult response.

As long as transactions are parallel—that is, parent-parent, child-child, or adult-adult—dialogue or transactions can go on indefinitely. Parallel transactions leave communication channels open for further exploration of the relationship or resolution of the matter being discussed, even if the initial response does not include all the information sought by the initiated transactions. But real communication is short-circuited whenever a cross-transaction occurs.

Central to any consideration of T.A. is the concept of stroking, or a need for recognition, which influences much of our activity in early life and influences our dominant ego states. Strokes may be either positive or negative, but whenever two or more persons are engaged in a transaction, they are, in T.A. language, exchanging strokes. The types of stroking we learn to accept early in life become established as patterns that stay with us throughout our lives. Understanding of these stroking patterns, according to supporters of T.A., is the first step toward changing them.

What opportunities are there for applying the concepts of T.A. to organizational development? As described in *Born to Win,* the transactional method is a personal method for analyzing and understanding behavior.[34] Although its pri-

---

34. Muriel James and Dorothy Jongeward, *Born to Win* (Reading, Mass.: Addison-Wesley, 1971).

mary concern is the discovery and fostering of awareness, self-responsibility, self-confidence, and sincerity, T.A. lays the foundations for changing dysfunctional behavior through the development of mutual trust between people. It promotes authentic interpersonal relationships and provides a means of opening up communication channels and of identifying, analyzing, and deciding on ways to eliminate communication barriers.

Responses to T.A. programs have generally been favorable. For example, all sixty-eight managers at the Bank of America who participated in a T.A. seminar believed that their adult ego states had been strengthened, and 86 percent believed that they were better able to handle difficult interpersonal problems.[35] The Bank of New York, which has trained about 250 of its first-line managers and about 50 middle and senior divisional managers in T.A., has been generally pleased with the effect of T.A.: "Transactional analysis is clearly not the salvation of the organization, so we've never introduced it as such. But we are convinced after nearly three years of experience with T.A. that it can be a useful tool for both personal and organizational growth."[36]

The above support for T.A. represents "intuitive feel" rather than substantive research. One of the few efforts to assess objectively the research on T.A. looked at over 100 reports. It was found that only 13 of these reports were valid research pieces and only 5 used any behavioral outcome measures.[37] Our position is that T.A. undoubtedly has a lot of supporters, but much of their enthusiasm has not yet been documented by valid research. Transactional Analysis may help people to understand others better and assist them in altering their responses so as to produce more effective results. However, there is little hard evidence at this time to corroborate such a conclusion.

IMPLICATIONS FOR PERFORMANCE AND SATISFACTION

Organizational Development has been an active applied area during the last two decades. It has provided specific structural and behavioral techniques for bringing about change, as well as offering suggestions on how the organization can better process change. Unfortunately, a lot of the supposed value of OD has to be taken on faith.[38] Case studies and anecdotal data abound, but there is an obvious lack of substantive performance data relating OD efforts to productivity, turnover, and absence. If we acknowledge that research in this area is far from flawless, what *can* we say about OD in its relation to attitudes and behavior?

35. "Business Tries Transactional Analysis," *Business Week,* January 12, 1974, pp. 74–75.

36. Harold M. F. Rush and Phyllis S. McGrath, "Transactional Analysis Moves into Corporate Training," *Conference Board Record,* July 1973, p. 42.

37. Mark J. Martinko and Fred Luthans, reported in *Training,* April 1979, p. 9.

38. See, for instance, Peggy Morrison, "Evaluation in OD: A Review and an Assessment," *Group and Organization Studies,* March 1978, pp. 42–70.

Many of the structural approaches have favorable impact on both attitudes and behavior. This was documented in Chapter 15. The human process approaches demonstrate a number of positive effects on attitudes, but there is little evidence "that organizational processes actually change, or that performance or effectiveness is increased."[39] One study, which used sixteen critical indices as somewhat questionable substitutes for organizational effectiveness, found that survey feedback was associated with statistically significant improvement on a majority of measures; process consultation was associated with improvement on a majority of measures; and sensitivity training was associated with a decline in two-thirds of the measures.[40]

FOR DISCUSSION

1. What is the relationship between OD and organizational adaptability?

2. What are the three stages of planned change?

3. What can be done to reduce resistance to change?

4. What are Theories X and Y, and what relevance do they have to OD?

5. What is MAPS?

6. What is sensitivity training? How effective is it in changing attitudes and job behavior?

7. Contrast survey feedback, process consultation, and team building.

8. Using OB Mod as an integrating concept, demonstrate the relationship between behavioral change, learning, motivation, and reward systems.

9. What is the goal of T.A.? How does T.A. work?

10. "OD techniques change attitudes and behavior." Discuss.

FOR FURTHER READING

BOWERS, D. G., "Organizational Development: Promises, Performances, Possibilities," *Organizational Dynamics,* Spring 1976, pp. 50–62. Promises of OD have generally gone unfulfilled; its performances are spotty. Suggests what went wrong and what should be done for OD to reach its potential.

BUCHANAN, P. C., "An OD Strategy at the IRS," *Personnel,* March-April 1979, pp. 44–52. Based on experience at the Internal Revenue Service, the author discusses what needs to be done in preparation for team building and suggestions to enhance follow-through.

CONNOR, P. E., "A Critical Inquiry into Some Assumptions and Values Characterizing OD," *Academy of Management Review,* October 1977, pp. 635–

39. Friedlander and Brown, "Organizational Development," p. 334.
40. Bowers, "O.D. Techniques."

44. Assumptions and values characteristic of OD are identified and discussed. Some implications of OD philosophy and practice are criticized.

FRENCH, W. L., and C. H. BELL, JR., *Organization Development: Behavioral Science Interventions for Organization Improvement,* 2nd ed. Englewood Cliffs, N.J.: Prentice-Hall, 1978. Popular introductory text that reviews OD theory and practice; including a section that assesses research on OD.

MIRVIS, P., and D. BERG, ed., *Failures in Organization Development and Change: Cases and Essays for Learning.* New York: John Wiley, 1977. Collection of cases and essays where OD failed. Also includes an analysis of why each OD effort failed and what was learned as a result.

WARRICK, D. D., and J. T. THOMPSON, "Still Crazy After All These Years," *Training and Development Journal,* April 1980, pp. 16–22. Notes discrepancies between traditional OD values and theories and what happens in practice.

POINT

LEVINSON

An assessment of OD practice

Adapted and edited from Harry Levinson, "The Clinical Psychologist as Organizational Diagnostician," Professional Psychology, *Winter 1972, pp. 34–40. Copyright © 1972 by the American Psychological Association. Reprinted/adapted by permission of the publisher and author.*

In recent years there has been considerable concern with organizational change and organizational development. Much of this concern has stemmed from the group dynamics movement, and those who have practiced organizational development have been largely social psychologists, sociologists, and others in a variety of disciplines who have applied variations of group dynamics techniques. A number of clinical psychologists have also been involved in this new direction.

Like nondirective therapy, organizational development practices concentrate largely on having people express themselves to each other about their mutual working interests and problems, on working together on the resolution of common problems, and on having people weigh out loud and with each other their organizational aspirations and goals. Often problem specific and frequently intuitive, these efforts are largely a-theoretical. It is presumed that the same general methods will apply to all organizations.

The field is presently in a fluid state, marked primarily by ad hoc problem-solving efforts and by a heavy emphasis on expedient techniques, ranging from games to confrontation, whose rationale frequently is poorly thought through and whose sometimes untoward consequences are ei-ther unrecognized or denied. However, as any skilled clinician knows, not all patients will prosper equally well with the same therapy, and there are severe limitations to that kind of clinical intervention which merely enables people to clarify their conscious feelings and to work on problems consciously perceived. For dealing with more complex problems at deeper levels, the clinician requires a comprehensive theory of personality and a range of therapies of choice.

Little of what is presently called organizational development involves anything like formal diagnosis. That is, while it is traditional for a responsible clinical psychologist to evaluate his client or patient both from the point of view of that person's problems and the capacity he has for dealing with them—and most psychologists would find it irresponsible to work with clients or patients otherwise—such processes are not within the purview of most people involved in organizational development. A psychologist cannot act responsibly in consultation, whether individual or organizational, unless he maintains a scientific point of view about what he does. This means that he must formulate a diagnosis which is essentially a working hypothesis about what he is dealing with, and then he must formulate methods (whether they be treatment, intervention, training experiences, or other devices) which will be effective tests of the hypothesis he proposes or which will compel him to revise his hypothesis and change his methods accordingly.

A diagnosis, whether of an individual or an organization, requires a comprehensive examination of the client's system. That examination of the individual client will frequently involve measures of intelligence and intellective or cognitive functions, defense and coping structures, modes of managing emotions, pinpointing focal conflicts, and understanding personal history as the context for character formation and styles of adaptation.

It is quite unfortunate that this process seems not to be an intrinsic part of contemporary organizational development. There are a number of reasons why this is so. There is no systematic body of professional knowledge about organizational development. Most books on the subject are piecemeal, made up of unintegrated papers. Most techniques are ad hoc, with limited rationale. Many, if not most, people who work with organization development have had limited training, some no more than having been in T-groups or, at best, having had T-group internship. Most have had no training in depth to understand the dynamics of individual personality, even those who have degrees in social psychology or sociology, let alone any sophisticated understanding of group processes. Many lean heavily on psychological clichés like "self-actualization" or "9-9, 5-5" or similar slogans derived from rubrics used in psychological research, without refining these rubrics into syndromes or formulations that create the conditions for intervention. Finally, much of OD seems to hinge on one device, T-group or confrontation, which, because it is the single technique for all problems, necessarily becomes merely a gimmick. With respect to organizational development, we are at that point in time comparable to the use of leeches in medicine. Just as they served the purpose of drawing bad blood, so the single technique in OD seems to be justified in terms of serving the purpose of drawing out bad feelings or emotions.

This state of affairs inevitably leads to certain kinds of failures, disillusionments, destructive consequences, and other negative outcomes which ultimately cause the public, in this case, the companies or other institutions, to withdraw, as many have, from group dynamics and encounter techniques. Here are some examples where the failure to diagnose led to untoward consequences.

1. A rigid, authoritarian company president, who built his organization into international prominence, was disappointed that he could not seem to retain a corps of young managers who had top management executive potential. While he hired many, they left after two or three years with the organization, usually moving up into high-level roles in other companies. He himself attributed this loss to an inadequate management development program and sought the help of a social scientist well-versed in the concept of confrontation. Certain that the problem was the executive himself, and equally certain that the executive would profit by attack by his subordinates, the social scientist arranged an organizational development program whose first steps included just that kind of confrontation. In the course of the experience, the president became livid with frustrated rage, angry that his paternalism was unappreciated, and abandoned his efforts to develop the company further. In impulsive anger, he sold it, a fact which ultimately cost him dearly and enmeshed his management in the adaptive problems of a merger which made them merely an appendage of a larger organization.

2. A major division of a large corporation undertook, with the help of a prominent and responsible consultant, an OD program intended to "open things up" to foster group cooperation. Shortly after this developmental effort, the division head was removed from his position when it was discovered that he had manipulated and exploited his subordinates, that he had sponsored orgies at sales meetings in violation of company ethics, and in various other psychopathic ways had acted irresponsibly and manipulatively. The consultant, however well-qualified in working with groups, knew nothing about individual psychology and, as a result, his efforts to "open people up" served only to make people potentially more vulnerable to exploitation. Under such circumstances, that group of managers would have been much better off to have learned ways of becoming more highly guarded and protected.

3. A major consulting organization undertook to advise on the drastic reorganization of a client firm. The consequence of this drastic reorganization was that many people who had previously held power were successfully deprived of their power, although they retained their positions. The

firm traditionally had insisted on and rewarded compliance so these men did not openly complain, but there was widespread depression and anger among them for which the consulting firm assumed no responsibility. In fact, it is doubtful whether their developmental efforts included any recognition of the psychological consequences of what they did.

4. As part of a developmental effort in a company, thought to be a wise course to "open people up," a trainer undertook encounter experiences which involved having the executives touch each other and engage in activities which brought them physically closer to each other. Two executives, whose latent homosexual impulses (unconscious and well-controlled) could not tolerate such closeness, had psychotic breaks and had to be hospitalized.

These are examples of destructive consequences of organizational consultation without diagnosis. I could offer many more examples, but these will suffice.

COUNTER POINT

SASHKIN

In defense of OD practices

Adapted and edited from Marshall Sashkin, "Organization Development Practices," Professional Psychology, *May 1973, pp. 187–94. Copyright © 1973 by the American Psychological Association. Reprinted/adapted by permission of the publisher and author.*

I share the concerns expressed by Levinson as to the adequacy of organization development (OD) practice. I further agree that clinical skills, training, and competence are of great import to effective OD work. Nonetheless, I believe that Levinson's extremely critical view of OD practices should be challenged and balanced, wtih particular reference to three points: (a) the state of the body of professional knowledge, (b) the variety and use of methodologies, and (c) the use of diagnostic methods.

Levinson feels that there is "no systematic body of professional knowledge about organizational development. Most books on the subject are piecemeal, made up of unintegrated papers. Most techniques are ad hoc, with limited rationale." Although these statements bear some truth, it seems far from the whole truth. Since the late 1940s, scholars have given us a substantial theoretical base, supplemented by further integrative schemas. There are now a number of texts on OD, and even books of integrated readings on the subject. In sum, one must conclude that there has been considerable progress toward a systematic body of professional knowledge about OD. While there is much more work needed, in both theory and practice, the state of integration of this body of knowledge is not much, if at all, behind that of other areas in psychology or psychology as a whole.

Levinson makes a gross overgeneralization in asserting that "much of OD seems to hinge on one device, T-group or confrontation, ... the single technique for all problems. . . ." Indeed, of the case examples given by Levinson, one involves a T-group; one, a confrontation design; one, an intergroup team development (it appears); and one is a structural change intervention. While it is true that some very successful practitioners rely on one preprogrammed "game plan," it is far from accurate to assert that any one technique or methodology dominates the field. One need only examine the literature to see this. One set of researchers described in detail a successful OD program which included only one T-group intervention, at an early stage, and utilized a great variety of very different techniques and interventions. An excellent review of the wide range of OD methodologies included such divergent methods as group therapy, survey feedback, and the balancing of the social with the technological system. Recently developed strategies, such as management by objectives, and human resources accounting can properly be called innovations in OD methodology. If any single factor in OD practice is most clear it is that an effective practitioner is familiar with and can use a variety of techniques and methods, selecting appropriate interventions on the basis of good diagnosis of the system.

We can all cite "horror stories" where a failure

to diagnose or an inaccurate diagnosis led to results damaging to the client system and sometimes to the OD practitioner. There is no argument that diagnosis is a crucial phase in an OD intervention. The argument that "little of what is presently called organizational development involves anything like formal diagnosis" is, however, debatable, and is not proven by a few case histories. The same is true, of course, for the opposite assertion. A few case histories involving extensive, well-designed diagnostic procedures will not prove that most of OD involves formal diagnostic efforts.

More as an example of what *current* OD can be like than as an attempt to prove that OD practitioners generally engage in extensive diagnosis, let us look briefly at a case example of a project now being carried out by researchers in the Center for Research on Utilization of Scientific Knowledge (CRUSK) of the Institute for Social Research at the University of Michigan. First, we should note that the project is a *team* effort, directly involving two psychologists and a communication researcher and assisted at points by others on the CRUSK staff. Thus the case of the OD practitioner working alone with his own favorite intervention method is not applicable here. The overall model being used by the CRUSK staff consists of four focus areas and five problem phases. Our concern here is only with the first two phases: *entry and familiarization,* a sort of prediagnostic phase; and *diagnostic evaluation* in a more formalized sense. The four focus areas, which extend through all time phases, are (a) how the organization plans for the future; (b) the organization's internal environment; (c) the organization's members—what they do and produce, their patterns of information exchange, factors in individual productivity, the structure of the reward system; and (d) the linkage between the organization and the clients it serves. These four focal areas made obvious the need for a team approach, in that no one individual could provide the required expertise in all areas.

The organization involved is a large government agency, with facilities spread across the United States. After making initial contact with top management and entering at this level, the CRUSK team spent the first year of the project in prediagnostic work: building an inside-outside team, getting a feel for the system (how it operates, what major problems exist), and letting those in the system get to know the researchers (how they operate, their methods, the kind of information and interventions they can proivde). After an initial meeting in Ann Arbor, the CRUSK team spent a day at the Washington office in meetings and small group interviews. During the year (seen by the CRUSK team as one of problem formulation and mutual learning), five visits were made to seven of the agency's regional facilities, ranging in time from one day to one week. Informal small group interviews were conducted (and recorded) at each facility. The data obtained were primarily for the purpose of learning what questions to ask in the later, more formal, diagnostic phase. In addition, the data indicate the diversity of viewpoints and, to some extent, some major problem areas (or areas for problem definition).

Concurrently, the CRUSK staff held meetings to pass information and feedback back to agency members. This planning, now in process, is being undertaken with constant reference to the detailed information collected during the first year with input from the inside team members, other agency personnel, and colleagues in CRUSK. The aim is to begin a more formal diagnostic phase, involving the determination by extensive data collection methods of the state of the system with regard to the specific problem areas and client needs identified earlier. This formal diagnostic phase is expected to take at least one year.

Neither Levinson's case examples nor the illustration given here tells us much about the actual diagnostic practices in general use of OD consultants. It may be relevant to note, however, that many published OD research studies begin with system diagnosis. One text, for instance, devoted more than two chapters to diagnostic orientation. Another developed an OD approach that includes both theory and action and that strongly emphasizes diagnosis.

In sum, although only a major survey investigation could determine the actual extent of diagnostic practice by OD practitioners (and the effectiveness of such diagnostic practice), it can be said that if the literature is any reflection of practice, there exists much concern for the use of effective diagnostic procedures and that the diagnostic process seems to be an intrinsic part of contemporary OD.

CASE IVA →

Who's in Charge Here?

Diane Fitzgerald has just submitted her two-week notice to Dr. Davis, the administrative director of the Toronto General Hospital. She explained her decision to resign.

"I can't take it here any longer, Dr. Davis," Diane began. "I've been a nursing supervisor in the maternity wing for four months, but I can't get the job done. How do you expect me to get the work done when I've got two or three bosses, each with different demands and priorities? Listen, Dr. Davis, I'm only human. Lord knows I've tried to do a decent job, but it can't be done. At least not by me. Let me give you an example. Believe me when I tell you that stories like this happen *every* day.

"I came into my office at 7:45 yesterday morning. I find a message on my desk from Penny Wright [the hospital's head nurse]. She tells me that she needs the bed-utilization report by 10 A.M. that day, so that she can make her presentation to the Board at the noon meeting. I knew the report would take me at least an hour and a half to prepare. But I got right to it. Thirty minutes later, Joyce [the nursing floor supervisor and Penny's immediate supervisor] comes in and asks me why two of my nurses aren't on duty. I told her that Dr. Lee [head of surgery] had taken them off my floor and was using them to handle an overload in the Emergency Surgical wing. I told Joyce that I had objected, but Lee said there were no other options. So what does Joyce say? She tells me to get those nurses back in the maternity section immediately. As Joyce is walking away, the phone rings. Who's on the other end? Karen Thompson [another supervisor who reports to Penny] is yelling at the top of her lungs that I'm five minutes late for the task force meeting on shift scheduling. I really like Karen and I think it was great for her to agree to chair the task force, but here she was chewing me out like *I* worked for *her!* I ask you, Dr. Davis, is this anyway to run a hospital?"

Questions

1. What is the formal chain of command?
2. Who has acted outside his or her authority?
3. What can Dr. Davis do to improve conditions?

CASE IVB → Easy Come, Easy Go!

Retail Credit Reports (RCR) operates out of Minneapolis, Minnesota. Employing approximately 115 people, the company supplies credit reports on individuals to department stores, oil companies, banks, and other organizations in Minnesota and western Wisconsin who utilize the information to make credit decisions. Firms pay a flat membership fee per year to use RCR's services plus a fee for each credit report, the cost varying with the amount of information desired.

RCR's personnel can basically be divided into one of four functions: management, secretarial support, service clerks, and investigators. In 1979, RCR employed 15 managers, 22 secretaries, 70 service clerks, and 8 investigators.

In February 1980, Jill Friedman, the senior manager in charge of the Minneapolis office, decided to implement a four-day workweek in the office. Ms. Friedman got the idea after hearing complaints from a number of the female office personnel that they wished they had more three-day weekends and after reading a recent article on the 4-40 week in *Fortune* magazine. A consultant was hired from a local university to help implement the program.

The consultant's strategy included tracking absence and satisfaction data before and after the shorter workweek was implemented. In this way, the consultant believed, it would be possible to assess the actual impact of the change.

The consultant had employees complete a questionnaire that assessed job satisfaction. He also reviewed employee personnel records to calculate absence figures. These became the base rates against which later figures could be compared.

Shortly after this information was obtained, employees were advised that RCR was moving to a four-day, forty-hour week. The announcement was made in a staff meeting. It was further announced that Mondays would be the extra day off. No mention was made of the criteria for deciding whether or not the program would be continued.

One month after the shorter workweek went into effect, the consultant made a follow-up survey of employee job satisfaction. Absence data was also obtained. However, unknown to the consultant, Jill Friedman was not pleased with how the change was working out. She was finding it increasingly difficult to schedule RCR's work activities. One month and three days after the 4-40 schedule was introduced, it was announced by Jill that RCR would be returning to the standard five-day week. The consultant, somewhat surprised, decided to make the best of the situation. He asked and received approval from Jill to do a third employee satisfaction survey. It was administered a month after the program was terminated. Absence data was also computed. This gave the consultant three sets of data. He had job satisfaction and absence data covering the period before the change was announced, a month after it had been implemented, and a month after it was terminated.

In June, the consultant provided a report to Jill giving the results he obtained. Job satisfaction improved significantly after the 4-40 week was implemented. After the program was discontinued, satisfaction dropped severely, to a level well below what it was before the shorter workweek was introduced. Absence date followed a similar pattern. Using the first set of data as a base (equal to 100), absenteeism dropped to 27 a month after 4-40 was introduced, but was up to 112 a month after 4-40 was terminated.

Questions

1. What factors should Jill have considered before implementing the 4-40 schedule?
2. How can a manager compare the added scheduling costs and difficulties associated with implementing a 4-40 program with savings from reduced absenteeism and other benefits?
3. Do you think the final job satisfaction and absentee data would have been different if the employees had been consulted before the 4-40 program was initiated? After it was initiated but before it was discontinued?
4. What are the implications from this case for instituting a structural change and then withdrawing it?

CASE IVC →

In Search of a 50 Percent Increase in Efficiency

Bill Richards was just beaming. An organizational analyst for a major oil company, he had just put the finishing touches on a report he was sure would save the corporation a lot of money and give him the kind of visibility at the head office that he felt he deserved.

Bill's proposal argued the current usage of secretaries at head office was inefficent. The report showed that in 1981, the corporation had 1,440 secretarial positions. This category had four subclasses—from entry-level typists (Secretary I) earning $810 to $1,240 a month, up to executive secretaries (Secretary IV), which paid $1,930 to $2,525 a month. The breakdown within classes found the following numbers at each level: Secretary I, 685; Secretary II, 517; Secretary III, 210; and Secretary IV, 28.

The total compensation cost, in 1981, for Secretary I through IV positions was $23.8 million. Bill's proposal basically restructures the use of secretaries. Secretaries III and IV would continue to be assigned to individual executives, but the first two levels would be reassigned from individual managers to a secretarial pool. Bill's analysis shows that a pool would increase efficiency by 50 percent. Specifically, he argues that the same amount of work could be handled by fewer than half of the 1,200 individuals currently at Secretary I and II levels. In dollars and cents, he calculates that the company would save between $8 and $9 million a year.

Bill's proposal and recommendations were received by his superiors with great enthusiasm. A three-month timetable was established in which the restructuring would occur. Consistent with company personnel policies, every effort would be made to protect all employees with more than one year of service. They would be offered transfers to one of the six production facilities or two marketing offices located within thirty miles of the company's head office.

Rumor of what soon became known as "The Richards Report" spread rapidly. Before top management even approved the document, detailed word of the report's contents had reached every secretary. The response by the secretaries was less than enthusiastic. Some said they would quit before being relegated to a secretarial pool. Many commented on losing the continuity of working for a single manager. Those with the lowest seniority complained of not wanting to be transferred to openings in the company's facilities out in the suburbs.

A year after restructuring began, Bill Richards submitted a follow-up report which included the following information:

> Secretarial compensation had been reduced by $8.7 million a year.
> 625 Secretary I and II employees were transferred or voluntarily resigned during the first three months of the program.
> Absences increased from an average of 0.7 days per employee per month before the restructuring to 1.8 afterward.
> Voluntary turnover increased from 1.7 per 100 employees per month before the restructuring to 6.1 afterward.
> Comments from management indicate no significant loss in quality of secretarial support, but a definite improvement in the speed in which requests are completed.

Questions

1. The savings due to restructuring are far less than $8.7 million. What other costs must be deducted to get a truer figure? Estimate these costs and compute the actual savings.
2. Explain how changes in technology may be able to offer insights into the secretaries' behavior.

CASE IVD →   What Happened to Team Effort?

Republic Avionics designs and manufactures sophisticated electronic devices for aerospace use. More than 90 percent of Republic's work evolves out of subcontracting for major aerospace firms like Boeing, General Dynamics, Lockhead, and McDonnell-Douglas. Founded in the late 1940s, the company grew to 1500 employees by the mid-1960s and has been stable at this size ever since.

Republic's organization is designed around projects. When a contract is obtained, it is assigned to a project manager who, in turn, is supported by one or more assistant project managers. A typical project manager may oversee five or six projects at a time. The actual manufacturing of the electronic devices is done in the company's manufacturing division which is headed by the director for manufacturing, Frank West. The director for manufacturing and project managers all report to a common boss—the vice-president for operations. Currently the vice-president for operations is Rob McDowell.

If each contract is to meet its time and quality objectives and come in within budget, the project manager must work closely with manufacturing. The importance of each is recognized at Republic. While the vice-president of manufacturing's annual salary of $120,000 is well above the average project manager's salary of $70,000, project managers earn more than second-level managers in the production function responsible for the manufacturing of the various components.

John Wilson had been hired by Republic in August 1981 to be a project manager. An engineer by training, he had established an impressive research record in the aerospace industry and Republic's top management considered itself lucky to have hired Wilson away from Zaron Industries, where he was a senior researcher in their electronic laboratories. Wilson was charged at Republic with supervising a number of projects, including a multimillion dollar subcontract for General Dynamics. Wilson was supported by Dave Brown, a twenty-six-year-old industrial engineer with an M.B.A. who had recently been hired out of a prestigous graduate school of business. Dave Brown impressed a large number of people at Republic as being bright and extremely ambitious.

In February 1982, Rob McDowell was informed by the auditing department that Wilson's project for General Dynamics was well behind schedule and running 14 percent over cost estimates. When McDowell confronted Wilson, the latter was obviously surprised. "I've had no knowledge that the project is off schedule. My assistant, Dave Brown, has mentioned that he's had to stay on top of the production people to make sure our project gets high priority. In fact, he's written several rather strong letters under my signature to Frank West to keep him aware of our concern. But Dave's always said everything was O.K., and that he just had to push those guys over in manufacturing a bit more than they have become accustomed to." An inquiry by McDowell to Frank West got a curt reply, "Tell John Wilson to get off my rear. I've got over three dozen manufacturing projects to get done and his letters and those nasty phone calls from his assistant have resulted in my people giving his projects lowest priority."

Questions

1. What is Wilson's responsibility? Has he done anything wrong?
2. What is Brown's responsibility? Has he done anything wrong?
3. How might organizational culture explain part of the current problems with the General Dynamic's project?
4. What can McDowell do to deal with the current problem?

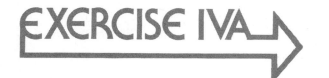

EXERCISE IVA

Bureaucratic Orientation Test

Instructions. For each statement, check the response (either mostly agree or mostly disagree) that best represents your feelings.

	MOSTLY AGREE	MOSTLY DISAGREE
1. I value stability in my job.	___	___
2. I like a predictable organization.	___	___
3. The best job for me would be one in which the future is uncertain.	___	___
4. The U.S. Army would be a nice place to work.	___	___
5. Rules, policies, and procedures tend to frustrate me.	___	___
6. I would enjoy working for a company that employed 85,000 people worldwide.	___	___
7. Being self-employed would involve more risk than I'm willing to take.	___	___
8. Before accepting a job, I would like to see an exact job description.	___	___
9. I would prefer a job as a freelance house painter to one as a clerk for the Department of Motor Vehicles.	___	___

10. Seniority should be as important as performance in determining pay increases and promotion. ___ ___
11. It would give me a feeling of pride to work for the largest and most successful company in its field. ___ ___
12. Given a choice, I would prefer to make $20,000 per year as a vice-president in a small company to $25,000 as a staff specialist in a large company. ___ ___
13. I would regard wearing an employee badge with a number on it as a degrading experience. ___ ___
14. Parking spaces in a company lot should be assigned on the basis of job level. ___ ___
15. If an accountant works for a large organization, he or she cannot be a true professional. ___ ___
16. Before accepting a job (given a choice), I would want to make sure that the company had a very fine program of employee benefits. ___ ___
17. A company will probably not be successful unless it establishes a clear set of rules and procedures. ___ ___
18. Regular working hours and vacations are more important to me than finding thrills on the job. ___ ___
19. You should respect people according to their rank. ___ ___
20. Rules are meant to be broken. ___ ___

Turn to page 536 for scoring directions and key.

Source: Andrew J. DuBrin, *Human Relations: A Job Oriented Approach* © 1978, pp. 687–88. Reprinted with permission of Reston Publishing Co., a Prentice-Hall Co., 11480 Sunset Hills Road, Reston, VA 22090.

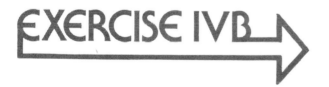

EXERCISE IVB

Rate Your Job's Motivating Potential

Utilizing your current job or one you have held in the past, rate its key dimensions on a scale from 1 to 7 (7 being the highest degree):

a. To what degree does your job require you to perform a variety of different work activities and allow you to use a wide range of your skills and talents? ___
b. To what degree does your job allow you to do something from beginning to end which results in a visible outcome? ___
c. To what degree does your job have a substantial impact on the lives or work of other people? ___

d. To what degree does your job provide you with freedom and discretion to schedule your own work and to determine how it will be done? ____

e. To what degree does your job itself provide you with clear and direct feedback on how effective you are in performing your job? ____

Turn to page 536 for scoring directions and key.

EXERCISE IVC ⟶

Rate Your Classroom Culture

Listed below are eight statements. Score each statement by indicating the degree to which you agree with it. If you strongly agree, give it a 5. If you strongly disagree, give it a 1.

1. My classmates are friendly and supportive. ____
2. My teacher is friendly and supportive. ____
3. I expect my final grade will accurately reflect the effort I make. ____
4. My teacher clearly expresses his/her expectations to the class. ____
5. My teacher encourages me to question and challenge him/her as well as other students. ____
6. I think the grading system used by my teacher is based on clear standards of performance. ____
7. My teacher makes me want to learn. ____
8. My teacher would give everyone in the class an "A" if we all earned it. ____

Turn to page 536 for scoring directions and key.

PART V

Organizational Dynamics

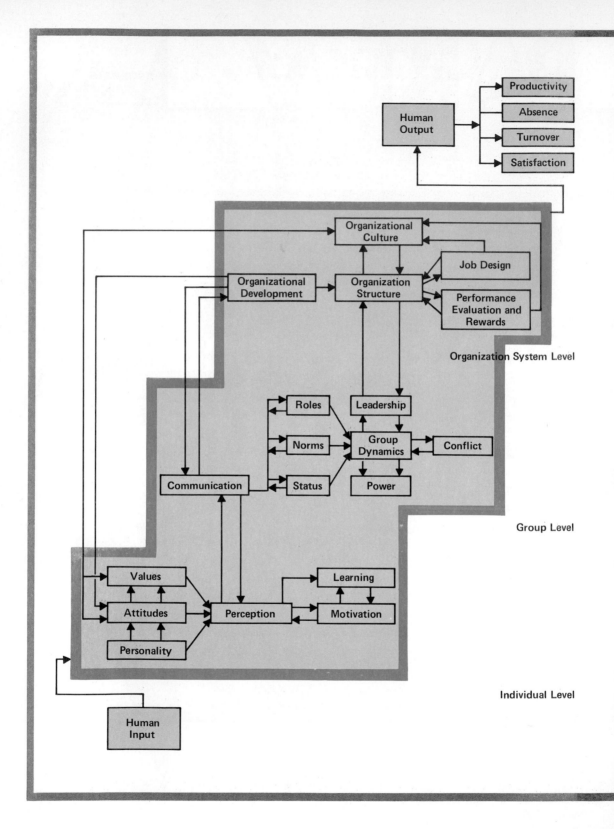

CHAPTER 19
Organizational Politics:
An Integrating Concept

AFTER STUDYING THIS CHAPTER, YOU SHOULD BE ABLE TO—

Define and explain the following key terms and concepts:

Dysfunctional political
  behavior
Functional political behavior

Organizational politics
Zero-sum reward practices

Understand:

Why all organizations are political systems
The difference between functional and dysfunctional political
  behavior
Why organizational politics is an integrating concept
Cultural factors that promote dysfunctional political behavior

> He who spits against the wind wets his shirt.
>
> —ANONYMOUS

It has only been in the last dozen years or so that organizational behavior researchers have come to acknowledge and accept what practitioners have long known: Organizations are political systems. Until very recently, OB scholars have neglected this aspect of organizational activities. They overemphasized the importance of supportive, harmonious, collaborative, and cooperative systems and underemphasized the often glaring discrepancy between behaviors that are in the organization's best interest and behaviors that are in the best interest of individuals or groups.

Organizations are made up of people who want "a niche from which to exert influence and be personally expressive, to earn just compensation, and to advance a career."[1] A nonpolitical perspective of organizational behavior can lead one to believe that employees will always behave in ways consistent with benefiting the organization. From such a perspective, when employees are seen to be pursuing their self-interest at the expense of the organization, it is assumed to be due to the employees' ignorance, miscalculation, or some failure on the part of management. A political view, however, can explain much of the seemingly irrational behavior in organizations. It can help explain, for instance, why employees withhold information, restrict output, attempt to build empires, publicize their successes, hide their failures, distort performance figures to make themselves look better, and similar actions that appear to be at odds with the organization's desire for effectiveness and efficiency. Only the naive can believe that the personal interests of individuals and the special interests that exist within the organization will be sublimated for the benefit of the organization. They will not be! For those who believe that organizations can be accurately described in terms of people demonstrating openness, trust, and cooperation, we offer you membership into what one author has called the "Buck Rogers school of organization theory."[2]

Organizations are political entities because they are staffed by people pur-

1. Samuel A. Culbert and John J. McDonough, *The Invisible War: Pursuing Self-Interest at Work* (New York: John Wiley, 1980), p. 6

2. Charles Perrow, "The Short and Glorious History of Organization Theory," *Organizational Dynamics*, Summer 1973, p. 3.

505

CHAPTER 19
*Organizational
Politics: An
Integrating
Concept*

suing self-interests. It would certainly be easier to predict behavior in organizations if this were not the case. What makes matters worse is that the smart people in organizations have learned to keep their self-interests hidden. They have found it is to their advantage that others not attribute their actions to the self-interest motive. So they couch what they do in terms of the best interests of the organization.[3] This, of course, only makes the explaining and predicting of organizational behavior harder. But "to ignore politicking is to ignore an integral facet of organizational behavior,"[4] and subsequently to reduce the accuracy of our explanations and predictions.

The theme of this chapter should now be evident: Viewing organizations as political arenas can help us in our goal of explaining and predicting behavior. We have not said that organizational politicking is right or wrong. We are only saying that this is the way it is!

WHAT IS ORGANIZATIONAL POLITICS?

Organizations require collective effort to attain their objectives, yet our discussion of individual motivation demonstrated that people are self oriented. Can we expect an individual to accept, for example, additional work that promises no personal gain, but that contributes to his or her departmental and organization's goals? No!

The fact that individuals behave in such ways as to enhance their own needs would not be as crucial a point were the organization's goals and the goals of individuals, as well as of groups within the organization, not at odds. What is best for a firm may not be best for employee John Smith. Similarly, what is good for the credit department can be detrimental to the sales department (i.e., the former attempts to keep losses low by authorizing credit only to substantial customers, while the latter seeks to sell as much as possible, regardless of the customer's credit worthiness).

The above examples lead us to our definition of organizational politics: any behavior by an organizational member that is self-serving. This behavior makes no reference to the goals or interests of the organization. When individuals act to enhance their own position, regardless of costs to the organization or to others, they are acting politically. Organizational politicking exists wherever people work together. It is "endemic to every organization, regardless of size, function, or character of ownership."[5]

Politicking may be a relatively new addition to the OB literature, yet we can find references to the importance of self-interest as an explanation of behavior in the writings of early philosophers and economists. The British social phi-

---

3. Dennis J. Moberg, "Organizational Politics: Perspective from Attribution Theory," paper presented to the American Institute of Decision Sciences, Chicago, 1977, p. 1

4. Andrew J. DuBrin, *Fundamentals of Organizational Behavior: An Applied Perspective* (Elmsford, N.Y.: Pergamon Press, 1974), p. 163.

5. John M. Pfiffner and Frank P. Sherwood, *Administrative Organization* (Englewood Cliffs, N.J.: Prentice-Hall, 1960), p. 311.

losopher, Jeremy Bentham, argued nearly 200 years ago that man behaves so as to maximize pleasure and minimize pain. Over two centuries ago, Adam Smith in his *Wealth of Nations,* said, "It is not from the benevolence of the butcher, the brewer, or the baker that we expect our dinner, but from their regard to their own interest." So the idea of behavior being based on self-interest is not new—it has just been overlooked or underemphasized.

If you remember our discussion of self-interest in the chapter on motivation, you may be asking: So what? We know that all behavior is based on self-interest! Therefore all behavior is political! How does this tautological conclusion help us to explain and predict organizational behavior?

Our answer lies in differentiating two types of political behavior: functional and dysfunctional. That is, it either assists in or deters the organization from attaining its goals. If, in acting in his or her own self-interest, a member behaves in ways that are compatible with the best interests of the organization, such behavior is functional. When this self-aggrandizement hinders the organization from achieving its goals, such actions are dysfunctional. This differentiation is depicted in Figure 19–1.

Our definition assumes that all employees are acting politically, but the act of being political means nothing until we determine the behavior's effect on the ends the organization seeks. Ideally, all employee behavior would be functional; that is, when they act so as to enhance their own self-interest they would be doing the same for the organization's interest. A sales commission compensation system that is well designed—giving the highest commission for sales of those products or services the organization wants most to sell—offers an illustration of where the interests of the organization are maximized by the salesperson pursuing his or her own self-interest (maximizing sales commissions). Unfortunately, these interests are not always complementary. This results in dysfunctional forms of behavior—the kind of activities that have given political behavior its negative connotations: scapegoating, passing the buck, red-herring tactics, discrediting others, sabotage, empire-building, falsification or withholding of important information, puffery (building up your contributions or accomplish-

Figure 19–1 Political Behavior

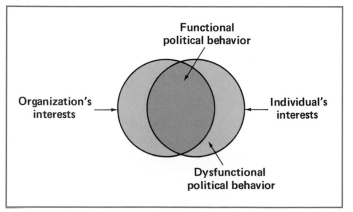

ments), and so forth (though these activities are not *always* dysfunctional). As students of organizational behavior, we should be aware of the detrimental impact that dysfunctional politicking can have on organizational effectiveness, and understand what conditions foster these undesirable outcomes.

WHY USE ORGANIZATIONAL POLITICS AS AN INTEGRATING CONCEPT?

Organizational politics may appear to be a strange integrating concept. Even to those students of organizational behavior who acknowledge its importance, politics may seem better placed in our discussion of group behavior, alongside power. But such a view ignores the fact that organizational politics embraces most of the concepts we have discussed throughout this book. Individual self-interest and its ramifications permeate the entire area of OB and can be used as an integrating theme to explain how individuals, groups, and structural components interact to create organizational behavior. In this chapter, we propose to demonstrate how the inclusion of organizational politics transforms the study of OB from a dry, static subject to a highly dynamic arena of action. Briefly, let us look at a few examples.

The Individual

Individuals act in what they believe to be their own self-interest. *Values* and *needs* determine what is in one's interest. This determination is an interpretation; that is, it represents what the individual *perceives* to be in his or her interest. Additionally, behavior is *learned* and conditioned by rewards. Since behavior is a function of its consequences, we recognize that what we learn and how we behave is closely linked to what we believe is personally desirable and consistent with our interests.

The Group

Whether an individual accepts a given *role,* adopts certain group *norms,* or joins a given group depends on the group's goals and how the individual perceives these goals aligning with his or her own goals. *Group decision making* is similarly a political process, influenced by an individual's desire for self-enhancement.

Who gains *power,* who exerts power, and who accepts power is also closely aligned to politics. Power is a valuable commodity in organizations because it is such an effective means to satisfying one's self-interest. Where it cannot be achieved individually, individuals resort to *coalitions* to achieve their ends. *Communication* requires the receiver to create meaning to cues initiated by the sender. One's self-interest will influence what one communicates and how one interprets others' communications. Looking at *leadership* as the adjudication of interests and the development of information and influence networks may provide more insights than concentrating on whether leaders use a task- or people-oriented style.[6] Similarly, a political perspective recognizes the inevitability of *conflict* as individuals and groups vie for scarce resources. Conflict resolution techniques that emphasize openness and trust have less applicability when the parties to the conflict are acknowledged as behaving in ways that are consistent with their self-interests.

The Organization System

Finally, politics affect organization system variables. As pointed out in Chapter 14, structural decisions are made by individuals, and these individuals cannot be expected to make decisions that will work against them or their constituencies. An *organization's structure* is, to a large degree, chosen by those in power in order that it will maintain and enhance their control. This power coalition also makes *job design* decisions, and they are likely to be strongly influenced by self-interest considerations. The fact that most jobs today are standardized and routine reflects that such designs fit nicely into the traditional hierarchial organization and provide those in power—management—with maximum control of employee behavior.[7]

Performance evaluation is a political process where objectivity can be only a standard. Since all actual evaluations contain some degree of subjective judgment, they are inherently influenced by the evaluator's self-interest. Reward distribution, too, is a political process. The basis upon which *rewards* are allocated is far from objective or devoid of the self-serving interests of the allocator, yet we know that rewards have an important effect on organizational behavior. We even find that *organizational development* is political. The decision to initiate change is a political decision. And, given the political perspective, the usefulness of OD is undoubtedly more limited or at least more complex than is usually conceived by OD proponents.[8] For example, intergroup development efforts are likely to be ineffective where the groups have divergent interests and are vying for scarce resources.

Summary

We have shown how organizational politics permeates and reshapes most of the concepts we have introduced in this book. The broad impact of politics at all three levels of analysis is dramatized in the following description of how some-

6. Michael Tushman, "A Political Approach to Organizations: A Review, Rationale, and Some Implications," Research Paper No. 114 (New York: Columbia University Graduate School of Business, 1976), pp. 36–38.

7. J. Richard Hackman, "The Design of Work in the 1980's," *Organizational Dynamics,* Summer 1978, p. 16.

8. Tushman, "Political Approach," p. 21.

509

CHAPTER 19
*Organizational
Politics: An
Integrating
Concept*

thing as basic as having people in the organization accept your contribution is entangled in a web of political actions:

—Third parties almost always view organization happenings from the vantage point of how events personally affect them and their own orientations to the organization.

—Whether or not third parties choose to value what is contributed depends on how well they see that contribution supporting and complementing that which they are self-conveniently pursuing.

—Whether or not third parties decide to take a stand and publicly support or criticize a contribution or perspective, depends on whether they think this can be done in a way that leaves their credibility intact and keeps their vested interests hidden.

—Since no definition of organizational reality fits all, people bargain and negotiate in their interpretations of each event, trying to find an interpretation that best serves a critical mass of self-interests, including their own.

—The large number of plausible organization realities makes it possible to find a perspective that devalues just about any contribution, and the constant threat that this might occur keeps people insecure and on the alert for others who may be out to push a meaning that renders their reality ineffective.

—In being ever sensitive to the meaning others attach to events, people constantly angle to support others whose orientations are compatible with their own and to block those whose orientations come at the expense of valuing that which they are trying to contribute.[9]

FACTORS CONTRIBUTING TO DYSFUNCTIONAL POLITICKING

Recent research and observation has identified a number of factors that appear to be associated with dysfunctional politics.

Individual Factors

At the individual level, researchers have identified certain personality characteristics and individual needs that are likely to be related to dysfunctional political behavior. Employees who are authoritarian, have a high-risking propensity, or possess an external locus of control have been shown to act politically with less regard for the consequences to the organization.[10] Additionally, a high need for

9. Culbert and McDonough, *Invisible War*, pp. 52–53.

10. See, for example, Bronston T. Mayes and Robert W. Allen, "Toward a Definition of Organizational Politics," *Academy of Management Review*, October 1977, pp. 672–78; Dennis J. Moberg, "Factors Which Determine the Perception and Use of Organizational Politics," paper presented at the 38th Annual Academy of Management Conference, San Francisco, 1978; and Lyman W. Porter, Robert W. Allen, and Harold L. Angle, "The Politics of Upward Influence in Organizations," in *Research in Organizational Behavior*, Vol. 3, ed. L L. Cummings, and B. M. Staw (Greenwich, Conn.: JAI Press, 1981) pp. 121–22.

power, autonomy, security, or status has been found to be a major contributor to an employee's tendency to engage in dysfunctional political behavior.[11]

Cultural Factors

Dysfunctional politicking, however, is probably more a function of the organization's culture than individual difference variables. Why? Because most organizations have a large number of employees with the characteristics we listed above, yet the presence of dysfunctional political behavior varies widely.

While we acknowledge the role that individual differences can play in fostering dysfunctional politicking, the evidence more strongly supports that certain cultures promote dysfunctional politics. Cultures characterized by role ambiguity, unclear performance evaluation systems, zero-sum reward allocation practices, democratic decision making, and high tolerance for conflict will create opportunities for dysfunctional political behavior.[12]

Role Ambiguity. Ambiguity in an employee's role fosters dysfunctional politicking. Ambiguity means that the prescribed behaviors of the employee are not clear. There are fewer limits, therefore, to the scope and functions of the employee's political actions. The clerical worker's role is usually unambiguous. When she acts to further her interests at the expense of the organization, it is usually quite obvious. The reason is that her role is clearly delineated. In contrast, personnel performing jobs such as researcher, analyst, or manager more typically have roles that lack clarity. Is a manager who appears to be deep in thought actually "thinking" or is she "daydreaming"? The first is important in the job; the second is a wasteful use of an organizational resource. But it is extremely difficult to know which is which. Similarly, many operative employees punch in on a time clock, clarifying when they are on the job and when they aren't. Professional and managerial personnel are usually excluded from such a practice. It is a lot easier, therefore, for the professional or manager to come in late, leave early, or exceed her alloted lunch hour. The more clearly one's tasks are defined, the more visible the deviations. Conversely, the more ambiguous the task requirements, the easier it is to satisfy one's self-interest and create a smoke screen that will cloud the dysfunctional aspects of an action upon the organization.

11. See, for example, J. E. Haas and T. E. Drabek, *Complex Organizations: A Sociological Perspective* (New York: Macmillan, 1973); Richard T. Mowday, "The Exercise of Upward Influence in Organizations," *Administrative Science Quarterly,* March 1978, pp. 137–56; and D. L. Madison, R. W. Allen, L. W. Porter, P. A. Renwick, and B. T. Mayes, "Organizational Politics: An Exploration of Manager's Perceptions," *Human Relations,* February 1980, pp. 79–100.

12. See, for example, Madison, et al., "Organizational Politics"; Porter et al., "The Politics of Upward Influence in Organizations," pp. 113–20; and Donald J. Vredenburgh and John G. Maurer, "A Process Framework of Organizational Politics," *Proceedings of the 41st Annual Academy of Management Conference,* San Diego, 1981, pp. 171–75.

511

CHAPTER 19
*Organizational
Politics: An
Integrating
Concept*

Unclear Performance Evaluation Systems. The practice of performance evaluation is far from a perfected science. The more that organizations use subjective criteria in the appraisal, emphasize a single outcome measure, or allow significant time to pass between the time of an action and its appraisal, the greater the likelihood that an employee can get away with dysfunctional politicking. Subjective performance criteria create ambiguity. The use of a single outcome measure encourages individuals to do whatever is necessary to "look good" on that measure but often at the expense of performing well on other important parts of the job that are not being appraised. The sales person who is appraised only on gross sales can be expected to do whatever is necessary to generate high sales in the immediate evaluation period. But in doing so, he is likely to ignore the small account that could be a large one in a few years, avoid providing feedback to the marketing research department on possible product changes, and the like. The amount of time that elapses between an action and its appraisal is also a relevant factor. The longer the time period, the more unlikely that the employee will be held accountable for his or her dysfunctional political behaviors. In many organizations, the performance feedback systems are slow. This is particularly true for management and professional positions. People are transferred or promoted to another position before their contribution on their current job can be fully evaluated. This creates a heightened need for employees to "look good" immediately and to do so in activities that are visible. Concern for immediacy of results can require members to engage in behaviors that have long-run dysfunctional impact on the organization. Similarly, emphasizing visible actions can be dysfunctional to the organization—*visible* activities are often not the same as *Important* activities.

Zero-Sum Reward Allocation Practices. The more than an organization's culture emphasizes the zero-sum or win-lose approach to reward allocations, the more employees will be motivated to engage in dysfunctional politicking. The zero-sum approach treats the reward "pie" as fixed so that any gain one person or group achieves has to come at the expense of another person or group. If I win, you must lose! If $10,000 in annual raises is to be distributed among five employees, then any employee who gets more than $2,000 takes money away from one or more of the others. Such a practice encourages making others look bad and increasing the visibility of what you do.

Democratic Decision Making. The last twenty years have seen a general move in North America toward making organizations less autocratic. While much of this move has been more in theory than in practice, it is undoubtedly true that in many organizations managers are being asked to behave more democratically. Managers are told that they should allow subordinates to advise them on decisions and that they should rely to a greater extent on group input into the decision process. Such moves toward democracy, however, are not necessarily desired by individual managers. Many managers sought their positions in order to have legitimate power so as to be able to make unilateral decisions. They fought hard and often paid high personal costs to achieve their influential positions. Sharing their power with others runs directly against their desires. The result is that managers may use the required committees, conferences, and group meetings in a superficial way—as arenas for maneuvering and manipulating.

High Tolerance for Conflict. If the organizational culture supports and encourages conflict, this can prompt individuals to engage in politicking. More importantly, if some conflict is viewed as functional in the organization, then the line where functional conflict ends and dysfunctional conflict begins is a perception which is open to interpretation. Like ambiguity, conflict can be used as a smoke screen to hide behaviors that do not align with the best interests of the organization.

PREDICTING DYSFUNCTIONAL POLITICKING

It would be useful to have some guidelines for explaining the influence politics can have in promoting suboptimized performance or redirecting behavior toward objectives that are not organizationally sanctioned. In other words, from our knowledge of political behavior, can we make any general predictions as to when people are more likely to engage in dysfunctional political behavior or what tactics they might use in attempting to further their personal interests? The following propositions offer some insights.

The more ambiguous (a) the formal role an individual is to fill or (b) his or her job-related goals, the greater the potential for that individual to engage in dysfunctional political behavior. Politicking intensifies with uncertainty or, contrarily, diminishes with certainty. Where organizational or departmental goals are unclear, or if a person's actual job assignment is vague or ambiguous, there is an increased tendency to engage in dysfunctional political behavior. Why? Because it is not clear what is functional or dysfunctional. Welding a bottle inside a door of a car on an automobile assembly line is clearly dysfunctional to the goal of producing trouble-free automobiles. Jobs on the assembly line are, for the most part, clearly defined. Management positions, on the other hand, are rarely so well demarcated. So too with college teaching positions. There is often considerable freedom for instructors to teach what they want within the very general course description written in the college catalogue. The college instructor therefore can "get away" with giving undue attention to pet topics or superficially discussing subjects that may be important but in which he or she is not particularly interested. The ambiguity surrounding the role of teachers in the classroom allows them considerable discretion. This may be functional when lectures compensate for omissions or weaknesses in the text, or take advantage of an instructor's special expertise in a topic. But it also allows instructors to engage in dysfunctional politics—teaching material that is irrelevant or that only marginally contributes to the goals of the course and the students' educational program.

The less objectivity in defining and measuring performance evaluation cri-

513

CHAPTER 19
*Organizational
Politics: An
Integrating
Concept*

teria, the greater potential for the individual to engage in dysfunctional political behavior. As we noted previously, people seek to know what is expected of them in their job and how they will be evaluated. Where performance can be measured objectively, individuals can satisfy the demands placed upon them by attempting to "look good" on the objective criteria. But few jobs fall into this category, and they become more scarce as one moves up the hierarchy.

Subjective evaluations encourage people to "look like" they are performing. When members are being judged on how closely they fit their evaluator's stereotypes of a "good employee" rather than on performance results, they engage in looking like good employees, whether appearances and actuality are correlated or not. This explains, incidentally, why employees may direct their energies into being on time, looking busy, dressing appropriately, and displaying traits of being friendly, cooperative, loyal, conscientious, and hard-working. In many organizations, these characteristics of a "good employee" are used as substitutes for objective performance data.

Where rewards are based on criteria other than performance, individuals will emphasize these "other" criteria even if it is at the expense of the organization. Consistent with our previous proposition, behavior will be a function of its consequences. Individuals "seek information as to what activities are rewarded, and then seek to do (or at least pretend to do) those things, often to the virtual exclusion of activities not rewarded."[13] If the organization's reward system pays off to those who "don't question the boss" or to those who "look busy," then people will agree with the boss and look busy, regardless of the dysfunctional impact of such behavior.

Individuals will seek to please their hierarchical superior in order to be looked upon favorably by him or her. To the extent that individuals help their superior to succeed, they are valued subordinates. Conversely, to the extent that they create problems for the superior, they are negatively evaluated.[14] Since superiors make *the* performance evaluation and given that individuals desire to be appraised favorably, individuals will act so as to contribute to the success of those immediately above them in the hierarchy. Such loyalty can be functional or dysfunctional. It becomes dysfunctional, for example, when individuals "cover" for their boss, defending him or her from outside attack when the attacks are legitimately based.

This proposition also indicates that organizational members are motivated to ingratiate themselves with their superiors. Attempting to win the boss's favor by "apple-polishing" has been demonstrated to result in more pay raises and more favorable performance evaluations, particularly where the superior has one or more hostile or disagreeable subordinates in addition to the compliant one.[15] Compliance appears to have its rewards, but of course it can become

13. Steven Kerr, "On the Folly of Rewarding A, While Hoping for B," *Academy of Management Journal,* December 1975, p. 769.

14. DuBrin, *Fundamentals of Organizational Behavior,* p. 150.

15. David Kipnis and B. A. Vanderveer, "Apple-Polishing Sometimes Pays Off," *OBI Interaction: The Management Psychology Newsletter,* July 16, 1971, pp. 5–6.

self-defeating if the superior perceives the compliant subordinate as a "yes-person" and the superior does not value such supportive behavior. In summary, individuals generally behave so as to please their boss.

Acquisition of power is the predominant manner in which self-interest is protected and promoted. As fully discussed in Chapter 12, influence will be sought to increase the probability of survival. Acquisition of power offers the most effective way to protect and promote one's self-interest.

The above propositions open the lid for looking into the organizational politics box. There is still a great deal that needs to be learned about the political process in organizations. Much of the theory at this time remains speculative. We can expect, however, that the next decade will change this as scholars begin actively to research the role and impact of politics on organizational behavior.

SOME CONCLUDING THOUGHTS

The end of a book frequently has the same meaning to an author that it has to the reader: It generates feelings of both accomplishment and relief. As both of us rejoice a bit at having nearly completed our journey through the field of organizational behavior, this is a good time to examine where we have been and what it all means. We have reviewed a lot of theories and, as Kurt Lewin is reported to have said, "There is nothing so practical as a good theory." Of equal importance is the truth that "there is nothing so *impractical* as a good theory that leads nowhere."[16]

Our major contention has been that organizational behavior is most easily understood by looking at it from three levels: the individual, the group, and the organization system. We started with the individual and attempted to review the major psychological contributions to understanding why individuals act as they do. We then looked at groups and argued that the understanding of group behavior is more complex than merely multiplying what we know about individuals by the number of members in the group. Beginning with our knowledge of individual behavior, we looked at how people act differently when in a group than when alone. Next, we overlaid organizational constraints upon our knowledge of individual and group behavior to improve our understanding of organizational behavior. Finally, to tap more fully the realities of organizational life, we noted how politics effect organizational behavior. This last chapter has sought to demonstrate that self-interests operate all the time and that an awareness of this reality can help you to more accurately explain and predict organizational behavior.

We are guilty of presenting a lot of theoretical concepts in these nineteen chapters, but hopefully there have been enough examples and illustrations to demonstrate that these theories can have practical value to you. Individually,

16. Newton Margulies and John Wallace, *Organizational Change: Techniques and Applications* (Glenview, Ill.: Scott, Foresman, 1973), p. vi.

515

CHAPTER 19
*Organizational
Politics: An
Integrating
Concept*

they offer some insights to behavior. Together, they provide a complex system to explain and predict organizational behavior.

A final comment: An understanding of OB can help you to be a more effective manager, but it offers no guarantee of success. The theories and techniques of OB are not unlike accounting principles or operations research techniques in that they all are tools in the operating manager's tool kit. However, no matter how high the quality of the tools, if the manager uses them incompetently, he or she is destined to fail.

Organizational behavior is not management. Rather, managers use their knowledge of OB to better understand why people do what they do, and to increase their ability to predict the effect of their actions on people's behavior and attitudes. You now have a basic set of OB tools that can provide insight as you observe and analyze the behavior of individuals in organizations. Hopefully, you will choose to use your tools to make more effective that institution upon which we depend in North America for satisfying our needs for goods and services—the Organization.

FOR DISCUSSION

1. Define organizational politics. How does it relate to motivation?
2. Why is organizational politics important in the study of OB?
3. "Politicking in organizations is bad." Do you agree or disagree? Discuss.
4. Differentiate between functional and dysfunctional political behavior.
5. What factors contribute to dysfunctional politicking?
6. Show how politics affect individual variables.
7. Show how politics affect group variables.
8. Show how politics affect organization system variables.
9. Describe cultural factors that contribute to dysfunctional political behavior.
10. What is the relationship between politics and power?

FOR FURTHER READING

Allen, R. W., D. L. Madison, L. W. Porter, P. A. Renwick, and B. T. Mayes, "Organizational Politics: Tactics and Characteristics of Its Actors," *California Management Review,* Fall 1979, pp. 77–83. Survey of eighty-seven managers looks at the tactics of organizational politics and the personal characteristics of those individuals who are most effective in using politics.

Gandz, J, and V. V. Murray, "The Experience of Workplace Politics," *Academy of Management Journal,* June 1980, pp. 237–51. Recent graduates of a business school report on the impact politics has in their organizations.

PETTIGREW, A. M., *The Politics of Organizational Decision-Making.* London: Tavistock Publications, 1973. Detailed study of the power and political factors involved in a computer equipment decision by a large British firm.

SCHEIN, V. E., "Individual Power and Political Behaviors in Organizations: An Inadequately Explored Reality," *Academy of Management Review,* January 1977, pp. 64–72. Looks at the bases of power and the intent and means of the powerholder to provide a starting point for research on political behaviors in organizations.

TUSHMAN, M., "A Political Approach to Organizations: A Review and Rationale," *Academy of Management Review,* April 1977, pp. 206–16. Considers why politics was ignored for so long, proposes a set of working assumptions as the basis for a political perspective, and reviews the OD literature from this political perspective.

ZALEZNIK, A., "Power and Politics in Organizational Life," *Harvard Business Review,* May-June, 1970, pp. 47–60. How the limitations of businessmen, in their cognitive and emotional capacities, play a major role in decision making.

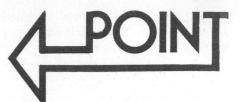

MAYES and ALLEN

Organizational politics goes beyond the simple performance of job tasks

Adapted and edited from Bronston T. Mayes and Robert W. Allen, "Toward a Definition of Organizational Politics," The Academy of Management Review, October 1977, pp. 672–78. With permission.

Anyone associated with almost any form of organization eventually becomes aware of activities that are described by employees as "political," but what is termed political by one observer may not be viewed as political by another. To understand the nature of political processes in organizations, some agreement as to what constitutes political behavior must be developed. This article attempts to shed light on the organizational political process by constructing a literature-derived definition of organizational politics (OP). Guiding this effort are the following assumptions:

1. Behavior referred to as politics takes place in varying degrees in all organizations.

2. Not all behavior in organizations can be categorized as political.

3. The organizational political process can be described in nonevaluative terms.

4. While many variables involved in describing organizational politics may be familiar to other organizational behavior concepts, a combination of these variables constitutes a unique process that cannot be described adequately by existing paradigms. This unique process is organizational politics.

Political behavior in an organization has been viewed as actions that make a claim against the organization's resource sharing system. Although some claims against an organization's resource sharing system may constitute political behavior, normally many of these claims would not be considered political. For example, an employee's asking for a salary raise, which constitutes a claim against the resource sharing system, would not be political behavior, but the use of threat to unionize to obtain a raise would be considered a political act. Circumstances surrounding the demand process must be considered in defining OP.

Wildavsky defines politics as conflict over whose preferences are to prevail in the determination of policy. To define politics as a form of conflict seems too narrow an approach, especially when one limits politics to the conflict over policy decisions. The administration of policy involves political activities in its own right. Thus, a suitable definition of OP must include the politics of policy implementation as well as the politics of policy determination.

In discussing power tactics used by executives, Martin and Sims state that politics is concerned with relationships of control or influence. Although control, power, and influence are key issues in the study of OP, this approach allows inclusion of behaviors and forms of influence not normally considered political. An example of a nonpolitical means of control in an organization is the periodic performance review when done in accordance with policy guidelines normally provided for this purpose. The review/appraisal constitutes a form of feedback to the ratee on his/her job performance and is a form of influence or control in that the employee is expected to correct performance deficiencies.

Some writers have considered politics as behavior directed toward personal gain. Although this approach is intuitively appealing, the argument can be made that all willful behavior ultimately serves some self-interest. If personal gain is the underlying motive for all calculated behavior, its inclusion in the definition of political activity adds nothing and may detract from definitional clarity. How is behavior classified if it is specified by the organization but also obtains rewards for the actor? Including self-interest in the definition of OP forces consideration of routine job performance as a political act. A suitable definition of OP must allow exclusion of routine job performance from consideration.

The definitions and research briefly presented above allow us to formulate a definition of OP that meets certain necessary conditions. First, a suitable definition would allow either micro or macro levels of analysis—consideration of both individual and organizational political phenomena. Second, it must allow for the use of politics in other than decision processes surrounding resource allocation. Third, any suitable definition of OP must clearly discriminate between political and nonpolitical behaviors. For example, routine job performance is not a political activity but could be considered so if earlier constructs are employed.

What, then, is an acceptable definition of organizational politics? A thread of continuity through the existing literature is best recognized as influence. If outcomes alone are not sufficient to define political behavior, the processes whereby outcomes are influenced must be examined. Thus the notion of influence is a necessary but not sufficient condition for the inference of political action. A supervisor making routine job assignments influences the behavior of subordinates, but this form of influence is not political. Likewise, some forms of influence may not be intentional. Politics implies calculated influence maneuvering. But even restricting politics to calculated influence is not a sufficient condition, in that some forms of calculated influence should also be excluded from the OP con-

struct. Is not the organization itself a form of influence calculated to restrict the behavior of its members? The organization structure as it exists at some given point in time should be excluded from the OP construct, although changes made to the existing structure could be politically relevant.

Therefore OP is a dynamic process of influence that produces organizationally relevant outcomes beyond the simple performance of job tasks. Common organizational practice is to provide each member of the organization with a description of duties that specifies the organizationally desired job outcome and the limits of discretionary behavior acceptable in attaining those outcomes. Thus, the existing organization delineates both acceptable outcomes and appropriate means to their attainment for each job position. Activities within these sanctioned boundaries must be considered nonpolitical. The considerations lead us to the following definition of OP:

Organizational politics is the management of influence to attain ends not sanctioned by the organization or to obtain sanctioned ends through nonsanctioned means.

This approach to a definition of OP is schematically represented in Table 1. Quadrant I, characterized by organizationally specified job behavior, is the only nonpolitical quadrant in the classification system. Quadrant II contains political activities recognized by some bureaucratic theorists as abuses of formal authority/power. Behavior in this quadrant is dysfunctional from the standpoint of the organization, in that organizational resources are being utilized to further nonorganizational objectives. The bureaucratic form of organization can be viewed as an attempt to eliminate this type of behavior.

Quadrant III defines political behavior undertaken to accomplish legitimate organizational objectives. The use of charisma or side-payments to accomplish sanctioned objectives would be included in behaviors assigned to this quadrant. Quadrant III activity could be functional to the organization if undesirable side effects did not occur. Indeed, some writers view organizationally functional Quadrant III behavior as leadership.

Quadrant IV behavior, like Quadrant II behavior, is dysfunctional from the organizational per-

Table 1 Dimensions of Organizational Politics

Influence means	Influence Ends	
	Organizationally sanctioned	Not sanctioned by organization
Organizationally sanctioned	I Nonpolitical job behavior	II Organizationally dysfunctional political behavior
Not sanctioned by organization	III Political behavior potentially functional to the organization	IV Organizationally dysfunctional political behavior

spective. It deviates from organization norms with respect to both outcomes and methods. This form of OP will not be tolerated if it is discovered. Due to the possibility of being dismissed from the or-ganization for such actions, individuals engaging in such behavior probably will be highly secretive, making Quadrant IV resistant to research attempts.

COUNTER POINT

ROBBINS

All job behaviors are political

Prepared especially for this volume by Stephen P. Robbins.

I share the concern of Professors Mayes and Allen as to the need to agree upon what constitutes political behavior in organizations. After reviewing their article, I find a number of points which we hold in common. However, I am going to argue that (1) Mayes and Allen have made explicit and implicit assumptions that prejudice the conclusions they reach and (2) their final definition is difficult, if not impossible, to operationalize. In the final analysis, Mayes and Allen have done little to clear a path through the organizational politics "jungle."

Every position paper is based on certain assumptions, and Mayes and Allen have explicitly stated four assumptions that guide their thinking. Yet, the charge can be made that Mayes and Allen have eliminated viable alternatives by creating unrealistic or unnecessary assumptions. Their assumptions that political behavior takes place in all organizations and that the organizational politics process is both unique and describable in nonevaluative terms are reasonable. But why do they assume that not all behavior in organizations can be categorized as political? Is this assumption necessary? More importantly, is there any evidence to support this assumption?

The authors have correctly noted that willful behavior ultimately serves some self-interest. Yet this bothers the authors when they say that: "If personal gain is the underlying motive for all cal-

culated behavior, its inclusion in the definition of political activity adds nothing and may detract from definitional clarity." This, too, is true, but it cannot be assumed away just to achieve clarity. Are accuracy and truth to be sublimated to expediency? I would hope not. Yet that is what the creation of this assumption imposes.

This assumption regarding the nonpervasiveness of political behavior arises again when Mayes and Allen argue that a suitable definition must clearly discriminate between political and nonpolitical behaviors. This would be nice if there was such a clear distinction. If it exists, I fail to find it. Even the examples that Mayes and Allen use in their article, which are meant to demonstrate actions that are not political, better illustrate my position than theirs.

An employee's asking for a salary raise is described as being nonpolitical. Against what criterion? Are all such requests justified? Will the requests be made by the most deserving? Do not most of us find the vying for salary increases one of the most active arenas for political maneuvering? Describing the request for a salary raise as nonpolitical fails the face validity test.

Mayes and Allen describe the periodic performance review when done in accordance with the organization's policy guidelines as another example of nonpolitical behavior. My previous argument holds. Decisions in organizations are not made against some irrefutable standard of objectivity. Management is an art, relying heavily on judgment. Performance appraisal is a *highly* subjective process and the literature demonstrates that nonperformance factors are major determinants of an individual's appraisal. So, of course, the performance review is far from an apolitical activity.

The making of routine job assignments by a supervisor has also been characterized as nonpolitical. Who among us, with a few years of working experience, cannot describe work assignments that have been given as having been politically determined? As long as some assignments are more desirable than others, there will be political jockeying among individuals to influence the outcome.

Mayes and Allen make it clear that their definition must exclude routine job performance from consideration. The problem that I see is the standard for determining what is routine job performance for each person in an organization. Mayes and Allen propose that each individual has a job description that specifies the organizationally desired job outcome and the limits of discretionary behavior acceptable in attaining those outcomes. Unfortunately, actual job behavior rarely looks anything like these job descriptions. When it does, it is often dysfunctional—as when union employees decide to "work to rule." A more accurate analysis suggests that the determination of what is sanctioned and what is not is far from clear in most jobs. It becomes increasingly vague as one moves from operative jobs, to middle-management positions, to the activities performed by top executives. For example, what is sanctioned behavior for the vice-president of marketing at General Foods? His or her job description will, by necessity, be written in such vague language as to make it impossible to appraise it against Mayes and Allen's "formally sanctioned" criterion. What is sanctioned will depend on who you ask. In fact, it could be argued that the bargaining and maneuvering over what is officially sanctioned by the organization in one's job is itself a hotly political process. People justify their own actions as being in the interest of the organization and perceive the actions of others as being political.

Let me conclude by proposing that all behavior in organizations is political. When people use legitimate power to achieve organizational objectives, this political behavior is functional. So, too, are those efforts to use other nonlegitimate power bases to achieve the organization's objectives. When power is used to achieve personal objectives that are not consistent with the organization's objectives, this is dysfunctional. Using Mayes and Allen's terminology, Quadrants I and III represent functional political behavior and Quadrants II and IV are dysfunctional.

I am in full agreement with Mayes and Allen's appraisal of Quadrants II and IV. These are clearly dysfunctional. But, I view all of Quadrant III to be functional since my perspective ignores means. If the ends are in the best interest of the organization, it is functional, not merely *potentially* functional. Finally, the major difference between Mayes and Allen's definition and mine lies in the evaluation of Quadrant I behavior. Since I argue that all behavior is political, it is my position that when individuals engage in behaviors that further the organization's attaining its objectives, such behavior is functional rather than nonpolitical. Such a definition emphasizes organizational goals—that is, is the individual's behavior aiding or hindering the organization in attaining its goals? It avoids the ambiguity in attempting to assess formally sanctioned role behavior. Of course, neither definition has successfully avoided the perception problem. In one, the problem is to determine if a behavior is formally sanctioned, in the other it is to determine if a behavior advances the organization toward its goals. I propose the latter is a more reliable standard.

CASE VA ➔ I Don't Make Decisions!

I met Ted Kelly for the first time at a cocktail party. As things happen, we got to talking about our work. When he found out I taught organizational behavior, he understood my interest in his job. Ted was the plant manager at a large chemical refinery in town. About ten minutes or so into our conversation, I asked him what type of leadership style he used.

Ted: "I don't make decisions at my plant."

Author: "You mean you use democratic leadership?"

Ted: "No. I said I don't make decisions! My subordinates are paid to make decisions. No point in my doing their jobs."

Ted went on to say that about five years ago he decided that his subordinate managers had become too dependent on him. After some deliberation, he made a decision—as he tells it, it was the last one he made on his job. He decided never to make a decision again.

I didn't really believe what I was hearing. I guess Ted sensed that, so he offered me an invitation to visit his plant. I wasn't going to miss the opportunity. I asked him when I could come over. "Any time you like, except Mondays between 1 and 3 P.M." "Anytime?" I questioned. "Yeah," he replied. "Ever since I decided not to decide, I've got nothing to keep me busy."

The middle of the next week, I popped in on Ted unannounced. I found his office by following the signs. He had no secretary. He was lying on his sofa, half asleep. My arrival seemed to jar him awake. He seemed glad to see me. He offered me a seat.

Our conversation began by my inquiring exactly what he did everyday. "You're looking at it. I sleep a lot. Oh yeah, I read the four or five memos I get from the head office every week." I couldn't believe what I was hearing. Here was a fifty-year-old, obviously successful, executive, probably earning better than $75,000 a year, telling me he doesn't do anything. He could tell, however, that I wasn't buying his story.

"If you don't believe what I'm saying, check with my subordinates," he told me. He said he had six department managers working for him. I asked him to choose one I could talk with.

"No, I can't do that. First, I don't make decisions. Second, when the one I chose confirmed what I've been telling you, you'd think it was a set-up. Here—these are the names and numbers of my department managers. You call them."

I did just that. I picked Pete Chandler, who headed up quality control. I dialed his number. He answered on the first ring. I told him that I

523

CHAPTER 19
*Organizational
Politics: An
Integrating
Concept*

wanted to talk to him about his boss's leadership style. He said "Come on over. I've got nothing to do anyway."

When I arrived at Pete's office, he was staring out the window. We sat down and he began to laugh. "I'll bet Ted's been telling you about how he doesn't make decisions." I concurred. "It's all true," he injected. "I've been here for almost three years and I've never seen him make a decision."

I couldn't figure out how this could be. "How many people do you have working here?" I asked.

Pete: "About 200."

Author: "How does this plant's operating efficiency stack up against the others?"

Pete: "Oh, we're number one out of the eighteen refineries. Been that way for years and years. Interesting thing is that this is the oldest refinery in the company, too. Our equipment may be outdated but we're as efficient as they come."

Author: "What does Ted Kelly do?"

Pete: "Beats me. He attends the staff meetings on Monday afternoons from 1 to 3 P.M., but other than that, I don't know."

Author: "I get it. He makes all the decisions at that once-a-week staff meeting?"

Pete: "No. Each department head tells what key decisions he made last week. We then critique each other. Ted says nothing. The only thing he does at those meetings is listen and pass on any happenings up at headquarters."

I wanted to learn more, so I went back to Ted's office. I found him clipping his fingernails.

"I told you I was telling the truth," was the first thing he said. What followed was a long conversation in which I learned the following facts:

The two-hour weekly staff meeting is presided over by one of the department heads. They choose among themselves who will be their leader. It's a permanent position. Any problem that has come up during the week, if it can't be handled by a manager, will first be considered by several of the managers together. Only if the problem is still unresolved will it be taken to the leader. All issues are resolved at that level. They are never taken to Ted Kelly's level.

The performance record at Kelly's plant is well known in the company. Three of the last four plant managers have come out of Kelly's plant. When asked by the head office to recommend candidates for a plant management vacancy, Ted always selects the department head who presides over the staff meetings. The result is that there is a great deal of competition to lead the staff meetings. Additionally, because of Kelly's plant record for breeding management talent, whenever there is a vacancy for a department manager at Kelly's plant, the best people in the company apply for it. Of course, the decision as to who is hired is made by the existing heads at their weekly staff meeting.

The three plant managers who previously worked under Kelly have instituted a similar leadership style. Their plants have also shown significant improvement as measured by the company-wide efficiency reports.

Even the department managers are practicing the Kelly method. They are forcing decision making down to their supervisors.

Questions

1. Why does Ted Kelly's "leadership style" work?
2. Draw a diagram of the formal plant authority structure. What is it like in reality?
3. How do rewards impact behavior in this case?
4. If Kelly's plant performance suddenly dropped off, what predictions would you make?

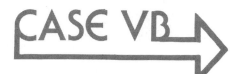

CASE VB

It's Performance Appraisal Time

Dana Ruff, manager for women's lingerie at the Macy's department store in San Francisco, always dreads November 1. That's the day that all managers are required to turn in performance appraisals on their employees. These appraisals become the major determinant of salary increases, decisions which are made in December and go into effect January 1.

"I can't think of any activity I dislike more in this job than doing the annual performance reviews," Dana related. "I see them as a no-win proposition. My poor performers fight the evaluations. They complain that I'm prejudiced, unobjective, overly picky. You name it, I've heard it all. They want to put the blame on anyone but themselves. And since I make the appraisals, I'm usually the target for most of the bitching. My good performers know they're doing a good job. There is nothing positive I can tell them that they don't expect. Their complaints are usually that I don't give them *enough* recognition. So, like I said, I can't win."

One of Dana's newer employees is one of her biggest problems. Shannon Hersch has been working for Dana and Macy's for seven months. In that short time, she has openly argued with Dana on a number of occasions, has bad-mouthed Dana within the department, and has made two formal complaints to the personnel office about the way Dana has treated her. As self-protection, Dana has taken to keeping a daily diary describing both the good and bad behaviors Shannon exhibits on the job.

525

CHAPTER 19
*Organizational
Politics: An
Integrating
Concept*

Dana has been getting complaints from several of her people about Shannon. They say she is disruptive. She's negative about her job and even comments negatively on Macy's as a place to work. But Shannon has several friends in the department and she appears to be having an impact on them. Based on what she sees and hears down on the floor, Dana believes that Shannon is developing a coalition of marginal workers—those who have received negative appraisals. She notices that Shannon and three peers in the department regularly take coffee breaks and lunch together.

Dana is aware that her boss is watching her more closely as a result of the complaints made to personnel. She has eight full-time and ten part-time employees. It's October 25. Dana's appraisals of her employees are due within the week. Of course, Dana's own appraisal by her boss is due at the same time.

Questions

1. How do performance appraisals effect behavior?
2. Should Dana talk with her boss?
3. Should Dana talk with Shannon?
4. What do you think Shannon's strategy is?
5. How can Dana find out what impact Shannon is having on departmental performance and morale?

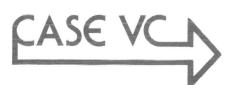

Games People Play
in the Shipping Department

The Science Fiction Book Club (SFBC) sells a large list of science fiction books, at discount prices, entirely by mail order. In 1980, the club shipped over 370,000 books and generated revenues of $3.4 million. Anyone familiar with the mail-order business realizes that it offers extremely high profit potential because, under careful management, inventory costs and overhead can be kept quite low. The biggest problems in mail-order businesses are filling orders, shipping the merchandise, and billing the customers. At SFBC, the Packing and Shipping (P&S) Department employs eight full-time people:

Ray, forty-four years old, has worked in P&S for seven years.
Al, forty-nine years old, has worked in P&S for nine years.
R.J., fifty-three years old, has worked in P&S for sixteen years. He had been head of the department for two years back in the mid-1970s but

stepped down voluntarily due to continuing stomach problems which doctors attributed to supervisory pressures.

Pearl, fifty-nine years old, was the original employee hired by the founder. She has been at SFBC for twenty-five years, and in P&S for twenty-one years.

Margaret, thirty-one years old, is the newest member of the department. She has been employed less than a year.

Steve, twenty-seven years old, has worked in P&S for three years. He goes to college at nights and makes no effort to hide that he plans on leaving P&S and probably SFBC when he gets his degree next year.

George, forty-six years old, is currently head of P&S. He has been with SFBC for ten years, and in P&S for six.

Gary, twenty-five years old, has worked in P&S for two years.

The jobs in a shipping department are uniformly dull and repetitive. Each person is responsible for wrapping, addressing, and making the bills out on anywhere from 100 to 200 books a day. Part of George's responsibilities are to make allocations to each worker and to ensure that no significant backlogs occur. However, George spends less than 10 percent of his time in supervisory activities. The rest of the time he wraps, addresses, and makes out bills just like everyone else.

Apparently to deal with the repetitiveness of their jobs, the department members have created a number of games that they play among themselves. At first glance, they seem almost childish. But it is obvious that the games mean something to these people. Importantly, each is played regularly. Some of the ones that will be described are done at least once a day. All are played a minimum of twice a week.

"The Stamp Machine Is Broken" is a game that belongs to Al. At least once a day, Al goes over to the postage meter in the office and unplugs it. He then proceeds loudly to attempt to make a stamp for a package. "The stamp machine is broken again," he yells. Either Ray or Gary, or both, will come over and spend thirty seconds or so trying to "fix it," then "discover" that it's unplugged. The one who finds it unplugged then says "Al, you're a mechanical spastic" and others in the office join in and laugh.

Gary is the initiator of the game "Steve, There's a Call for You." Usually played in the late afternoon, an hour or so before everyone goes home, Gary will pick up the phone and pretend that there is someone on the line. "Hey, Steve, it's for you," he'll yell out. "It's Mr. Big [the president of SFBC]. Says he wants you to come over to his office right away. You're going to be the new vice-president!" The game is an obvious sarcastic jab at Steve's going to college and his frequent comments about someday being a big executive.

At least two or three times a day, Ray will go out of his way to walk by Margaret's desk. As he walks by, he sensuously runs his hand down

527

CHAPTER 19
*Organizational
Politics: An
Integrating
Concept*

her back and blows in her ear. She always jumps, though she knows he's coming. Ray's desk is two ahead of Margaret's and to get behind her he has to walk by her. The irony of this little flirtatious game is that Margaret obviously loves the attention, though she always plays "upset" by Ray's actions. In fact, when Ray was on vacation for two weeks last month, everyone noticed how Margaret seemed depressed. Could she actually be missing Ray?

R.J., though fifty-three years old, has never married and lives with his mother. The main interests in his life are telling stories and showing pictures of last year's vacation and planning for this year's vacation. Without exception, everyone finds R.J.'s vacation talk boring. But that doesn't stop Pearl or George from "setting him up" several times a week. "Hey R.J., can we see those pictures you took last year in Oregon, again?" That question always gets R.J. to drop whatever he's doing and out come 75 to 100 pictures from his top drawer. "Hey, R.J., what are you planning to do on your vacation this year?" always gets R.J.'s eyes shining and invariably leads to the unfolding of maps he also keeps in his top drawer.

George's favorite game is "What's It Like to Be Rich?" which he plays with Pearl. Pearl's husband had been a successful banker and had died a half-dozen years earlier. He left her very well off financially. Pearl enjoys everyone knowing that she doesn't have to work, has a large lovely home, buys a new car every year, and includes some of the city's more prominent business people and politicians among her friends. George will mention the name of some big shot in town and Pearl never fails to take the bait. She proceeds to tell how he is a close friend of hers. George might also bring up money in some context in order to allow Pearl to complain about high taxes, the difficulty in finding good housekeepers, the high cost of traveling to Europe, or some other concern of the affluent.

Questions

1. Analyze the group dynamics going on in P&S.
2. How do these games effect the department's performance?
3. Relate the actions in this case to job design and motivation theory.

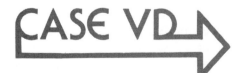

CASE VD — United Manufacturing Company

United Manufacturing Company is a closely held, family corporation located in a small midwestern town of about 7,000 people. It employs 1,000, of which 50 are managers and the rest shop employees. The shop is divided into fifteen departments with each department responsible for a different product. Each department has a department head and one foreman.

United has been very profitable the last five years, earning over 20 percent on sales. This profitability corresponds to the length of time the piece rate incentive plan has been in effect. United has a Wage and Salary Department and employs well-trained industrial engineers to analyze and improve production methods, standardize operations, and set time standards for operations. Base rates for every job are bargained with the union, but management sets the piece rate and uses past performance as one criteria along with time studies.

In the incentive plan, the earnings of the employee are directly proportionate to his output. For every 1 percent increase in output, the worker is given a 1 percent increase in wages. In the past few years, wages have risen steadily to the point where they are high for their type of industry, and the highest in that immediate part of the country. The plant has a record of good labor relations. Turnover and absenteeism are also low.

One of the fifteen departments is Department 551, which makes electronic relays that are added to the final product in the later stages of production. These relays are also sold throughout the country to other manufacturers in the same line. This accounts for approximately 25 percent of United's profits.

Six months ago a time study was initiated by the Wage and Salary unit of activities in Department 551. Although they told no one, word spread quickly throughout the department. Absenteeism soared from 5 percent to 20 percent. Employee concern was visible through a large increase in Department 551 grievances.

The Wage and Salary unit, on the basis of past performance and their time study, made the recommendation to top management that a new procedure be instituted in Department 551 that would make the job less complicated. At the same time, they recommended that the piece rate standard be raised. This effectively increased the standard approximately 15 percent. Top management accepted the recommendation and sent a directive to Fred Wilson, the Department Head of 551, ordering him to initiate the change. Wilson carried out the request and posted the new piece rate standards on the departmental bulletin board. The foreman, who aligns himself with Wilson, made sure the workers followed the new procedure by spot checking each worker five or six times a day during the first month and, more recently, two or three times a day. He also counted the output of each worker and reported this to Wilson at the end of each week.

But the change is affecting production and worker pay. Until six months ago, the employees in Department 551 were averaging $350 a month incentive pay and working at approximately 50 percent above

529

CHAPTER 19
*Organizational
Politics: An
Integrating
Concept*

standard. As soon as the Wage and Salary people started their time study, production dropped to 20 percent above standard and incentive pay dropped proportionally. When the new procedure was introduced and the new standard announced, production dropped initially to 70 percent of the former output. It then rose steadily to 85 percent, but has stagnated at this level. Management attributed the initial drop to the new procedure but could not see why it did not rise again to the old level. The Production Department Manager believed some workers might be "holding back" production and instructed Wilson to fire anyone found "restricting" their output. This led to the threatening of three top producers. Although their individual output went up, the department still averaged only 87 percent of the old standard.

Following the threat of discharge to these three men, grievances nearly doubled for the week and continued at 50 percent above normal for the remainder of the month. The shop steward that handled these grievances was very aggressive, and management believed he was partly to blame for the dissent. On the other hand, workers obviously felt he was representing them very well, as he had just been reelected for his fifth consecutive six-month term as steward. Most of these grievances were being directed at the new standard. The foreman's response has been to demonstrate to the workers who complain that the standards are easily attainable. He has done this by taking over a job and working fervently for about ten minutes, then announcing that he has no trouble meeting the standard.

Things have grown worse during the past few weeks. The employees of Department 551 have started wearing black arm bands and at times have worn their employee number pinned to their backs, in prison fashion. On these occasions they have marched up and down the aisles yelling at each other. On one occasion, about thirty people sat in the cafeteria until the precise time they were to return to their jobs. Then they jumped up, in the process knocking over chairs and spilling trays to the floor, yelling in unison "GO! GO! GO!" and marched out the door counting cadence. This obviously upset the entire cafeteria, which had about 200 people in it at the time. One startled man suffered a mild heart attack and was taken to the hospital.

Another time, fifty employees from Department 551 brought toy whistles to work and blew the whistles all the time they were at their desks. The foreman took all the names of those involved and turned the list over to Wilson. This list eventually reached the president of the company. The rumor around the shop is that the president intends to "dock" all the employees involved.

Lately, the workers in 551 have resorted to much more drastic tactics. One day they all sat at their work benches with their arms folded and refused to work the last hour of their work day. On another day, they all walked off the job at noon, after one of the workers got into an argument with the foreman. They have also taken out a full-page ad in the local newspaper accusing United of unfair labor practices.

Management is becoming increasingly alarmed about the turn of events. Sympathizers from the rest of the company are growing in number and the grapevine is carrying the report that if the workers in Department 551 call a strike, 60 percent of the other employees will follow in support. Production in Department 551 has reached the level where they are no longer supplying enough relays to fill the needs of United, much less the demands from outsiders. Also, because the employees took out the newspaper ad last week, several prominent businessmen from the area have inquired into the matter.

There are also other factors to consider: (1) the general economy is strong, with nationwide unemployment at a low 5.5 percent, (2) the local unemployment rate is only 3.8 percent, (3) and it takes approximately four weeks to train a person to do the job in Department 551, with another eight to ten week wait before the new worker normally reaches 80 percent efficiency.

Questions

1. Analyze this case by assessing the effect of each of the following concepts on employee behavior: (a) perception; (b) motivation; (c) group dynamics; (d) leadership; (e) power; (f) communication; (g) conflict; (h) job design; (i) culture; (j) organizational development.
2. As a consultant, what recommendations would you make to management?

Scoring Keys for Activity Exercises

Exercise II—A. Value Assessment

Each item in the Value Assessment exercise is coded in the following manner:

A = theoretical dimension
B = economic-political dimension
C = aesthetic dimension
D = social dimension

Total scores for each dimension are calculated by adding the number associated with the response on the dimension items for each "Yes" response. For example, in the B items (economic-political), if you replied "Yes" only to 31, 34, and 76, your total score on the economic-political dimension would be 23 (5 + 8 + 10). When a sample of 389 females and 352 males was taken, the following percentile norms were developed.

	% PERCENTILE	THEORETICAL	ECONOMIC-POLITICAL	AESTHETIC	SOCIAL
	100	110	110	110	110
	90	74	70	96	96
	80	60	54	88	88
	70	48	46	79	82
	60	40	39	69	77
Female	50	32	32	62	72
(N = 389)	40	25	25	54	67
	30	19	21	46	59
	20	14	17	36	52
	10	8	11	22	39
	1	0	1	3	0

	% PERCENTILE	THEORETICAL	ECONOMIC-POLITICAL	AESTHETIC	SOCIAL
	100	110	110	110	110
	90	85	89	83	90
	80	74	76	69	80
	70	66	67	60	73
	60	54	56	47	65
Male	50	45	49	39	56
(N = 352)	40	39	38	32	47
	30	31	30	26	39
	20	21	21	20	33
	10	11	12	12	25
	1	0	0	0	4

If you scored high on any dimension, the meaning is indicated below.*

Theoretical. A high score indicates that you prefer and consider most worthwhile those activities that involve a problem-solving attitude and are related to investigation, research, and scientific curiosity.

Economical-Political. A high score indicates that you prefer and consider most worthwhile those activities that involve the accumulation of money and the securing of executive power.

Aesthetic. A high score indicates that you prefer and consider most worthwhile those activities that involve art, music, dance, and literature.

Social. A high score indicates that you prefer and consider most worthwhile those activities that involve service and help to people; you exhibit a definite desire to respond and be with people socially.

Exercise II–B. Attitude Measure of Women as Managers

Items 1, 3, 6, 7, 15, 16, 17, 18, 20, and 21 should be reversed so that a high scale score is associated with a favorable attitude toward women

There is a possible score of 147 points on this twenty-one-item scale. The higher your score, the more favorable your attitude toward women as managers. A study of 180 male and 100 female full-time employees in an international distributing company found females to average 119 on this test. Males averaged 102.

Business students, many of whom aspire to managerial positions, should score above these averages. Your score should provide you with insights into your attitude toward women as managers.

Exercise II–C. Needs Test

Growth needs are items 2, 5, 8, 11.

Relatedness needs are items 1, 4, 7, 10.

Existence needs are items 3, 6, 9, 12.

Add the scores for each need set (for example, the summation of your scores on items 2, 5, 8, and 11 represent your growth need total). If you considered all four items within a need category to be very important, you would obtain the maximum total of 20 points.

College students typically rate growth needs highest. However, you may currently have little income and consider existence needs as most important. For instance, one student of mine scored 20, 10, and 15 for growth, relatedness, and existence needs, respectively. This should be interpreted to mean that her

*The scoring instruction information was taken from John R. Robinson and Phillip R. Shaver, *Measures of Social Psychological Attitudes*, rev. ed. (Ann Arbor, Mich.: Institute for Social Research, 1973), pp. 510–11.

relatedness needs are already substantially satisfied. Her growth needs, on the other hand, are substantially unsatisfied.

Note that a low score may imply that a need is unimportant to you or that it is substantially satisfied. The implication, however, is that *everyone* has these needs. So a low score is usually taken to mean that this need is substantially satisfied.

Exercise III—A. Status Ranking Task

The "correct" ranking is:*

1. U.S. Supreme Court Justice
2. Physician
3. Scientist
4. State governor
5. College professor
6. Lawyer
7. Dentist
8. Psychologist
9. Banker
10. Sociologist
11. Public school teacher
12. Author of novels
13. Undertaker
14. Newspaper columnist
15. Policeman

Score your individual worksheets by adding up the differences between your ranks and the key, regardless of sign. That is, make all differences positive and add them up. Low scores, of course, are better than high ones. Do the same with the group ranking.

Compute the average score of the individual members and compare it with the group score. Was the group score lower? Relate this exercise (both process and outcome) to the topics of group decision making, status, conflict, and leadership.

*Note that this ranking is time-bound. It represents occupational status at least twenty years ago. In the interim years, certain occupations may have increased in ranking (i.e., dentist, author of novels, newspaper columnist), while others have declined (i.e., lawyer, public school teacher).

Exercise III—B. Leadership Questionnaire

In order to find your leadership style:

1. Circle the item numbers for items 8, 12, 17, 18, 19, 30, 34, and 35.
2. Write a "1" in front of the *circled items* to which you responded S (seldom) or N (never).
3. Write a "1" in front of *items not circled* to which you responded A (always) or F (frequently).
4. Circle the "1's" which you have written in front of the following items: 3, 5, 8, 10, 15, 18, 19, 22, 24, 26, 28, 30, 32, 34, and 35.
5. Count the circled "1's." This is your score for concern for people. Record the score in the blank following the letter "P" at the end of the questionnaire.

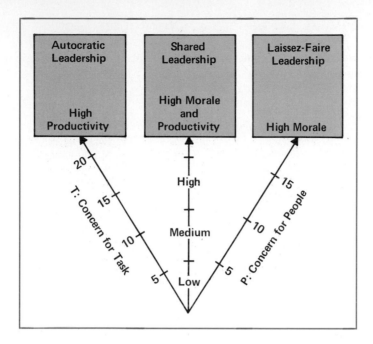

6. Count the uncircled "1's." This is your score for concern for task. Record this number in the blank following the letter "T."

7. Now, refer to the diagram below. Find your score on the *concern for task* dimension (t) on the left-hand arrow. Next, move to the right-hand arrow and find your score on the *concern for people* dimension (p). Draw a straight line that intersects the P and T score. The point at which that line crosses the *shared leadership* arrow indicates your score on that dimension.

Exercise III—C. Power-Orientation Test

This test is designed to compute your Machiavellianism (Mach) score. To obtain your score, add the number you have checked on questions 1, 3, 4, 5, 9, and 10. For the other four questions, reverse the numbers you have checked: 5 becomes 1, 4 is 2, 2 is 4, 1 is 5. Total your ten numbers to find your score. The National Opinion Research Center, which used this short form of the scale in a random sample of American adults, found that the national average was 25.

The results of research using the Mach test have found that: (a) men are generally more Machiavellian than women; (b) older adults tend to have lower Mach scores than younger adults; (c) there is no significant difference between high Machs and low Machs on measures of intelligence or ability; (d) Machiavellianism is not significantly related to demographic characteristics such as educational level or marital status; and (e) high Machs tend to be in professions that emphasize the control and manipulation of individuals—for example, managers, lawyers, psychiatrists, and behavioral scientists.

Exercise IV—A. Bureaucratic Orientation Test

Give yourself one point for each statement for which you responded in the bureaucratic direction:

1.	Mostly agree	11.	Mostly agree
2.	Mostly agree	12.	Mostly disagree
3.	Mostily disagree	13.	Mostly disagree
4.	Mostly agree	14.	Mostly agree
5.	Mostly disagree	15.	Mostly disagree
6.	Mostly disagree	16.	Mostly agree
7.	Mostly agree	17.	Mostly disagree
8.	Mostly agree	18.	Mostly agree
9.	Mostly disagree	19.	Mostly agree
10.	Mostly agree	20.	Mostly disagree

A very high score (15 and over) would suggest that you would enjoy working in a bureaucracy. A very low score (5 or lower) would suggest that you would be frustrated by working in a bureaucracy, especially a large one.

Exercise IV—B. Rate Your Job's Motivating Potential

Place the scores for questions "a" through "e" into the following formula:

$$MPS = \frac{a + b + c}{3} \times d \times e$$

A high or low score on "d" or "e" will carry a heavy weight. A total MPS of 200 or higher suggests high motivating potential. Scores below 50 suggest very low potential.

Exercise IV—C. Rate Your Classroom Culture

Add up your score on the eight items. Your score will lie somewhere between 8 and 40.

A high score (30 or above) describes an open, warm, human, trusting, and supportive culture. A low score (20 or below) describes a closed, cold, task-oriented, autocratic, and tense culture.

Compare your score against the ones tabulated by your classmates. How close do they align? Discuss perceived discrepancies.

Glossary

Absenteeism. Failure to report to work.

Absolute evaluation standards. Employees are compared against an absolute standard rather than against each other.

Accommodation. The willingness of one party in a conflict to place his opponent's interests above his own.

Achievement need. The drive to do things better.

Activities. The physical movements that individuals make that can be observed by others.

Adhocratic structure. A structure that is flexible, adaptive, and responsive; organized around unique problems to be solved by groups of relative strangers with diverse professional skills.

Affiliation need. The desire for friendly and close interpersonal relationships.

Anxiety. Tension.

Assertiveness. A power tactic; setting deadlines, giving orders, and demanding compliance with requests.

Assumed similarity. Judging other people to be like you.

Attitudes. Evaluative statements or judgments concerning objects, people, or events.

Attribution theory. When individuals observe behavior, they attempt to determine whether it is internally or externally caused.

Authoritarianism. The belief that there should be status and power differences among people in organizations.

Authority. The right, inherent in one's formal position, to act or command others to act.

Autocratic leader. One who dictates decisions down to subordinates.

Autonomous work team. A group that is free to determine how the goal assigned to it is to be accomplished and how tasks are to be allocated.

Autonomy. The degree to which a job provides substantial freedom and discretion to the individual in scheduling the work and in determining the procedures to be used in carrying it out.

Avoidance. Withdrawing from or suppressing conflict.

Behavioral theories of leadership. Theories proposing that specific behaviors differentiate leaders from nonleaders.

Behavioral view of conflict. The belief that conflict is a natural and inevitable outcome in any group.

Blocking. A power tactic: engaging in a work slowdown or threatening to discontinue working.

Bureaucratic structure. A structure characterized by high complexity, high formalization, impersonality, career tracks, employment decisions based on merit, and separation of members' organizational and personal lives.

Causality. The implication that the independent variable causes the dependent variable.

Caused behavior. Behavior that is directed toward some end; not random.

Centralization. The degree to which decision making is concentrated at a single point in the organization.

Channel. The medium through which a communication message travels.

Classical conditioning. A type of conditioning where an individual responds to some stimulus that would not invariably produce such a response.

Coalitions. Two or more individuals who combine their power to push for or support their demands.

Coercive power. Power that is based on fear.

Cognitive dissonance. Any incompatibility between two or more attitudes, or between behavior and attitudes.

Cognitive evaluation theory. Extrinsic rewards allocated for behavior that had been previously intrinsically rewarded tends to decrease the overall level of motivation.

Cohesiveness. Degree to which group members are attracted to each other and share common goals.

Collaboration. A situation where the parties to a conflict each desire to satisfy fully the concern of all parties.

Command group. A manager and his or her immediate subordinates.

Communication. The transference and understanding of meaning.

Communication networks. Channels by which information flows.

Communication process. The steps between a source and a receiver that result in the transference of meaning.

Compensation. A defensive behavior characterized by the expenditure of an unusual amount of energy on one activity to make up for a deficiency in another.

Competition. A situation where one party seeks to achieve his goals or further his interests, regardless of the impact of this behavior on others.

Complexity. The degree of vertical, horizontal, and spatial differentiation in an organization.

Conditioning. Developing a behavior pattern through association.

Conflict. A process in which an effort is purposely made by A to offset the efforts of B by some form of blocking that will result in frustrating B in attaining his goals or furthering his interests.

Conformity. Adjusting one's behavior to align with the norms of the group.

Consideration. The extent to which a person is likely to have job relationships that are characterized by mutual trust, respect for subordinate's ideas, and regard for their feelings.

Contingency variables. Those variables that moderate the relationship between the independent and dependent variables and improve the correlation.

Continuous reinforcers. Reinforce a desired behavior each and every time it is demonstrated.

Decentralization. Low centralization; decision making is concentrated low in the organization.

Decoding. Retranslating a sender's communication message.

Delphi Technique. A group decision method in which individual members, acting separately, pool their judgment in a systematic and independent fashion.

Democratic leader. One who shares decision making with subordinates.

Dependence. A's relationship to B when B possesses something that A requires but that B alone controls.

Dependent variable. The response that is measured; the outcome.

Dysfunctional conflict. Conflict that hinders group performance.

Ectomorph. Thin body build; inclined to be fine-boned and fragile.

Effectiveness. Achievement of goal.

Efficiency. The ratio of effective output to the input required to achieve it.

Elasticity of power. The relative responsiveness of power to change in available alternatives.

Emergent behavior. Behavior that is in addition to what is required.

Employee-oriented leader. One who emphasizes interpersonal relations.

Encoding. Converting a communication message to symbolic form.

Encounter stage. The stage in which a new employee sees what the organization is really like and confronts the likelihood that expectations and reality may diverge.

Endomorph. Fleshy body build; inclined toward fatness.

Environment. Anything outside the organization itself.

Equity theory. Individuals compare their job inputs and outcomes with those of others.

Exchange of benefits. A power tactic; the trading of favors.

Expectancy theory. The strength of a tendency to act in a certain way depends on the strength of an expectation that the act will be followed by a given outcome and on the attractiveness of that outcome to the individual.

Expert power. Influence based on special skills or knowledge.

Expressives. People who desire jobs for the intrinsic satisfaction that the work itself provides.

Extrinsic motivators. Rewards received from the environment surrounding the context of work.

Extroversion. Outgoing and expressive personality.

Fantasy. A defensive behavior characterized by daydreaming.

Feedback. The degree to which carrying out the work activities required by a job results in the individual obtaining direct and clear information about the effectiveness of his performance.

Feedback loop. The final link in the communicative process; puts message back into the system as a check against misunderstandings.

Felt conflict. Emotional involvement in a conflict creating anxiety, tenseness, frustration, or hostility.

Fixed-interval schedule. Rewards are spaced at uniform time intervals.

Fixed-ratio schedule. After a fixed or constant number of responses are given, a reward is initiated.

Flex-time. Employees work during a common core time period each day but have discretion in forming their total workday from a flexible set of hours outside the core.

Formal group. A designated work group defined by the organization's structure.

Formalization. The degree to which jobs within the organization are standardized.

Friendship group. Those brought together because they share one or more common characteristics.

Functional conflict. Conflict that supports the goals of the group and improves its performance.

Functional structure. A structure characterized by grouping similar and related occupational specialties together.

Goal-setting theory. Specific and difficult goals lead to higher performance.

Grapevine. The informal communication channel.

Group. Two or more individuals, interacting and interdependent, who come together to achieve particular objectives.

Groupthink. Phenomenon in which the norm for consensus overrides the realistic appraisal of alternative courses of action.

Growth need strength. A measure of an employee's desire for self-esteem and self-actualization.

Halo effect. Drawing a general impression about an individual based on a single characteristic.

Higher-order needs. Needs that are satisfied internally; needs for love, esteem, and self-actualization.

Horizontal differentiation. The degree of differentiation between units based on the orientation of members, the nature of the tasks they perform, and their education and training.

Identification. A defensive behavior characterized by modeling oneself after another.

Independent variable. The presumed cause of the dependent variable.

Informal group. A group that is neither structured nor organizationally determined; appears in response to the need for social contact.

Informational cues. Words, actions, silence, or inaction that individuals need to derive meaning from communication.

Ingratiation. A power tactic; nonobtrusive behaviors like acting humble or making others feel important.

Initiating structure. The extent to which a leader is likely to define and structure his or her role and those of subordinates in the search for goal attainment.

Instrumentals. People who see their work as a means to another end.

Integrated work team. A group that decides the specific allocation of the tasks assigned to it.

Interaction analysis. A technique of group analysis based on observed interaction patterns between individuals.

Interactionist view of conflict. The belief that conflict is not only a positive force in a group but that it is absolutely necessary for a group to perform effectively.

Interactions. The verbal and nonverbal communication and contacts that actually take place between people.

Interest group. Those working together to attain a specific objective with which each is concerned.

Intergroup development. OD efforts to improve interactions between groups.

Intermittent reinforcers. Reinforcers given often enough to make the behavior worth repeating but not every time it is demonstrated.

Intrinsic motivators. The pleasure or value associated with the content of a work task.

Introversion. Withdrawn and quiet personality.

Intuition. A feeling not necessarily supported by research.

Jargon. Specialized vocabulary.

Job characteristics model. Identifies five job characteristics and their relationship to personal and work outcomes.

Job design. The way that tasks are combined to form complete jobs.

Job enlargement. The horizontal expansion of jobs.

Job enrichment. The vertical expansion of jobs.

Job involvement. The degree to which a person identifies with his job, actively participates in it, and considers his performance important to his sense of self-worth.

Job redesign. The changing of job tasks.

Job rotation. The periodic shifting of a worker from one task to another.

Job satisfaction. An attitude toward work; how one feels toward his or her job.

Kinesics. The study of body motions.

Knowledge power. The ability to control unique and valuable information.

LPC. Least Preferred Co-Worker questionnaire that measures task- or relationship-oriented leadership style.

Leader-participation model. Provides a sequential set of rules to be followed in determining the form and amount of participation in decision making.

Leadership. The ability to influence a group toward the achievement of goals.

Learning. Any relatively permanent change in behavior that occurs as a result of experience.

Leniency error. The tendency to evaluate a set of employees too high (positive) or too low (negative).

Line authority. The right to command.

Locus of control. The degree to which people believe they are masters of their own fate.

Low differentiation. The use of a limited range of the rating scale when evaluating performance.

Lower-order needs. Needs that are satisfied externally; physiological and safety needs.

Machiavellianism. Degree to which an individual is pragmatic, maintains emotional distance, and believes that means can justify ends.

Management. A field of study devoted to determining how best to attain goals in organizations.

Managerial grid. A nine-by-nine matrix outlining eighty-one different leadership styles.

MAPS. Multivariate analysis, participation, and structure; a structural OD technique.

Matrix. A structure that creates dual lines of authority, combines the functional and product structures.

Maturation theory. Proposes that all healthy people seek situations that offer autonomy, wide interests, treatment as an equal, and the opportunity to exhibit their ability to deal with complexity.

Mechanistic structure. A structure characterized by high complexity, high formalization, and centralization.

Merit. A reward criterion; deserving and/or excellent.

Mesomorph. Athletic body build; inclined to be muscular.

Message. What is communicated.

Metamorphosis stage. The stage in which a new employee adjusts to his work group's values and norms.

Model. An abstraction of reality; a simplified representation of some real-world phenomena.

Moderating variable. Abates the effect of the independent variable on the dependent variable; a contingency variable.

Motivating potential score. A predictive index suggesting the motivation potential in a job.

Motivation. The willingness to do something, conditioned by this action's ability to satisfy some need for the individual.

nAch. Need to achieve or continually strive to do things better.

Need. Some internal state that makes certain outcomes appear attractive.

Negative reinforcers. Stimuli whose withdrawal strengthens and increases the probability that a behavior will be repeated.

Nominal Group Technique. A group decision method in which individual members meet face-to-face to pool their judgments in a systematic but independent fashion.

Norms. Acceptable standards of behavior within a group that are shared by the group's members.

Objectives. Specific goals against which actual performance is compared.

OB Mod. Use of reinforcement techniques to shape and change organizational behavior.

Operant conditioning. A type of conditioning in which desired voluntary behavior leads to a reward or prevents a punishment.

Opportunity power. Influence obtained as a result of being in the right place at the right time.

Organic structure. A structure characterized by low complexity, low formalization, and decentralization.

Organization. The planned coordination of the activities of two or more people in order to achieve some common and explicit goal through division of labor and a hierarchy of authority.

Organizational behavior. A field of study that investigates the impact that individuals, groups, and structure have on behavior within organizations for the purpose of applying such knowledge toward improving an organization's effectiveness.

Organizational commitment. An individual's orientation toward the organization in terms of loyalty, identification, and involvement.

Organizational culture. An organization's personality; a relatively uniform perception held of the organization.

Organizational development. Change-oriented activities.

Organizational politics. Any behavior by an organizational member that is self-serving.

Organization size. The number of people employed in an organization.

Path-goal model of leadership. Emphasizes the influence of the leader on subordinate goals and the paths to these goals.

Perceived conflict. Awareness by one or more parties of the existence of conditions that create opportunities for conflict to arise.

Perception. A process by which individuals organize and interpret their sensory impressions in order to give meaning to their environment.

Performance evaluation. The process by which an organization obtains data about an employee's effectiveness.

Personality. How a person affects others, how he understands and views himself, and his pattern of inner and outer measurable traits.

Personality traits. Enduring characteristics that describe an individual's behavior.

Personal power. Influence attributed to one's personal characteristics.

Persuasive power. The ability to allocate and manipulate symbolic rewards.

Position power. Influence inherent in one's formal position in the organization.

Positive reinforcement. A reward that strengthens a desired behavior.

Power. A capacity that A has to influence the behavior of B so that B does something he would not otherwise do.

Power-control view of structure. The belief that an organization's structure is the result of a power struggle by internal constituencies who are seeking to further their interests.

Power need. The desire to make others behave in a way that they would not otherwise have behaved in.

Prearrival stage. The period of learning that occurs before a new employee joins the organization.

Primary reinforcers. Reinforcers that are rewarding in and of themselves.

Problem solving. Bringing about change or resolving conflict through interpersonal discussions; seeks to identify differences.

Process consultation. Consultant gives a client insights into what is going on around him, within him, and between him and other people; identifies processes that need improvement.

Product structure. A structure characterized by grouping activities together that relate to a specific product.

Production-oriented leader. One who emphasizes technical or task aspects of the job.

Productivity. A performance measure including effectiveness and efficiency.

Projection. A defensive behavior characterized by attributing one's own problems or motives to someone else.

Psychological contract. An unwritten agreement that sets out what management expects from the employee and vice versa.

Punishment. Stimuli that weaken behavior and reduce the probability of repetition.

Quality circles. A voluntary work group of employees who meet regularly to discuss their quality problems, investigate causes, recommend solutions, and take corrective actions.

Rationality. A power tactic; presenting information in a logical manner.

Rationalization. A defensive behavior characterized by developing untrue but credible explanations to justify inconsistent behaviors or attitudes.

Reaction formation. A defensive behavior characterized by acting contrary to one's real feelings.

Referent power. Influence held by A based on B's admiration and desire to model himself after A.

Regression. A defensive behavior characterized by reverting back to an earlier and less mature level.

Reinforcement. Any stimulus that acts to strengthen a response.

Reinforcement theory. Behavior is a function of its consequences.

Relative evaluation standards. Employees are compared against each other.

Repression. A defensive behavior characterized by withholding threatening information from the conscious.

Required behavior. The activities, interactions, and sentiments defined by the group's formal leaders and assigned to the members as their specified roles.

Reward power. The ability to distribute anything of value.

Ringelmann effect. Increases in a group's size are inversely related to individual performance.

Risky-shift phenomenon. Group decisions may contain a greater degree of risk than many of the members would have been willing to take on their own.

Role. A set of expected behavior patterns attributed to someone occupying a given position in a social unit.

Role conflict. A situation in which an individual is confronted by divergent role expectations.

Role expectations. How others believe a person should act in a given situation.

Role identity. Certain attitudes and behavior consistent with a role.

Role perception. An individual's view of how he or she is supposed to act in a given situation.

Sanctions. A power tactic; withholding or threatening to withhold a reward.

Scientific management. A body of literature developed in the early 1900s concerned with incentives, selection, training, and the design of jobs to eliminate time and motion waste.

Secondary reinforcers. Conditioned needs that we have learned to value.

Selective perception. People interpret what they see based on their background and experiences.

Self-actualization. The drive to become what one is capable of becoming.

Sensitivity training. Training groups that seeks to change behavior through unstructured group interaction.

Sentiments. The values, attitudes, and beliefs held by a person.

Shaping behavior. Systematically reinforcing each successive step that moves an individual closer to the desired response.

Sharing. A situation where each party to a conflict must give up something, resulting in a compromised outcome.

Shorter workweek. Typically a four-day week, with employees working ten hours a day.

Similarity error. Giving special consideration when rating others to those qualities that the evaluator perceives in himself.

Simple structure. A structure characterized by low complexity, low formalization, and authority centralized in a single person.

Skill variety. The degree to which a job requires a variety of different activities.

Socialization. The process that adapts employees to the organization's culture.

Sociogram. A graphic representation of the attractiveness and interaction rankings and patterns derived from sociometry.

Sociometry. A technique of group analysis based on identifying whom members like and dislike.

Sociotechnical systems. A job design philosophy emphasizing both the technical and social aspects of work.

Spatial differentiation. The degree to which the location of an organization's offices, plants, and personnel are geographically dispersed.

Span of control. The number of subordinates who report directly to a manager.

Staff authority. The right to support and advise.

Status. A prestige grading, position, or rank within a group.

Status equity. The degree to which group members perceive that the status hierarchy is equitable.

Status hierarchy. A prioritizing of individuals by their relative rank.

Stereotyping. Judging someone on the basis of the perception of the group to which that person belongs.

Stress. A dynamic condition in which an individual is confronted with an opportunity, constraint, or demand related to what he or she desires and for which the outcome is perceived to be both uncertain and important.

Structure. The degree of complexity, formalization, and centralization in the organization.

Survey feedback. The use of questionnaires to identify discrepancies among member perceptions; discussion follows and remedies are suggested.

Systematic study. Looking at relationships, attempting to attribute causes and effects, and drawing conclusions based on scientific evidence.

Task group. Those working together to complete a job task.

Task identity. The degree to which the job requires completion of a whole and identifiable piece of work.

Task significance. The degree to which the job has a substantial impact on the lives or work of other people.

Team building. High interaction among group members to increase trust and openness.

Technology. How an organization transfers its inputs to outputs.

Theory X. The assumption that employees dislike work, are lazy, dislike responsibility, and must be coerced to perform.

Theory Y. The assumption that employees like work, are creative, seek responsibility, and can exercise self-direction.

Traditional view of conflict. The belief that all conflict must be avoided.

Trait theories of leadership. Personal characteristics differentiate leaders from non-leaders.

Transactional analysis. Defines and analyzes communication interactions between people; a theory of personality.

Turnover. Voluntary and involuntary permanent withdrawal from the organization.

Type A behavior. Aggressive involvement in a chronic, incessant struggle to achieve more and more in less and less time, and, if necessary, against the opposing efforts of other things or other persons.

Type B behavior. Rarely harried by the desire to obtain a wildly increasing number of things or to participate in an endlessly growing series of events in an ever-decreasing amount of time.

Uncertainty. Doubt about future outcomes due to unplanned change.

Upward appeal. A power tactic; making a formal appeal to a higher level.

Value systems. A prioritizing of individual values according to their relative importance.

Values. Basic convictions that a specific mode of conduct or end-state of existence is personally or socially preferable to an opposite or converse mode of conduct or end-state of existence.

Variable-interval schedule. Rewards are distributed in time so that reinforcements are unpredictable.

Variable-ratio schedule. The reward varies relative to the behavior of the individual.

Vertical differentiation. The number of hierarchial levels in the organization.

Work modules. The creation of two-hour time task units, four of which equal an eight-hour day; can be allocated in ways to give workers diverse tasks.

Name Index

A

Aaagaard, A.K., 415
Adams, J.S., 148
Adorno, T., 84
Aiken, M., 375
Ajzen, I., 65
Albrecht, K., 91
Alderfer, C.P., 137, 253, 479
Allen, R.W., 509, 510, 515, 517, 520, 521
Allport, G.W., 52, 72, 76, 100
Andrews, F., 345
Angle, H.L., 509
Anthony, S.B., 287
Ardrey, R., 18
Arensberg, C.M., 15, 200
Argyris, C., 80, 277
Arnold, H.J., 146
Asch, S.E., 120, 214–15
Atkinson, J.W., 110

B

Bachman, J.G., 327
Bachrach, S.B., 314, 316, 317
Badin, I.J., 136
Baker, H., 245
Bales, R.F., 234
Bannister, B.D., 297
Barnes, L.B., 291

Barnlund, D.C., 245
Barrett, D., 274
Barrow, J.C., 292
Bartley, S., 124
Baruch, B., 4
Bass, B.M., 126
Bavelas, A., 274
Beaumont, E.F., 435
Beehr, T.A., 93
Behling, O., 96
Bell, C.H., Jr., 487
Bem, D.J., 246
Benne, K.D., 480
Bennett, A.C., 444, 446
Bennis, W.G., 89, 277, 394, 396, 480
Berg, D., 487
Berger, C.J., 386
Berger, J., 224
Berkowitz, L., 148, 251
Berlew, D.E., 89
Berlo, D.K., 263, 264
Berman, H.J., 61
Bernardin, J.J., 99
Bickman, L., 221
Binzen, P., 345
Birdwhistell, R.L., 266
Bischof, L.J., 100
Black, J.S., 60
Blackburn, R.S., 407
Blake, R.R., 290, 291, 303, 482
Blau, P.M., 373, 435
Bonnano, J., 287
Bouchard, T., 103–3
Bower, G.H., 180

Bowerman, B., 250
Bowers, D.G., 327, 479, 486
Boxx, W.R., 415
Brayfield, A.H., 62, 63, 68
Brenner, S.N., 207
Bretton, G.E., 279
Bridwell, L.G., 136
Brief, A.P., 95
Broadwater, G., 150
Brown, C.A., 63
Brown, L.D., 476, 479, 482
Bruner, J.S., 120
Bryant, P., 286
Buchanan, B., II, 57, 464
Buchanan, P.C., 486
Buchwald, A., 234
Buckley, W.F., 271
Bulian, P.V., 64
Bunker, A., 205
Bunker, D.R., 478
Burke, R.J., 433
Burke, W.W., 479
Burnham, D.H., 139, 330
Burns, T., 378
Butterfield, D.A., 465
Byrne, D., 100

C

Calder, B.J., 145, 146
Caldwell, D.F., 269, 270
Calvasina, E.J., 415
Campbell, D.J., 145
Campbell, J.P., 246, 451, 477, 478
Campbell, K.M., 145
Cantril, H., 108
Capone, A., 314
Capwell, D.F., 62
Carrell, M.R., 149
Carson, J., 217, 218
Cartwright, D., 253, 290, 314
Cascio, W.F., 126
Cass, E.L., 212, 226, 228, 412
Cattell, R.B., 76, 77
Chadwick-Jones, J.K., 63
Chávez, C., 287
Chemers, M.M., 308

Cherrington, D.J., 55
Child, J., 373, 377
Chin, R., 480
Christie, R., 84, 328, 364
Chung, K.H., 158
Clark, R.D., III, 246
Coates, C.H., 140
Coch, L., 473
Cohen, A.R., 419
Colby, F.M., 262
Colby, J., 443
Cole, D., 452
Cole, E., 452
Condie, S.J., 55
Connolly, T., 158
Connor, P.E., 486
Coons, A.E., 289
Cooper, C.L., 92, 93, 95
Cooper, M.R., 65
Costello, T.W., 125, 173
Costigain, R., 415
Craft, R.E., Jr., 63
Crockett, W.H., 62, 63, 68
Crow, W.J., 128
Crozier, M., 323
Culbert, S.A., 504, 509
Cummings, L.L., 144, 386, 419, 509
Cyert, R.M., 323

D

Dalton, D.R., 386
Dalton, G.W., 443
Darrow, C.N., 80
Daughen, J.R., 345
Davis, C., 443
Davis, K., 274, 275
Davis, L.E., 419
Dearborn, D.C., 117
DeCharms, R., 144
Deci, E.L., 144, 145
Delbecq, A.L., 247, 375
DeLorean, J., 265, 452–53
DeMontes, A.I., 179
Desoto, C.B., 100
Deutsch, M., 348
DeVries, D.L., 180

Dillinger, J., 317
Distefano, M.K., Jr., 63
Dittrich, J.E., 149
Dominguez, B., 179
Drabek, T.E., 510
Drexler, J.A., Jr., 451, 468
DuBrin, A.J., 499, 505, 513
Duncan, R.B., 376
Dunham, R.B., 400, 406, 407
Dunnette, M., 63, 84, 85, 93, 343, 451, 477, 478

E

England, J.L., 55
Epstein, S., 100
Erikson, E.H., 80
Etzioni, A., 316
Evan, W., 455
Evans, M.G., 417
Eysenck, H.J., 77

F

Farber, S.L., 104
Fast, J., 266
Faulkner, W., 118
Feeney, E.J., 177
Fein, M., 419
Feldman, D.C., 456, 462, 464
Ferriss, R., 479
Festinger, L., 58–59
Fiedler, F.E., 286, 294–97, 299, 301, 302, 304, 308
Fielding, G.J., 386
Filley, A.C., 293, 348, 350, 352, 354
Fine, G.A., 275
Fink, C.F., 240, 249, 336
Fishbein, M., 65
Flippo, E.B., 14
Foley, P.M., 65
Fonzerelli, A., 315
Ford, D.L., Jr., 391
Ford, G.R., 331

Ford, H., 454
Forehand, G.A., 451
Fournet, G.P., 63
Fox, R., 18
Francis, A., 443
Franke, R.H., 224
Franklin, J.L., 454
French, J.R.P., Jr., 314, 316, 473
French, W.L., 472, 474, 487
Freud, S., 80
Friedlander, F., 476, 479, 482
Friedman, A., 149
Friedman, M., 95, 97
Funkhouser, G.R., 450

G

Gadon, H., 419
Galenson, W., 163
Gandhi, M., 287
Gandz, J., 515
Geis, F., 328, 364
Geis, R.L., 84
Gergin, T.G., 329
Gerwin, D., 375
Ghiselli, E.E., 137, 306
Gillespie, D.F., 373
Gilmer, B.V.H., 451
Glass, D.C., 91
Glube, R., 301, 304
Golembiewski, R.T., 416
Goodale, J.C., 415
Goodman, P.S., 148, 149
Gordon, F.E., 119
Gough, H., 84
Gould, R., 80
Granovetter, M., 455
Graves, C.W., 53
Graves, J., 241
Gray, J.L., 183
Greene, C.N., 63, 82
Greenhaus, J.H., 136
Greiner, L.E., 291
Guetzkow, H., 214, 278
Gullahorn, J.T., 249
Gustafson, D.H., 247

H

Haas, J.E., 373, 510
Hackman, J.R., 93, 253, 269, 400,
    401, 404, 405, 406, 407, 410,
    420, 422, 456, 508
Hage, J., 375
Haire, M., 108, 137
Hall, D.T., 57, 136
Hall, J., 278, 345
Hall, R.H., 310
Hammer, T.H., 443
Hamner, E.P., 483
Hamner, W.C., 54, 61, 83, 293–94,
    483
Hampton, D.R., 258
Handelsman, M., 200
Haney, W.V., 278
Harkins, S., 241
Harlan, A., 212
Harriman, M.C., 426
Harrison, F., 348
Hartley, E.L., 473
Harvey, J.B., 245
Hayakawa, S.I., 265
Heberlein, T.A., 60
Hegel, G., 11
Hellriegel, D., 463
Hellweg, S.A., 276
Hemingway, E., 118
Henderson, A.M., 381
Heneman, H.G., III, 152
Hermann, J.A., 179
Herzberg, F., 62, 141–44, 160
Hilgard, E.R., 180
Hill, J.W., 156, 158
Hill, R.E., 345
Hill, V.S., 65
Hitler, A., 287
Hoffman, R.L., 242, 345
Hogan, R., 100
Hohenfeld, J.A., 149
Holden, C., 102
Holder, J.J., Jr., 255
Holland, J.L., 86, 87
Holt, R.P., 74
Hom, P.W., 64
Homans, G.C., 235–39, 252, 253

Hoover, J.E., 454
Hope, B., 217
Hopkins, B.L., 179
Hornstein, H.A., 479
Hosek, J., 57
Hougland, J.G., Jr., 34
House, R.J., 144, 156, 225, 293, 297,
    304, 305
House, W.C., 254
Hulin, C.L., 64
Hunt, J.G., 156, 158, 224, 306
Hunt, R.G., 101
Hunter, J.E., 137

I

Ingham, A.G., 241
Inkeles, A., 61, 224
Insko, C., 249
Ivancevich, J.M., 327, 328, 415
Ivy, T.T., 65

J

Jablonsky, S.F., 180
Jago, A.G., 301
James, L.R., 386, 464
James, M., 484
Janis, I.L., 74, 85, 243–45, 344
Janson, R., 410
Jefferson, T., 454
Jermier, J.M., 302
Jewell, L.N., 254
Johnson, B.M., 278
Johnson, E., 320–21
Johnson, F.R., 453
Johnson, L.B., 244, 319
Johnson, M.P., 61
Johnson, R.D., 178
Jones, A.R., 386, 464
Jones, J.E., 361, 363
Jongeward, D., 484
Jung, C., 77

K

Kagan, J., 74
Kahle, L.R., 61
Kahn, R.L., 95, 223, 225, 290, 348, 392, 408
Kaplan, L.B., 65
Karmel, B., 14, 303, 419
Katerberg, R., Jr., 64
Katz, D., 66, 95, 225, 290, 348, 392
Kaul, J.D., 224
Kearns, D., 319
Kearny, W.J., 443
Keller, R.T., 93
Kelley, H.H., 114, 124
Kelly, J., 73, 90, 205, 210
Kelman, H.C., 65
Kennedy, J.F., 244–45
Kerlinger, F., 23
Kerr, J., 212
Kerr, S., 212, 289, 293, 302, 513
Kess, T., 145
Key, W.B., 124
Keyes, R., 204, 216
Kilmann, R.H., 349, 476
Kimberly, J., 393
King, M.L., Jr., 287, 291
Kipnis, D., 116, 139, 314, 317, 323, 324, 513
Klien, E.B., 80
Koch, J.L., 34
Kochman, T., 272
Koenig, R., Jr., 375
Kogan, N., 85, 246
Korda, M., 329
Korman, A.K., 136
Kotter, J.P. 206, 329
Kraft, W.P., 410
Kreitner, R., 173, 175, 483
Kursh, C.O., 282

L

LaFollette, W.R., 464
Lair, J., 72
Land, E., 454

Larson, L.L., 306
Latané, B., 241
Latham, G.P., 150
Lawler, E.E., III, 5, 14, 68, 121, 136, 157, 158, 386, 419, 438, 443, 451, 478
Lawler, E.J., 314, 316, 317
Lawless, D.J., 223
Lawrence, P.R., 376, 482
Lazarus, R.S., 98
Leavitt, H.J., 50, 226, 332
Leblebici, H., 455
Lee, D., 34
Lenk, H., 345
Levinger, G., 241
Levinson, D.J., 80
Levinson, H., 488, 491, 492
Levinson, M.H., 80
Lewin, K., 16, 291, 473, 514
Lewis, J., 102
Libo, L., 249
Lichtman, C.M., 101
Lieberman, M.A., 477
Lieberman, S., 204
Likert, R., 66, 277
Lindzey, E., 120
Lindzey, G., 52
Lipman-Blumen, J., 332
Lippert, F.G., 14
Lippitt, R., 291
Lipset, S.M., 163
Lirtzman, S.I., 225
Litterer, J.A., 373
Litwin, G.H., 454
Locke, E.A., 63, 64, 150, 152, 155, 159, 181, 183, 184, 185
Lord, R.G., 149
Lorenz, C., 18
Lorsch, J.W., 34, 376, 463, 482
Louis, M.R., 464
Luce, R.D., 336
Luthans, F., 145, 173, 175, 176, 177, 483

M

McCaskey, M.B., 278
McCauley, C., 124

McClelland, D.C., 110, 137–39, 140, 157, 330
McDonough, J.J., 504, 509
McGehee, W., 167
McGrath, J.E., 93
McGrath, P.S., 485
McGregor, D., 160, 277, 306, 475
McGuire, J.W., 14, 287, 308
Machiavelli, N., 84, 329
McKee, B., 80
McKelvey, B., 476
McNamara, R., 245
McPherson, J.W., 126
Madison, D.L., 510, 515
Maher, J.R., 410
Mahl, G.F., 74
Maier, N.R.F., 160, 242, 345
Mann, L., 85
Mannheim, B.F., 373
Mansfield, R., 373
March, J.G., 265, 323
Marcus, P.M., 327
Margerison, C., 301, 304
Margulies, N., 481, 514
Marshall, J., 92, 93
Martindale, D., 95
Martinko, M., 145, 485
Marx, K., 11
Maslow, A., 134–36, 137, 139, 140, 156, 160
Massengil, D., 419
Maurer, J.G., 510
Mausner, B., 62, 141
Mawhinney, T.C., 180
Mayes, B.T., 509, 510, 515, 517, 520, 521
Mayo, E., 212
Mealiea, L.W., 34
Michela, J.L., 124
Miewald, R.D., 396
Miles, M.B., 477
Miles, M.G., 480
Miles, R.E., 15
Miles, R.H., 393
Mileti, D.S., 373
Milken, M., 320
Miner, J.B., 83, 136, 139, 146, 157, 180, 296, 306
Mintzberg, H., 377, 379, 392
Mirvis, P., 487

Mitchell, T.R., 82, 269, 270, 297, 299, 304
Moberg, D.J., 34, 505, 509
Moede, W., 240
Molander, E.A., 207
Molloy, J.T., 221–22
Mommsen, W., 397
Money, M.H., 297
Montes, F., 179
Moore, L.F., 34
Moreno, J.L., 232, 234
Morgan, B.S., 65
Morris, D., 18
Morrison, P., 485
Morse, J.J., 463
Mouton, J.S., 290, 291, 303, 482
Mowday, R.T., 64, 99, 510
Moyer, W.W., 83
Moyers, B., 244
Muchinsky, P.M., 156, 276
Mullin, B.J., 92
Munson, J.M., 65
Murphy, C.J., 289
Murray, V.V., 349, 515
Myers, M.S., 53
Myers, S.S., 53

N

Nader, R., 291
Neilsen, E.H., 482
Nemiroff, P.M., 391
Newcome, T.M., 473
Newman, J.E., 93
Nichols, J., 368
Nicholson, N., 63
Nightingale, F., 133
Nixon, R.M., 244, 245, 331
Nollen, S.D., 416
Nongaim, K.E., 136
Nord, W.R., 98, 114, 178, 415
Norton, D.D., 419

O

Odbert, H.S., 76
Oldham, G.R., 35, 93, 400, 404, 405, 410

Olsen, L.O., 444, 446
O'Reilly, C.A., III, 86, 269, 270, 279
Organ, D.W., 54, 82, 83, 293–94
Organt, G.J., 438
Ottemann, R., 483

P

Packard, V.O., 65
Parsons, T., 381
Patterson, B., 203–4, 207
Pavlov, I., 169–70
Payne, R., 95
Peckham, V., 241
Pellegrin, R.J., 140
Pelz, D.C., 345
Perrow, C., 323, 374, 504
Peter, L.J., 232
Petterson, R.O., 62
Pettigrew, A.M., 516
Pfeffer, J., 157, 310, 311, 329, 374,
    376, 377, 455
Pfeiffer, J.W., 361, 363
Pfiffner, J.M., 505
Phillips, S.L., 276
Pierce, J.L., 400, 406, 407
Pinder, C.C., 34
Pizam, A., 431
Pondy, L.R., 342
Porter, H., 245
Porter, L.W., 62, 63, 64, 68, 75, 98,
    99, 124, 136, 137, 140, 151,
    155, 159, 250, 275, 279, 299,
    386, 438, 509, 510, 515
Posner, B.Z., 65
Powell, G.N., 465
Pritchard, R.D., 145
Proehl, C.W., Jr., 416
Pryer, M.W., 63
Pugh, D.S., 377
Purdy, K., 410

R

Rabinowitz, S., 57
Raiffa, H., 336

Rauschenberger, J., 137
Raven, B., 314, 316
Reagan, R., 434
Reddin, W.J., 291, 307
Redding, W.C., 268
Reinharth, L., 152
Reitz, H.J., 254
Renwick, P.A., 510, 515
Reynolds, B., 217
Rhode, J.G., 5, 121, 157
Rhodes, S.R., 27
Rice, R.W., 297
Riker, W.H., 326
Ringelmann, 240–41, 252
Ritti, R.R., 450
Rizzo, J.R., 225
Robbins, S.P., 20, 207, 220, 265, 337,
    352, 392, 400, 520
Roberts, K.H., 279
Robinson, J.R., 533
Roethlisberger, F.J., 280
Rogers, C.R., 38, 280
Rogers, M., 438
Rokeach, M., 50, 55
Ronan, W.W., 438
Rosenholtz, S.J., 224
Rosenman, R.H., 95, 97
Rosenzweig, M.R., 75, 124, 136, 155,
    250, 299
Rosnow, R.L., 275
Rossman, M., 210
Rotter, J.B., 82
Rousseau, D.M., 406
Rowan, R., 275
Roy, D.F., 225
Ruch, F.L., 28, 72
Runyon, K.E., 82
Rush, H.M.F., 485
Rushing, W.A., 373
Rusk, D., 245
Russell, B., 12, 314

S

Safire, W., 272
Salaman, G., 454
Salancik, G.R., 145, 146, 149, 157,
    311, 376

Saleh, S.D., 57
Salk, J., 218
Samuel, Y., 373
Sashkin, M., 491
Sayles, L.R., 160, 162, 200
Schein, E.H., 14, 89, 206, 296, 303, 452, 456, 461, 480
Schein, V.E., 516
Schlesinger, A., 244
Schmidt, S.M., 314, 324
Schmidt, W.H., 262, 293
Schmitt, N., 137
Schneider, B., 451, 464
Schneider, H.L., 419
Schneier, C.E., 180
Schoenherr, R.A., 373
Schotters, F.J., 410
Schrank, R., 419
Schriesheim, C.A., 62, 289, 297
Schuler, R.S., 91, 92, 95
Schuman, H., 61
Schuster, J.R., 438
Schwab, D.P., 144, 152
Schweitzer, A., 133
Scott, W.E., 145
Scott, W.G., 392
Scully, M., 431
Seashore, S.E., 251
Sechrest, L., 75, 97
Segal, M., 124
Selye, H., 92
Shakespeare, W., 203
Shapiro, H.J., 156
Shaver, P.R., 533
Shaw, G.B., 50, 132
Shaw, M.E., 239, 242
Sheehy, G., 80–82
Sheldon, W.H., 77, 78, 79
Shepard, J.M., 34
Sherwood, F.P., 505
Silverman, R.E., 78
Simon, H.A., 117, 265, 278
Skinner, B.F., 36, 38, 39, 170, 180, 181, 182, 183
Slesinger, J.A., 327
Slocum, J.W., Jr., 463
Sloma, R.L., 482
Smigel, E.O., 455
Smith, A., 402
Smith, C.G., 327

Smith, F., 61
Smyser, C.M., 82
Snow, C.C., 15
Snyder, R.A., 451
Snyderman, B., 141
Soat, D.M., 479
Solano, C., 100
Spendolini, M.J., 386
Springer, J., 102
Stalker, G.M., 378
Stanley, D., 435
Staw, B.M., 35, 145, 146, 149, 386, 452, 509
Steele, F.I., 89
Steers, R.M., 27, 62, 63, 64, 98, 151, 159
Stein, A., 250
Stengel, C., 336
Stevens, R.E., 65
Stitt, C.L., 124
Stogdill, R.M., 254, 288, 289, 307
Stöhr, O., 102–3
Stone, E.F., 99
Strauss, G., 15, 160, 162, 266
Strickland, L.H., 111
Strober, M.H., 119
Student, K., 327
Summer, C.E., 258
Suttle, J.L., 136, 253, 269, 401, 456
Sutton, H., 275
Swanson, G.E., 473
Sweigenhaft, R.L., 211
Swinth, R.L., 92

T

Tagiuri, R., 53, 120, 454
Tannenbaum, A.S., 15, 327, 346
Tannenbaum, R., 293
Taylor, F.W., 402
Taylor, K.F., 153
Taylor, R.N., 85
Tedeschi, J.T., 139
Thomas, E.J., 240, 249
Thomas, K.W., 262, 343, 349
Thompson, J.D., 374, 393
Thompson, J.T., 487
Thompson, P.H., 443

Thompson, V.A., 345
Tiger, L., 18
Timm, P.R., 268
Tragash, H.J., 126
Tudor, W.D., 386
Tushman, M., 508, 516

V

Van den Berghe, P.L., 14
Vanderveer, B.A., 513
Van deVen, A.H., 247, 375
Van Maanen, J., 452, 456, 458
Van Sell, M., 95
Van Zelst, R., 233
Vernon, P.E., 52
Vleeming, R.G., 84
Vredenburgh, D.J., 510
Vroom, V.H., 63, 69, 152, 287,
        299–302, 304, 305

W

Wahba, M.A., 136, 152, 156
Waldo, D., 368
Wallace, J., 481, 514
Wallace, R., 443
Wallach, M.A., 85, 246
Wallin, J.A., 178
Walton, R.E., 228, 412
Warren, J.R., 74
Warrick, D.D., 487
Watson, J.B., 166
Watson, T., 454
Weaver, C.N., 144
Webber, R.A., 124, 258
Weber, M., 381, 396, 397
Webster, E.C., 116
Weed, S.E., 82
Week, E.D., 410

Weeks, D.A., 438, 439
Weick, K.F., 451, 478
Westhead, P., 320–21
Whetton, D.A., 393
White, S.E., 269
Whyte, W.F., 217
Wicker, A.W., 60
Wigdor, L.A., 144
Wilensky, H.L., 15
Wilkens, P.L., 268
Wilkinson, I., 314, 324
Williams, K., 241
Williams, K.L., 410
Williams, M.S., 345
Wilson, E.O., 17
Wilson, M., 249
Winthrop, J., 210
Witkin, H.A., 110
Woodward, J., 374
Wright, J.P., 453

Y

Yager, E., 414
Yalom, I.D., 477
Yankelovich, D., 55
Yetton, P., 299–302, 304, 305
Yufe, J., 102–3
Yukl, G.A., 150

Z

Zald, M.N., 310, 323, 329
Zaleznik, A., 516
Zalkind, S.S., 125, 173
Zander, A., 250, 253, 290
Zelditch, M., 224
Zimbardo, P.G., 28
Zimmer, F.G., 212, 226, 228, 412

Subject Index

A

Absenteeism, 27
Absolute standards, in evaluation, 428–29
Abstract models, 22
Achievement:
  motive, 138–39
  orientation, 83
Activities in group model, 235
Adhocracy (*see* Adhocratic structure)
Adhocratic structure, 383
Affiliation, 138–39, 202
Alienation, 162–63
Anthropology, 10
Anxiety, 76–77
Attitudes:
  changing, 58–60, 472–74
  consistency of, 57–60
  defined, 55
  as an independent variable, 28
  influence on perception, 109–10
  relationship to behavior, 60–61
  sources of, 56
  types of, 56–57
  vs. values, 55–56
  women manager's exercise, 194–96
Attribution theory, 113–15
Authoritarianism, 84
Authority (*see* Position power)
Autocratic-democratic continuum leadership model, 292–94
Autonomous work teams, 412–13
Autonomy, 405, 451

B

Behavior (*see* Organizational behavior)
Behavioral:
  conflict view, 338
  control, 36–39
  leadership theories, 288–92
  modification, 181–85, 483–84
Birth order and personality, 74
Body language, 266–67
Body type and personality, 78–79
Bureaucracy (*see* Bureaucratic structure)
Bureaucratic structure, 380–81, 394–97, 498–99

C

Case exercises, 40–45, 186–92, 355–60, 493–98, 522–30
Cattell's trait theory of personality, 76–77
Causality, 24–25
Caused behavior, 5
Centralization, 371–72, 389
Change:
  organizational (*see* Organizational development)
  process, 473–74
Changing behavior (*see* Learning *and* Organizational development)
Classical conditioning, 169–70

Coalitions, 325–26
Coercive power, 317
Cognitive:
  dissonance, 58–60
  evaluation theory, 144–46
Cohesiveness, group, 249–52
Command group, 200
Communication:
  barriers, 264–66, 280–81
  defined, 262
  grapevine, 274–75
  as an independent variable, 30
  networks, 272–75
  nonverbal, 266–67
  perception, 267–70
  process, 262–64
Compensation, 89
Complexity, 368–69
Conditioning, 169–71
Conflict:
  behavioral view of, 338
  in culture, 451
  defined, 336–37
  dysfunctional, 338–39, 346
  functional, 338–39, 344–46
  as an independent variable, 30
  interactionist view of, 338
  paradox of, 339
  process, 340–46
  resolution techniques, 343–44,
    350–54
  role of, 207
  sources of, 340–42
  traditional view of, 337–38
Conformity, 214–15
Consensus in decisions, 255–57
Consideration, 289, 451
Contingency:
  conditions, 12
  model of OB, 33
Continuous reinforcers, 173–75
Controlling behavior, 36–39
Culture (*see* Organizational culture)

D

Debate, value of, 12–13
Decentralization, 371–72, 389

Decision making:
  group, 242–48, 255–59, 299–302
  individual, 85, 115–17, 427–32,
    435–39
  organizational, 450–55, 504–14
Defensive behaviors, 87–90
Delphi technique, 247–48
Democratic leaders, 292–94
Dependency (*see* Power)
Dependent variables, 23, 26–28
Descriptive models, 22
Differentiation:
  horizontal, 369, 388
  low, 431
  spatial, 369–70
  vertical, 369, 389
Discretionary time, as a reward
    criterion, 437–38
Dissonance (*see* Cognitive dissonance)
Diversity, member, as a group
    contingency, 241–42
Dress and group behavior, 221–22
Dynamic models, 21–22

E

Education, objectives of, 11
Effectiveness, 26–27
Efficiency, 26–27
Effort:
  in motivation, 152–56
  perception of, 116
  as a reward criterion, 436–37
Elasticity of power, 321–22
Emergent behavior in group model,
    236
Employee-oriented leaders, 290
Environment:
  as a determinant of structure, 376–77
  and personality, 74
Equity theory, 147–50, 268–69
ERG theory, 136–37
Esteem need, 135
Ethics of behavioral control, 38–39
Existence need, 137
Expectancy:
  defined, 152
  theory, 152–56

Expectations:
  influence on perception, 111–12
  role, 205–6
Experience, influence on perceptions, 111
Expert power, 318
Expressive orientation, 85–86
Extrinsic motivators, 141–46
Extroversion-introversion personality, 77–78

F

Fantasy, 89
Feedback, 263–64, 405
Fiedler contingency model of leadership, 294–97
Figure-ground perception, 112
Flex-time, 416–17
Formal groups, 200–204
Formalization, 370–71
Friendship group, 201
Functional structure, 381–82

G

Genetics and behavior, 17–18, 102–5
Goal-setting theory, 150–51
Goals, group, 203
Grapevine, 274–75
Group(s):
  analysis, 232–34
  behavior, 8–10, 25–26, 30
  behavior model, 235–39
  cohesiveness, 248–52
  decision making, 242–48, 255–59
  defined, 200
  designing organizations around, 226–29
  dynamics, 232–53
  formal, 200–201
  goals, 201–3
  as an independent variable, 30
  informal, 200–201
  think, 243–45
  types of, 200–201
Growth need, 137, 405, 406

H

Halo effect, 119–20, 430
Hawthorne studies, 212–14
Hedonism, 133
Hegelian dialectic, 11
Heredity and personality, 73, 102–5
Hierarchy of needs, 134–36
Higher-order needs, 135–36
Humanistic values, 28
Human relations, 15
Human relations specialist, 234

I

Identification, 89
Identity:
  group, 202
  role, 204–5
Incentives (*see* Motivation *and* Rewards)
Independent variables, 23, 28–33
Individual behavior, 8, 25–26, 29
Individual differences, 5
Individual needs vs. the organization, 160–63
Inflation in evaluations, 431–32
Influence (*see* Power)
Informal groups, 200–201
Informal organization, 274–75
Informational cues, 269–70
Initiating structure, 289
Instrumentality, 152
Instrumental orientation, 85–86
Integrated work teams, 412
Interaction analysis, 234
Interactionist view of conflict, 338
Interactions in group model, 235–36
Interest group, 201
Interests, influence on perception, 110–11
Intergroup development, 482
Intermittent reinforcers, 173–75
Interviews and perception, 115–16
Intrinsic motivators, 141–46
Introversion-extroversion personality, 77–78
Intuition, 4–6

J

Jargon, 270–72
Job:
  characteristics model, 404–7, 417
  design, 31, 237, 401–17
  difficulty, as a reward criterion, 437
  enlargement, 403
  enrichment, 403, 409–12
  involvement, 57
  redesign, 401, 420–23 (*see also* Job
    design)
  rotation, 408
  satisfaction, 56–57, 66–69

K

Kinesics, 266
Knowledge power, 318

L

Language (*see* Jargon)
Leader-member relations, 295
Leader-participation model, 299–302
Leadership:
  behavioral theories, 288–92
  contingency theories, 292–303
  defined, 286
  importance of, 308–9
  as an independent variable, 30
  integration of theories, 303–4
  Managerial Grid, 290–91
  Michigan studies, 289–90
  Ohio State studies, 289
  participative, 292–94, 299–302
  path-goal model, 297–99
  substitutes for, 302–3
  test, 362–63
  trait theories, 287–88
  Vroom-Yetton model of, 299–302
Learning:
  defined, 167
  importance of, 168–69
  as an independent variable, 29
  and motivation, 166–67

Least preferred coworker (LPC), 294
Legitimate power, 316 (*see also*
    Position power)
Leniency error, 430
Line-staff, 387–88
Locus of control, 82–83
Love need, 135
Lower-order needs, 135–36
Loyalty and perception, 117

M

Machiavellianism, 84–85
Management and OB, 11
Managerial Grid, 290, 291
MAPS, 476
Matrix structure, 383, 386
Maturation theory, 80
Mechanistic structure, 378–79
Merit, as a reward criterion, 435
Michigan leadership studies, 289–90
Models:
  abstract, 22
  components of, 22–25
  defined, 20–21
  descriptive, 22
  dynamic, 21–22
  normative, 22
  objective, 21
  physical, 22
  static, 21–22
  subjective, 21
  value of, 21
Moderating variables, 24, 33
Modern synthesis, 17–18
Money and motivation, 136, 142–43,
    144–46, 147–50, 151–56,
    439–41
Morale (*see* Job satisfaction)
Motivating potential, job, 406–7,
    499–500
Motivation:
  defined, 132
  extrinsic, 141–46
  hygiene theory, 141–44
  as an independent variable, 29
  intrinsic, 141–46
  by job design, 401–7, 417

need theories, 134–41
and performance evaluation, 427–28
process theories, 146–56
Motives, influence on perception, 110

N

Needs test, 196
Need theories, 134–41
Negative reinforcement, 172
Networks, communication, 272–75
Nominal group technique, 247
Nonverbal communication, 266–67
Normative models, 22
Norms: (*see also* Conformity *and*
    Groupthink)
    defined, 211–12
    as an independent variable, 29–30
    influence on behavior, 222–23

O

OB (*see* Organizational behavior)
Objective models, 21
Objectives:
    of education, 11
    in evaluation, 429
    of a model, 23
OB Modification, 483–84
OD (*see* Organizational development)
Ohio State leadership studies, 289
Operant conditioning, 170–71 (*see also*
    Behavioral modification)
Opportunity power, 318–19
Organic structure, 378–79
Organization, defined, 6
Organizational behavior (OB):
    as a biological science, 17–18
    contributors to, 8–10
    defined, 6–7
    education in, 11–12
    and management, 11
    model, 32
    reasons for studying, 7–8
    as a social science, 15–16
Organizational change (*see*
    Organizational development)

Organizational climate (*see*
    Organizational culture)
Organizational commitment, 57
Organizational culture:
    defined, 450–52
    in groups, 237
    as an independent variable, 31, 33
    and politics, 510–12
    source of, 454–55
    test, 500
Organizational development:
    defined, 472
    human process techniques,
        477–85
    as an independent variable, 33
    objectives, 474–75, 488–92
    structural techniques, 476
Organizational politics:
    defined, 505–7, 517–21
    dysfunctional, 509–14
Organization chart, 20–21
Organization structure:
    classification of, 378–83
    in culture, 451
    defined, 368–72
    determinants of, 372–78
    as an independent variable, 31
    model, 390
Organization systems, 25–26, 31

P

Participative leadership, 292–94,
    299–302
Passages theory, 80–82
Path-goal model of leadership, 297–99
Perception:
    and communication, 267–70
    defined, 109
    distortion in, 109–13
    factors influencing, 109–13
    as an independent variable, 29
    of person, 113–20
    vs. reality, 108–9
    and rewards, 434–35
    role of, 205
    selective, 117–18
    training to improve, 126–29

Performance:
as a dependent variable, 26–28
as a reward criterion, 436
satisfaction relationship, 62–64
Performance evaluation:
errors in, 429–32
as an independent variable, 31
methods, 428–29
and motivation, 427–28
and perception, 116
purpose of, 427
sharing results of, 432–33
standards, 428
Personality:
defined, 72–73
determinants of, 73–75
development theories of, 80–82
as group contingency, 240
as an independent variable, 28
influence on perception, 110
vs. organization hypothesis, 160–63
traits, 76
types, 76–79, 86–87
Personal power, 318
Persuasive power, 317–18
Physical models, 22
Physiological needs, 135
Point-Counterpoint, use of, 12–13
Political science, 10
Politics (*see* Organizational politics)
Position power, 295, 318
Positive reinforcement (*see*
Reinforcement)
Power:
bases of, 316–19
coalitions, 325–26
coercive, 317
control, as determinant of structure,
377–78
defined, 314–15
dependency on, 315, 320–23
elasticity of, 321–22
expert, 318
group, 202–3, 325–26
as an independent variable, 30
knowledge, 318
and leadership, 315–16
legitimate, 316
motives, 138–39
opportunity, 318–19

oriented managers, 330–31
position, 295, 318
referent, 316
reward, 317
sources of, 316–19
tactics, 324–35
test of, 363–64
uncertainty, 323
Prediction of behavior, 4–6, 7
Primary reinforcers, 171–72
Principles, 11–12
Problem solving, 350–51
Process consultation, 480
Production-oriented leaders, 290
Productivity, 26–27
Product structure, 382–83
Projection, 90
Proximity, influence on perception of,
112–13
Psychology, 8
Punishment, 172

Q

Quality circles, 413–14

R

Rationalization, 90
Reaction formation, 90
Reality vs. perception, 108–9
Referent power, 316
Regression, 89
Reinforcement, 151–52, 171–75 (*see
also* Operant conditioning *and*
Behavioral modification)
Relatedness needs, 137
Relational manager, 332–33
Relationships in a model, 24–25
Relative standards, in evaluation, 429
Repression, 89
Required behavior in group model,
236, 238
Reward(s): (*see also* Motivation *and*
Reinforcement)
in culture, 451

determinants, 435–39
extrinsic, 441
group, 237
as an independent variable, 31
intrinsic, 441
in learning, 171–75, 434
perception of, 434–35
power, 317
types of, 439–42
Risk taking, 85
Risky-shift phenomenon, 245–47
Role(s):
  conflict, 207
  defined, 203–4
  expectations, 205–6
  identity, 204–5
  as an independent variable, 29–30
  influence on behavior of, 222
  perception of, 205
Rumors (*see* Grapevine)

S

Safety needs, 135
Satisfaction (*see* Job satisfaction)
Scientific management, 402
Secondary reinforcers, 171–72
Security, need for, 201–2
Self:
  actualization need, 135
  assessment of performance, 433
  concept, 87–90
  interest, 133–34, 505–7
Seniority, as a reward criterion, 437
Sensitivity training, 477–78
Sentiments in group model, 236
Sex, as group contingency, 239–40
Shaping behavior, 171–75 (*see also*
    Reinforcement *and* Behavioral
    modification)
Shorter workweek, 414–15
Similarity:
  error, 430
  in perception, 113, 118
Simple structure, 379–80
Situation: (*see also* Contingency)
  perception, 113
  personality, 75

Size:
  as determinant of structure, 372–73,
    387
  as group contingency, 240–41
Skills, as a reward criterion, 437
Skill variety, 404–5
Social desirability (*see* Conformity)
Socialization:
  defined, 455–56
  methods, 457–62
  process, 456–57
Social psychology, 10
Social system, 8, 10
Sociobiology, 17–18
Sociogram, 233
Sociology, 8, 10
Sociometry, 232–34
Sociotechnical systems, 403–4
Span of control, 388
Spatial arrangements, 210–11
Standardization, 370–71
Static models, 21–22
Status:
  defined, 215–17
  equity, 217–223
  group, 202
  as an independent variable, 29–30
  influence on behavior of, 223
  ranking test, 361
  sources of, 217–22
Stereotypes, 118–19
Stress, 90–97
Structure (*see* Organization structure)
Subjective models, 21
Substitutes for performance, 432
Survey feedback, 478–80
Systematic study of OB, 5–6, 7, 16

T

Task:
  design (*see* Job design)
  groups, 200–201
  identity, 404–5
  significance, 405
  specialist, 234
  structure, 295
Team building, 480–82

Technology, as determinant of
    structure, 373–75
Theory X, 475
Theory Y, 475
Traditional view of conflict, 337–38
Training to improve perception, 126–29
Trait approach to personality, 76
Trait theories of leadership, 287–88
Transactional analysis (TA), 484–85
Turnover, 27–28
Type A personality, 95–97
Type approach to personality, 76–79,
    86–87
Type B personality, 95–97

sources of, 51–52
Values:
    assessment test, 192–94
    defined, 50
    importance of, 51
    as an independent variable, 28
    influence on perception of, 109–10
    types of, 54
Variables:
    defined, 23
    dependent, 23
    independent, 23
    moderating, 24, 33
Vocational Preference Inventory, 86

V

Valence, 152
Value systems:
    defined, 50–51

W

Women managers, attitude measure
    exercise, 194–96
Work modules, 408–9